Clinical Reasoning in Musculoskeletal Practice

For Elsevier

Content Strategist: Poppy Garraway, Serena Castelnovo
Content Development Specialist: Sally Davies, Veronika Watkins
Senior Project Manager: Manchu Mohan
Designer/Design Direction: Bridget Hoette
Illustration Manager: Nichole Beard

Clinical Reasoning in Musculoskeletal Practice

SECOND EDITION

MARK A JONES BSc(Psych) PT GradDipManipTher MAppSc

Senior Lecturer, Program Director, Master of Advanced Clinical Physiotherapy, School of Health Sciences, University of South Australia, Adelaide, Australia

DARREN A RIVETT BAppSc(Phty) GradDipManipTher MAppSc(ManipPhty) PhD

Professor, School of Health Sciences, University of Newcastle, Callaghan, New South Wales, Australia

FOREWORD BY

ANN MOORE CBE

Professor Emerita, School of Health Sciences, University of Brighton, Brighton, UK
Director of the Council for Allied Health Professions Research (CAHPR)

ELSEVIER

Edinburgh   London   New York   Oxford   Philadelphia   St Louis   Sydney   Toronto   2019

ELSEVIER

First edition 2004
Second edition 2019

ISBN 978-0-7020-5976-6
e-ISBN 978-0-7020-5977-3

British Library Cataloguing in Publication Data
A catalogue record for this book is available from the British Library

Library of Congress Cataloging in Publication Data
A catalog record for this book is available from the Library of Congress

---

ELSEVIER your source for books, journals and multimedia in the health sciences

www.elsevierhealth.com

 Working together to grow libraries in developing countries

www.elsevier.com • www.bookaid.org

The publisher's policy is to use paper manufactured from sustainable forests

Printed in Great Britain

Last digit is the print number: 10 9 8 7 6 5 4

Contents

SECTION 3
Learning and Facilitating Clinical Reasoning   561

Foreword

This book, *Clinical Reasoning in Musculoskeletal Practice,* is the second edition of a book published in 2004 by Mark Jones and Darren Rivett. The title of the first version was *Clinical Reasoning for Manual Therapists.* It is very welcome to see the development of this title – recognizing the spread of approaches that musculoskeletal physiotherapists now take in addition to manual therapy which is still an important and fundamental approach. The book is of extreme relevance and importance to all practitioners dealing with musculoskeletal issues in clinical practice on a daily basis. The book is also highly relevant for clinical educators; academics focused on musculoskeletal science and practice in educational, as well as clinical settings; and, of course, for students, whether at undergraduate or postgraduate level.

It is exciting to see how clinical reasoning and decision-making theories have developed over the last 15 years or so, and this book captures these theoretical developments and also captures the clinical relevance and applications of these theories. Mark Jones and Darren Rivett have very successfully brought together 52 authors who are well known in the field of musculoskeletal physiotherapy. Importantly, the authors are based in 12 countries from across the world, which thus represents an international perspective on clinical reasoning.

The book contains three sections. Section 1 contains five chapters which focus on key theories which inform clinical reasoning in musculoskeletal practice. This section is a fundamental read before moving on into the next section: 'Clinical Reasoning in Action: Case Studies From Musculoskeletal Practitioners'. Section 2 consists of 25 chapters with each one focusing on a different musculoskeletal condition and demonstrating considerable complexities. Each case study includes a history of the patient's condition, examination findings, their treatment approaches, and their outcomes. In addition Mark Jones and Darren Rivett worked with the lead author of each of these chapters to explore their clinical reasoning throughout the case study, and finally, they provide a clinical reasoning commentary which links the clinician's reasoning to the five theoretical chapters in Section 1.

Finally, Chapter 31 (Section 3) is a very useful chapter on strategies to facilitate clinical reasoning development, and readers will also find the two appendices very helpful in practice, as they contain a clinical reflection form and a clinical reasoning reflection worksheet.

This book is certainly a must-read for all those interested in musculoskeletal practice, and I would like to thank Mark and Darren for producing such a valuable contribution to the musculoskeletal field. I would also like to thank all the contributors to the book, who provide important insights and inspiration for us all.

Professor Emerita Ann P Moore CBE PhD FCSP FMACP Dip TP Cert Ed.
School of Health Sciences, University of Brighton, Brighton, UK

Preface

We published our first edition of *Clinical Reasoning for Manual Therapists,* focused on making expert clinical reasoning explicit through case studies, in 2004. Clearly there was a great need for such a resource, both in formal musculoskeletal educational programs and as a stimulus for informal professional development in clinical reasoning, as the book has been widely adopted internationally and has stood the test of time. Since then, however, there has been significant continued growth in the research evidence musculoskeletal clinicians are expected to know and use and an increase in the understanding of pain science. Associated with this growth in empirical research and understanding of pain has been a parallel increase in the emphasis on psychosocial assessment, pain education and cognitive-behavioural management. Of course, the clinical reasoning theory has also accordingly adapted and progressed in this time.

The political pressure for research- and evidence-based practice is greater than ever, increasingly in an attempt to justify cost-cutting measures in health care. This is despite the plethora of systematic reviews now available concluding, more often than not, that there is insufficient high-level research to judge what managements are best. Similarly, the relatively recent rise in musculoskeletal practice of clinical prediction rules – statistically derived clinical tools designed to assist in decision making – has generated much interest, particularly amongst less experienced clinicians and those not well versed in clinical reasoning. However, there is growing concern that clinical prediction rules are being adopted as a 'lazy man's' substitute for clinical reasoning and are being prematurely adopted by clinicians and required by funding bodies despite usually not having been fully validated and scientifically demonstrated to have a positive impact.

Conversely, pain science and chronic pain or disability research convincingly highlight the importance of musculoskeletal practitioners increasing their skills in psychosocial assessment and management. Although formal classroom education in these areas is increasing at the pre- and post-professional levels, it is still arguably less developed and often not well integrated into the clinical practice components of the curriculum. A key challenge to musculoskeletal education and clinical practice is to strengthen this important area without diminishing the knowledge and procedural skills essential to 'hands-on' physical assessment and treatment. Indeed, physiotherapy 'hands-on' procedural skills may be under threat from those who promote education (e.g. in pain management) as a *replacement* for established physical therapies, rather than something that needs to be *integrated* with those same therapies (Jull and Moore, 2012; Edwards and Jones, 2013). Arguably, skilled clinical reasoning is more important than ever because of the external pressures for greater efficiency and quality patient outcomes.

In this book, the theory underpinning clinical reasoning has been significantly expanded from the previous edition to include the following completely new chapters:

Chapter 1: Clinical reasoning: fast and slow thinking in musculoskeletal practice
Chapter 2: Understanding pain in order to treat patients in pain
Chapter 3: Influence of stress, coping and social factors on pain and disability in musculoskeletal practice
Chapter 4: Assessment, reasoning and management of psychological factors in musculoskeletal practice
Chapter 5: Clinical prediction rules: their benefits and limitations in clinical reasoning
Chapter 31: Strategies to facilitate clinical reasoning development

Aside from these six theory chapters, the bulk of the book is comprised of 25 new case study chapters of real patients, presented from their initial appointment through to discharge. In each case chapter, Mark and/or Darren worked with the clinical authors to explore their clinical reasoning throughout the case, then provided a Clinical Reasoning Commentary that links aspects of the clinical authors' reasoning to the theory chapters. The overarching aim is to 'bring to life' the clinical reasoning theory and underpinning sciences in the context of a real-world clinical problem. Contributing clinical authors were invited on the basis of their world-renowned expertise in the case area, with representation of both spinal and peripheral musculoskeletal cases, multiple clinical approaches and authors from around the globe. Although the 'hypothesis categories' framework presented in Chapter 1 was used as the basis for the majority of questions asked of clinical authors, they were not provided with this or any of the other theory chapters when writing their cases or answering the Reasoning Questions – that is, they were not prompted or required to conform to any of the theory presented in the first five chapters.

With such a diverse group of contributing clinical authors, there are, understandably, differences in the examination information obtained and forms of treatment used. However, despite this variability, there is considerable similarity across the cases with respect to their thoroughness in examination, scope of clinical reasoning and individually tailored management, informed by both research and experience-based evidence. Although the language used to report the cases and answer the Reasoning Questions also varies somewhat across the cases, consistent with the clinical reasoning promoted in the theory chapters, the reasoning presented throughout the cases is also holistic, biopsychosocial, collaborative and patient centred. Attention to both the physical and the psychosocial presentation is consistently evident, along with management that promotes patient understanding and self-efficacy.

It should be apparent by now to the discerning reader why we have modified the title of the book from the original *Clinical Reasoning for Manual Therapists* to *Clinical Reasoning in Musculoskeletal Practice* in this edition. The breadth of clinical practice in the musculoskeletal field has clearly changed significantly since 2004, and the title change is an attempt to reflect just that while still embracing manual therapy as a core skill for the musculoskeletal practitioner.

Finally, we would like to express our sincere gratitude to the many contributing authors, both of the theoretical chapters and of the clinical reasoning cases. Although the gestation of this second edition has been rather more protracted than anticipated, they have uniformly demonstrated great patience and ongoing enthusiasm for this new edition of the book.

Mark A. Jones
Adelaide, Australia, 2019

Darren A. Rivett
Newcastle, Australia, 2019

REFERENCES

Edwards, I., Jones, M., 2013. Movement in our thinking and our practice. Manual Ther 18 (2), 93–95.
Jull, G., Moore, A., 2012. Hands on, hands off? The swings in musculoskeletal physiotherapy practice. Man Ther 17 (3), 199–200.

Contributors

Jason M. Beneciuk DPT PhD MPH
Research Assistant Professor, Department of Physical Therapy, College of Public Health and Health Professions, University of Florida, Gainesville, Florida; Clinical Research Scientist, Brooks Rehabilitation, Jacksonville, Florida, USA

Kim L. Bennell BAppSci(Physio) PhD
Redmond Barry Distinguished Professor, Centre for Health, Exercise and Sports Medicine, Department of Physiotherapy, University of Melbourne, Melbourne, Victoria, Australia

Mark J. Catley BPhysio(Hons) PhD
Lecturer, School of Health Sciences, University of South Australia, Adelaide, Australia

Nicole Christensen BS BA PT MAppSc PhD
Professor and Chair, Department of Physical Therapy, Samuel Merritt University, Oakland, California, USA

Helen Clare DipPhty GradDipManipTher MAppSc DipMD&T PhD FACP
Director of Education, McKenzie Institute International, Sydney, New South Wales, Australia

Joshua A. Cleland PT PhD
Professor, Franklin Pierce University, Physical Therapy Program, Manchester, New Hampshire, USA

Chad E. Cook PT PhD FAAOMPT
Professor and Program Director, Duke Doctor of Physical Therapy Program, Duke University School of Medicine, Duke Clinical Research Institute, Durham, North Carolina, USA

Gray Cook MSPT OCS CSCS
Founder, Functional Movement Systems, Chatham, Virginia, USA

Jill Cook BAppSci(Phty) PGDip(Manips) PhD GradCertHigherEd
Professor, La Trobe University Sport and Exercise Medicine Centre, La Trobe University, Bundoora, Victoria, Australia

Michel W. Coppieters PT PhD
Professor, Menzies Foundation Professor of Allied Health Research, Griffith University, Brisbane and Gold Coast, Queensland, Australia; Professor, Amsterdam Movement Sciences, Faculty of Behavioural and Movement Sciences, Vrije Universiteit Amsterdam, Amsterdam, The Netherlands

Margot De Kooning PhD
Researcher, Department of Physiotherapy, Human Physiology and Anatomy (KIMA), Faculty of Physical Education and Physiotherapy, Vrije Universiteit Brussel (VUB), Brussels, Belgium; Physiotherapist, Department of Physical Medicine and Physiotherapy, University Hospital Brussels, Brussels, Belgium; Member, Pain in Motion International Research Group

Ina Diener BSc(Physio) PhD
Part-Time Senior Lecturer, Stellenbosch University, Stellenbosch and University of the Western Cape, Cape Town, South Africa

Sean Docking BHSc(Hons) PhD
Postdoctoral Research Fellow, La Trobe University Sport and Exercise Medicine Centre, La Trobe University, Bundoora, Victoria, Australia

Bill Egan PT DPT OCS FAAOMPT
Associate Professor of Instruction, Department of Physical Therapy, College of Public Health, Temple University, Philadelphia, Pennsylvania, USA

Timothy W. Flynn PT PhD OCS FAAOMPT FAPTA
Professor of Physical Therapy, South College, Knoxville, Tennessee; Owner & Clinician, Colorado In Motion, Fort Collins, Colorado, USA

Steven Z. George PT PhD FAPTA
Professor and Director of Musculoskeletal Research, Duke Clinical Research Institute and Vice Chair of Clinical Research, Department of Orthopaedic Surgery, Duke University School of Medicine, Durham, North Carolina, USA

Alison Grimaldi BPhty MPhty(Sports) PhD
Adjunct Research Fellow, University of Queensland, Brisbane, Queensland; Practice Principal, Physiotec, Brisbane, Australia

Toby Hall PT PHD MSc FACP
Adjunct Associate Professor, School of Physiotherapy and Exercise Science, Curtin University, Perth; Senior Teaching Fellow, The University of Western Australia, Perth, Australia

Amy S. Hammerich PT DPT PhD OCS GCS FAAOMPT
Associate Professor, School of Physical Therapy, Regis University, Denver, Colorado, USA

Robin Haskins BPhty(Hons) PhD
Physiotherapist, John Hunter Hospital, Newcastle, New South Wales; Conjoint Lecturer, School of Health Sciences, University of Newcastle, Callaghan, New South Wales, Australia

Eric J. Hegedus PT DPT PhD OCS
Professor and Chair, High Point University, Department of Physical Therapy, High Point, North Carolina, USA

Mark A. Jones BSc(Psych) PT GradDipManipTher MAppSc
Senior Lecturer, Program Director, Master of Advanced Clinical Physiotherapy, School of Health Sciences, University of South Australia, Adelaide, Australia

Gwendolen Jull AO MPhty PhD FACP
Emeritus Professor, Physiotherapy, School of Health and Rehabilitation Sciences, University of Queensland, Brisbane, Australia

Roger Kerry PhD FMACP
Associate Professor, Division of Physiotherapy and Rehabilitation Sciences, University of Nottingham, Nottingham, UK

Kyle Kiesel PT PhD
Professor and Chair of Physical Therapy, College of Education and Health Sciences, University of Evansville, Evansville, Indiana, USA

Diane G. Lee BSR FCAMT CGIMS
Clinician and Consultant, Diane Lee & Associates, Surrey, British Columbia; Curriculum Developer and Lead Instructor, Learn with Diane Lee, Surrey, British Columbia, Canada

Jeremy Lewis PhD FCSP
Professor of Musculoskeletal Research, University of Hertfordshire, Hertfordshire, UK; Consultant Physiotherapist, MSK Sonographer and Independent Prescriber, Central London Community Healthcare NHS Trust, London, UK

Adriaan Louw PT PhD
Owner and CEO, International Spine and Pain Institute, Story City, Iowa, USA

Anneleen Malfliet PT MSc
Physiotherapist, Research Foundation – Flanders (FWO), Brussels; PhD Researcher, Vrije Universiteit Brussel (VUB), Brussels, and Ghent University, Ghent; Physiotherapist, University Hospital Brussels, Brussels, Belgium; Member, Pain in Motion International Research Group

Ricardo Matias PT PhD
Researcher, Champalimaud Research, Champalimaud Centre for the Unknown, Lisbon; Lecturer, Physiotherapy Department, School of Health, Polytechnic Institute of Setúbal, Setúbal, Portugal

Kyle A. Matsel PT DPT SCS CSCS
Assistant Professor of Physical Therapy,
University of Evansville, Evansville,
Indiana, USA

Mark Matthews MPhty(Musc) BPhty
PhD candidate, University of Queensland,
Brisbane, Australia

Stephen May MA MSc PhD FCSP
Reader in Physiotherapy, Sheffield Hallam
University, Sheffield, South Yorkshire, UK

**Christopher McCarthy
PGDip(Biomech) PGDip(ManTher)
PGDip(Phty) PhD FMACP FCSP**
Clinical Fellow, Manchester School of
Physiotherapy, Manchester Metropolitan
University, Manchester, UK

**Jenny McConnell AM BAppSci(Phty)
GradDipManTher MBiomedEng FACP**
Practice Principal, McConnell
Physiotherapy Group, Mosman,
New South Wales, Australia

**Rebecca Mellor BPhty(Hons)
MPhty(Musc) PhD**
NHMRC Senior Academic Research
Officer, School of Health and
Rehabilitation Sciences, University of
Queensland, Brisbane, Queensland,
Australia

**G. Lorimer Moseley DSc PhD FAHMS
FACP HonFPMANZCA HonMAPA**
Professor of Clinical Neuroscience and
Foundation Chair in Physiotherapy,
University of South Australia, Adelaide;
NHMRC Principal Research Fellow

Robert J. Nee PT PhD MAppSc
Professor, School of Physical Therapy and
Athletic Training, Pacific University,
Hillsboro, Oregon, USA

**Patricia Neumann DipPhysio PhD
FACP**
Lecturer, School of Health Sciences,
University of South Australia, Adelaide,
Australia

Jo Nijs PT MT PhD
Professor of Physiotherapy and
Physiology, Department of Physiotherapy,
Anatomy and Human Physiology, Faculty
of Physical Education and Physiotherapy,
Vrije Universiteit Brussel (VUB), Brussels,
Belgium; Member, Pain in Motion
International Research Group

**Peter G. Osmotherly BSc
GradDipPhty MMedSci(ClinEpi) PhD**
Senior Lecturer in Physiotherapy,
University of Newcastle, Callaghan,
New South Wales, Australia

**Peter O'Sullivan DipPhysio
GradDipManipTher PhD FACP**
Professor, School of Physiotherapy and
Exercise Science, Curtin University, Perth,
Australia

**Ebonie Rio BAppSci BPhysio(Hons)
MSportsPhysio PhD**
Postdoctoral Research Fellow, La Trobe
University Sport and Exercise Medicine
Centre, La Trobe University, Bundoora,
Victoria, Australia

**Darren A. Rivett BAppSc(Phty)
GradDipManipTher
MAppSc(ManipPhty) PhD**
Professor, School of Health Sciences,
University of Newcastle, Callaghan,
New South Wales, Australia

Mariano Rocabado PT DPT PhD
Professor, Faculty of Dentistry, University
of Chile; Director, Rocabado Institute,
Santiago, Chile

Susan A. Scherer PT PhD
Professor, Rueckert-Hartman College of
Health Professions, Regis University,
Denver, Colorado, USA

**Jochen Schomacher PT OMT MCMK
DPT BSc MSc PhD**
Freelance teacher of physiotherapy and
manual therapy, Erlenbach ZH,
Switzerland

Christopher R. Showalter PT DPT OCS FAAOMPT
Owner and Program Director, MAPS Fellowship in Orthopedic Manual Therapy, Mattituck, New York, USA

Chris R. Showalter PT DPT OCS FAAOMPT
Program Director, MAPS Fellowship in Orthopedic Manual Therapy, Mattituck, New York, USA

Michele Sterling BPhty MPhty GradDipManipPhysio PhD FACP
Director, NHMRC Centre of Research Excellence in Road Traffic Injury Recovery; Associate Director, Recover Injury Research Centre, University of Queensland, Herston, Queensland, Australia

Alan J. Taylor MSc MCSP
Assistant Professor, Physiotherapy and Rehabilitation, Faculty of Medicine & Health Sciences, University of Nottingham, Nottingham, UK

Judith Thompson DipPhysio PGDip(Continence & Women's Health) PhD FACP
Lecturer, Faculty of Health Sciences, School of Physiotherapy and Exercise Science, Curtin University, Perth, Australia

Rafael Torres Cueco PT PhD
Professor, Department of Physiotherapy, University of Valencia, Spain; Director of Master's Program on Manual Therapy, University of Valencia; President and founder of the Spanish Society of Physiotherapy and Pain (Sociedad Española de Fisioterapia y Dolor SEFID); Facilitator, WCPT Physical Therapy Pain Network; Instructor, Neuro Orthopaedic Institute (NOI); Member of the Spanish Pain Society

Bill Vicenzino BPhty GradDipSportsPhty MSc PhD
Professor of Sports Physiotherapy, School of Health and Rehabilitation Sciences, University of Queensland, Brisbane, Queensland, Australia

Harry J. M. von Piekartz BSc MSc PT MT PhD
Professor of Physiotherapy and Study Director, Master of Science musculoskeletal Programm, University of Applied Science, Osnabrück, Germany; Senior Lecturer in Musculoskeletal Therapy, International Maitland Teacher Association (IMTA), Cranial Facial Therapy Academy (CRAFTA) and Neuro Orthopaedic Institute (NOI); private practitioner in specialized musculoskeletal therapy, Ootmarsum, the Netherlands

Jodi L. Young PT DPT OCS FAAOMPT
Associate Professor of Physical Therapy, A.T. Still University, Mesa, Arizona, USA

Introduction

This new edition of our book is intended for all clinicians in musculoskeletal practice who wish to improve their skills in clinical reasoning and decision-making by learning from the reasoning of some of the most acclaimed clinicians in the world and by ensuring the knowledge supporting their reasoning is comprehensive and contemporary. Musculoskeletal practitioners all along the spectrum of clinical expertise and experience will benefit from integrating the latest theory and science as they engage in reasoning through detailed and varied clinical cases. The book can stand alone as a resource or can be used in a complementary manner with other learning materials, and it lends itself to both individual study and group learning activities designed to promote the learning of clinical reasoning.

Transformative learning theory (Cranton, 2006; Mezirow 2009, 2012) refers to the process by which we use critical reflection to transform prior, taken-for-granted understandings to make them more inclusive, open, reflective and discriminating. For the focus in this book on improving your clinical reasoning skills, this requires an awareness of your current understanding of reasoning and a critical reflection on clinical reasoning in practice as a means of transforming your clinical understanding and potentially your clinical practice.

The initial new theory chapters on clinical reasoning; pain science; stress, coping and social factors; psychological factors; and clinical prediction rules provide important knowledge to underpin contemporary biopsychosocially based clinical reasoning in musculoskeletal practice. As discussed in Chapters 1 and 5, human bias can undermine our judgements. To reduce bias and improve clinical reasoning, it is critical to first understand your own clinical reasoning, including the processes involved, different foci of reasoning attended to and factors influencing clinical reasoning proficiency. In addition to the theory chapters, the 25 new cases throughout this book should promote reflection and improve your understanding of your own clinical reasoning as you compare your reasoning as each case unfolds to that of the expert clinical authors, with accompanying reasoning commentary linking back to the theory chapters. This should facilitate an improved breadth, depth and accuracy of your clinical reasoning and clinical decisions, with the final chapter providing further strategies to develop your clinical reasoning skills in an ongoing manner. We see clinical reasoning as an essential professional competency and believe we need to study and practice clinical reasoning alongside our other professional competencies.

Practising clinical reasoning, by reading the cases and reasoning explored through the cases in this book (along with other strategies for facilitating clinical reasoning discussed in Chapter 31), will improve your underpinning understanding and hopefully your own clinical reasoning skills in actual clinical practice. To optimize that learning, the cases should not simply be read passively. As Mezirow (2012) highlights, transformative learning requires participation in constructive discourse to use the experience (and reasoning) of others to elicit reflection and awareness of your own reasoning and associated assumptions. Constructive discourse can occur by attempting to answer the Reasoning Questions posed throughout the cases prior to reading the expert clinicians' Answers to Reasoning Questions and by comparing and critiquing your reasoning with the reasoning put forward during the case. Even more stimulating and probably more beneficial is to engage in constructive discourse of a case and its associated reasoning in small groups of two or more practitioners or students.

Clinical reasoning in musculoskeletal practice is not an exact science with absolute correct and incorrect judgements. That is, it is not essential to agree with all the reasoning explained throughout the cases. What is important is that all cases present their assessment and management with explicit reasoning for what is done. When comparing your own reasoning to the case reasoning of the expert clinical authors, especially where differences exist, readers should consider assumptions being made (both in the case reasoning and your own) in assessments (e.g. information obtained versus not obtained), assessment analysis (e.g. hypothesis substantiation and alternative hypotheses), management (e.g.

clinical and research support provided, and alternative management options) and outcome re-assessment (e.g. breadth of self-report and physical measures informing treatment progression and success generally). Rather than simply attempting to pick holes in the clinical approach taken and the reasoning provided, readers are encouraged to suspend judgement and 'try on' the different points of view put forward. This sort of open-minded constructive discourse is important to both consolidating and varying your own perspectives. Practising clinical reasoning through the cases in this manner will assist your application of the theory covered in Chapters 1–5 and 31, to your reasoning in clinical practice, improving both your integration of that theory and your clinical reasoning proficiency.

REFERENCES

Cranton, P., 2006. Understanding and Promoting Transformative Learning: A Guide for Educators of Adults, second ed. Jossey-Bass Wiley, San Francisco, CA.

Mezirow, J., 2009. Transformative learning theory. In: Mezirow, J., Taylor, E.W., Associates (Eds.), Transformative Learning in Practice: Insights From Community, Workplace, and Higher Education. Jossey-Bass Wiley, San Francisco, CA, pp. 18–31.

Mezirow, J., 2012. Learning to think like an adult. Core concepts of transformative theory. In: Taylor, E.W., Cranton, P., Associates (Eds.), The Handbook of Transformative Learning: Theory, Research, and Practice. Jossey-Bass, San Francisco, CA, pp. 73–95.

SECTION 1

Key Theory Informing Clinical Reasoning in Musculoskeletal Practice

1

Clinical Reasoning: Fast and Slow Thinking in Musculoskeletal Practice

Mark A. Jones

Introduction

In this chapter clinical reasoning in musculoskeletal practice is presented as being multi-dimensional and involving fast, intuitive first impressions and slow, more analytical deliberations. It is hypothesis oriented, dialectic, collaborative and reflective. Skilled clinical reasoning contributes to clinicians' learning and to the transformation of existing perspectives. The scope of clinical reasoning is presented through discussion of three key frameworks: (1) biopsychosocial philosophy of practice, (2) clinical reasoning strategies and (3) hypothesis categories. Cognitive processes involved in clinical reasoning (e.g. deduction, induction, abduction) are explained, and key factors influencing skilled clinical reasoning and expertise are discussed, including critical thinking, metacognition, knowledge organization, data collection and procedural skills, and patient–therapist therapeutic alliance. Lateral thinking is proposed as important to the generation of new ideas.

Why do we need to study and practice clinical reasoning? Nobel Laureate Daniel Kahneman highlights the numerous biases of human judgment that occur due to quick judgments and a lack of analytical thinking. He describes two broad forms of thinking: fast (System 1) thinking characterized by automatic and effortless first impressions and intuition (as with tacit pattern recognition) and slow (System 2) thinking characterized by analytical deliberations requiring more attention, time and effort (Kahneman, 2011). Both of these fictitious[1] systems operate together, with System 1 running automatically and System 2 normally in a low-effort mode. Our System 1 quick impressions receive minimal scrutiny from our slower System 2 analysis, and if endorsed, those initial impressions and intuitions turn into beliefs that lead to actions. More simply, you accept your fast impressions as representing a prior belief without further scrutiny (note that this is true for patients as well as clinicians). However, when System 1 runs into difficulty, as when the representativeness of a finding (e.g. within a patient's story, physical assessment or outcome re-assessment) is unclear, contradictory or not what you expected, System 2 is called upon for more attentive processing.

A wide range of errors (e.g. poor, inaccurate judgments) can be attributed to quick first impressions and decisions based on insufficient information and lack of further deliberation. For example, consider the following puzzle (Kahneman, 2011, p. 44) and your first impression/intuition (without formally trying to solve it):

A bat and ball cost $1.10.
The bat costs one dollar more than the ball.
How much does the ball cost?

---

[1]Kahneman highlights that his Systems 1 and 2 are fictitious in the sense that they are not systems in the convention of entities with interacting aspects that can be simply attributed to one part of the brain or another. He explains that the value of this distinction relates to the aptitude of our mind to better understand constructs presented as stories with active agents, in this case Systems 1 and 2.

The quick, intuitive and wrong answer is 10 cents[2] (50% of Harvard, MIT and Princeton students studied got this wrong; 80% of students from less prestigious universities) (Kahneman, 2011). Although heuristics, or shortcuts in thinking, work well in many circumstances, if they go unchecked by more deliberative thinking, as with this example, errors will occur.

When you consider that every patient cue perceived (verbal, visual, kinaesthetic) undergoes some level of System 1 and/or System 2 processing, it is easy to appreciate the potential for analogous errors in musculoskeletal clinical reasoning. For example:

Acromioclavicular joint (ACJ) pain is provoked with shoulder movement into horizontal flexion.
Horizontal flexion provokes ACJ-area pain on active-movement testing.
The patient's pain is due to nociception in the ACJ.

The patient reports mid-thoracic pain consistently provoked after sitting to eat lunch.
The patient reports sitting in fully slouched position when eating lunch.
Mid-thoracic pain is due to nociception associated with slouched sitting at lunch.

Inappropriate pain beliefs and cognitions contribute to nociplastic pain sensitization.
A patient has inappropriate pain beliefs and cognitions.
The patient has nociplastic pain sensitization.

These examples illustrate errors of deduction. Nociception from other structures can be responsible for ACJ-area pain (e.g. subacromial tissues); other predisposing factors than slouched sitting can precipitate mid-thoracic pain (e.g. gallbladder nociception secondary to eating fatty foods); and inappropriate pain beliefs and cognitions can also exist with nociceptive dominant pain. Although you may believe your System 2 would not uncritically endorse these System 1 conclusions without obtaining further supporting information, it is a bit disheartening to contemplate the large number of biases evidenced in health-related and non-health-related human judgment that Kahneman and others (e.g. Croskerry, 2003; Hogarth, 2005; Kahneman et al., 1982; Lehrer, 2009; Schwartz and Elstein, 2008) report. Some examples easily recognizable in clinical practice include the following:

- The 'priming' influence of prior information (e.g. diagnosis provided in a referral, imaging findings, influence of a recent publication or course)
- 'Confirmation bias', or the tendency to attend to and collect data that confirm existing hypotheses
- 'Memory bias' of a spectacular successful outcome
- 'Overestimation of representativeness', as with the probability of a diagnosis given a finding being confused with the probability of a finding given a diagnosis
- 'Conservatism or stickiness', where initial impressions and hypotheses are not revised in the face of subsequent non-supporting information

The greater the coherence of our fast-thinking impressions, the more likely we are to jump to conclusions without further System 2 analysis. Unfortunately, humans are prone to find and accept coherence on the basis of limited information, so much so that Kahneman (2011, p. 86) has characterized this trait associated with many of our biases as 'What You See Is All There Is', that is, the assumption or acceptance that the information at hand is all that is available. You build a story (explanation) from the information you have, and if it is a good, coherent story, you believe it. Paradoxically, coherent stories are easier to construct when there is less information to make sense of.

Although fast thinking is the source of many of our errors, ironically, it is also the source of most of what we do right. When you break down the overall synthesis and analysis of a patient's presentation and consider the vast number of first-impression, fast-thinking judgments that lead up to and inform our understanding of patients and their

---

[2]If a ball is 10 cents and a bat is one dollar more ($1.10), then together they would be $1.20, not $1.10. The ball is 5 cents.

problems (e.g. quick recognition of when a patient's telling of his or her story requires clarification; patient discomfort and emotions; observed postural, movement and control impairments; when additional physical testing is required for physical differentiation, etc.), the ubiquity of our fast thinking is obvious. With appropriate training and experience, we learn to effectively use our fast thinking to recognize potentially significant cues, interpret contextualized meanings, recognize when clarification and further testing are required to refine interpretations, and identify appropriate actions and solutions. The key is not to deny the use of initial impressions and fast thinking but to build our skill with this through quality practice and to be aware of the pitfalls and common errors of bias. One of the foremost researchers in problem solving, Herbert Simon (also a Nobel Laureate), perhaps best known for his seminal problem-solving research with chess masters, explains intuition as 'nothing more and nothing less than recognition' (Simon, 1992, p. 155). That is, accurate intuitions of experts are best explained by the effects of prolonged practice.

Although we articulate our judgments and make decisions through our analytical thinking, that is not to say this system is without error. Our slow analytical thinking will often simply endorse or rationalize ideas generated through our fast thinking (Kahneman, 2011). Research has demonstrated that experts function largely on pattern recognition (e.g. Boshuizen and Schmidt, 2008; Jensen et al., 2007; Kaufman et al. 2008; Schwartz and Elstein, 2008) and that overanalyzing also leads to errors in judgment (Lehrer, 2009; Schwartz and Elstein, 2008). However, although not flawless, our slow analytical thinking provides a backup, a check for our fast first impressions and pattern recognition that reduces error and as such needs to be understood and developed, especially in areas of uncertainty and complexity.

Kahneman concludes that humans need help to make more accurate judgments and better decisions. We need to study and practice clinical reasoning, alongside our other professional competencies, to improve the accuracy of both our fast and slow thinking.

Key Point

All thinking, including musculoskeletal clinical reasoning, involves a combination of fast System 1 first impressions, inductions or pattern recognition and slow System 2 deliberations, testing of hypotheses and deductions. Although errors occur in both fast and slow thinking, bias in human judgment necessitates the use of slow analytical thinking, particularly in areas of uncertainty and complexity, to minimize error. An understanding of clinical reasoning and practice doing clinical reasoning are needed to improve clinical reasoning proficiency and enhance the application of core musculoskeletal-associated theory to clinical practice.

The Scope of Clinical Reasoning

Clinical reasoning can be defined as a reflective process of inquiry and analysis carried out by a health professional in collaboration with the patient with the aim of understanding the patient, the patient's context and the patient's clinical problem(s) in order to guide evidence-based practice (Brooker, 2013, supplied by Mark Jones). Although more extensive definitions are available (see Christensen and Nordstrom, 2013; Higgs and Jones, 2008), this captures the broad essence of what we hope to promote in this book.

Musculoskeletal clinicians work with a multitude of problem presentations in a variety of clinical practice environments (e.g. outpatient clinics, private practices, hospital- or outpatient-based rehabilitation and pain unit teams, sports settings, home care and industrial work sites). The clinical presentations they encounter are, therefore, varied, ranging from discrete, well-defined problems amenable to technical solutions to complex, multifactorial problems with uniqueness to the individual that defy the technical rationality of simply applying a 'proven' protocol of management. Schön (1987, p. 3) characterizes this continuum of professional practice as existing between the 'high, hard ground of technical rationality' and 'the swampy lowland' where 'messy, confusing problems defy technical solution'. To practise at both ends of the continuum clinicians must have good propositional (scholarly, research based) and non-propositional (professional craft) knowledge as well as advanced technical skills to solve problems of a discrete, well-defined nature. However, to understand and manage successfully the 'swampy lowland' of complex patient problems requires a rich blend of biopsychosocial knowledge and professional know-how, combined with personal awareness of your own philosophy of practice, potential biases and diagnostic, procedural and teaching skills. Contemporary musculoskeletal clinicians must have a high level of knowledge and skills across a comprehensive range of competencies, including assessment, management, communication (including teaching, negotiating, counselling), documentation and professional, legal and ethical comportment. Effective performance within and across these competencies requires a broad perspective of what constitutes health and disability and equally broad skills in both diagnostic and non-diagnostic clinical reasoning.

Clinical Reasoning in a Biopsychosocial Framework

The biopsychosocial framework was originally put forward by Engel (1977). As depicted in the World Health Organization (WHO) International Classification of Functioning, Disability and Health (ICF) model (WHO, 2001) (Fig. 1.1) the biopsychosocial perspective recognizes that disability is the result of the cumulative effects of the biological health condition (disease, illness, pathology, disorder), external environmental influences (e.g. physical, social, economic, political, etc.) and internal personal influences (e.g. age, gender, education, beliefs, culture, coping style, self-efficacy, etc.). This is in contrast to the reductionist biomedical model that previously dominated medicine and musculoskeletal practice where disease and illness were primarily attributed to pathogens, genetic or developmental abnormalities or injury. By understanding disability as also being socially constructed, the health professions, including musculoskeletal practice, expanded or made more explicit the need for clinicians to understand all potential biopsychosocial influences and integrate that understanding into their existing assessments, reasoning and management (e.g. Borrell-Carrió et al., 2004; Edwards and Jones, 2007a, 2007b; Epstein and Borrell-Carrió, 2005; Imrie, 2004; Jones et al., 2002; Jones and Edwards, 2008).

The contribution of psychosocial factors to the development, and particularly the maintenance, of patients' pain and disability and clinicians' assessments of their patients' psychosocial status is the focus of Chapters 3 and 4. For the purpose of this chapter, the biopsychosocial framework illustrated in Fig. 1.1 is used to highlight the scope of knowledge, skills and clinical reasoning required to fully understand our patients' problems and our patients themselves (i.e. the person behind the problem). The boxes across the middle of the diagram depict the patient's clinical presentation, incorporating physical impairments of body functions and structures, restrictions and capabilities in functional activities and restrictions and capabilities in the patient's ability to participate in life situations (e.g. work, family, sport, leisure) that collectively make up the patient's disability. Bidirectional arrows between the clinical presentation and the biomedical, environmental and personal influences

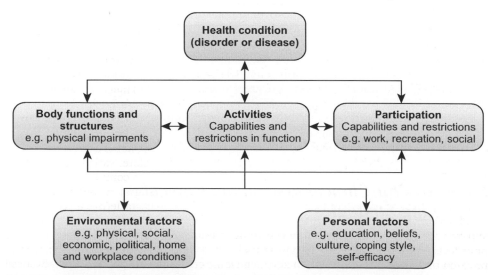

Fig. 1.1 Adaptation of World Health Organization (WHO) International Classification of Functioning, Disability and Health (ICF) framework. *(Reproduced with permission [WHO, 2001, p. 18].)*

reflect the reciprocal relationship whereby each has the potential to influence the other (Borrell-Carrió et al., 2004; Duncan, 2000; Pincus, 2004). For example, where traditionally functional restrictions, physical impairments and pain would have been conceptualized as the end result of a specific injury/pathology or syndrome, the reciprocal arrows highlight that these also can be associated with and even maintained by environmental and personal influences. A holistic understanding of a patient's clinical presentation therefore necessitates attention and analysis of the patient's physical health, environmental and personal factors. Although musculoskeletal clinicians are generally well educated to assess and manage the physical and many environmental dimensions of the patient's health condition, formal education and experience assessing, analysing and managing psychological and social factors contributing to both acute and chronic pain is often less developed and less structured (e.g. Barlow, 2012; Bishop and Foster, 2005; Foster and Delitto, 2011; Main and George, 2011; Overmeer et al., 2005; Sanders et al., 2013; Singla et al., 2014). The sociological dimension of psychosocial in particular is generally given less attention as a factor contributing to the pain experience (Blyth et al., 2007). A growing body of literature is now available informing musculoskeletal clinicians' psychosocial assessment and management (e.g. French and Sim, 2004; Hasenbring et al., 2012; Johnson and Moores, 2006; Jones and Edwards, 2008; Keefe et al., 2006; Main et al., 2008; Muncey, 2002; Schultz et al., 2002; also see Chapters 3 and 4) with literature also explicitly relating the WHO ICF to categorization of clinical problems, clinical reasoning and management (e.g. Allet et al., 2008; Childs et al., 2008; Cibulka et al., 2009; Edwards and Jones, 2007a; Escorpizo et al., 2010; Jette, 2006; McPoil et al., 2008; Steiner et al., 2002).

Being able to practice within a biopsychosocial framework requires different sets of knowledge and clinical skills to be able to understand both the biological problems and the environmental and personal factors that may predispose to the development or contribute to the maintenance of the patient's pain and disability experiences. As such, a distinction can be made between understanding and managing the biological problem to effect change versus understanding and interacting with the person to effect change. To assist clinicians' application of biopsychosocial practice, we have promoted our evolving use of two frameworks for guiding the focus of clinical reasoning required (clinical reasoning strategies) and the categories of decisions required (hypothesis categories) (Edwards et al., 2004a; Jones, 1987, 2014; Jones et al., 2008).

Key Point

Conceptualizing disability as the cumulative effects of the biological health condition (disease, illness, pathology, disorder), environmental influences (e.g. physical and social) and personal influences (e.g. beliefs, culture, socio-economic, education) highlights the scope of knowledge, skills and clinical reasoning required to practice in a biopsychosocial framework. Musculoskeletal clinicians are traditionally well educated in the assessment and management of physical and environmental factors contributing to patients' disabilities; however, formal education and experience assessing, analysing and managing psychological and social factors are often less developed and less structured. Psychosocial assessment and management feature in varying degrees within the case studies of this book. Attention to how psychosocial factors are screened, the reasoning used to determine their contribution to individual patients' clinical presentations and how they are addressed in management will assist clinicians in further developing this important component of their biopsychosocial practice.

Focus of Our Clinical Reasoning: Clinical Reasoning Strategies

When students first consider clinical reasoning in musculoskeletal practice, they typically only focus on diagnosis, with diagnosis itself often limited to categorizing the type of problem, injury or pathology. When all potential influences present in the biopsychosocial perspective (Fig. 1.1) are considered, as well as the reasoning required in the corresponding management of identified influences, then clearly reasoning about diagnosis represents only a portion of the reasoning that actually occurs in clinical practice. Research and theoretical propositions across a range of health professions (e.g. physiotherapy, medicine, nursing, occupational therapy) have identified explicit foci of clinical reasoning, including diagnostic reasoning, narrative reasoning, procedural reasoning, interactive reasoning, collaborative reasoning, predictive reasoning, ethical reasoning and teaching as reasoning (Higgs and Jones, 2008). Edwards and colleagues (Edwards, 2000; Edwards et al., 2004a) investigated the clinical reasoning of expert physiotherapists in three different fields of physiotherapy (musculoskeletal, neurological and domiciliary/home health care) and found that these physiotherapists employed a range of 'clinical reasoning strategies' despite the differing emphases of their examinations and management. The following clinical reasoning strategies were each associated with a range of diverse clinical actions:

Diagnostic reasoning: Reasoning underpinning the formation of a musculoskeletal practice diagnosis related to functional limitation(s) and associated physical and movement impairments with consideration of pain type, tissue pathology and the broad scope of potential contributing factors.

Narrative reasoning: Reasoning associated with understanding patients' pain, illness and/or disability experiences. This incorporates their understanding (including personal meaning) of their problem(s) and effects on their lives; their expectations regarding management; associated cognitions and emotions; their ability to cope; and the effects these personal perspectives have on their clinical presentation, particularly whether they are facilitating or obstructing their recovery.

Reasoning about procedure: Reasoning underpinning the selection, implementation and progression of treatment procedures. Although clinical guidelines provide broad direction, typically focusing only on diagnostic categorization, practising clinicians need to adaptively reason how best to apply those guidelines to patients' individual presentations and goals. Progression of treatment is mostly then guided by judicious outcome re-assessment that attends to impairment and function-/disability-related outcomes.

Interactive reasoning: Reasoning guiding the purposeful establishment and ongoing management of clinician–patient rapport (discussed further under Factors Influencing Reasoning).

Collaborative reasoning: The shared decision-making between patient and clinician (and others) as a therapeutic alliance in the interpretation of examination findings, setting of goals and priorities, and implementation and progression of treatment (see Edwards et al. [2004b] and Trede and Higgs [2008] for further detail).

Reasoning about teaching: Reasoning associated with the planning, execution and evaluation of individualized and context sensitive strategies to facilitate change, including facilitating motivation for change, facilitating conceptual change in understanding and beliefs (e.g. regarding medical and musculoskeletal diagnosis and pain), facilitation of constructive coping strategies, and facilitation of improved physical performance, activity and participation capabilities (e.g. rehabilitative exercises, conditioning, sport technique, activity pacing and graded exposure).

Predictive reasoning: Reasoning utilized in judgments regarding effects of specific interventions and overall prognosis. Although prognostic judgments regarding whether musculoskeletal therapy can help and expected time frame are not precise, a thorough reasoning consideration of biological, environmental and personal factors that recognizes both facilitators and barriers (i.e. positives and negatives in a patient's presentation), as well as what is and isn't modifiable, will assist this reasoning strategy.

Ethical reasoning: Reasoning underpinning the recognition and resolution of ethical dilemmas which impinge upon patients' ability to make decisions concerning their health and upon the conduct of treatment and its desired goals (see Edwards et al. [2005] and Edwards and Delany [2019] for further detail).

Consideration of these diagnostic and non-diagnostic foci of reasoning assist by highlighting the broad scope of clinical reasoning we should be aware of, critique and strive to improve. The complexity of our reasoning is further evident in the finding that expert physiotherapists have been shown to dialectically move in their reasoning between contrasting biological and psychosocial poles in a fluid and seemingly effortless manner (Edwards, 2000; Edwards et al., 2004a). For example, a diagnostic test may elicit a patient response reflecting fear of movement underpinned by inappropriate beliefs and cognitions regarding their diagnosis, pathology and/or pain. Sensitivity, specificity and likelihood ratios of the diagnostic test inform the likelihood of having that condition. At the same time, the expert clinician perceives the more qualitative patient expressions of fear, tempering their diagnostic analysis and dialectically shifting their reasoning from biological to psychosocial.

Attending to patients' psychosocial status alongside physical/diagnostic findings is essential. It is not possible to fully understand a patient's pain and disability experience without a comprehensive physical examination that reveals the extent of physical impairment and disability they have to cope with. Similarly, psychosocial assessment will not only inform diagnostic reasoning, but it also enables identification of unhelpful perspectives that need to be addressed in management for both acute and chronic presentations. Although the clinical reasoning strategies provide a framework to assist students and practicing clinicians recognize the different foci of reasoning required, it is also helpful to recognize the different categories of clinical decisions required within these different reasoning strategies.

Key Point

> Diagnostic reasoning represents only one focus of clinical reasoning in musculoskeletal practice. Expert clinicians have been shown to employ a range of 'clinical reasoning strategies' incorporating different foci of reasoning including diagnostic reasoning, narrative reasoning, reasoning about procedure, interactive reasoning, collaborative reasoning, reasoning about teaching, predictive reasoning and ethical reasoning. Experts are able to dialectically move in their clinical reasoning between the biological and psychosocial poles of the biopsychosocial framework in accordance with emerging patient information. Awareness, critique and practice in all areas of clinical reasoning are important to developing expertise in clinical practice.

Categories of Clinical Decisions Required: Hypothesis Categories

It seems obvious that clinicians should know the purpose of every question they ask their patients and every physical assessment they conduct. That is, what do you want to find out, and what decision will that information inform? It is not necessary or even appropriate to stipulate a definitive list of decisions all clinicians must consider, as this would only stifle the independent and creative thinking important to the evolution of our professions. However, a minimum list of categories of decisions that can/should be considered is helpful to those learning and reflecting on their clinical reasoning because it provides them with initial guidance to understand the purpose of their questions and physical assessments, encourages breadth of reasoning beyond diagnosis and creates a framework in which clinical knowledge can be organized as it relates to decisions that must be made (i.e. diagnosing, understanding psychosocial influences, determining therapeutic interventions, establishing rapport/therapeutic alliance, collaborating, teaching, prognosis and managing ethical dilemmas). What follows is a list of 'hypothesis categories' initially proposed by Jones (1987) that has continued to evolve through professional discussion to this current format (Table 1.1). Research evidence regarding musculoskeletal clinicians' focus of clinical reasoning, including reasoning across and within these different categories, is available (e.g. Barlow, 2012; Doody and McAteer, 2002; Edwards et al., 2004a; Jensen, 2007; Rivett and Higgs, 1997; Smart and Doody, 2006). This, combined with reflective discourse from experienced clinicians and clinical educators, broadly supports the relevance and use of these particular hypothesis categories. Nevertheless, these specific hypothesis categories are not being recommended for uncritical use by all clinicians, and whatever categories of decisions are adopted should continually be reviewed to ensure they reflect contemporary health care and musculoskeletal practice.

TABLE 1.1

HYPOTHESIS CATEGORIES

- Activity and participation capability and restriction
- Patients' perspectives on their experiences and social influences (psychosocial status)
- Pain type
- Sources of symptoms
- Pathology
- Impairments in body function or structure
- Contributing factors to the development and maintenance of the problem
- Precautions and contraindications to physical examination and treatment
- Management/treatment selection and progression
- Prognosis

Activity and Participation Capability and Restriction

Patients' activity capabilities and restrictions directly relate to the ICF framework of health and disability presented in Fig. 1.1 and refer to the patient's functional abilities and restrictions (e.g. walking, lifting, sitting, etc.) that are volunteered and further screened for. To gain a complete picture, it is important the clinician identifies those activities the patient is capable of alongside those that are restricted.

Patients' participation capabilities and restrictions refer to the patient's abilities and restrictions to participate in life situations (e.g. work, recreation/sport, family, etc.). Again, determining participation capabilities, including modified participation (e.g. modified work duties), is important because this will contribute to other decisions such as prognosis and management. Note that identifying patients' activity and participation restrictions and capabilities, either through interview or through questionnaire, does not really qualify as formulating 'hypotheses' in the sense that these are not clinicians' judgments or deductions; rather, they are simply essential information to obtain in order to understand the extent of the patient's disability and quality of life. They are included in the hypothesis categories framework simply to facilitate attention to these critical aspects of the patient's pain/disability experience. Later, when making judgments about pain type, the proportionality of activity and participation restrictions and the physical impairments/pathology identified through examination will need to be considered. When activity and participation restrictions are out of proportion to identified physical impairments and pathology, then it may reflect a nociplastic pain type (IASP Taxonomy 2017; Nijs et al., 2015; Smart et al., 2012c; Woolf, 2011), and it is likely the patient's psychosocial status will be negatively contributing to the patient's disability.

Patient Perspectives on Their Experiences and Social Influences (Psychosocial Status)

Patients' perspectives on their experiences and social influences relate to the patient's psychosocial status, which the clinician needs to assess and understand. Musculoskeletal clinicians' psychosocial assessment is discussed in more detail in Chapters 3 and 4. But briefly, psychosocial assessment incorporates such things as:

- What are the patient's perspectives of their pain/disability experience?
  - Understanding / beliefs regarding their problem, its diagnosis, about pain (for example, with respect to: seriousness, changeability and controllability) AND what is the basis of those beliefs (i.e. why do they think that)?
  - What are their expectations and beliefs about management and their role in management? What are their specific goals?
  - How they are coping, emotionally (e.g., anger, depressive symptoms, feelings of vulnerability, etc.) and behaviorally? Do they have any specific coping strategies (e.g. medication, rest, alcohol, exercise, avoidance), and if so, are they effective?

- What are the patient's social circumstances (e.g. education / health literacy, culture, living, work, friends, etc.) and what is their perception of support:
  - How does the patient think they are perceived by their partner, workmates and employer, and how does this affect their self-concept, self-efficacy and pain/disability experience?
- Is change important to the patient? What is their self-efficacy to positively contribute to change? What tasks do they currently believe they can perform? What tasks do they believe they will be able to return to following management?

In the clinical reasoning strategies framework presented earlier, hypotheses regarding psychosocial status fit within narrative reasoning focused on understanding patients' pain, illness and/or disability experiences. When assessing understanding of their problem (e.g. diagnosis, pain), this is not simply their superficial understanding (e.g. what the doctor told them or what they have read); rather, it refers to what meaning they attach to that understanding (e.g. likely recovery, fear of further damage, etc.).

Pain Type

Understanding pain, including types of pain, differences between acute and chronic pain, referred pain and the associated neurophysiology, is essential knowledge to musculoskeletal clinicians. For this knowledge to be useful in clinical practice, it then must be linked to clinical reasoning, for example, clinical patterns of different pain types and the implications to precautions in assessment and management, management strategies and prognosis. Chapter 2 provides an overview of contemporary pain science understanding linked to clinical reasoning. For the purposes of this chapter, pain type is discussed as a hypothesis category because of its overarching importance to these other reasoning decisions, especially management.

The three main types of pain musculoskeletal clinicians need to be able to assess for and recognize include nociceptive pain (with and without inflammation), neuropathic pain and nociplastic pain[3] (e.g. Gifford et al., 2006; IASP Taxonomy 2017; Nijs et al., 2014b; Woolf, 2011, 2014). Nociceptive pain is protective and refers to pain that is associated with actual or threatened damage to non-neural tissue and involves activation of peripheral nociceptors (IASP Taxonomy 2017). Nociceptive inflammatory pain occurs with tissue damage, and/or immune cell activation in the case of systemic inflammation, facilitating repair by causing pain hypersensitivity until healing occurs (Woolf, 2010). Neuropathic pain refers to pain arising as a direct consequence of a lesion or disease affecting the somatosensory system and can be further differentiated into peripheral or central neuropathic pain depending on the anatomic location of the lesion (IASP Taxonomy 2017; Jensen et al., 2011; Treede et al., 2008). Nociplastic pain is dysfunctional pain associated with altered nociceptive processing in the central nervous system in the absence of overt peripheral drivers such as tissue injury or neuropathy. Nociplastic pain has been demonstrated in a wide range of conditions commonly treated by musculoskeletal clinicians, including non-specific chronic back pain, complex regional pain syndrome, chronic fatigue syndrome, fibromyalgia, post-surgical pain, and visceral pain hypersensitivity syndromes (Ashina et al., 2005; Clauw 2015; Coombes et al., 2012; Fernandez-Carnero et al., 2009; Lluch Girbés et al., 2013; Meeus et al., 2012; Nijs et al., 2012a; Perrotta et al., 2010; Price et al., 2002; Roussel et al., 2013; Woolf, 2011). The hypersensitivity manifests as increased responsiveness to a variety of stimuli, including mechanical pressure, chemical substances, light, sound, cold, heat, stress and electrical, with links to a range of CNS dysfunctions, as discussed in Chapter 2.

Although both subjective and physical clinical features of pain types have been reported (Bielefeldt and Gebhart, 2006; Mayer et al., 2012; Nijs et al., 2010; Nijs et al. 2015; Schaible, 2006; Smart et al., 2012a, 2012b, 2012c; Treede et al., 2008; Woolf, 2011), diagnostic criteria and biomarkers of nociplastic pain are still not definitive (Kosek et al.,

---

[3]Through most of the writing of this book this third pain type was called "maladaptive central nervous system sensitization". This was changed to "nociplastic" in the final stages of writing to be consistent with the IASP change in terminology. However, it is acknowledged the new term is controversial and may change again in the future.

2016; Vardeh, Mannion & Woolf, 2016; Woolf, 2011, 2014). As such, when clinical features of different pain types co-exist, differentiation is challenging. This is particularly true for initial appointments where the full picture of the patient's presentation (subjective, imaging, physical findings) is still emerging. For example, the full pain experience, including initial screening for adverse psychosocial factors by interview and/or questionnaire, often is not fully revealed at the first appointment. As clinician–patient rapport develops and time allows for questionnaire responses to be explored and clarified, a fuller picture will usually become available. Both physical and psychosocial stress can contribute to neuroimmune system dysregulation and thus contribute to pain hypersensitization. Clarification of apparent overlap in pain mechanisms (e.g. nociception with and without sensitization) may be assisted through outcome re-assessments of targeted treatment interventions over a defined period of time. That is, nociplastic pain occurs in response to both internal and external inputs, including cognitive and emotional modulation (e.g. thoughts, beliefs, fears, anxiety) and can be triggered, but not maintained, by nociception from pathological, inflamed or overloaded tissues if present, enabling increased sensitivity (or decreased load tolerance) to co-exist with somatic and visceral nociception. While pain type informs management, the mechanisms and contributors that underpin pain type can differ and change over time. As such, hypotheses about the dominant pain type may change as further information comes to light. Short-term treatments and re-assessments to potentially relevant physical impairments may assist in establishing how much an apparent sensitization is being driven by the symptomatic physical impairments or other co-existing cognitions, emotions and life stressors. Although interventions directed at musculoskeletal tissues have central modulatory influences (e.g. Cagnie et al., 2013; Nijs et al., 2011a, 2012a; Schmid et al., 2008; Smith et al., 2013, 2014; Vincenzino et al., 2007b; Zusman, 2008), they are unlikely to be sufficient on their own to resolve persistent nociplastic pain. However, when physical impairments and associated disability underpin psychological stress and negative cognitions, skilled physical and environmental management would be expected to improve if not resolve negative psyche and disability. When both physical and cognitive/affective factors appear to contribute to maintained pain and disability, management would logically address both. In contrast, successful management for dominant nociplastic pain and persistent pain memories maintained by psychosocial factors will likely require combinations of pharmacotherapy and cognitive-behavioural strategies through pain neuroscience education, facilitation of active coping strategies, graded activity and exercise (Louw et al., 2011; Moseley, 2004; Moseley & Butler, 2017; Nijs et al., 2011a, 2011b, 2012b, 2014a; Turk and Flor, 2006; Zusman, 2008) and is unlikely to be helped by traditional tissue-based approaches. The importance of recognizing clinical features of nociplastic pain is also evident when hypothesizing about potential nociceptive tissue pathology or sources based on joint, muscle and soft tissue assessments. Nociplastic pain can create local false-positive provocation of symptoms suggestive of tissue pathology (Gifford, 1998; Nijs et al., 2010) illustrating the influence of one hypothesis category (e.g. pain type) on another (e.g. source of symptoms) and the complexity of clinical reasoning required.

Source of Symptoms

Although the majority of patients with musculoskeletal problems present with pain as a symptom, they also present with other symptoms such as hyper-/hypoesthesias, paraesthesias, dysesthesias, vascular associated symptoms, stiffness, weakness, joint sensations (e.g. instability, clicking, locking) and urinary urgency and incontinence, among others. Patients in other areas of clinical practice (e.g. neurological, cardiorespiratory) present with additional symptoms characteristic of disorders of those systems. Consequently, as discussed under General Health Screening, it is important thorough screening occurs for other symptoms beyond the patient's main complaint to ensure that relevant symptoms not spontaneously volunteered and that relevant health comorbidities are not missed.

When patients do present with pain, and when a nociceptive 'pain type' is hypothesized, then it is appropriate to reason further regarding potential sources of nociception. Although validation of the source of nociception on the basis of a clinical examination alone is often limited, biological and clinical knowledge of pain distribution, patterns of provocation and relief and common mechanisms of onset enables clinicians to hypothesize about the likely sources of nociception. The accuracy of this aspect of diagnosis is significantly better with some types of problems (e.g. muscle and ligament injuries) than others (e.g. low back pain). However, even when a specific tissue cannot be confirmed, broader hypotheses about body regions (e.g. spine versus shoulder or hip) are still helpful in differential questioning and testing through the subjective and physical examination.

As an example of generating hypotheses regarding possible sources of nociception for a patient's symptoms based on the area of symptoms, consider the body chart in Table 1.2 depicting a common area of shoulder pain and the potential nociceptive, neuropathic and visceral sources of nociception that should be considered.

TABLE 1.2

BODY CHART DEPICTING AN EXAMPLE OF SYMPTOM LOCATION AND THE POTENTIAL NOCICEPTIVE, NEUROPATHIC AND VISCERAL SOURCES THAT SHOULD BE CONSIDERED FOR THAT SYMPTOM AREA

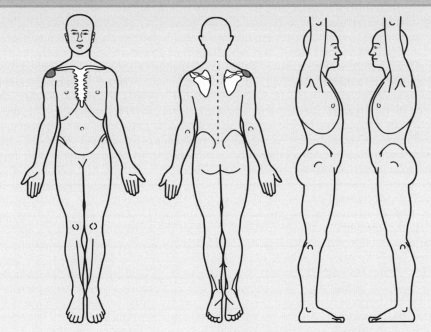

Potential Local Nociceptive Sources	Potential Neuropathic Sources	Potential Nociceptive Sources of Somatic Referral	Potential Nociceptive Sources of Visceral Referral
• Glenohumeral periarticular (rotator interval structures, capsule and ligaments) • Glenohumeral intra-articular (glenoid labrum, biceps attachment, joint surface) • Subacromial space (rotator cuff, biceps, bursa, coraco-acromial ligament, acromion) • Acromioclavicular joint	• Axillary nerve • Suprascapular nerve • C3–C7 nerve roots	• Any C5/C6 motion segment structures (muscle, posterior intervertebral joint) • Any somatic structure sharing the C5–C6 innervation	• Visceral structures with common innervation to shoulder (e.g. phrenic nerve C3–C5 innervates diaphragm, pericardium, gallbladder, pancreas) • Visceral structures capable of irritating diaphragm (heart, spleen [L], kidneys, pancreas, gallbladder [R], liver [R])

Considering potential structures involved within the suggested columns assists a thorough generation of hypotheses that can then be 'tested' with further questioning through the behaviour of symptoms (aggravating and easing factors), history, general health screening and physical examination–treatment–re-assessment. As alluded to earlier, hypotheses about specific tissue sources of nociception for the patient's symptoms must be made with consideration of the dominant pain type hypothesized. Although clinical examination cannot always confirm the actual nociceptive source of a patient's nociceptive-dominant symptoms, clues from the area and behaviour of symptoms, history, physical examination and treatments/re-assessments, combined with knowledge of common clinical patterns, will enable the clinician to hypothesize the likely structures at fault and possibly their pathology.

Pathology

Pathology is defined as the structural and functional changes in the body caused by disease or trauma (Goodman and Fuller, 2009). Although it is often not possible for musculoskeletal clinicians to confirm pathology clinically, similar to the limitation of clinically confirming the source of nociception, it is still important to hypothesize about pathology for consideration of implications to other hypothesis categories, particularly precautions to physical examination and treatment, management and prognosis. Some suspected pathologies require further investigation and possibly medical or surgical management (e.g. fracture, dislocation, compartment syndrome, cauda equine, visceral referred symptoms), whereas others simply require more caution in physical examination and treatment (e.g. neuropathic pain, seronegative spondyloarthropathies). Research regarding management for different pathologies informs broad management strategies, and understanding of known or suspected pathology also enables better estimation of prognosis (e.g. post-traumatic sprained wrist versus painful wrist associated with rheumatoid arthritis).

Pathology should be considered with respect to characteristic morphological changes of the structures and tissues involved and with respect to the associated pathogenesis or pathophysiological processes underpinning those changes. Symptom presentation alone can be insufficient to guide safe and effective examination and treatment. For example, hypotheses regarding suspected acute muscle or ligament injury and knowledge of the associated inflammatory healing process significantly guide the stages of management based on pathophysiology. However, although pathology can be a source of nociception and can correlate with activity and participation restrictions as well as physical impairments found on examination, pathology also can be asymptomatic, similar pathology can present quite differently in different patients and patients can present with tissue nociception without detectable pathology. Even when pathology is symptomatic, it may not correlate with activity and participation restrictions, physical impairment or improvement in symptoms. As such, pathology is not a good outcome measure, and over-focus on pathology can lead to errors of reasoning. Skilled clinical reasoning necessitates that the clinician must avoid simply administering prescribed pathology-focussed treatments. Practice guidelines and research- and theory-supported literature on management for different disorders and pathologies (e.g. tendinopathy – Cook and Purdam [2009]; intervertebral disc – Adams et al. [2010]; exercise for tissue repair – Khan and Scott [2009]; lateral epicondylalgia – Coombes et al. [2009]; see also Goodman and Fuller [2009]) provide excellent resources so long as application of their recommendations and principles are tailored to each patient's presentation (see Chapter 5). Hypotheses regarding pathology are particularly critical for identifying possible sinister and non-musculoskeletal conditions that require further investigation (discussed further under Precautions and Contraindications). A balance in reasoning between sources of symptoms (e.g. nociception), pathology and impairment is important. Known sources of symptoms and pathology must be seriously considered and unknown sources and pathology cautiously hypothesized. Adverse psychosocial influences and physical impairments should all be considered for their contribution to the development and maintenance of the patient's pain and disability. Although physiological effects of manual therapy and exercise can positively affect tissue healing (e.g. Khan and Scott, 2009) and pain neuromodulation (Nijs et al., 2012b, 2014a; Schmid et al., 2008; Vicenzino et al., 2007b; Voogt et al., 2015; Zusman, 2008), pathology is usually an ineffective or inefficient outcome measure to monitor on its own, and hence treatment interventions are best directed to negative psychosocial influences, function and associated physical impairments with due consideration of the pathology and pain type categories.

Impairments in Body Function or Structure

Impairment in the context of a patient's health condition is a loss or abnormality of body structure or of a physiological or psychological function (WHO, 2001). In musculoskeletal practice, psychological impairments typically manifest as elevated and functionally maladaptive psychological reactions to symptoms (i.e. 'yellow flags') and are explicitly targeted within the hypothesis category of patients' perspectives on their experience and social influences. Physiological impairments can exist in any body system (e.g. musculoskeletal, neurologic, psychologic, cardiovascular, respiratory, hematologic, gastrointestinal, genitourinary, gynaecologic, immunologic, endocrine), which may be closely associated with presenting musculoskeletal symptoms and impairments, may masquerade as 'musculoskeletal' and may have comorbid implications to musculoskeletal management such as exercise and fitness prescription. Although musculoskeletal clinicians are not qualified to diagnose outside their area of training, thorough screening of symptoms and general health, as discussed further in this section, is essential to identify previously diagnosed and potential undiagnosed non-musculoskeletal problems within different body systems for consideration of relevance to the patient's 'musculoskeletal' presentation and possible referral and further investigation (Goodman, Heick & Lazaro, 2017).

Common musculoskeletal-associated physical impairments hypothesized from the subjective examination and confirmed in the physical examination include impairments in posture, active and passive movement, soft tissue, neurodynamics and motor function (e.g. cognitive and proprioceptive awareness, control, balance and coordination, strength, etc.). Like pathology, physical impairments may be symptomatic and directly associated with the nociceptive source of the patient's symptoms or asymptomatic but still contributing by altering stress/load elsewhere causing other structures to be symptomatic (e.g. tight scalene muscles compromising neurovascular structures). Asymptomatic physical impairments must be analyzed with regard to the structures and processes responsible (e.g. restricted passive hip extension due to hip joint hypomobility, hip flexor tightness/tone and/or anterior neural irritation; or lower extremity weakness and trophic changes secondary to vascular claudication and peripheral vascular disease). Judging whether an impairment is contributing to other structures being symptomatic can sometimes be done through assessment of the effect of kinematic correction on symptom provocation (e.g. Mobilizations With Movement, scapular correction/assistance during movement, lumbopelvic postural correction during movement) but still must be critically evaluated through ongoing management and re-assessment.

Symptomatic physical impairments in a nociceptive-dominant presentation also have to be analyzed as to the structures, pathology and processes involved. Qualitative and quantitative description of symptomatic impairments with respect to pain (e.g. Visual Analogue Scale), mobility (e.g. active and passive range of movement and relationship to symptoms) and dynamic control (e.g. patterns of activation and kinematics) assist in the selection and progression of treatment, as well as the sensitivity of re-assessments.

Contributing Factors

Hypotheses regarding potential contributing factors represent the predisposing or associated factors involved in the development or maintenance of the patient's problem. Both intrinsic and extrinsic factors should be considered, including environmental, psychosocial, behavioural, physical/biomechanical and hereditary.

The potential physical contributing factors that can create excessive strain causing another structure to be symptomatic are quite varied. Examples here include hip extension stiffness causing increased lumbar spine strain during walking and weakness of the scapular upward rotators causing increase subacromial strain during shoulder elevation. Just as physical impairments commonly exist without becoming symptomatic, physical impairments can also cause increased strain without those tissues becoming symptomatic. Although these impairments still represent risk factors for musculoskeletal symptoms later (analogous to dietary risk factors for heart disease), establishing their relevance in a patient's current pain presentation requires systematic intervention to alter the impairment and re-assessment of the effect. Often this can be established relatively quickly with procedures that immediately address the impairment (e.g. manual assistance or taping of the scapula) or brief trial treatments to assess their benefit.

Even with the same pathology, different patients can have different physical, environmental and psychosocial contributing factors necessitating quite different management. For example, three patients can present with similar subacromial bursitis pathology causing subacromial nociception but quite different predisposing contributing factors necessitating quite different management. Patient one, for example, may present with a tight posterior glenohumeral joint capsule causing increased anterio-superior humeral head translation during overhead activities that result in bursal irritation. Patient two has good posterior capsule mobility, as reflected in the patient's good range of humeral internal rotation and horizontal flexion, but this patient has poor control/strength of the scapular force couples required to upwardly rotate the scapula, resulting in inadequate rotation, a narrowed subacromial outlet during overhead activities and bursal irritation. Patient three also has a motor control/strength problem but not of the scapula; instead, the rotator cuff force couples responsible for maintaining humeral head depression during elevation are ineffective resulting in increased superior translation and, again, bursal irritation. Knowledge of common contributing factors to different clinical problems combined with skilled reasoning to establish their relevance is essential. Although treatment directed to the hypothesized source of the patient's nociception is often effective in relieving symptoms, contributing factors must be addressed in order to minimize reoccurrence.

Precautions and Contraindications to Physical Examination and Treatment

Patient safety is paramount, and there is a range of decisions within this hypothesis category that clinicians must consider, including the following:

- Whether a physical examination should be carried out at all (versus immediate referral for further medical consultation/investigation) and if so, the extent of examination that can be safely performed that will minimize the risk of aggravating the patient's symptoms
- Whether specific safety tests are indicated (e.g. cervical arterial dysfunction testing, neurological examination, blood pressure/heart rate, instability tests, etc.)
- Whether any treatment should be undertaken (versus referral for further consultation/investigation)
- The appropriate dose/strength of any physical interventions planned

A number of factors will contribute to determining the extent of physical examination and treatment that is safe to perform, including the following:

- Presence of symptoms that have known association with more serious pathologies (e.g. cervical arterial dysfunction, aortic aneurysm, spinal cord, cauda equina, cancer, fracture, acute compartment syndrome, etc.)
- Dominant pain type (neuropathic and nociplstic pain types typically require more caution in not flaring up symptoms and caution with the patient's potential over-focus on symptoms and pathology)
- Patient's perspectives (anxious, fearful, angry patients, particularly with negative past medical/physiotherapy experiences require more caution)
- Severity and irritability of symptoms (Hengeveld and Banks, 2014)
- Nature of known pathologies (e.g. rheumatoid arthritis or osteoporosis require caution due to weakened tissues)
- Progression of the presentation (e.g. worsening problems require more caution)
- Presence of other medical conditions that may masquerade as a musculoskeletal problem or co-exist and require consideration and monitoring so that musculoskeletal interventions do not compromise the patient's other health problems (e.g. cardiac and respiratory conditions).

General Health Screening

General health screening for other health problems is essential to hypotheses regarding pre-cautions and contraindications. This requires knowledge of the body systems and common features of medical conditions, particularly those that overlap with neuromusculoskeletal problems. This form of screening is not for the purpose of assigning a medical diagnosis; rather medical/general health screening by musculoskeletal clinicians is for the purpose of identifying patients who may have medical conditions that require further investigation and medical consultation. This is particularly important to first-contact practitioners who see patients who have not previously been evaluated by a medical practitioner, but it is also important to clinicians practicing under referral because non-musculoskeletal conditions may have been missed or developed since the patient last saw a doctor. Clinicians should be familiar with recognized 'red flags', which are symptoms and signs that may indicate the presence of systemic or more sinister pathology / disease and non-musculoskeletal disorders masquerading as musculoskeletal that require further medical investigation. Red flag screening has poor diagnostic utility in patients with low back pain (e.g. Cook et al., 2017; Downie et al., 2013) highlighting the importance of integrating red flag screening into a reasoning process. Although some patient presentations warrant immediate medical attention (e.g. clinical features of cervical arterial dissection or cauda equina), single red flags (or even a cluster of red flags) do not necessarily necessitate medical referral (Goodman, Heick & Lazaro, 2017). The inevitable costs from further investigations on the basis of red flags with poor diagnostic utility is not justified (Cook et al., 2017). Instead, red flags must be interpreted in the context of the patient's full presentation with recognition of what constitutes a medical emergency and when "watchful waiting" is advised where red flags are monitored as treatment progresses (Cook et al., 2017). If physiotherapy and other management does not produce the expected improvement and when non-investigated red flags persist or worsen then medical consultation is warranted. There are different lists of red flags available in the literature, and the texts by Boissonnault (2011), Sebastian (2015), and Goodman, Heick & Lazaro (2017) are excellent resources written for musculoskeletal clinicians.

Management and Treatment

Management in this context refers to the overall health management of the patient, including consultation and referral to other health professionals, health promotion interventions (e.g. fitness assessment and management) and patient advocacy as required (e.g. with insurers or employers). Treatment refers to the specific therapeutic interventions (educational and physical) carried out during an appointment and the underlying reasoning required to determine what to address first, the strategy/procedure to use, the content and delivery of education, the dosage of the intervention, the outcome measures to reassess and the 'homework' or self-management appropriate for optimizing change (in understanding, impairment, activity and participation).

Most important to skilled reasoning is that there are no recipes! Health care in general and musculoskeletal practice in particular are not an exact science. Although clinical trials, clinical guidelines, clinical prediction rules and theory extrapolated from basic science all provide helpful guides to management for different problems, these should not be taken as prescriptions (Greenhalgh et al., 2014). Instead, clinicians must judge how the patient matches the population in the research reported and then tailor management to the individual patient's unique lifestyle, goals, activity and participation restrictions, perspectives and social circumstances, pain type, potential pathology and physical impairments. Because research-supported management efficacy is still lacking for most clinical problems, skilled reasoning is the clinician's best tool to minimize the risk of mismanagement and over-servicing.

The biopsychosocial model highlights the need for management to be holistic (i.e. addressing physical, environmental, psychosocial as required) with systematic and thorough re-assessments to determine inter-relationships between different physical impairments (e.g. presence of a neurodynamic impairment secondary to a soft tissue interface impairment) and between physical impairments and psychosocial factors (e.g. education to improve understanding leading to a decrease in patient fear and concurrent improvement in movement impairments). Management of contributing factors is essential to minimize the risk of reoccurrence, and patient understanding and active involvement are critical to promoting self-efficacy, self-management and long-term success.

Prognosis

Clinical judgment about prognosis refers to the therapist's informed hypotheses regarding the natural course of musculoskeletal problems, the efficacy of therapeutic interventions addressing their patient's unique presentation, and an estimate of how long this will take. Whether a patient's problem can be resolved, improved or the patient can be assisted to live with it depends in part on whether the factors underpinning the problem are modifiable or not. Prognostic research in low back pain explains less than 50% of the outcome variability due to methodological shortcomings in prognostic research and the multifactorial nature of patients' pain and disability (Hayden et al., 2010). In addition, there is insufficient understanding around the relative influence factors such as genetics, pathology, physiology and psychosocial influences. Musculoskeletal clinicians therefore need to be aware of the broad range of factors that may influence prognosis and recognise those that may be modified. Broadly, a patient's prognosis is determined by the nature and extent of the patient's problem(s), the natural course of the problem, the efficacy of therapeutic interventions and his or her ability and willingness to make the necessary changes (e.g. in lifestyle, psychosocial and physical contributing factors) to facilitate recovery or improved quality of life. Clues will be available throughout the subjective and physical examination and the ongoing management including the following:

- Patient's perspectives and expectations (including readiness, motivation and confidence to make changes)
- External incentives (e.g. return to work) and disincentives (e.g. litigation, lack of employer support)
- Extent of activity/participation restrictions
- Nature of problem (e.g. systemic disorder such as rheumatoid arthritis versus local ligamentous such as ankle sprain)
- Extent of 'pathology' and physical impairments
- Social, occupational and economic status
- Dominant pain type present
- Stage of tissue healing when overt injury has occurred
- Irritability of the disorder
- Length of history and progression of disorder
- Patient's general health, age and pre-existing disorders

Although prognostic decisions also are not an exact science, it is helpful to consider a patient's prognosis by reflecting on the positives and negatives from this list.

How to Use the Hypothesis Categories Framework

The decisions required in clinical practice will determine the information sought (e.g. safety information considered important necessitates safety-oriented questions and physical tests). However, the hypothesis category framework is not intended to direct the order in which information is obtained or the precise inquiries and physical tests utilized to obtain that information. Rather, simultaneous with thorough questioning and listening to understand a patient's story, followed by thorough screening of physical function, clinical reasoning within the hypothesis category framework involves consideration of the different categories of decisions as information unfolds. Although examinations must occur with immediate interpretation and ongoing synthesis of findings, narrow formulation of the problem into limited lists of hypotheses generated by the 'diagnosis', symptoms or duration of problem that are then ticked off through select testing lead to errors of omission (see Chapter 31). It is not possible or desirable to stipulate what hypothesis categories a clinician should be considering at any given point in time (e.g. it is not realistic or cognitively efficient to consider every hypothesis category after every new piece of information is obtained). However, equally, the clinician should not simply be obtaining information without thinking. In fact, by the end of the subjective examination, the clinician will typically have opinions (hypotheses) in most hypothesis categories in order to judge how much physical examination can be safely performed and which physical examination procedures are most important to prioritize at the first appointment. Clues to each category of hypothesis are available throughout the examination and ongoing management, with decisions eventually reached on the strength of supporting versus negating evidence.

Initial hypotheses generated (in any category) are 'tested' against further information obtained, which may also elicit consideration of a new, previously unconsidered hypothesis. Hypothesis generation and testing occurs through routine questions and physical assessments but may also be hypothesis driven as with the question asked or physical assessment performed with a specific hypothesis in mind (e.g. specific questioning regarding back versus hip postures and movements for a patient with groin pain; or clinical testing for instability in the patient with subjective features of instability). Clinical reasoning is therefore a dynamic, cyclic process that is 'hypothesis-oriented' (hypothesis generation, testing, reformulation) that leads to an evolving understanding of both the patient and the patient's problem(s). Although the physical examination is not limited to hypotheses formulated in the subjective examination as with a checklist, existing hypotheses logically still inform physical testing and prioritizing which tests are most important at the first appointment. That is, a structured physical examination is important to screen all relevant systems (e.g. articular, neural, muscular, soft tissue, fitness, etc.), but not every physical test is necessary for every patient, and a clear rationale (as opposed to following a rigid routine without reasoning) is needed for all assessments. Physical examination findings, including patient perspectives elicited during the physical such as fear of pain and movement, are then synthesized with existing hypotheses resulting in an evolving understanding sufficient for initial decisions on management and treatment. It is this ability to think on your feet through the examination and ongoing management that leads to variations in subjective questioning (e.g. qualification of patient responses and aspects of stories explored further) and physical assessments. Explicit consideration of different categories of clinical judgment or hypotheses and the scope of information informing each may assist in minimizing the 'What You See Is All There Is' and associated biases (Kahneman, 2011) described at the start of this chapter.

Key Point

> Understanding the scope of clinical judgments required across the different foci of clinical reasoning in a biopsychosocial framework assists comprehensive analysis of patient information obtained (e.g. answers to questions, physical findings, medical tests and treatment re-assessments). 'Hypothesis categories' proposed include activity capability/restriction, participation capability/restriction, patient's perspectives on their experience and social influences, pain type, sources of nociception and associated pathology, physical impairments and associated body structures/tissues involved, contributing factors to the development and maintenance of the problem, precautions and contraindications to physical examination and treatment, management/treatment selection and progression, and prognosis. Clues to each category of judgment are available throughout the examination and ongoing treatment re-assessments. Hypotheses generated are 'tested' against further information obtained, providing support, no support or consideration of new hypotheses, with ongoing evolution of understanding.

Inferences Within the Different Hypothesis Categories: Deduction, Induction/Pattern Recognition and Inference to the Best Explanation (Abduction)

When established criteria exist for making decisions and those criteria are fulfilled within the patient assessment, the judgment or inference made can be considered a deduction based on the premises or criteria. In logic, a correct deduction is simply judged on whether the criteria have been met or not, regardless of whether the original criteria themselves are correct. Given that the criteria on which we base the majority of our clinical decisions have not been explicitly validated and should constantly be critiqued for their accuracy, it is best to keep these deductions as hypotheses rather than fixed conclusions, thereby encouraging openness to revision.

When judgments are made that generalize from limited information (i.e. without checking all criteria normally expected), this inference represents an induction as when a clinical pattern is quickly recognized on the basis of limited key features. Inductive pattern recognition is not limited to diagnostic pathology or syndrome categorization, as such generalizations are also common regarding psychosocial status, pain type, precautions/contraindications and prognosis. In fact, research in medical education (e.g. Boshuizen and Schmidt, 2008) has demonstrated that experienced clinicians' pattern retention, and hence recognition, is more inclusive, incorporating enabling or predisposing factors, pathobiological and psychosocial processes and the resulting consequences or disability:

- Enabling conditions: conditions or constraints under which a disease or problem occurs, such as personal, social, medical, hereditary and environmental factors
- Fault: the pathobiological and psychosocial processes associated with any given disease or disability
- Consequences of the fault: signs and symptoms of the particular problem as well as its functional impact on the patient's life

Such patterns can exist generically (e.g. tendinopathy, spinal stenosis, etc.) but will also be recalled as specific cases of past patients that facilitate diagnoses with new patients ('instantiated scripts'; Boshuizen and Schmidt, 2008). Clearly, inductive pattern recognition relies on a good organization of biopsychosocial knowledge linked to clinical presentations. Although inductive reasoning or pattern recognition is common in experienced clinicians who typically possess a large repertoire of patterns to draw from (Edwards et al., 2004a; Edwards and Jones, 2007b; Kaufman et al., 2008; Marcum, 2012; Norman, 2005; Schwartz and Elstein, 2008), like all 'fast thinking', it is prone to error and ideally should therefore be supported by slower, analytical deductive hypothesis testing, particularly in more complex presentations and by less experienced clinicians.

But how can we explain the theorizing, typically regarding causal mechanisms, we regularly engage in when confronted with unexpected or unfamiliar information that cannot be deduced from established or accepted prior knowledge? What occurs prior to criteria having been developed on which deductions and later inductions are made? Inference to the best explanation (also called abduction) is a creative explanation used when clear deductions are not available (Lipton, 2004). Clinically, this is required when trying to account for what may initially present as disparate, unclear information or situations. It is essentially an unproven explanatory hypothesis that best explains the evidence, much like the detective who must entertain the best explanation that could account for a crime. Although inference to the best explanation may emerge through slow analytical reflection of competing explanations, it can also come as an unexpected flash of insight (Råholm, 2010). This real and frequently used form of inference used without further critique (clinical as well as research) is fraught with error and likely to only result in self-confirming beliefs (analogous to Kahneman's 'associative coherence' System 1 bias). Bias can be minimized through critique – both your own, through critical application of personal theory to other patients, and from the profession, through discussion, debate and research. However, the creative insight of seeing patterns (explanations) in previously unlinked information through inference to the best explanation is an inevitable and necessary first stage to understanding unfamiliar phenomena and to generate new ideas.

Key Point

Generating, testing and accepting hypothesis judgments in clinical reasoning within established medical and musculoskeletal specific knowledge frameworks involves a combination of deductive inference as to whether established criteria for the judgment have been met and inductive inference to recognize clinical patterns on the basis of limited information. Clinical patterns exist and can be learned for pathology/syndrome, pain type, precautions/contraindications and prognosis. Experienced clinicians possess a large repertoire of patterns to draw from that include both generic patterns typical across patients and 'instantiated' patterns, or recall of the key features, or stories, about individual patients they have seen and learned from. When confronted with unexpected and unfamiliar information, where established criteria for deductive and inductive inferences don't apply, clinicians theorize about the 'best explanation' through abductive inference. Inference to the best explanation, typically about causal mechanisms, is important to the discovery of new ideas. However, to avoid the human bias of simply following self-confirming beliefs, it is important to subject personal theories of explanation to critique – both your own, through critical application to other patients, and from the profession, through discussion, debate and research.

Thinking on Your Feet: Interpreting Information Across Different Hypothesis Categories

Patient information will inform several hypothesis categories at the same time. Just as the clinician may be asking a pathology-/impairment-oriented question but receive a patient answer that sheds light on the patient's perspectives (i.e. psychosocial status), a question directed at understanding the patient's activity capability and restrictions will often provide clues to other hypothesis categories at the same time. Consider, for example, a 72-year-old patient's response to a question regarding what aggravates his back and bilateral leg pains:

Walking, I'm afraid to even try anymore. Even short 5- to 10-minute walks make the back and legs worse, and then I have to sit down to ease it off. Sitting is good but I can't sit all day! I can't even help out around the house anymore or get over to see the grandchildren. I'm really worried it might be something serious.

This one answer provides information regarding multiple hypothesis categories:

- Activity restriction: walking
- Activity capability: sitting
- Participation restrictions: helping around house and seeing grandchildren
- Patient Perspectives: afraid to try walking, worried it may be serious
- Pain type: behaviour of symptoms clues to nociceptive and/or neuropathic pains
- Sources of nociception and associated pathology: back and leg symptoms related; lumbar joints and nerve roots implicated; consistent with spinal stenosis clinical pattern (age and behaviour of symptoms)
- Contributing factors: age
- Precautions: age, easily aggravated, bilateral leg pain, patient's fears/worry
- Prognosis: (-'s) age, disability, extent of symptoms, neurogenic, perspectives; (+'s) easing factor

Having a clear framework of the categories of judgments needed to understand patients and their problems for the purpose of guiding management enables clinicians to pick up cues beyond the intent of their question or physical assessment and relate judgments in one area to others. In the end, the clinician gains clues to the different hypothesis categories throughout the whole examination and ongoing management that must be interpreted, weighed for significance and analyzed with other supporting and negating information. The hypothesis categories also provide a biopsychosocially oriented organizing framework to link academic knowledge to clinical reasoning through the patient examination-treatment-re-assessment process, facilitating the learning of clinical patterns.

Key Point

Awareness of the different categories of judgments needed to understand patients and their problems for the purpose of guiding management, such as the proposed hypothesis categories framework, enables clinicians to be alert to patient information forthcoming that was beyond the intent of their question or physical assessment. Although clinicians will follow their own structured patient examination, it is important that information obtained from both the subjective and physical examination is interpreted and synthesized as it unfolds. Generally, most patient information obtained will have relevance to more than one hypothesis category, and decisions eventually made should be linked to the cumulative information (often incorporating both supporting and non-supporting information to a decision) synthesized over the full examination (and later re-assessment of treatment interventions).

Factors Influencing Clinical Reasoning

Understanding the cognitive processes used in clinical reasoning (including abductive inference to the best explanation theorizing; fast System 1 first impressions, inductions or pattern recognition; and slow System 2 deliberations, testing of hypotheses and deductions) assists critique and focused practice to improve reasoning. Although it is tempting to reduce clinical reasoning to these cognitive processes, this fails to recognize other dimensions that are also parts of the gestalt or whole of clinical reasoning. Simply understanding the cognitive processes will not ensure skilled reasoning. Numerous factors influence proficiency in clinical reasoning, including associated attributes of critical thinking, higher-order metacognition, knowledge organization, data-collection and procedural skills, and patient–therapist therapeutic alliance – incorporating communication effectiveness, emotional intelligence and skills in 'interactive', 'collaborative' and 'ethical' reasoning.

Critical Thinking

Although generic thinking skills are themselves insufficient for expertise in clinical practice (Boshuizen and Schmidt, 2008; Elstein et al., 1978), skilled clinical reasoning incorporates the fundamentals of critical thinking. Critical thinking generally involves analyzing and assessing information, issues, situations, problems, perspectives and thinking processes (Paul and Elder, 2007). It underpins the different forms of inference. Rather than unquestionably accepting information, critical thinking fosters a sort of healthy scepticism that appraises information for its accuracy, completeness and relevance to facilitate understanding and identification of solutions. Inherent in critical thinking is reflection and awareness of the assumptions under which we, and others, think and act (Brookfield, 2008). Assumptions are taken-for-granted beliefs acquired through life and through formal education that are often tacit and hence typically not considered or challenged. Uncritically accepted assumptions often emerge from professional philosophies or approaches to practice or from personal experiences that have shaped one's views. Without scrutiny, such assumptions place us at risk of reasoning on the basis of inaccurate and biased 'knowledge' (i.e. unsubstantiated views and popular opinions), making us vulnerable to misinterpretations, inaccurate judgments and, ultimately, less effective health care. Unjustified assumptions in clinical practice can be minimized through a range of safeguards, including the following:

- Qualifying patients' meaning
- Screening to ensure information is not missed
- Testing for competing hypotheses
- Attending to 'negatives' or features of a presentation that do not fit favoured hypotheses and explanations
- Openly subjecting and comparing your own reasoning to that of others

Examples of screening topics that optimize thoroughness and avoid clinical assumption include the following:

- Screening for additional symptoms not spontaneously volunteered (e.g. other body areas, vascular, neuropathic, psychological, etc.)
- Screening for additional activity and participation restrictions and capabilities not volunteered
- Screening for psychosocial factors and their relationship to the clinical presentation
- Screening for general health comorbidities and red flags

Metacognition

Metacognition is a form of self-awareness that incorporates monitoring of yourself (e.g. your thinking, your knowledge, your performance) as though you are outside yourself observing and critiquing your practice. There is an integral link between cognition, metacognition and knowledge acquisition that facilitates learning from clinical practice experience (Higgs et al., 2008a; Marcum, 2012; Schön, 1987). This self-awareness is not limited to the formal hypotheses considered and treatments selected; metacognitive awareness of performance is also important. This, for example, underpins the experienced clinician's immediate recognition that a particular phrasing of a question or explanation was not clear. Similarly, metacognitive awareness of the effectiveness of a physical procedure enables immediate recognition that the procedure needs to be adjusted or perhaps should be abandoned as, for example, when cues such an increase in muscle tone or the patient's expression signal the procedure was not achieving its desired effect. Lastly, metacognition is important to recognizing limitations in knowledge. The student or clinician who lacks awareness of his or her own knowledge limitations will learn less. Experts not only know a lot in their area of practice, they also know what they don't know. That is, experts are typically very quick to recognize a limitation in their knowledge (e.g. a patient's medication they are unfamiliar with, a medical condition, a peripheral nerve sensory and motor distribution) and act on it by consulting a colleague or appropriate resource.

Knowledge Organization

Well-structured knowledge is essential to domain competence (Glaser and Bassok, 1989; Ruiz-Primo et al., 2001). Research studies in cognitive psychology and artificial intelligence (e.g. Greeno and Simon, 1986), categorization (e.g. Hayes and Adams, 2000), expertise (e.g. Boshuizen and Schmidt, 2008; Jensen et al., 2007) and education (e.g. Pearsall et al., 1997) have collectively demonstrated the importance of well-developed knowledge to successful performance. Well-structured knowledge is not simply how much an individual knows but how that knowledge is organized, including the differentiation and relationships between core concepts. All forms of knowledge are important, including clinicians' broader worldview, their philosophy of practice and their medical and profession-specific knowledge. Knowledge emerges from what we believe or hold to be true (Higgs et al., 2008b). Clinicians utilize a combination of propositional knowledge ('knowing that') generated formally through research and scholarship and non-propositional knowledge ('knowing how') generated primarily through practice experience. Non-propositional knowledge can be divided further into professional craft knowledge and personal knowledge. Craft knowledge comprises professional knowledge such as procedural, communication and teaching knowledge and skills, based on academic propositional knowledge (e.g. anatomy, biomechanics, neurophysiology, learning theory, psychology, sociology, etc.) that has been refined and contextualized through clinical experience. Personal knowledge includes that knowledge acquired through personal life experiences (including community and cultural) that contributes to shaping a person's beliefs, values and attitudes. Clinicians who are alert to both community and their own attitudes (i.e. personal knowledge) regarding, for example, different population subgroups (e.g. ethnic, workers compensation, substance abuse) are better able to safeguard against their own assumptions, biases or prejudices leading to premature or incorrect judgments. Understanding and successfully managing patients' problems requires a rich organization of all three types of knowledge. Propositional knowledge provides us with theory and research substantiation on which to base our practice, whereas non-propositional professional craft knowledge provides us with the means to use that theory and research evidence in the clinic.

Data-Collection and Procedural Skills

Given clinical reasoning is based on information obtained from and about the patient, the accuracy and effectiveness of our clinical judgments is influenced by the quality of information (e.g. patient interview, physical examination, outcome re-assessments) on which those judgments are based. Within the patient interview clarification for meaning is essential to enhance accuracy, completeness and relevance of information obtained.

There are many situations where the patient makes a general statement that requires clarification to accurately understand the meaning. Examples include such things as constancy of symptoms (where clarification of 'constant' reveals daily symptoms but not every moment of the day), area of symptoms (where, for example, the patient's perception of the 'shoulder' is clarified to actually be the supraspinous fossa) and aggravating factors (where, for example, 'walking' requires clarification regarding what aspect of the walking is a problem – time, speed, distance, surface, phase of gait, etc.). Screening questions such as other symptoms, aggravating or easing factors and general health represent clarification for completeness. Clarification of meaning to establish relevance is always needed to establish relationships between symptoms and predisposing and aggravating factors established through the history and behaviour of symptoms. This is particularly important to judgments regarding patient perspectives and social factors (psychosocial status). Clarifying relationships between beliefs, cognitions, emotions, perceived and actual support, and behaviours to the history and behaviour of the patient's symptoms assists recognition of unhelpful beliefs and stressors that are contributing to one patient's pain and disability experience versus co-existing but not adversely affecting another's. The importance of clarification for meaning and relevance is also evident with questions regarding a patient's understanding of his or her problem that often only elicit superficial accounts of what the patient's doctor or others have told the patient but not necessarily what it means to the patient with respect to the cause, management and the future. Because patient perspectives cannot be judged on face value as normal versus abnormal (or maladaptive) in the same way physical health (e.g. blood pressure, range of movement, strength) can be judged, it is essential that perspectives are clarified and explored further. For example, the persistent pain patient who volunteers praying as a coping strategy may be erroneously judged to be passively relying on others and lacking in motivation to take an active role. If that statement is clarified and explored further, there will be some patients for whom praying functions as a motivating source of support and conviction to do all they can to help themselves, further highlighting the need for continual clarification.

The quality of physical assessment data (as influenced by procedural skills) to clinical reasoning judgments is equally important. Errors in subjective assessments of physical tests (e.g. posture, range of active and passive movement, kinematics, judgments regarding stiffness, laxity/instability, motor performance and soft tissue, etc.) underpin the importance of using reliable objective measures wherever possible and diagnostic procedures with the greatest validity. When objective measurement is not available, findings should be re-checked for consistency, related to other findings (e.g. passive accessory movement findings considered for congruence with physiological movement findings), and cautiously integrated with more objective findings for guiding reasoning judgments.

Patient–Clinician Therapeutic Alliance

The patient–clinician therapeutic alliance encompasses rapport, emotions (Marcum, 2013; Pinto et al., 2012), patient–clinician collaboration (Barr and Threlkeld, 2000; Edwards et al., 2004b, Pinto et al., 2012; Trede and Higgs, 2008) and ethical deliberations (Edwards and Delany, 2019).

Rapport

The manner in which an examination and therapy is provided with respect to patient rapport and the level of clinician interest, empathy and confidence conveyed influences patients' information volunteered, motivation for change, willingness to participate in self-management and their outcomes in general (Ferreira et al., 2013; Hall et al., 2010; Klaber Moffett and Richardson, 1997). Despite specific questions and sequence of questions asked varying according to education and personal experience, the aim should be the same, that is, to understand the patient's problems and his or her individual pain/disability experience in order to inform effective, collaborative management. Although the patient interview and examination are largely about gaining information to understand the patient and his or her problems, the nature and manner (e.g. tone, non-verbal behaviours, time allowed) of the clinician's questions, instructions and responses to patient questions and answers will influence the interest the patient perceives the clinician has in him or her, the confidence the patient has in the clinician and the success of the therapeutic relationship in general (Ferreira et al., 2013; Hall et al., 2010; Klaber Moffett and Richardson, 1997). That is, our questions and responses (verbal and non-verbal) are interpreted by patients as conveying our thoughts. Many patients report negative experiences with medical and other health professionals who they felt didn't listen or believe them (e.g. Johnson, 1993; Matthias et al., 2014; Payton et al., 1998). Without good rapport, the patient is less likely to collaborate in providing the necessary information or in the management, potentially compromising clinical reasoning and jeopardizing the eventual outcome.

Emotions

Perceptual judgments are influenced by emotions (Kahneman, 2011; Langridge, Roberts and Pope, 2016; Lehrer, 2009; Marcum, 2013). One only needs to recall the negative emotions elicited from an unpleasant encounter with a patient, or perhaps a patient you felt showed no interest in getting better, to reflect on whether emotions influence your own reasoning. The ability to accurately perceive, appraise and express emotions and to recognize emotion-elicited thoughts and judgments has been characterized as 'emotional intelligence' influencing clinical reasoning (Marcum, 2013). This metacognitive awareness and strategies for optimizing communication in difficult patient–clinician interactions are important to minimizing the adverse effects of emotions on clinical reasoning (Langridge, Roberts and Pope, 2016). For example, interactive reasoning, defined earlier as reasoning associated with purposeful establishment and management of rapport, underpins many successful communicators' abilities to effectively interact with difficult patients. Although no single communication strategy works for every circumstance, finding and fostering common ground (e.g. sports, movies, children, etc.) will often facilitate rapport. Better rapport generally leads to better provision of information and better collaboration. Better rapport may also enhance patient understanding of education and advice offered as 'the insecure and threatened self appears to disable understanding' (Osborn, 2014, p. 753).

Perception and Empathy

Clinical reasoning is largely grounded in human perception (tacit and conscious) that precedes inferential judgments. As such, perception could be considered to initiate clinical reasoning as with recognizing and responding to perceived cues in patients' answers and physical presentations. Such perceptions are influenced by prior knowledge and philosophy of practice biasing what is attended to. Strategies such as screening questions, explained earlier, or looking at posture and movement from different perspectives can minimize the error of only perceiving (hearing, seeing, feeling) what you are looking for. A unique form of perception (that can also be associated with emotion) important to understanding the person behind the problem (i.e. their pain experience), and also integral to developing rapport and therapeutic alliance, is empathy. Empathy in a clinical context refers to clinicians' cognitive abilities to understand what their patients are experiencing and clinicians' affective abilities to imaginatively project themselves into their patients' situations (Braude, 2012). Having and conveying empathy probably constitute a personal skill acquired through life, but when applied in practice, patients are more likely to feel they have been given a voice, have been heard and have been believed, all of which strengthen the therapeutic alliance.

Patient–Clinician Collaboration

The importance of 'collaborative reasoning' as a reasoning strategy is underscored by the evidence that patients who have been given an opportunity to share in the decision-making take greater responsibility for their own management, are more satisfied with their health care and have a greater likelihood of achieving better outcomes (Arnetz et al., 2004; Edwards et al., 2004b, Trede and Higgs, 2008). Rather than promoting passive patient compliance, patient-centred health care promotes motivation for change and active patient participation in decision-making requiring collaboration in assessment, goal-setting and management. Patient self-efficacy to contribute to change, learning (i.e. altered understanding and improved health behaviour), and shared responsibility in management are primary outcomes sought in a collaborative reasoning approach. Specific strategies for involving patients in their health care, including when differences in opinion exist, and motivating patients to make changes are addressed by Edwards et al. (2004b), Trede and Higgs (2008) and Miller and Rollnick (2012).

Ethical Reasoning

On the surface 'ethical reasoning' as a strategy or focus of thinking and decision-making mostly brings to mind the formal codes of practice (i.e. ethics) each country's professional associations have in place. Although the four principles that underpin traditional codes of practice (i.e. autonomy, non-maleficence, beneficence and justice; Beauchamp and Childress, 2013) retain their importance, contemporary literature in ethics highlights the challenges of applying black-and-white principles in actual practice and argue for a broader perspective on ethics. Because ethics and ethical reasoning have historically not been prominent in professional education, it is not surprising many clinicians either lack the moral sensitivity to recognize ethical issues or lack the knowledge of ethics theory to critically apply ethical reasoning in practice. Edwards and Delany (2019) make the point that just as clinical educators should not accept students' diagnostic clinical reasoning based simply on personal inclination (without sound theory and research supported rationale linked to the patient's presentation), similarly, ethical reasoning, as required, for example, in understanding cultural influences on decisions made by patients regarding their health, needs to be based on ethics theory applied to the particulars of the patient's circumstances. Readers are referred to the work of Edwards (Edwards and Delany [2019] regarding ethical reasoning in clinical practice generally; Edwards et al. [2014] regarding ethical reasoning as it relates to chronic pain) for overviews of ethics theory and recommendations for applying that theory to practice.

Key Points

- Numerous factors influence proficiency in clinical reasoning, including associated attributes of critical thinking, higher-order metacognition, knowledge organization, data-collection and procedural skills, and patient–clinician therapeutic alliance – incorporating communication effectiveness, emotional intelligence and skills in 'interactive', 'collaborative' and 'ethical' reasoning.
- The critical thinking attribute of 'healthy scepticism' ensures information is scrutinized for its accuracy, completeness and relevance and assumptions within your own and others' perspectives are critically examined. Unjustified assumptions in clinical practice can be minimized through regular qualification of patient meaning, screening to ensure information is not missed, testing for competing hypotheses, attending to 'negatives' when judging hypotheses and openly subjecting and comparing your reasoning to that of others.
- Metacognition, or self-awareness of your own thinking, knowledge and performance, facilitates learning in clinical practice.
- Clinical reasoning is informed by a broad range of knowledge, including the propositional biological and psychosocial knowledge within health, personal know-how or craft knowledge of musculoskeletal practice, and self-knowledge of your own beliefs, values and attitudes.
- Clinical reasoning is only as good as the information (data) on which it is based, necessitating regular use of strategies to avoid assumptions such as clarification of patient meaning, screening questions, objective measurement where possible, and cautious use of subjective assessments.
- Clinician interest, empathy and confidence all contribute to developing rapport important to the therapeutic alliance and patient participation in therapy, including information provided and motivation for change. 'Emotional intelligence' to accurately perceive, appraise, and express emotions, while safeguarding your own emotions do not unfairly bias your clinical judgments, combined with 'interactive reasoning' skills to optimize rapport will indirectly contribute to better clinical reasoning.
- Patient–clinician collaboration in assessment, goal-setting and management facilitates patient responsibility in self-management (and consequently self-efficacy), patient satisfaction and better outcomes.
- Clinicians need to expand on their knowledge of the traditional principles of ethics underpinning formal codes of practice (i.e. autonomy, non-maleficence, beneficence, justice) to include greater understanding of ethics theory, greater recognition of ethical issues, and greater ability to critically apply ethical reasoning in practice.

Skilled Clinical Reasoning Contributes to Clinicians' Learning

Critical reflection is unanimously promoted as necessary throughout the critical thinking, clinical reasoning and education literature to perceive, critique, discuss and revise our research- and experience-based knowledge and actions (e.g. Brookfield, 1987; Clouder, 2000; Cranton, 2006; Higgs and Jones, 2008; Mezirow, 2000; Mezirow, 2012; Rodgers, 2002; Schön, 1983, 1987; Taylor and Cranton, 2012). Constructivist learning theory broadly recognizes learning as experiential and individual, involving the processes of reflection, experimentation and evaluation that ultimately result in personal change. Within this philosophy of learning, knowledge is constructed by the individual through the transformation of experience (e.g. Cranton, 2006; Mezirow, 2000; Taylor and Cranton, 2012). When clinical reasoning is supported by metacognitive awareness of knowledge (e.g. biomedical, psychosocial, professional, clinical beliefs and research evidence), clinical judgments and proficiency in management skills and is subjected to regular critical reflections, both clinical reasoning and learning through clinical reasoning are facilitated. Learning theory and strategies for facilitating clinical reasoning are discussed in detail in Chapter 31. Although System 2 critical reflection provides a safeguard to our fast, intuitive, first impression System 1 thinking that will also lead to learning, it is not the only means by which new ideas, perspectives and professional directions are created.

Creative, Lateral Thinking

In his seminal text *The Structure of Scientific Revolutions*, Thomas Kuhn (1970) points out that many of the major breakthroughs in science did not occur due to carefully controlled scientific research; rather, they often emerged from accidents or the lone insight of an individual. If we only encourage logical thinking and practice within the realm of what is 'known' or substantiated by research evidence we limit the variability and creativity of thinking that is important to the generation of new ideas. Where logical thinking encourages making justified deductions, lateral thinking involves restructuring and escape from old patterns and looking at things in different ways (DeBono, 2014). The logical thinker attends only to what is obviously relevant, whereas the lateral thinker recognizes that sometimes seemingly irrelevant information assists in viewing the problem from a different perspective. Strategies for facilitating both logical and lateral thinking in clinical reasoning are reviewed in Chapter 31.

Summary

Musculoskeletal clinicians need to be able to think fast and slow in clinical practice. Reasoning across the full spectrum of straightforward/common to more complex problem presentations requires a rich blend of biopsychosocial knowledge, professional know-how, and skilled diagnostic and non-diagnostic clinical reasoning. Understanding different foci of reasoning (i.e. diagnostic, narrative, procedural, interactive, collaborative, predictive, ethical, and teaching as reasoning) and key categories of clinical decisions required across these reasoning strategies (i.e. hypothesis categories) assists clinical reasoning in a biopsychosocial framework. Numerous factors influence how well clinicians reason in practice, including the cognitive processes they use (e.g. abductive inference to the best explanation theorizing; fast System 1 first impressions, inductions or pattern recognition; and slow System 2 deliberations, testing of hypotheses and deductions), their 'critical thinking', their higher-order metacognition, their knowledge and knowledge organization, their data-collection and procedural skills and their patient–therapist therapeutic alliance. As clinical reasoning skills improve, learning from clinical practice improves. Equipped with skills in deductive and inductive inference, critical thinking to minimize bias and abductive inference to contemplate new explanations, logical thinkers can and should also look at problems from different perspectives to discover new patterns and ideas through lateral thinking.

The clinical reasoning theory presented here provides the foundation for the clinical reasoning discussed in the other theory chapters and the Reasoning Questions and Commentary integrated throughout each of the 25 cases of the book. Improvement in clinical reasoning requires practice in clinical reasoning, and to optimize that learning, the cases should not simply be read passively; rather, readers should attempt to answer Reasoning Questions posed prior to reading the case Answers, and then compare and critique their reasoning with the reasoning put forward through the case.

REFERENCES

Adams, M.A., Stefanakis, M., Dolan, P., 2010. Healing of a painful intervertebral disc should not be confused with reversing disc degeneration: implications for physical therapies of discogenic back pain. Clin. Biomech. (Bristol, Avon) 25, 961–971.

Allet, L., Burge, E., Monnin, D., 2008. ICF: clinical relevance for physiotherapy? a critical review. Adv. Physiother. 10, 127–137.

Arnetz, J.E., Almin, I., Bergström, K., et al., 2004. Active patient involvement in the establishment of physical therapy goals: effects on treatment outcome and quality of care. Adv. Physiother. 6, 50–69.

Ashina, S., Bendtsen, L., Ashina, M., 2005. Pathophysiology of tension-type headache. Curr. Pain Headache Rep. 9, 415–422.

Barlow, S.E., 2012. The barriers to implementation of evidence-based chronic pain management in rural and regional physiotherapy outpatients. Realising the potential. HETI Report. Rural research capacity building program. NSW Ministry of Health. Available from: www.aci.health.nsw.gov.au.

Barr, J., Threlkeld, A.J., 2000. Patient/practitioner collaboration in clinical decision making. Physiother. Res. Int. 5, 254–260.

Beauchamp, T., Childress, J., 2013. Principles of Biomedical Ethics, seventh ed. Oxford University Press, Oxford.

Bielefeldt, K., Gebhart, G.F., 2006. Visceral pain: basic mechanisms. In: McMahon, S.B., Koltzenburg, M. (Eds.), Wall and Melzack's Textbook of Pain, fifth ed. Elsevier, China, pp. 721–736.

Bishop, A., Foster, N.E., 2005. Do physical therapists in the United Kingdom recognize psychosocial factors in patients with acute low back pain? Spine 11, 1316–1322.

Blyth, F.M., Macfarlane, G.J., Nicholas, M.K., 2007. The contribution of psychosocial factors to the development of chronic pain: the key to better outcomes for patients? Pain 129, 8–11.

Boissonnault, W.G., 2011. Primary care for the physical therapist. In: Examination and Triage, second ed. Elsevier, St. Louis.

Borrell-Carrió, F., Suchman, A.L., Epstein, R.M., 2004. The biopsychosocial model 25 years later: principles, practice, and scientific inquiry. Ann. Fam. Med. 2, 576–582.

Boshuizen, H.P.A., Schmidt, H.G., 2008. The development of clinical reasoning expertise. In: Higgs, J., Jones, M.A., Loftus, S., Christensen, N. (Eds.), Clinical Reasoning in the Health Professions, third ed. Butterworth Heinemann Elsevier, Amsterdam, pp. 113–121.

Braude, H.D., 2012. Conciliating cognition and consciousness: the perceptual foundations of clinical reasoning. J. Eval. Clin. Pract. 18, 945–950.

Brooker, C., 2013. Mosby's Dictionary of Medicine, Nursing and Health Professions, ninth ed. Elsevier, Edinburgh.

Brookfield, S., 2008. Clinical reasoning and generic thinking skills. In: Higgs, J., Jones, M.A., Loftus, S., Christensen, N. (Eds.), Clinical Reasoning in the Health Professions, third ed. Butterworth Heinemann Elsevier, Amsterdam, pp. 65–75.

Brookfield, S.D., 1987. Developing critical thinkers. In: Challenging Adults to Explore Alternative Ways of Thinking and Acting. Jossey-Bass, San Francisco.

Cagnie, B., Dewitte, V., Barbe, T., et al., 2013. Physiologic effects of dry needling. Curr. Pain Headache Rep. 17, 348–355.

Childs, J.D., Cleland, J.A., Elliott, J.M., et al., 2008. Neck pain: clinical practice guidelines linked to the International Classification of Functioning, Disability, and Health from the Orthopaedic Section of the American Physical Therapy Association. J. Orthop. Sports Phys. Ther. 38, A1–A34.

Christensen, N., Nordstrom, T., 2013. Facilitating the teaching and learning of clinical reasoning. In: Jensen, G.M., Mostrom, E. (Eds.), Handbook of Teaching and Learning for Physical Therapists, third ed. Elsevier Butterworth Heinemann, St. Louis, pp. 183–199.

Cibulka, M.T., White, D.M., Woehrle, J., et al., 2009. Hip pain and mobility deficits–hip osteoarthritis: clinical practice guidelines linked to the International Classification of Functioning, Disability, and Health from the Orthopaedic Section of the American Physical Therapy Association. J. Orthop. Sports Phys. Ther. 39, A1–A25.

Clauw, D.J., 2015. Diagnosing and treating chronic musculoskeletal pain based on the underlying mechanism(s). Best Pract. Res. Clin. Rheumatol. 29 (1), 6–9.

Clouder, L., 2000. Reflective practice in physiotherapy education: a critical conversation. Stud. High. Educ. 25, 211–223.

Cook, C., George, S., Reiman, M., 2017. Red flag screening for low back pain: nothing to see here, move along: a narrative review. Br. J. Sports Med. http://dx.doi.org/10.1136/bjsports-2017-098352.

Cook, J.L., Purdam, C.R., 2009. Is tendon pathology a continuum? A pathology model to explain the clinical presentation of load-induced tendinopathy. Br. J. Sports Med. 43, 409–416.

Coombes, B.K., Bisset, L., Vicenzino, B., 2009. A new integrative model of lateral epicondylalgia. Br. J. Sports Med. 43, 252–258.

Coombes, B.K., Bisset, L., Vicenzino, B., 2012. Thermal hyperalgesia distinguishes those with severe pain and disability in unilateral lateral epicondylalgia. Clin. J. Pain 28, 595–601.

Cranton, P., 2006. Understanding and Promoting Transformative Learning: A Guide for Educators of Adults, second ed. Jossey-Bass, San Francisco.

Croskerry, P., 2003. The importance of cognitive errors in diagnosis and strategies to minimize them. Acad. Med. 78 (8), 775–780.

De Bono, E., 2014. Lateral Thinking, An Introduction. Vermilion, New York.

Doody, C., McAteer, M., 2002. Clinical reasoning of expert and novice physiotherapists in an outpatient orthopaedic setting. Physiotherapy 88, 258–268.

Downie, A., Williams, C.M., Henschke, N., et al., 2013. Red flags to screen for malignancy and fracture in patients with low back pain: systematic review. Br. Med. J. 347, 7095, 1–9.

Duncan, G., 2000. Mind-body dualism and the biopsychosocial model of pain: what did Descartes really say? J. Med. Philos. 25, 485–513.

Edwards, I., Braunack-Mayer, A., Jones, M., 2005. Ethical reasoning as a clinical-reasoning strategy in physiotherapy. Physiotherapy 91, 226–236.

Edwards, I., Delany, C., 2019. Ethical reasoning. In: Higgs, J., Jensen, G., Loftus, S., Christensen, N. (Eds.), Clinical Reasoning in the Health Professions, fourth ed. Elsevier, Edinburgh, pp. 169–179.

Edwards, I., Jones, M., 2007a. Clinical reasoning and expertise. In: Jensen, G.M., Gwyer, J., Hack, L.M., Shepard, K.F. (Eds.), Expertise in Physical Therapy Practice, second ed. Elsevier, Boston, pp. 192–213.

Edwards, I., Jones, M., 2007b. The role of clinical reasoning in understanding and applying the International Classification of Functioning, Disability and Health (ICF). Kinesitherapie 71, e1–e9.

Edwards, I., Jones, M., Carr, J., et al., 2004a. Clinical reasoning strategies in physical therapy. Phys. Ther. 84, 312–335.

Edwards, I., Jones, M., Higgs, J., et al., 2004b. What is collaborative reasoning? Adv. Physiother. 6, 70–83.

Edwards, I., Jones, M., Thacker, M., Swisher, L.L., 2014. The moral experience of the patient with chronic pain: bridging the gap between first and third person ethics. Pain Med. 15, 364–378.

Edwards, I.C., 2000. Clinical Reasoning in Three Different Fields of Physiotherapy - A Qualitative Case Study Approach. PhD Thesis, University of South Australia, Adelaide, SA, Australia. Available at: http://www.library.unisa.edu.au/adt-root/public/adt-SUSA-20030603-090552/index.html.

Elstein, A.S., Shulman, L., Sprafka, S., 1978. Medical Problem Solving: An Analysis of Clinical Reasoning. Harvard University Press, Cambridge.

Engel, G.L., 1977. The need for a new medical model: a challenge for biomedicine. Science 196, 129–136.

Epstein, R.M., Borrell-Carrio, F., 2005. The biopsychosocial model: exploring six impossible things. Fam. Syst. Health 23, 426–431.

Escorpizo, R., Stucki, G., Cieza, A., et al., 2010. Creating an interface between the International Classification of Functioning, Disability and Health and physical therapist practice. Phys. Ther. 90, 1053–1067.

Fernandez-Carnero, J., Fernandez-de-Las-Penas, C., de la Llave-Rincon, A.I., et al., 2009. Widespread mechanical pain hypersensitivity as sign of central sensitization in unilateral epicondylalgia: a blinded, controlled study. Clin. J. Pain 25, 555–561.

Ferreira, P.H., Maher, C.G., Refshauge, K.M., et al., 2013. The therapeutic alliance between clinicians and patients predicts outcomes in chronic low back pain. Phys. Ther. 93, 470–478.

Foster, N.E., Delitto, A., 2011. Embedding psychosocial perspectives within clinical management of low back pain: integration of psychosocially informed management principles into physical therapist practice–challenges and opportunities. Phys. Ther. 91, 790–803.

French, S., Sim, J., 2004. Physiotherapy: A Psychosocial Approach. Elsevier, Edinburgh.

Gifford, L., 1998. Central mechanisms. In: Gifford, L. (Ed.), Topical Issues in Pain: Whiplash – Science and Management. Fear-avoidance Beliefs and Behaviour, CNS Press, Falmouth, pp. 67–80.

Gifford, L., Thacker, M., Jones, M.A., 2006. Physiotherapy and pain. In: McMahon, S.B., Koltzenburg, M. (Eds.), Wall and Melzack's Textbook of Pain, fifth ed. Elsevier, pp. 603–617.

Glaser, R., Bassok, M., 1989. Learning theory and the study of instruction. Annu. Rev. Psychol. 40, 631–666.

Goodman, C.C., Fuller, K.S., 2009. Pathology, Implications for the Physical Therapist, third ed. Saunders/Elsevier, St. Louis.

Goodman, C.C., Heick, J., Lazaro, R.T., 2017. Differential Diagnosis for Physical Therapists, Screening for Referral, sixth ed. Elsevier, St. Louis.

Greenhalgh, T., Howick, J., Maskrey, N., 2014. 2014 Evidence based medicine: a movement in crisis? BMJ 348, g3725. doi:10.1136/bmj.g3725. (Published 13 June 2014).

Greeno, J.G., Simon, H.A., 1986. Problem solving and reasoning. In: Atkinson, R.C., Hersteing, R., Lindsey, G.L., Luce, R.D. (Eds.), Steven's Handbook of Experimental Psychology, vol. 2, second ed. Learning and Cognition. Lawrence Erlbaum Associates, Hillsdale, NJ, pp. 572–589.

Hall, A.M., Ferreira, P.H., Maher, C.G., et al., 2010. The influence of the therapist-patient relationship on treatment outcome in physical rehabilitation: a systematic review. Phys. Ther. 90, 1099–1110.

Hasenbring, M.I., Rusu, A.C., Turk, D.C., 2012. From acute to chronic back pain. In: Risk Factors, Mechanisms and Clinical Implications. Oxford University Press, Oxford.

Hayden, J.A., Dunn, K.M., van der Windt, D.A., Shaw, W.S., 2010. What is the prognosis of back pain? Best Pract. Res. Clin. Rheumatol. 24, 167–179.

Hayes, B., Adams, R., 2000. Parallels between clinical reasoning and categorization. In: Higgs, J., Jones, M. (Eds.), Clinical Reasoning in the Health Professions. Butterworth-Heinemann, Oxford, pp. 45–53.

Hengeveld, E., Banks, K., 2014. Maitland's vertebral manipulation. In: Management of Neuromusculoskeletal Disorders – Volume One, eighth ed. Churchill Livingstone Elsevier, Edinburgh.

Higgs, J., Jones, M.A., 2008. Clinical decision making and multiple problem spaces. In: Higgs, J., Jones, M.A., Loftus, S., Christensen, N. (Eds.), Clinical Reasoning in the Health Professions, third ed. Butterworth Heinemann Elsevier, Amsterdam, pp. 3–18.

Higgs, J., Fish, D., Rothwell, R., 2008a. Knowledge generation and clinical reasoning in practice. In: Higgs, J., Jones, M.A., Loftus, S., Christensen, N. (Eds.), Clinical Reasoning in the Health Professions, third ed. Butterworth Heinemann Elsevier, Amsterdam, pp. 163–172.

Higgs, J., Jones, M.A., Titchen, A., 2008b. Knowledge, reasoning and evidence for practice. In: Higgs, J., Jones, M.A., Loftus, S., Christensen, N. (Eds.), Clinical Reasoning in the Health Professions, third ed. Butterworth Heinemann Elsevier, Amsterdam, pp. 151–161.

Hogarth, R.M., 2005. Deciding analytically or trusting your intuition? The advantages and disadvantages of analytic and intuitive thought. In: Betsch, T., Haberstroh, S. (Eds.), The Routines of Decision Making. Lawrence Erlbaum Associates, Mahwah, NJ, pp. 67–82.

IASP Taxonomy, 2017. IASP Publications, Washington, D.C., viewed December 2017, http://www.iasp-pain.org/Taxonomy.

Imrie, R., 2004. Demystifying disability: a review of the International Classification of Functioning, Disability and Health. Sociol. Health Illn. 26, 287–305.

Jensen, G.M., 2007. Expert practice in orthopaedics: competence, collaboration, and compassion. In: Jensen, G.M., Gwyer, J., Hack, L.M., Shepard, K.F. (Eds.), Expertise in Physical Therapy Practice, second ed. Saunders Elsevier, St. Louis, pp. 125–144.

Jensen, G.M., Gwyer, J., Hack, L.M., Shepard, K.F., 2007. Expertise in Physical Therapy Practice, second ed. Saunders Elsevier, St. Louis.

Jensen, T.S., Baron, R., Haanpaa, M., et al., 2011. A new definition of neuropathic pain. Pain 152, 2204–2205.

Jette, A.M., 2006. Toward a common language for function, disability, and health. Phys. Ther. 86, 726–734.

Johnson, R., 1993. Attitudes just don't hang in the air…' disabled people's perceptions of physiotherapists. Physiotherapy 79, 619–626.

Johnson, R., Moores, L., 2006. Pain management: integrating physiotherapy and clinical psychology in practice. In: Gifford, L. (Ed.), Topical Issues in Pain 5. CNS Press, Falmouth, pp. 311–319.

Jones, M.A., 1987. The clinical reasoning process in manipulative therapy. In: Dalziel, B.A., Snowsill, J.C. (Eds.), Proceedings of the Fifth Biennial Conference of the Manipulative Therapists Association of Australia. Melbourne, VIC, Australia, pp. 62–69.

Jones, M.A., 2014. Clinical reasoning: from the Maitland Concept and beyond. In: Hengeveld, E., Banks, K. (Eds.), Maitland's Vertebral Manipulation, Management of Neuromusculoskeletal Disorders – Volume One, eighth ed. Churchill Livingstone/Elsevier, Edinburgh, pp. 14–82.

Jones, M.A., Edwards, I., 2008. Clinical reasoning to facilitate cognitive-experiential change. In: Higgs, J., Jones, M.A., Loftus, S., Christensen, N. (Eds.), Clinical Reasoning in the Health Professions, third ed. Butterworth Heinemann Elsevier, Amsterdam, pp. 319–328.

Jones, M.A., Edwards, I., Gifford, L., 2002. Conceptual models for implementing biopsychosocial theory in clinical practice. Man. Ther. 7, 2–9.

Jones, M.A., Jensen, G., Edwards, I., 2008. Clinical reasoning in physiotherapy. In: Higgs, J., Jones, M.A., Loftus, S., Christensen, N. (Eds.), Clinical Reasoning in the Health Professions, third ed. Butterworth Heinemann Elsevier, Amsterdam, pp. 245–256.

Kahneman, D., 2011. Thinking, Fast and Slow. Allen Lane, London.

Kahneman, D., Slovic, P., Tversky, A., 1982. Judgment Under Uncertainty: Heuristics and Biases. Cambridge University Press, New York.

Kaufman, D.R., Yoskowitz, N.A., Patel, V.L., 2008. Clinical reasoning and biomedical knowledge: implications for teaching. In: Higgs, J., Jones, M.A., Loftus, S., Christensen, N. (Eds.), Clinical Reasoning in the Health Professions, third ed. Butterworth Heinemann Elsevier, Amsterdam, pp. 137–149.

Keefe, F., Scipio, C., Perri, L., 2006. Psychosocial approaches to managing pain: current status and future directions. In: Gifford, L. (Ed.), Topical Issues in Pain 5. CNS Press, Falmouth, pp. 241–256.

Khan, K.M., Scott, A., 2009. Mechanotherapy: how physical therapists' prescription of exercise promotes tissue repair. Br. J. Sports Med. 43, 247–251.

Klaber Moffett, J.A., Richardson, P.H., 1997. The influence of the physiotherapist-patient relationship on pain and disability. Physiother. Theory Pract. 13, 89–96.

Kosek, E., Cohen, M., Baron, R., Gebhart, G.F., Mico, J.A., Rice, A.S.C., et al., 2016. Do we need a third mechanistic descriptor for chronic pain states? Pain 157 (7), 1382–1386.

Kuhn, T.S., 1970. The Structure of Scientific Revolutions, second ed. University of Chicago Press, Chicago.

Langridge, N., Roberts, L., Pope, C., 2016. The role of clinician emotion in clinical reasoning: Balancing the analytical process. Man. Ther. 21, 277–281.

Lehrer, J., 2009. How We Decide. Houghton Mifflin Harcourt, Boston.

Lipton, P., 2004. Inference to the Best Explanation, second ed. Routledge, London.

Lluch Girbés, E., Nijs, J., Torres-Cueco, R., Lopez Cubas, C., 2013. Pain treatment for patients with osteoarthritis and central sensitization. Phys. Ther. 93, 842–851.

Louw, A., Diener, I., Butler, D.S., Puentedura, E.J., 2011. The effect of neuroscience education on pain, disability, anxiety, and stress in chronic musculoskeletal pain. Arch. Phys. Med. Rehabil. 92, 2041–2056.

Main, C.J., George, S.Z., 2011. Psychologically informed practice for management of low back pain: future directions in practice and research. Phys. Ther. 91, 820–824.

Main, C.J., Sullivan, M.J.L., Watson, P.J., 2008. Pain Management. Practical Applications of the Biopsychosocial Perspective in Clinical and Occupational Settings. Churchill Livingstone Elsevier, Edinburgh.

Marcum, J.A., 2012. An integrated model of clinical reasoning: dual-processing theory of cognition and metacognition. J. Eval. Clin. Pract. 18, 954–961.

Marcum, J.A., 2013. The role of emotions in clinical reasoning and decision making. J. Med. Philos. 38, 501–519.

Matthias, M.S., Krebs, E.E., Bergman, A.A., et al., 2014. Communicating about opioids for chronic pain: a qualitative study of patient attribution. Eur. J. Pain 18, 835–843.

Mayer, T.G., Neblett, R., Cohen, H., et al., 2012. The development and psychometric validation of the central sensitization inventory. Pain Pract. 12, 276–285.

McPoil, T., Martin, R., Cornwall, M., et al., 2008. Heel pain–plantar fasciitis: clinical practice guidelines linked to the International Classification of Function, Disability, and Health from the Orthopedic Section of the American Physical Therapy Association. J. Orthop. Sports Phys. Ther. 38, A1–A18.

Meeus, M., Vervisch, S., De Clerck, L.S., et al., 2012. Central sensitization in patients with rheumatoid arthritis: a systematic literature review. Semin. Arthritis Rheum. 41, 556–567.

Mezirow, J., 2000. Learning to think like an adult: core concepts of transformation theory. In: Mezirow, J. (Ed.), Learning as Transformation: Critical Perspectives on a Theory in Progress. Jossey-Bass, San Francisco, pp. 3–33.

Mezirow, J., 2012. Learning to think like an adult. Core concepts of transformation theory. In: Taylor, E.W., Cranton, P., Associates (Eds.), The Handbook of Transformative Learning. Theory, Research and Practice. Jossey-Bass, San Francisco, pp. 73–95.

Muncey, H., 2002. Explaining pain to patients. In: Gifford, L. (Ed.), Topical Issues in Pain 4. CNS Press, Falmouth, pp. 157–166.

Miller, W.R., Rollnick, S., 2012. Motivational Interviewing: Helping People Change, third ed. The Guilford Press, New York.

Moseley, G.L., 2004. Evidence for a direct relationship between cognitive and physical change during an education intervention in people with chronic low back pain. Eur. J. Pain 8, 39–45.

Moseley, G.L., Butler, D.S., 2017. Explain Pain Supercharged. The clinician's handbook. Noigroup Publications, Adelaide, South Australia.

Nijs, J., Kosek, E., Van Oosterwijck, J., Meeus, M., 2012b. Dysfunctional endogenous analgesia during exercise in patients with chronic pain: to exercise or not to exercise? Pain Physician 15, ES205–ES213.

Nijs, J., Lluch Girbés, E., Lundberg, M., et al., 2015. Exercise therapy for chronic musculoskeletal pain: innovation by altering pain memories. Man. Ther. 20 (10), 216–220.

Nijs, J., Meeus, M., Cagnie, B., 2014a. A modern neuroscience approach to chronic spinal pain: combining pain neuroscience education with cognition-targeted motor control training. Phys. Ther. 94, 730–738.

Nijs, J., Meeus, M., Van Oosterwijck, J., et al., 2011a. Treatment of central sensitization in patients with 'unexplained' chronic pain: what options do we have? Expert Opin. Pharmacother. 12, 1087–1098.

Nijs, J., Meeus, M., Van Oosterwijck, J., et al., 2012a. In the mind or in the brain? scientific evidence for central sensitization in chronic fatigue syndrome. Eur. J. Clin. Invest. 42, 203–212.

Nijs, J., Van Houdenhove, B., Oostendorp, R.A., 2010. Recognition of central sensitization in patients with musculoskeletal pain: application of pain neurophysiology in manual therapy practice. Man. Ther. 15, 135–141.

Nijs, J., van Wilgen, C.P., Lluch Girbés, E., et al., 2014b. Applying modern pain neuroscience in clinical practice: criteria for the classification of central sensitization pain. Pain Physician 17, 447–457.

Nijs, J., van Wilgen, P.C., Van Oosterwijck, J., et al., 2011b. How to explain central sensitization to patients with 'unexplained' chronic musculoskeletal pain: practice guidelines. Man. Ther. 16, 413–418.

Norman, G., 2005. Research in clinical reasoning: past history and current trends. Med. Educ. 39, 418–427.

Osborn, M., 2014. More than just being nice: the importance of rapport to understanding. Eur. J. Pain 18, 753–754.

Overmeer, T., Linton, S.J., Holmquist, L., et al., 2005. Do evidence-based guidelines have an impact in primary care? a cross-sectional study of Swedish physicians and physiotherapists. Spine 30, 146–151.

Paul, R., Elder, L., 2007. A Guide for Educators to Critical Thinking Competency Standards. Foundation for Critical Thinking, Dillon Beach, CA.

Payton, O.D., Nelson, C.E., Hobbs, M.S.C., 1998. Physical therapy patients' perceptions of their relationships with health care professionals. Physiother. Theory Pract. 14, 211–221.

Pearsall, N.R., Skipper, J.E.J., Mintzes, J.J., 1997. Knowledge restructuring in the life sciences: a longitudinal study of conceptual change in biology. Sci. Educ. 81, 193–215.

Perrotta, A., Serrao, M., Sandrini, G., et al., 2010. Sensitisation of spinal cord pain processing in medication overuse headache involves supraspinal pain control. Cephalalgia 30, 272–284.

Pincus, T., 2004. The psychology of pain. In: French, S., Sim, K. (Eds.), Physiotherapy: A Psychosocial Approach. Elsevier, Edinburgh, pp. 95–115.

Pinto, R., Ferreira, M., Oliveira, V., et al., 2012. Patient-centred communication is associated with positive therapeutic alliance: a systematic review. J. Physiother. 58, 77–87.

Price, D.D., Staud, R., Robinson, M.E., et al., 2002. Enhanced temporal summation of second pain and its central modulation in fibromyalgia patients. Pain 99, 49–59.

Råholm, M.B., 2010. Abductive reasoning and the formation of scientific knowledge within nursing research. Nurs. Philos. 11, 260–270.

Rivett, D.A., Higgs, J., 1997. Hypothesis generation in the clinical reasoning behavior of manual therapists. J. Phys. Ther. Educ. 11, 40–45.

Rodgers, C., 2002. Defining reflection: another look at John Dewey and reflective thinking. Teach. Coll. Rec. 104, 842–866.

Roussel, N.A., Nijs, J., Meeus, M., et al., 2013. Central sensitization and altered central pain processing in chronic low back pain: fact or myth? Clin. J. Pain 29, 625–638.

Ruiz-Primo, M.A., Shavelson, R.J., Schultz, S.E., 2001. On the validity of cognitive interpretations of scores from alternative concept-mapping techniques. Educational Assessment 7, 99–141.

Sanders, T., Foster, N.E., Bishop, A., Ong, B.N., 2013. Biopsychosocial care and the physiotherapy encounter: physiotherapists' accounts of back pain consultations. BMC Musculoskelet. Disord. 14, 65. http://www.biomedcentral.com/1471-2474/14/65.

Sebastian, D., 2015. Differential Screening of Regional Pain in Musculoskeletal Practice. Jaypee Brothers Medical Publishers, New Delhi.

Schaible, H.G., 2006. Basic mechanisms of deep somatic pain. In: McMahon, S.B., Koltzenburg, M. (Eds.), Wall and Melzack's Textbook of Pain, fifth ed. Elsevier, pp. 621–633.

Schmid, A., Brunner, F., Wright, A., Bachmann, L.M., 2008. Paradigm shift in manual therapy? evidence for a central nervous system component in response to passive cervical joint mobilisation. Man. Ther. 13, 387–396.

Schön, D.A., 1983. The Reflective Practitioner. Basic Books, New York.

Schön, D.A., 1987. Educating the Reflective Practitioner: Toward a New Design for Teaching and Learning in the Professions. Jossey-Bass, San Francisco.

Schultz, I.Z., Crook, J.M., Berkowitz, J., et al., 2002. Biopsychosocial multivariate predictive model of occupational low back disability. Spine 27, 2720–2725.

Schwartz, A., Elstein, A.S., 2008. Clinical reasoning in medicine. In: Higgs, J., Jones, M.A., Loftus, S., Christensen, N. (Eds.), Clinical Reasoning in the Health Professions, third ed. Butterworth Heinemann Elsevier, Amsterdam, pp. 223–234.

Simon, H., 1992. What is an "explanation" of behavior? Psychol. Sci. 3, 150–161.

Singla, M., Jones, M., Edwards, I., Kumar, S., 2014. Physiotherapists' assessment of patients' psychosocial status: Are we standing on thin ice? A qualitative descriptive study. Man. Ther. http://dx.doi.org/10.1016/j.math.2014.10.004.

Smart, K., Doody, C., 2006. Mechanisms-based clinical reasoning of pain by experienced musculoskeletal physiotherapists. Physiotherapy 92, 171–178.

Smart, K.M., Blake, C., Staines, A., et al., 2012a. Mechanisms-based classifications of musculoskeletal pain: part 3 of 3: symptoms and signs of nociceptive pain in patients with low back (+/- leg) pain. Man. Ther. 17, 352–357.

Smart, K.M., Blake, C., Staines, A., et al., 2012b. Mechanisms-based classifications of musculoskeletal pain: part 2 of 3: symptoms and signs of peripheral neuropathic pain in patients with low back (+/- leg) pain. Man. Ther. 17, 345–351.

Smart, K.M., Blake, C., Staines, A., et al., 2012c. Mechanisms-based classifications of musculoskeletal pain: part 1 of 3: symptoms and signs of central sensitisation in patients with low back (+/- leg) pain. Man. Ther. 17, 336–344.

Smith, A.D., Jull, G., Schneider, G., et al., 2013. A comparison of physical and psychological features of responders and non-responders to cervical facet blocks in chronic whiplash. BMC Musculoskelet. Disord. 14, 313.

Smith, A.D., Jull, G., Schneider, G., et al., 2014. Cervical radiofrequency neurotomy reduces central hyperexcitability and improves neck movement in individuals with chronic whiplash. Pain Med. 15, 128–141.

Steiner, W.A., Ryser, L., Huber, E., et al., 2002. Use of the ICF model as a clinical problem-solving tool in physical therapy and rehabilitation medicine. Phys. Ther. 82, 1098–1107.

Taylor, E.W., Cranton, P., 2012. The Handbook of Transformative Learning. Theory, Research, and Practice. Jossey-Bass, San Francisco.

Trede, F., Higgs, J., 2008. Collaborative decision making. In: Higgs, J., Jones, M.A., Loftus, S., Christensen, N. (Eds.), Clinical Reasoning in the Health Professions, third ed. Butterworth Heinemann Elsevier, Amsterdam, pp. 31–41.

Treede, R.D., Jensen, T.S., Campbell, J.N., et al., 2008. Neuropathic pain: redefinition and a grading system for clinical and research purposes. Neurology 70, 1630–1635.

Turk, D.C., Flor, H., 2006. The cognitive-behavioural approach to pain management. In: McMahon, S.B., Koltzenburg, M. (Eds.), Wall and Melzack's Textbook of Pain, fifth ed. Elsevier, pp. 339–348.

Vardeh, D., Mannion, R.J., Woolf, C.J., 2016. Toward a mechanism-based approach to pain diagnosis. J. Pain 17 (9), T50–T69.

Vicenzino, B., Cleland, J.A., Bisset, L., 2007a. Joint manipulation in the management of lateral epicondylalgia: a clinical commentary. J. Man. Manip. Ther. 15, 50–56.

Vicenzino, B., Paungmali, A., Teys, P., 2007b. Mulligan's mobilization-with-movement, positional faults and pain relief: current concepts from a critical review of literature. Man. Ther. 12, 98–108.

Voogt, L., de Vries, J., Meeus, M., Struyf, F., Meuffels, D., Nijs, J., 2015. Analgesic effects of manual therapy in patients with musculoskeletal pain: a systematic review. Man. Ther. 20 (2), 250–256.

Woolf, C.J., 2010. What is this thing called pain? J. Clin. Invest. 120, 3742–3744.

Woolf, C.J., 2011. Central sensitization: implication for diagnosis and treatment of pain. Pain 152, s2–s15.

Woolf, C.J., 2014. What to call the amplification of nociceptive signals in the central nervous system that contribute to widespread pain? Pain 155 (10), 1911–1912.

World Health Organization, 2001. International Classification of Functioning, Disability and Health. World Health Organization, Geneva.

Zusman, M., 2008. Associative memory for movement-evoked chronic back pain and its extinction with musculoskeletal physiotherapy. Phys. Ther. Rev. 13, 57–68.

2

Understanding Pain in Order to Treat Patients in Pain

Mark J. Catley • G. Lorimer Moseley • Mark A. Jones

Pain is not the only reason people seek the care of musculoskeletal practitioners, but it is clearly one of the most common symptoms patients report. Pain-associated musculoskeletal conditions are the leading cause of global disability and, despite advances in knowledge and an exponential increase in healthcare costs, the problem only appears to be worsening (Vos et al., 2012). Given the prevalence of pain in the community, it is remarkable that pain is rarely the focus of medical and allied health graduate programs (Briggs et al., 2011, 2013; Jones and Hush, 2011).

Understanding pain, and the factors that contribute to it, is an important first step toward effectively treating and managing patients with pain. Knowledge of pain theory and biology enables clinicians to better understand and explain the full spectrum of pain presentations they encounter, from simple to complex (Moseley, 2003). It affords them an ability to reason through the potential contributors to a patient's pain, informing hypotheses regarding diagnosis, management and prognosis (see Chapter 1 for a full discussion of the hypothesis category clinical reasoning framework) (Jones et al., 2002). Importantly, an understanding of pain ensures all of the hypothesized contributors to pain are appropriately managed or addressed.

In this chapter, we review the complexity of pain from a theoretical perspective and briefly describe the biological and pathobiological processes associated with it. We introduce pain type as an important hypothesis category and attempt to link the clinical signs and symptoms observed in patients with pain to the mechanisms that may underpin them. In conclusion, we consider how reasoning about the contributors to pain can potentially improve patient outcomes.

Understanding Pain

With rare exception, we have all experienced pain, and these experiences influence our understanding of pain. That a small scratch generally hurts less than a deep graze and that pain seemingly lessens as an injury heals imply that the degree of pain we feel relates directly to the extent of an injury. Pain is thus usually interpreted as a symptom indicative of damage to the body. If pain persists, the intuitive explanation is that the injury or disease process that initiated it has failed to resolve.

Unfortunately, the training many clinicians receive reinforces intuitive understandings of pain. Pathoanatomical models of pain that depict pain as a marker of tissue damage remain influential. Most undergraduate textbooks inadvertently portray pain as an inevitable consequence of the activation of a specialized three-neurone 'pain pathway' – pain is considered a symptom of pathology that resolves only after an injury has healed (Martini, 2006; Snell, 2010). Rarely is it acknowledged that such depictions are not fact but trivializations that reflect the ideas of antiquated pain theories that do not stand up to scrutiny (Gatchel et al., 2007; Moayedi and Davis, 2013).

Misunderstandings regarding pain are unhelpful for patients and clinicians alike. Patients who view pain as a marker of the state of the tissues may be reluctant to participate in treatment and activities of daily life (George et al., 2006; Pincus et al., 2002). In acute pain presentations, these patients may rely on passive treatment strategies alone and not see a need to address predisposing and contributing factors that are relevant to both immediate outcome and minimization of recurrence. In persistent pain presentations, these patients may adopt maladaptive pain-escape coping strategies such as rest or altering the way they move or position themselves in an attempt to protect the painful body part (Darlow et al., 2015; Waddell, 1998) (see Chapter 3 for further discussion of stress and coping theory). They may seek passive treatment strategies that provide only temporary relief, perhaps trying one therapy after another in the search for relief or an explanation for their pain that makes sense (Watson, 2013). Clinicians who view pain as a symptom of pathology will approach the management of people in pain from a purely biomedical perspective – one that focuses solely on the tissues. They may misinform patients about the meaning and source of their symptoms or unintentionally reinforce negative attitudes toward pain in their patients (Bishop et al., 2008; Coudeyre et al., 2006; Darlow et al., 2013). In cases of persistent pain, some clinicians might rely only on passive treatments that offer temporary pain relief but do not address contributing factors. Failure to understand the biopsychosocial nature of all pain may result in some clinicians stigmatizing patients with persistent pain, who do not respond to treatment based on a biomedical model, as having 'psychogenic pain' or being malingerers – adding to the suffering of these patients rather than relieving it (Synnott et al., 2015).

There are compelling arguments as to why solely tissue-based understandings of pain must be rejected. Stories abound of people who sustained serious injuries but felt no pain – for example, soldiers who report horrific yet painless injuries in the midst of battle, shark-attack victims who report painless amputations and sportspeople who play on through injury without pain (Butler and Moseley, 2013; Melzack and Wall, 1996). Everyday experiences such as those scratches or bruises we notice on our bodies but are unable to recall when they occurred attest to this too. Such examples demonstrate that injury, and the sensory information it generates, can occur independent of pain. Conversely, the accounts of phantom limb pain highlight that pain can be felt in the clear absence of pathology and sensory information (Melzack, 1999; Ramachandran and Blakeslee, 1999).

The relationship between pain and pathology is also unclear. One in two people with moderate to severe radiographic osteoarthritic changes in their knees is asymptomatic, whereas 1 in 10 people with severe knee pain will have no evidence of radiographic arthritis (Bedson and Croft, 2008). A similar discordance is noted in spinal pain, where imaging findings of degeneration are highly prevalent in asymptomatic people and appear to be a normal part of aging (Brinjikji et al., 2015). The same holds true for neuropathies. In a large-scale study of patients with diabetes, only 60% of those with severe neuropathy reported pain (Abbott et al., 2011). Indeed, it has been stated that no study to date, for any pain-related condition, has demonstrated a direct relationship between pathology and pain (Clauw, 2015). That is, neither the presence or absence of pain nor the intensity of pain can be accurately predicted by the presence or absence of pathology.

Every pain, whether associated with significant injury or a momentary feeling that facilitates protection, is dependent on meaning and context. Experiments that manipulate the meaning of a noxious stimuli or the mood of the participants receiving the stimulus directly influence the intensity of pain (Arntz et al., 1994; Butler and Moseley, 2013; Moseley and Arntz, 2007). Clinically, the severity of pain has been shown to vary depending on the perceived cause. Soldiers injured in battle report less pain and require less analgesia than civilians undergoing procedures of comparable impact (Melzack and Wall, 1996), and mastectomy patients who attribute pain to returning cancer report higher levels of pain than those who do not (Smith et al., 1998). These examples seemingly suggest that the meaning of pain, survival versus a potentially life-changing event in the first instance and expectations of mortality in the second, influence how much pain is experienced. A growing clinical literature demonstrates that both pain intensity and duration are associated with mood factors, catastrophization, fear and poor expectation of recovery (Chapman and Vierck, 2017; Edwards et al., 2016).

Rather than an accurate marker of tissue pathology, pain is an unpleasant feeling (Moseley and Butler, 2017) that has both sensory and emotive aspects that cannot be extricated (Merskey and Bogduk, 1994). Pain is influenced by factors from the biological, psychological and social domains (Gatchel et al., 2007) and urges the protection (whether it is needed or not) of the body part in which it is felt. In the next section, we consider how the brain theoretically determines the need for protection and how it constructs a pain experience.

We also briefly describe some of the key mechanisms that underpin pain, extrapolating from the basic and clinical sciences.

Key Point

> Pain is not an accurate marker of the presence or extent of tissue injury. Patients who view it as such may be reluctant to participate in treatment and activities of daily life. Clinicians who view it as such will approach the management of people in pain from a purely biomedical perspective.

The Biology of Pain – A Brief Primer

Pain Is a Feeling

Pain is a feeling – it occurs in consciousness. It is an unpleasant feeling, and it has a location. These characteristics separate it from 'senses', which are engaged whether or not they are felt, and separate it from emotions, which conventionally refer to automatic bodily responses. Pain is perhaps best considered as a protective feeling, alongside other feelings such as hunger, thirst and dyspnoea – all unpleasant and all compelling triggers for whole-organism behaviour. When we consider 'pain-related mechanisms', we must consider mechanisms by which feelings emerge into consciousness – arguably 'the difficult problem' of life science; we must consider the detection of potentially dangerous tissue events; we must consider everything that occurs in between.

Despite a vast amount of thinking, humans have not yet discovered how consciousness emerges. There are metaphorical accounts, and there are frameworks and even guiding principles, but the notion of hardware – neural and immune cells in the brain – producing such things as feelings remains in the 'magic' category and may well remain there for some time to come. Although we do not know *how* feelings emerge, we do have some solid frameworks that can explain much of *when, why and to what extent* they emerge.

Neurotags

Contemporary theory regarding how the brain produces the wide array of outputs it does is captured to some extent by a model of the brain as a massive collection of neuroimmune networks, or representations, that are in a constant state of collaboration and competition. In modern pain parlance, these representations are often referred to as 'neurotags' (Butler and Moseley, 2013). Neurotags can be thought of as the pain-related mechanism most 'proximal' to pain – the last thing that happens. A full account of neurotags is beyond the scope of this chapter – the reader is referred elsewhere for this (see Moseley and Butler [2017]) – but understanding the main principles that govern the operation of neurotags will allow the reader to integrate the diverse range of factors, covered in theory Chapters 3 and 4 and the case study chapters through this book, that need to be considered when one analyzes why someone is hurting.

A neurotag can be labelled according to the output it generates. For example, a neurotag that results in a given movement command can be labelled as the neurotag for that movement command. A neurotag that results in back pain can be labelled 'back pain neurotag'. The likelihood that back pain will occur at any given point in time can be considered according to the influence of the back pain neurotag. Factors that govern the influence of a neurotag include the efficacy of its synaptic (neuro-neural and neuro-immune) connections, the number of cells involved (its 'mass') and the precision of its connection. One can readily see that the longer one has back pain, the more efficacious its connections become ('neuroplasticity') and the greater its influence. Clinically, this would manifest as allodynia (pain due to a stimulus that does not normally provoke pain) and hyperalgesia (increased pain from a stimulus that normally provokes pain).

The truly biopsychosocial nature of pain is also captured by this neurotag model. Each neurotag is under the influence of a potentially infinite number of other neurotags. For example, a noxious event in the back may well lead to activation of a 'back nociception' neurotag, which is highly influential over the 'back pain' neurotag; if the patient believes he or she has a back that 'goes out', is 'worn' or is 'degenerated', then each of these beliefs will be held by neurotags. Each of these neurotags will exert some influence over the back pain neurotag. The magnitude of that influence will be determined by the synaptic efficacy, mass and precision of those neurotags.

This idea that neurotags compete and collaborate for influence offers sensible explanations for many observations that are not easily explained by previous models. For example, intriguing perceptual experiments such as those showing very cold stimuli feeling hot, and more painful, when they coincide with a red visual cue (Moseley and Arntz, 2007), more expensive wines tasting better (and activating brain reward circuits) and a raft of visual illusions are all consistent with competing influences of neurotags on other neurotags. Consider also that fear tends to trump pain: the fear neurotag and the back pain neurotag *compete* for priority; any cue that suggests the entire organism is in danger and needs to take protective action will increase the probability of activating the fear neurotag; any cue that suggests a particular body part should be protected will increase the probability of activating the pain neurotag. This makes ecological and evolutionary sense: given the option to protect one's life, or protect one's arm, for example, it would seem most beneficial to do the former. The interactions of diverse neurotags and the individual nature of neurotags, corresponding to patients' unique biopsychosocial makeup, highlight the need for explicit and comprehensive assessment of biological, psychological and social factors (see Chapters 3 and 4 for further discussion of psychological and social factors).

Danger Detection Is Important

It is sensible, when thinking about pain-related mechanisms, to have a sound understanding of how danger is detected and transmitted to the brain. This capacity to detect, transmit and represent danger is called nociception. According to what we currently know about brain activity associated with nociception, nociceptive neurotags are large and have high synaptic efficacy, which means they will be highly influential over pain neurotags.

Nociception is well studied. The tissues of the body are by and large very well innervated by free nerve endings. These free nerve endings are primarily small-diameter and thinly myelinated (Aδ) or unmyelinated (C) fibres, although some are wide-diameter myelinated (Aβ) fibres. Free nerve endings vary in many ways. For example, some have a low threshold, some high; some adapt quickly, some slowly; some have small receptive fields, and some have large ones. In a normal physiological state, it is the high-threshold free nerve endings that function most like nociceptors (or 'danger detectors') – they only respond to large and rapid changes in the tissue environment.

Free nerve endings terminate in the spinal cord, where they enter a complex matrix of neurones, interneurons and immune cells. Contemporary neurophysiological models of the grey matter of the spinal cord relate most closely to those of the brain. We can apply the neurotag idea here as well, conceptualizing the spinal cord as a long tube of brain-like neuroimmune networks, or neurotags, surrounded by the white matter 'freeways' via which messages travel quickly and without interruption to and from higher centres (Moseley and Butler, 2017). The output of spinal neurotags will be to either influence other spinal neurotags or activate projection neurones that terminate in the body (these are motor neurones, which emerge from the ventral horn of the spinal cord) or supraspinally (these are spinal nociceptors, which emerge from the dorsal horn and join the ascending 'freeway' to the thalamus). This complex matrix within the spinal cord offers a mechanism by which massive computational capacity can occur at a spinal level. Indeed, contemporary pain theory rejects the idea of the dorsal horn working as a relay station for nociceptive input, endorsing instead the idea of the dorsal horn working as a processing station that determines the spatial and temporal features of any further signals of danger that are transmitted to the brain.

Danger detectors have a wide variety of sensors in their walls – ion channels that respond to chemical, thermal or mechanical changes in the tissues or to a shift in the voltage across the cell membrane (Ringkamp et al., 2013) (for full review in accessible language, see Moseley and Butler [2017]). The response profile of a given danger detector will reflect the mix of ion channels in its membrane – some respond to small and innocuous changes in the tissue environment (including one sub-class of nociceptors that responds to light, 'sensual' touch – coined 'C-aress fibres' [Abraira and Ginty, 2013; McGlone et al., 2014]); some have such high thresholds that they are effectively silent in the absence of inflammation.

Peripheral Sensitization, Primary Allodynia and Hyperalgesia

One remarkable characteristic of danger detectors is their response to inflammation. Injury triggers inflammation – the first stage of tissue repair. A range of sensors on danger detectors triggers a series of events that occur *inside* the neurone and render its chemical, thermal, mechanical and voltage-driven sensors more sensitive. The effect of this response is to sensitize the danger detectors and to 'bring online' those very high-threshold danger detectors that are normally silent. These adaptations in the stimulus–response profile of danger detectors is called peripheral sensitization.

The effect of peripheral sensitization on spinal nociception obeys the mass-based principle of neurotags: more spinal neurotags activated equates to more influence over spinal nociceptors. As such, the stimulus–response advantage mediated at the tissue level by inflammation is replicated in the spinal cord. All things being equal (which they never really are), the clinical result will be a reduced pain threshold (allodynia) and an increased response to a given noxious stimulus (hyperalgesia). Peripheral sensitization will follow the inflammatory state of the tissues, and as such, nociceptive sensitivity is closely tied to immune activity. A full review is well beyond the scope of this chapter, but suffice it here to suggest that under normal conditions, inflammation will begin to recede within a week of injury, a process that usually triggers the resolution of sensitivity.

Spinal Sensitization, Secondary Allodynia and Hyperalgesia

Activation of spinal neurotags triggers learning within the dorsal horn. According to the synaptic efficacy principle of neurotags, this learning, or enhanced synaptic efficacy, increases the influence of spinal neurotags and therefore further enhances the stimulus–response adaptations. The mechanisms by which this learning occurs include transient shifts in baseline voltage across post-synaptic membranes, increased production of post-synaptic receptors and a shift in the immune-mediated 'set point' of the synapse. This process was for some time referred to as central sensitization (as distinct from peripheral sensitization) but is probably better labelled 'spinal sensitization'. It produces a shift in stimulus–response profiles and increased receptive fields of spinal nociceptors, which manifests clinically as reduced pain thresholds to mechanical input ('secondary allodynia') and increased response to a given noxious stimulus ('secondary hyperalgesia'). These effects can be so profound that the spinal neurotags associated with tactile input can gain access to spinal nociceptive neurotags. Clinically, this can manifest as pain on light touch, a cardinal sign of neural disease or injury (neuropathic pain).

Descending Modulation of Nociception

The nociceptive system is a two-way system. Spinal neurotags are under a wide range of descending modulatory inputs. Projection neurones from midbrain nuclei (most famously the periaqueductal gray, or PAG), terminate in the grey matter of the spinal cord. These descending projections can exert facilitatory influences or inhibitory influences, categorized as 'descending facilitation' or 'descending inhibition'. Midbrain nuclei receive projections from many different brain areas, providing the hardware for potent and diverse brain-driven modulation of spinal nociception. This capacity brings the truly biopsychosocial nature of pain and protection into relevance for any painful episode, acute or longstanding, because of the clear capacity for any cue from across the biological, psychological and social domains to influence activity and learning in the spinal cord.

Whereas the function of the nociceptive system is affected by activity, inflammation and modulatory influences, the integrity of the nociceptive system can be affected by damage or disease of the hardware – the peripheral nerves, dorsal root ganglia, nerve roots or central nervous system components. Disruption of the capacity of wide-diameter neurones to transmit messages will compromise sensibility or strength – so-called negative signs. Perhaps counterintuitively, disruption of free nerve endings, or spinal nociceptors, to transmit messages can result in more sensitivity, not less – so-called positive signs (Nee and Butler, 2006). Peripheral mechanisms include problems with the cell wall, resulting in abnormal impulse generating sites (AIGSs), which are usually mechanically sensitive such that mechanical stimulation triggers a discharge that outlasts the stimulus itself by up to 2 minutes. Even for very slowly adapting free nerve endings, this time frame is very abnormal. Such a disruption can result in pain of a similar time profile. AIGSs can also result in spontaneous firing, which will enhance synaptic efficacy upstream, thereby replicating the spinal sensitization effects described earlier. Disruption of free nerve endings, or central nociceptive neurotags, can also result from disease, for example, diabetic neuropathy or multiple sclerosis; severe trauma, for example, gunshot-related wounds or amputation; excessive sustained or repetitive mechanical loading, for example, compartment syndrome; and chemical irritation or blood flow compromise, for example, nerve root irritation or tumour.

Central Sensitization – Tertiary Allodynia and Hyperalgesia

The mechanisms by which spinal neurotags become more influential – learning (synaptic efficacy principle) and collaboration (mass principle) – also apply to cortical neurotags. However, when the cortical neurotags that represent nociception undergo these changes, the effects are, predictably, more widespread. Moreover, when the neurotags that produce protective outputs (including pain but also protective motor, endocrine, descending modulatory, autonomic and immune responses) undergo these changes, the effects now increase the influence of any cues related to protection. Considering the biopsychosocial nature of pain, sensitivity in these protective neurotags will result in reduced pain thresholds for any combination of cues from across biological, psychological and social (importantly capturing context here) domains and increased pain for a given combination of those cues. The manifestation of these changes can be conceptualized as tertiary allodynia (reduced pain thresholds) and tertiary hyperalgesia (increased pain in normally painful situations).

There are other changes that occur in spinal and cortical function when pain persists. These changes are well studied from a clinical and behavioural perspective and from a brain-imaging and neurophysiology perspective. Several groups are working to integrate these two fields. Many of the more 'bizarre' presentations of people with persistent pain, for example, the feeling of swelling when none exists or the feeling that one no longer 'owns' a painful body part, can be explained by those changes in function. One model that seeks to make sense of that wider body of literature is the cortical body matrix, and the reader is referred elsewhere for more information pertaining to that subject (Moseley et al., 2012).

Key Point

> Pain is a feeling; it is unpleasant, localizable in the body and serves to protect when protection is needed. Pain is one of several protective responses (motor, endocrine, descending modulatory, autonomic and immune responses) that are initiated when the 'best guess' computation concludes that body tissue is in danger; together, these responses normally ensure the optimal conditions for escaping injury or recovering after injury. In addition, the nervous system adapts in its ability to detect danger by becoming more sensitive, and this sensitization serves to increase the likelihood of pain. Sometimes, however, pain persists when protection is no longer required. Biological, psychological and contextual factors can each influence the persistence of pain and nervous system sensitization and lead to dysregulation of the other protective systems.

Classifying Pain

Pain is typically categorized in terms of where it is felt, how it is described (e.g. aching, burning) and how long it has persisted. *Acute* refers to pain of recent onset, whereas *chronic* refers to pain which has persisted past the normal time of healing (Bonica, 1953), which, in practice, may be less than 1 month or more than 6 months, depending on the extent of injury and the bodily tissues affected (Treede et al., 2015).

Pain is also categorized in terms of why it might occur, and this underpins the notion of *pain type* (Butler, 2000; Gifford, 1998; Jones et al., 2002). Pain type is an attempt to categorize pain by the mechanisms hypothesized to be contributing to it. These contributors are deduced from clinical findings and associated investigations. Although multiple mechanisms are inevitably present in every pain presentation, clinicians can make informed hypotheses regarding which contributors are dominant and likely to be driving a pain state. The reasoning process is informed by a comprehensive understanding of pain-related mechanisms and the symptoms and signs that are thought to infer their presence.

The types considered here are those most widely discussed in the literature – nociceptive, inflammatory, neuropathic, mixed, nociplastic and augmented pain. It has been acknowledged, however, that this list is not exhaustive, and other contributors, including autonomic, neuroendocrine and neuroimmune, may dominate some presentations (Smart et al., 2011). Nonetheless, the categories discussed in this chapter incorporate these other contributors in principle, thus accounting for the majority of clinical presentations. Here, we review the symptoms and signs associated with each type, referencing the biological mechanisms they likely infer.

Nociceptive Pain

Nociceptive pain refers to pain that is associated with actual or threatened damage to non-neural tissue and involves the activation of peripheral nociceptors (*IASP Taxonomy*, 2015). It is important to note that the term *nociceptive pain*, which is widely accepted in the literature, does not imply causation (i.e. nociception equals pain) because every pain experience involves cognitive, contextual and mood factors. Rather, it suggests that tissue-based nociceptive mechanisms are dominant contributors to the experience. Nociceptive pain is clearly advantageous because it facilitates protection. It may occur with excessive strain or a shift in chemical environment, without overt injury, for example, posture-associated nociception triggered by a local increase in lactic acid. In the event of injury, *inflammatory* (i.e. inflammation-related) *pain*, a subtype of nociceptive pain (Loeser and Treede, 2008), ensures behaviours that optimize recovery are adopted and usually resolves as injured tissues heal (Costigan et al., 2009). In some conditions, for example, osteoarthritis or rheumatoid arthritis, nociceptive pain may persist, although such cases are also associated with spinal and cortical sensitization (see following discussion of nociplastic pain). Notably, radiological findings do not constitute evidence of inflammatory pain.

Because nociceptive pain suggests a significant contribution of free nerve endings, it may be associated with evidence of pathology, such as the cardinal signs of inflammation or radiographic findings that are in accord with the clinical presentation and, where appropriate, the reported mechanism of injury (Costigan et al., 2009; Woolf, 2010). Pain severity in this pain type is reasoned to be 'proportionate' (but not equal) to the extent of the injury (Nijs et al., 2014; Smart et al., 2010), suggesting that psychological or contextual factors, although relevant, are not augmenting pain to any great degree. Nociceptive pain may be associated with some somatic referral but is generally localized to the area of injury. The presence of inflammation infers the development of both peripheral and spinal sensitization; hence, some localized allodynia and hyperalgesia around the injured region would be expected but 'proportionate' to the suspected pathology.

In keeping with the hypothesis of peripheral sensitization, it is reasonable to expect nociceptive pain presentations to have clear mechanical patterns of aggravation and easing factors and a recognizable mechanism of onset (history), for example, overt trauma or some form of overuse or excessive strain (Smart et al., 2010). Movement and palpation tests that assess injured tissue should reliably elicit pain and reproduce the patient's symptoms. Nociceptive pain, when associated with acute injury, should resolve well within normal tissue healing times (Costigan et al., 2009).

Neuropathic Pain

Neuropathic pain refers to pain that is associated with a lesion or disease of the somatosensory nervous system (Treede et al., 2008). It can be further categorized by location depending on whether the lesion affects the peripheral or central nervous system (Merskey and Bogduk, 1994), but here we limit our discussion to peripheral neuropathic contributors. To be classified as neuropathic pain, clear evidence of a neuropathic lesion or disease is required (Jensen et al., 2011), and a grading system of certainty has been proposed (Finnerup et al., 2016). The requirement of evidence prevents painful conditions with proposed but undetectable neuropathic contributors, for example, small-fibre neuropathic contributors, from being included in this category (Jensen et al., 2011). It also excludes conditions characterized by signs of spinal or central sensitization in the absence of demonstrable neuropathic drivers. It is worth iterating here that neuropathy is not necessarily painful, and of those acute nerve injuries associated with pain, the majority resolve. As with nociceptive pain, neuropathic pain infers neuropathic mechanisms are the dominant, but not the only, contributors to the experience.

Although sophisticated neurophysiological techniques have been described, a thorough patient interview and physical examination is still considered most appropriate (Haanpää et al., 2011). A patient's mechanism of injury, past medical history or surgical history may infer neural tissues have been injured, mechanically compromised or diseased.

Neuropathic pain is generally localized to the distribution of the nerve thought to be affected (although spinal processing may lead to non-dermatomal variations [Schmid et al., 2013]) and may be accompanied by the other signs indicative of neuronal dysfunction, such as pins and needles, numbness and weakness. Indicative of AIGS formation, neuropathic pain may be described as burning, shooting, sharp, aching or like an electric shock (Smart et al., 2010). It may be triggered mechanically by movement or may be spontaneous in nature with a lingering aftersensation. Hence, neuropathic pain can be easily irritated. Provocation of pain with neurodynamic tests (e.g. straight leg raise) that physically load neural tissue or direct palpation of nerves in the area thought to be compromised (e.g. Tinnel's test) may reproduce patients' symptoms (Nee and Butler, 2006).

If neuropathic pain is hypothesized, a thorough neurological assessment should be included as part of the physical examination. Assessment of tactile sensation, pinprick, vibration, cold and warmth provides evidence of the positive and negative signs associated with neuropathy (Haanpää et al., 2011).

Several questionnaire-based screening tools have been devised to assist clinicians in screening for potential neuropathic contributors. Although alone they are considered inferior to clinical assessment, they can assist non-clinicians to differentiate between the likely dominance of nociceptive and neuropathic contributors. They also provide a measure of pain type along a continuum for reporting purposes and can be facilitated over the telephone or Internet if patients are treated from remote locations (Haanpää et al., 2011). Some recommended tools, including painDETECT (Freynhagen et al., 2006) and Douleur neuropathique (DN4) (Bouhassira et al., 2005), consist solely of self-report items, whereas others, such as the Leeds assessment of neuropathic symptoms and signs (LANSS) (Bennett, 2001), include both self-report items and physical assessment items.

Mixed Pain

Mixed pain refers to presentations that include evidence of both neuropathic and nociceptive contributors. Although every presentation includes multiple contributors, mixed pain as a category is reserved for those cases that have clear nociceptive and neuropathic contributors that may be directly or indirectly related and require equal consideration in management.

Nociplastic Pain

How to define the type of pain that persists in the absence of overt tissue or nerve pathology is a contentious issue because it is a category based on inference rather than evidence (Hansson, 2014; Woolf, 2014). Several descriptors have been put forward, including maladaptive algopathic, nocipathic and central sensitization pain (Kosek et al., 2016; Nijs et al., 2014). What they share in common is reference to functional changes within the central nociceptive pathways, although, as noted previously, such changes are associated with nociceptive and neuropathic pain also. Here, we refer to this category of pain as nociplastic; a term endorsed by the IASP (International Association for the Study of Pain) Task Force on Taxonomy that captures the nociceptive plasticity (Kosek et al., 2016). Nociplastic pain is clearly dysfunctional as it serves no protective benefit to the people experiencing it.

Nociplastic pain is significantly disproportionate to any plausible tissue contributions, persists beyond expected tissue healing times and may be recurrent in nature. It is characterized by widespread allodynia and hyperalgesia that persist in the absence of overt neuropathic or tissue-based drivers. It is thus inferred that sensitization is maintained due to alterations in the descending modulatory pathways and dysregulation of the other protective systems. In the absence of reliable biomarkers, it is, however, a clinical category of exclusion (Vardeh et al., 2016).

Nociplastic pain is often associated with psychological distress (Smart et al., 2010); maladaptive beliefs; poor self-efficacy; disproportionate physical impairment; disrupted family, work and social life; and disturbed sleep (Edwards et al., 2016). These factors are both consequences of, and contributors to, pain. Conceptualized as neurotags, unhelpful beliefs, for example, may influence and contribute to the persistence of pain while facilitating sensitivity in spinal neurotags via the descending pathways. Psychological stressors or mood factors may activate protective systems, indirectly influencing peripheral and spinal sensitization. Conditions such as fibromyalgia, non-specific chronic back pain, complex regional pain syndrome (type 1) or irritable bowel syndrome are examples of this pain type (Clauw, 2015; Woolf, 2011).

Nociplastic pain may be disproportionately severe, diffuse in nature and vary in response physical or functional tests. Patients may have difficulty localizing their pain or may report it having a migratory nature. Pain may be reported in multiple body regions, and it may be reflected on the contralateral limb. Allodynia may be widespread and not follow a logical anatomical distribution (Smart et al., 2010). Patients may also report perceptual disturbances such as feelings of swelling or neglect-like symptoms (Bray and Moseley, 2011; Moseley et al., 2006; Stanton et al., 2012).

The Central Sensitization Inventory (CSI) has been developed to assist clinicians in screening for symptoms indicative of central sensitization (Mayer et al., 2012). It contains 25 items that assess pain- and health-related symptoms, providing a total score between 0 and 100. Scores greater than 40 have been shown to correctly differentiate patients with and without central sensitization-related syndromes (Neblett et al., 2013). An algorithm approach, incorporating the CSI, has been described to specifically identify those patients with nociplastic pain (Nijs et al., 2014). The approach prioritizes the exclusion of neuropathic contributors, then looks to differentiate nociplastic pain from nociceptive pain. Two criteria are considered key: pain disproportionate to the injury or pathology and pain that is diffusely distributed. The former is considered essential, whereas the presence of the latter either confirms the verdict or advises further interrogation via the CSI (Nijs et al., 2014) (see also case Chapter 25 where this algorithm is applied in the reasoning differentiation of pain type). Specific tools to detect the presence of pain-related perceptual disturbance have been developed and validated for some pain populations. The Fremantle Back Awareness Questionnaire (Wand et al., 2016) and Neurobehavioral Questionnaire for patients with complex regional pain syndrome (Galer and Jensen, 1999) are examples.

Augmented pain, a subtype of nociplastic pain, refers to nociceptive or neuropathic presentations whereby pain and pain-related behaviours are clearly disproportionate to the contributions of peripheral drivers. As with nociplastic pain, augmented pain is associated with psychological distress and expectations of poor recovery. It is well documented that the likelihood of successful recovery diminishes the longer pain persists (Costa et al., 2009; Itz et al., 2013; Waddell, 1998). For this reason, we have chosen to differentiate augmented pain from nociplastic pain to highlight the need to identify acute patients who are at significant risk of chronicity. Augmented pain thus presents with clinical signs and symptoms indicative of tissue or neural pathology in conjunction with psychological, social and environmental risk factors, so-called yellow flags (see case Chapter 14 for an example of a patient presentation hypothesized to represent augmented pain).

Yellow flags were developed as guidelines to assist clinicians in identifying risk factors in patients with low back pain (Kendall et al., 1997) and have since been adapted to other chronic pain conditions. They are categorized broadly under the following headings: beliefs (including appraisals and judgements), behaviours and emotional responses (Nicholas et al., 2011). Beliefs include, but are not limited to, patients' understanding of pain (Moseley and Butler, 2015), catastrophising (Sullivan et al., 2001), perceived control (Jensen et al., 2002; Nicholas et al., 2011) and expectations of recovery (Iles et al., 2008). Behaviours include avoidance activities (Leeuw et al., 2007) and passive coping strategies such as resting at times of pain, medication seeking and withdrawal from physical activity (Watson, 2013). Assessment and treatment require attention to the patient's understanding of his or her condition, including the patient's threat appraisal, and management of expectations. Ensuring patients understand conflicting or complex diagnoses and results of further investigations is essential, as is the avoidance or clarification of diagnostic jargon. As noted previously, many different emotions are expressed by patients in pain, the majority being negative. These include depression and anxiety, but also frustration and anger (Gatchel et al., 2007). Ensuring patients can express these emotions freely and that each is considered in the management plan is essential. Although they are unhelpful and potential barriers to recovery, yellow flags should be considered normal psychological reactions to musculoskeletal symptoms that can be amenable to change by trained members of the multidisciplinary team when identified early (Nicholas et al., 2011).

Other colours that have been introduced to the flag system include orange, blue and black. Orange flags distinguish psychological risk factors that are considered abnormal – psychiatric factors that meet the criteria for psychopathology and require specialist mental health referral (e.g. clinical depression, personality disorder) (Main, 2013; Nicholas et al., 2011). Blue and black flags that relate to the perception (e.g. perceived time pressures, lack of job satisfaction, employer support, stressful work environment) and the characteristics (e.g. rates of pay, working conditions) of the patient's workplace, respectively, should also be considered and addressed (Main and Spanswick, 2000).

Other risk factors worthy of note include high levels of pain, age and gender, where older persons and females are at higher risk. Also of note are social isolation, relationships (overly supportive and unsupportive), a primary language different from that of the country of residency, low levels of education and longer duration of pain or a greater period of reduced activity before consultation (Costa et al., 2009; Flor et al., 1987; Henschke et al., 2008; Nicholas et al., 2011; Romano et al., 1995; van Hecke et al., 2013) (also see discussion under Social Relationships and Health in Chapter 3).

Several screening tools have been devised to assist clinicians in identifying yellow flags associated with augmented or nociplastic pain presentations, and these have been discussed in more detail elsewhere (see the discussion of psychological factor screening by questionnaire in Chapter 4 of this book). Noteworthy examples include the Orebro Musculoskeletal Pain Questionnaire (Linton and Halldén, 1998), the Pain Catastrophizing Scale (Sullivan et al., 1995), Pain Self-Efficacy Questionnaire (Nicholas, 2007), Neurophysiology of Pain Questionnaire (Moseley, 2003) and the Depression, Anxiety and Stress Scale (Lovibond and Lovibond, 1995), with each showing reasonable psychometric properties (Catley et al., 2013; Di Pietro et al., 2014; Parkitny et al., 2012; Walton et al., 2013; Westman et al., 2008).

If a nociplastic or augmented pain type is reasoned, a multifaceted and often multidisciplinary management approach that targets each hypothesized contributor is indicated. In augmented pain, reduction of pain intensity is a treatment priority. However, for nociplastic pain, the emphasis usually shifts toward function.

Key Points

> Pain type refers to the categorization of pain in terms of the mechanisms hypothesized to be contributing to it. Categories include nociceptive, inflammatory, neuropathic, mixed, nociplastic and augmented pain. Because multiple mechanisms are present in every pain presentation, these descriptors do not infer cause but rather describe or qualify the dominant contributing mechanism. The contributing mechanisms are deduced from clinical findings and associated investigations.

Implications of Pain Type Categorization

Consideration of pain type encourages a biopsychosocial approach to patient care. It is informed by a comprehensive patient interview and physical examination. Understanding patients' symptom(s) presentation, their activity and participation capabilities and restrictions, their perspectives on their pain and disability experiences (see Chapter 4 for suggested categories of information to screen regarding patients' perspectives) and their social circumstances (i.e. "narrative reasoning") provides a holistic overview that enables pain type to be hypothesized for further 'testing'/inference through the physical examination and ongoing re-assessments of intervention strategies.

Reasoning through the plausible contributors to pain informs diagnosis, prognosis and management. Note that in this text, diagnostic reasoning is not limited to the traditional medical categorization of pathology or disease. Instead, as discussed in Chapter 1, musculoskeletal practice diagnosis encapsulates the clinician's analysis of the patient's functional limitation(s) and associated physical and movement impairments with consideration of pain type, tissue pathology and the broad scope of potential contributing factors. Contributing factors to the development and maintenance of the patient's problem(s) can be psychological, social, environmental, physical and hereditary. For example, in some conditions such as acute back pain, tissue contributions to pain may be unclear, but reasoning through the likely sources can inform clinical decisions regarding management and the advice provided to patients. Early identification of an augmented or nociplastic pain will ensure the treatment strategy is adapted appropriately to accommodate potential psychosocial barriers to recovery. It also informs prognosis, as patients with significant yellow flags will likely take longer to recover.

Consideration of pain type, however, must ensure red flags – signs suggestive of sinister pathology – are thoroughly investigated and not mistakenly attributed to nervous system sensitization (Koes et al., 2010). Around 50 red flags have been reported, and when considered in isolation, many have high false-positive rates (Henschke et al., 2009; Williams et al., 2013). If acted upon uncritically, red flags could unnecessarily increase the cost of management and perhaps impede a patient's recovery; for example, there is a growing appreciation of the negative impact the overuse of imaging can have (Brinjikji et al., 2015; Darlow et al., 2017). Nonetheless, the presence of some factors may indicate that immediate action should be taken (e.g. features of cauda equina syndrome), and a combination of red flags (e.g. trauma, age and sex) or the failed resolution of a flag (e.g. fever) may indicate the need for further investigations (Henschke et al., 2009).

Although pain type is an important consideration, there are several limitations of categorization that should be noted. First, pain type informs the reasoning process but is not a diagnosis. Any hypotheses regarding pain and therefore its management should be considered in the greater context of the patient presentation (Rabey et al., 2015) (see Chapter 1 for discussion of pain type in the context of other hypothesis categories). Second, the mechanisms underpinning pain are complex and individual mechanisms, inferred by examination, are not necessarily unique to any particular pathological process (Woolf and Mannion, 1999). In a similar manner, pain contributors, especially those psychological and contextual contributors, vary continually on a moment-by-moment basis and may differ in influence over time, indicating that the reasoning process is a continuing one. Third, pain type categorization is dependent on the knowledge, expertise and experience of the clinician. Because the pain sciences are continually evolving as new knowledge surfaces, it is imperative clinicians keep up-to-date with the literature and continue to develop their clinical skills. Fourth, pain type categories are yet to be comprehensively validated against 'gold-standard' neurophysiological techniques, such as quantitative sensory testing in any pain condition (Rabey et al., 2015). Rather, they are inferred by expert opinion on the basis of extrapolation of basic science evidence (Smart et al., 2010). Finally, clinical evidence to support the categorization of patients according to pain type to improve patient outcome is currently scant (Hensley and Courtney, 2014).

Conclusions

Pain is a feeling. It is influenced by a multitude of factors and is always about protection of the body. Understanding pain as a protective feeling rather than an accurate marker of tissue damage enhances clinician confidence when confronted with complex presentations, improves the therapeutic alliance between clinician and patient and facilitates a truly biopsychosocial patient-centred approach to management. Although the mechanisms underpinning pain are complex and not fully understood, informed clinicians are able to make hypotheses regarding the dominant contributors to pain through inference of the presenting signs and symptoms. Pain type, as a hypothesis category, reflects these dominant contributors whereby pain presentations can be broadly categorized as nociceptive, neuropathic and nociplastic. Although further research is needed to validate the profiling of patients and to determine whether categorization improves patient outcomes, when considered in the context of a reasoning framework, hypotheses regarding pain type inform decisions of diagnosis, management and prognosis and encourage a multifaceted and often multidisciplinary management approach, as recommended in most contemporary clinical guidelines.

REFERENCES

Abbott, C.A., Malik, R.A., van Ross, E.R.E., Kulkarni, J., Boulton, A.J.M., 2011. Prevalence and characteristics of painful diabetic neuropathy in a large community-based diabetic population in the U.K. Diabetes Care 34 (10), 2220–2224.
Abraira, V.E., Ginty, D.D., 2013. The sensory neurons of touch. Neuron 79 (4), 618–639.
Arntz, A., Dreesson, L., De Jong, P., 1994. The influence of anxiety on pain: attentional and attributional mediators. Pain 56, 307–314.
Bedson, J., Croft, P.R., 2008. The discordance between clinical and radiographic knee osteoarthritis: A systematic search and summary of the literature. BMC Musculoskelet. Disord. 9 (1), 116.
Bennett, M., 2001. The LANSS pain scale: the Leeds Assessment of Neuropathic Symptoms and Signs. Pain 92, 147–157.
Bishop, A., Foster, N.E., Thomas, E., Hay, E.M., 2008. How does the self-reported clinical management of patients with low back pain relate to the attitudes and beliefs of health care practitioners? A survey of UK general practitioners and physiotherapists. Pain 135 (1), 187–195.
Bonica, J.J., 1953. The Management of Pain. Lea & Febiger, Philadelphia.
Bouhassira, D., Attal, N., Alchaar, H., Boureau, F., Brochet, B., Bruxelle, J., et al., 2005. Comparison of pain syndromes associated with nervous or somatic lesions and development of a new neuropathic pain diagnostic questionnaire (DN4). Pain 114 (1), 29–36.
Bray, H., Moseley, G.L., 2011. Disrupted working body schema of the trunk in people with back pain. Br. J. Sports Med. 45 (3), 168.
Briggs, E.V., Carrl, E.C.J., Whittakerl, M.S., 2011. Survey of undergraduate pain curricula for healthcare professionals in the United Kingdom. Eur. J. Pain 15 (8), 789–795.
Briggs, A.M., Slater, H., Smith, A.J., Parkin-Smith, G.F., Watkins, K., Chua, J., 2013. Low back pain-related beliefs and likely practice behaviours among final-year cross-discipline health students. Eur. J. Pain 17 (5), 766–775.
Brinjikji, W., Luetmer, P.H., Comstock, B., Bresnahan, B.W., Chen, L.E., Deyo, R.A., et al., 2015. Systematic literature review of imaging features of spinal degeneration in asymptomatic populations. AJNR Am. J. Neuroradiol. 36 (4), 811–816.
Butler, D.S., 2000. The Sensitive Nervous System. Noigroup Publications, Unley, South Australia.
Butler, D.S., Moseley, G.L., 2013. Explain Pain, second ed. Noigroup Publications, Adelaide, South Australia.
Catley, M.J., O'Connell, N.E., Moseley, G.L., 2013. How good is the Neurophysiology of Pain Questionnaire? A Rasch analysis of psychometric properties. J. Pain 14 (8), 818–827.
Chapman, C.R., Vierck, C.J., 2017. The transition of acute postoperative pain to chronic pain: an integrative overview of research on mechanisms. J. Pain 18 (4), 359.e1–359.e38.
Clauw, D.J., 2015. Diagnosing and treating chronic musculoskeletal pain based on the underlying mechanism(s). Best Pract Res Clin Rheumatol 29 (1), 6–19.
Costa, L.D.C.M., Maher, C.G., McAuley, J.H., Hancock, M.J., Herbert, R.D., Refshauge, K.M., et al., 2009. Prognosis for patients with chronic low back pain: inception cohort study. BMJ 339 (b3829).

Costigan, M., Scholz, J., Woolf, C.J., 2009. Neuropathic pain: a maladaptive response of the nervous system to damage. Annu. Rev. Neurosci. 32, 1–32.

Coudeyre, E., Rannou, F., Tubach, F., Baron, G., Coriat, F., Brin, S., et al., 2006. General practitioners' fear-avoidance beliefs influence their management of patients with low back pain. Pain 124 (3), 330–337.

Darlow, B., Dean, S., Perry, M., Mathieson, F., Baxter, G.D., Dowell, A., 2015. Easy to harm, hard to heal: patient views about the back. Spine 40 (11), 842–850.

Darlow, B., Dowell, A., Baxter, G.D., Mathieson, F., Perry, M., Dean, S., 2013. The enduring impact of what clinicians say to people with low back pain. Ann Fam Med 11 (6), 527–534.

Darlow, B., Forster, B.B., O'Sullivan, K., O'Sullivan, P., 2017. It is time to stop causing harm with inappropriate imaging for low back pain. Br. J. Sports Med. 51, 414–415.

Di Pietro, F., Catley, M.J., McAuley, J.H., Parkitny, L., Maher, C.G., Costa, L.D.C.M., et al., 2014. Rasch analysis supports the use of the pain self-efficacy questionnaire. Phys. Ther. 94 (1), 91–100.

Edwards, R.R., Dworkin, R.H., Sullivan, M.D., Turk, D.C., Wasan, A.D., 2016. The role of psychosocial processes in the development and maintenance of chronic pain. J. Pain 17 (9 Suppl.), T70–T92.

Finnerup, N., Haroutounian, S., Kamerman, P., Baron, R., Bennett, D., Bouhassira, D., et al., 2016. Neuropathic pain: an updated grading system for research and clinical practice. Pain 157 (8), 1599–1606.

Flor, H., Kerns, R.D., Turk, D.C., 1987. The role of spouse reinforcement, perceived pain, and activity levels of chronic pain patients. J. Psychosom. Res. 31 (2), 251–259.

Freynhagen, R., Baron, R., Gockel, U., Tölle, R., 2006. painDETECT: a new screening questionnaire to identify neuropathic components in patients with back pain. Curr Med Res Opin 22 (10), 1911–1920.

Galer, B.S., Jensen, M.P., 1999. Neglect-like symptoms in complex regional pain syndrome: results of a self-administered survey. J. Pain Symptom Manage. 18 (3), 213–217.

Gatchel, R.J., Peng, Y.B., Peters, M.L., Fuchs, P.N., Turk, D.C., 2007. The biopsychosocial approach to chronic pain: scientific advances and future directions. Psychol. Bull. 133 (4), 581.

George, S.Z., Fritz, J.M., McNeil, D.W., 2006. Fear-avoidance beliefs as measured by the fear-avoidance beliefs questionnaire: change in fear-avoidance beliefs questionnaire is predictive of change in self-report of disability and pain intensity for patients with acute low back pain. Clin. J. Pain 22 (2), 197–203.

Gifford, L., 1998. Pain, the tissues and the nervous system: a conceptual model. Physiotherapy 84 (1), 27–36.

Haanpää, M., Attal, N., Backonja, M., Baron, R., Bennett, M., Bouhassira, D., et al., 2011. NeuPSIG guidelines on neuropathic pain assessment. Pain 152 (1), 14–27.

Hansson, P., 2014. Translational aspects of central sensitization induced by primary afferent activity: what it is and what it is not. Pain 155 (10), 1932–1934.

Henschke, N., Maher, C.G., Refshauge, K.M., Herbert, R.D., Cumming, R.G., Bleasel, J., et al., 2008. Prognosis in patients with recent onset low back pain in Australian primary care: inception cohort study. BMJ 337 (a171).

Henschke, N., Maher, C.G., Refshauge, K.M., Herbert, R.D., Cumming, R.G., Bleasel, J., et al., 2009. Prevalence of and screening for serious spinal pathology in patients presenting to primary care settings with acute low back pain. Arthritis Rheum. 60 (10), 3072–3080.

Hensley, C.P., Courtney, C.A., 2014. Management of a patient with chronic low back pain and multiple health conditions using a pain mechanisms–based classification approach. J Orthop Sports Phys Ther 44 (6), 403–C402.

IASP Taxonomy 2015, IASP Publications, Washington, D.C., viewed December 2015, <http://www.iasp-pain.org/Taxonomy>.

Iles, R.A., Davidson, M., Taylor, N.F., 2008. Psychosocial predictors of failure to return to work in non-chronic non-specific low back pain: a systematic review. Occup. Environ. Med. 65 (8), 507–517.

Itz, C.J., Geurts, J.W., Kleef, M., Nelemans, P., 2013. Clinical course of non-specific low back pain: a systematic review of prospective cohort studies set in primary care. Eur. J. Pain 17 (1), 5–15.

Jensen, T.S., Baron, R., Haanpää, M., Kalso, E., Loeser, J.D., Rice, A.S.C., et al., 2011. A new definition of neuropathic pain. Pain 152 (10), 2204–2205.

Jensen, M.P., Ehde, D.M., Hoffman, A.J., Patterson, D.R., Czerniecki, J.M., Robinson, L.R., 2002. Cognitions, coping and social environment predict adjustment to phantom limb pain. Pain 95 (1), 133–142.

Jones, M., Edwards, I., Gifford, L., 2002. Conceptual models for implementing biopsychosocial theory in clinical practice. Man. Ther. 7 (1), 2–9.

Jones, L.E., Hush, J.M., 2011. Pain education for physiotherapists: is it time for curriculum reform? Journal of Physiotherapy 57, 207–208.

Kendall, N.A., Linton, S.J., Main, C.J. 1997. Guide to assessing psychosocial yellow flags in acute low back pain: Risk factors for long-term disability and work loss, Accident Rehabilitation and Compensation Insurance Corporation of New Zealand and the National Health Committee, Wellington, New Zealand.

Koes, B.W., van Tulder, M., Lin, C.W.C., Macedo, L.G., McAuley, J., Maher, C., 2010. An updated overview of clinical guidelines for the management of non-specific low back pain in primary care. Eur. Spine J. 19 (12), 2075–2094.

Kosek, E., Cohen, M., Baron, R., Gebhart, G.F., Mico, J.A., Rice, A.S.C., et al., 2016. Do we need a third mechanistic descriptor for chronic pain states? Pain 157 (7), 1382–1386.

Leeuw, M., Linton, S.J., Goossens, M.E.J.B., Vlaeyen, J.W., Boersma, K., Crombez, G., 2007. The fear-avoidance model of musculoskeletal pain: current state of scientific evidence. J. Behav. Med. 30, 77–94.

Linton, S.J., Halldén, K., 1998. Can we screen for problematic back pain? A screening questionnaire for predicting outcome in acute and subacute back pain. Clin. J. Pain 14 (3), 209–215.

Loeser, J.D., Treede, R.D., 2008. The Kyoto protocol of IASP Basic Pain Terminology. Pain 137 (3), 473–477.

Lovibond, S.H., Lovibond, P.F. 1995. Manual for the depression anxiety stress scales, Psychology Foundation, Sydney.

Main, C.J., 2013. The importance of psychosocial influences on chronic pain. Pain Management 3 (6), 455–466.

Main, C.J., Spanswick, C.C., 2000. Pain management: an interdisciplinary approach. Anaesth. Intensive Care 29 (4), 441.

Martini, F., 2006. Fundamentals of Anatomy & Physiology, seventh ed. Pearson Education Limited, San Francisco.

Mayer, T.G., Neblett, R., Cohen, H., Howard, K.J., Choi, Y.H., Williams, M.J., et al., 2012. The development and psychometric validation of the central sensitization inventory. Pain Pract. 12 (4), 276–285.

McGlone, F., Wessberg, J., Olausson, H., 2014. Discriminative and affective touch: sensing and feeling. Neuron 82 (4), 737–755.

Melzack, R., 1999. From the gate to the neuromatrix. Pain 82, S121–S126.

Melzack, R., Wall, P.D., 1996. The Challenge of Pain, second ed. Penguin Books, London, England.

Merskey, H., Bogduk, N., 1994. Classification of Chronic Pain, IASP Task Force on Taxonomy, second ed. IASP Press, Seattle.

Moayedi, M., Davis, K.D., 2013. Theories of pain: from specificity to gate control. J. Neurophysiol. 109, 5–12.

Moseley, G.L., 2003. Unraveling the barriers to reconceptualization of the problem in chronic pain: the actual and perceived ability of patients and health professionals to understand the neurophysiology. J. Pain 4 (4), 184–189.

Moseley, G.L., Arntz, A., 2007. The context of a noxious stimulus affects the pain it evokes. Pain 152, S2–S15.

Moseley, G.L., Butler, D.S., 2015. Fifteen years of explaining pain: the past, present and future. J. Pain 16 (9), 807–813.

Moseley, G.L., Butler, D.S., 2017. Explain Pain Supercharged. Noigroup Publications, Adelaide, South Australia.

Moseley, G.L., Gallace, A., Spence, C., 2012. Bodily illusions in health and disease: physiological and clinical perspectives and the concept of a cortical 'body matrix. Neurosci. Biobehav. Rev. 36 (1), 34–46.

Moseley, G.L., McCormick, K., Hudson, M., Zalucki, N., 2006. Disrupted cortical proprioceptive representation evokes symptoms of peculiarity, foreignness and swelling, but not pain. Rheumatology 45 (2), 196–200.

Neblett, R., Cohen, H., Choi, Y., Hartzell, M.M., Williams, M., Mayer, T.G., et al., 2013. The Central Sensitization Inventory (CSI): establishing clinically significant values for identifying central sensitivity syndromes in an outpatient chronic pain sample. J. Pain 14 (5), 438–445.

Nee, R.J., Butler, D.S., 2006. Management of peripheral neuropathic pain: integrating neurobiology, neurodynamics, and clinical evidence. Physical Therapy in Sport 7 (1), 36–49.

Nicholas, M.K., 2007. The pain self-efficacy questionnaire: taking pain into account. Eur. J. Pain 11 (2), 153–163.

Nicholas, M.K., Linton, S.J., Watson, P.J., Main, C.J., 2011. Early identification and management of psychological risk factors ("yellow flags") in patients with low back pain: a reappraisal. Phys. Ther. 91 (5), 737–753.

Nijs, J., Torres-Cueco, R., Van Wilgen, C.P., Girbes, E.L., Struyf, F., Roussel, N., et al., 2014. Applying modern pain neuroscience in clinical practice: criteria for the classification of central sensitization pain. Pain Physician 17 (5), 447–457.

Parkitny, L., McAuley, J.H., Walton, D., Costa, L.O.P., Refshauge, K.M., Wand, B.M., et al., 2012. Rasch analysis supports the use of the depression, anxiety, and stress scales to measure mood in groups but not in individuals with chronic low back pain. J. Clin. Epidemiol. 65 (2), 189–198.

Pincus, T., Burton, A.K., Vogel, S., Field, A.P., 2002. A systematic review of psychological factors as predictors of chronicity/disability in prospective cohorts of low back pain. Spine 27 (5), E109–E120.

Rabey, M., Beales, D., Slater, H., O'Sullivan, P., 2015. Multidimensional pain profiles in four cases of chronic non-specific axial low back pain: An examination of the limitations of contemporary classification systems. Man. Ther. 20 (1), 138–147.

Ramachandran, V.S., Blakeslee, S. 1999. Phantoms in the brain: Human nature and the architecture of the mind. Fourth Estate, London.

Ringkamp, M., Raja, S.N., Campbell, J.N., Meyer, R.A., 2013. Peripheral mechanisms of cutaneous nociception. In: McMahon, S.B., et al. (Eds.), Wall and Melzack's Textbook of Pain, sixth ed. Elsevier, Philadelphia.

Romano, J.M., Turner, J.A., Jensen, M.P., Friedman, L.S., Bulcroft, R.A., Hops, H., et al., 1995. Chronic pain patient-spouse behavioral interactions predict patient disability. Pain 63 (3), 353–360.

Schmid, A.B., Nee, R.J., Coppieters, M.W., 2013. Reappraising entrapment neuropathies: mechanisms, diagnosis and management. Man. Ther. 18 (6), 449–457.

Smart, K.M., Blake, C., Staines, A., Doody, C., 2010. Clinical indicators of 'nociceptive', 'peripheral neuropathic' and 'central' mechanisms of musculoskeletal pain. A Delphi survey of expert clinicians. Man. Ther. 15 (1), 80–87.

Smart, K.M., Blake, C., Staines, A., Doody, C., 2011. The discriminative validity of "nociceptive," "peripheral neuropathic," and "central sensitization" as mechanisms-based classifications of musculoskeletal pain. Clin. J. Pain 27 (8), 655–663.

Smith, W.B., Gracely, R.H., Safer, M.A., 1998. The meaning of pain: cancer patients' rating and recall of pain intensity and affect. Pain 78 (2), 123–129.

Snell, R.S., 2010. Clinical Neuroanatomy, seventh ed. Lippincott Williams & Wilkins, Philadelphia.

Stanton, T.R., Lin, C.W.C., Smeets, R.J.E.M., Taylor, D., Law, R., Moseley, G.L., 2012. Spatially defined disruption of motor imagery performance in people with osteoarthritis. Rheumatology 51 (8), 1455–1464.

Sullivan, M.J.L., Bishop, S.R., Pivik, J., 1995. The pain catastrophizing scale: Development and validation. Psychol. Assess. 7 (4), 524–532.

Sullivan, M.J.L., Thorn, B., Haythornthwaite, J.A., Keefe, F., Martin, M., Bradley, L.A., et al., 2001. Theoretical perspectives on the relation between catastrophizing and pain. Clin. J. Pain 17, 52–64.

Synnott, A., O'Keeffe, M., Bunzli, S., Dankaerts, W., O'Sullivan, P., O'Sullivan, K., 2015. Physiotherapists may stigmatise or feel unprepared to treat people with low back pain and psychosocial factors that influence recovery: a systematic review. J Physiother 61 (2), 68–76.

Treede, R.D., Jensen, T.S., Campbell, J.N., Cruccu, G., Dostrovsky, J.O., Griffin, J.W., et al., 2008. Neuropathic pain redefinition and a grading system for clinical and research purposes. Neurology 70 (18), 1630–1635.

Treede, R.D., Rief, W., Barke, A., Aziz, Q., Bennett, M.I., Benoliel, R., et al., 2015. A classification of chronic pain for ICD-11. Pain 156 (6), 1003–1007.

van Hecke, O., Torrance, N., Smith, B.H., 2013. Chronic pain epidemiology and its clinical relevance. Br. J. Anaesth. 111 (1), 13–18.

Vardeh, D., Mannion, R.J., Woolf, C.J., 2016. Toward a mechanism-based approach to pain diagnosis. J. Pain 17 (9), T50–T69.

Vos, T., Flaxman, A.D., Naghavi, M., Lozano, R., Michaud, C., Ezzati, M., et al., 2012. Years lived with disability (YLDs) for 1160 sequelae of 289 diseases and injuries 1990–2010: a systematic analysis for the Global Burden of Disease Study 2010. The Lancet 380 (9859), 2163–2196.

Waddell, G., 1998. The Back Pain Revolution. Churchill Livingstone, Edinburgh.

Walton, D.M., Wideman, T.H., Sullivan, M.J.L., 2013. A Rasch analysis of the Pain Catastrophizing Scale supports its use as an interval-level measure. Clin. J. Pain 29 (6), 499–506.

Wand, B.M., Catley, M.J., Rabey, M.I., O'Sullivan, P.B., O'Connell, N.E., Smith, A.J., 2016. Disrupted Self-Perception in People With Chronic Low Back Pain. Further Evaluation of the Fremantle Back Awareness Questionnaire. J. Pain 17 (9), 1001–1012.

Watson, P., 2013. Psychosocial predictors of outcome from low back pain. In: Gifford, L. (Ed.), Topical Issues in Pain 2: Biopsychosocial assessment and management; Relationships and pain. CNS Press, Kestrel, UK, pp. 85–111.

Westman, A., Linton, S.J., Öhrvik, J., Wahlén, P., Leppert, J., 2008. Do psychosocial factors predict disability and health at a 3-year follow-up for patients with non-acute musculoskeletal pain? A validation of the Örebro Musculoskeletal Pain Screening Questionnaire. Eur. J. Pain 12 (5), 641–649.

Williams, C.M., Henschke, N., Maher, C.G., van Tulder, M.W., Koes, B.W., Macaskill, P., et al., 2013. Red flags to screen for vertebral fracture in patients presenting with low-back pain. Cochrane Database Syst. Rev. (1), CD008643.

Woolf, C.J., 2010. What is this thing called pain? J. Clin. Invest. 120 (11), 3742.

Woolf, C.J., 2011. Central sensitization: implications for the diagnosis and treatment of pain. Pain 152, S2–S15.

Woolf, C.J., 2014. What to call the amplification of nociceptive signals in the central nervous system that contribute to widespread pain? Pain 155 (10), 1911–1912.

Woolf, C.J., Mannion, R.J., 1999. Neuropathic pain: aetiology, symptoms, mechanisms, and management. The Lancet 353 (9168), 1959–1964.

Influence of Stress, Coping and Social Factors on Pain and Disability in Musculoskeletal Practice

Amy S. Hammerich • Susan A. Scherer • Mark A. Jones

Like individuals with any other health condition, individuals with either acute or chronic and recurring musculoskeletal conditions may need to adjust their behaviours and lifestyles while trying to maintain basic physical, social, vocational and recreational activities. To manage their musculoskeletal condition, individuals must try to understand the nature of their problem, create or learn self-care strategies for dealing with pain, manage and attempt to overcome functional problems and identify and utilize available support and resources wisely. Chapter 4 reviews some of the psychological factors needed by individuals to influence positive treatment outcomes (e.g. self-efficacy) and reduce fears that may hinder outcomes. Individual coping characteristics are evidenced by the behaviours patients demonstrate in order to manage their condition. To date, the general musculoskeletal literature lacks a strong theoretical foundation for understanding health behaviours, particularly in comparison with research in other areas of chronic disease (Painter et al., 2008; Allegrante and Marks, 2003; Taal et al., 1993; Andersen, 2002; Black and White, 2005; Blank and Bellizzi, 2008).

This chapter explores behavioural factors associated with the two main sources of stress in individuals with musculoskeletal disorders: pain and disability. The theoretical framework of this chapter is guided by the stress and coping model (Lazarus and Folkman, 1984b) and focuses on both individual-level and social-level factors that influence the experience of disability in patients with musculoskeletal conditions.

Theoretical Framework

A theoretical framework can help identify beliefs and behaviours used by patients who experience stressors and need to engage in coping in order to adjust to a musculoskeletal disorder. Two primary stressors have often been identified in the previous musculoskeletal literature: pain and disability. Differing experiences with a musculoskeletal disorder can result in different appraisals of the stressors of pain and disability by patients. Often individuals with similar musculoskeletal disorders have different outcomes related to the experience of pain and disability even with similar treatment approaches. We have many examples in practice of patients who may have similar musculoskeletal conditions and even may have similar testing results or scores on outcome measures, such as the Oswestry Disability Index or the Lower Extremity Functional Scale, yet one will do well with coping with the condition, and the other will be significantly limited in many life activities and participation. Prognostic factors may provide a predictive indication of which patients we may observe a positive outcome (regardless of treatment), whereas treatment effect moderators provide an indication of which patients will beneficially respond to specific treatments. Understanding psychosocial factors and coping behaviours may add additional insights into patient responses to treatments and potential for improved outcomes. In order to understand the overall experiences of pain and disability, we examine two frameworks important to musculoskeletal clinicians' assessment, reasoning and management: the stress-diathesis model (Shanahan and Macmillan, 2008; Elder, 1994) and the International Classification of Functioning, Disability and Health (ICF) model (World Health Organization [WHO], 2001) framework of health and disablement (Shanahan and Macmillan, 2008; Rowland, 1989). Both models include identifying contributing factors and modifying resources that are available to patients that also influence outcomes.

The stress and coping model (Lazarus and Folkman, 1984b) is used to identify what coping behaviours preserve well-being in patients with musculoskeletal disorders while facing stressful experiences with acute or chronic conditions. Integrating the new lens of health as described by the ICF framework introduced in Chapter 1 requires consideration of the larger personal and environmental influences around the individual. Finally, this chapter explores self-rated health and self-efficacy from the perspective of social cognitive theory (Bandura, 1977b; Bandura, 1977a) and social support as a social resource for health in the stress and coping model (Lazarus and Folkman, 1984a, 1984b). Understanding both individual-level and social-level concepts will serve to broaden the understanding of health behaviours that influence patients with musculoskeletal disorders and ultimately influence treatment and related outcomes in caring for individuals with musculoskeletal disorders.

Behavioural Factors in Musculoskeletal Disorders

Individuals with musculoskeletal disorders often report decreases in physical health (Weinstein et al., 2008; Fritz et al., 1998; Whitman et al., 2003). Decreased physical health, either real or perceived, can impact an individual in many ways. Overall, it is known that those who have decreased physical health reduce or eliminate participation in daily living, physical, social and recreational activities. A lack of activity has been shown to lead to other stressors such as obesity and general physical deterioration that may eventually result in further disability with the onset of cardiovascular and other serious health problems (Pinsky et al., 1990). Activity restrictions may also lead to low self-confidence, fear-avoidance behaviours, depression and other psychological problems that further restrict the person with a musculoskeletal disorder from participation in activities of daily living (ADLs), physical activities, recreational activities, social activities and community functions (Shakil et al., 1999; Kirkaldy-Willis and Bernard, 1999; Hirsch and Liebert, 1998). Chapter 4 further explains how psychological factors such as maladaptive cognitions (e.g. pain and 'illness' representations or beliefs, catastrophizing), distress, fear based beliefs and related avoidance behaviours are negative influences on the stressors of pain and disability and result in declines in treatment success in musculoskeletal disorders in general (Waddell et al., 1993; Flynn et al., 2002; Buer and Linton, 2002). Psychological distress, from frustrations to anxiety and depression, and fear-avoidance behaviours correlate with reduced participation in functional daily tasks, indicating a higher risk for disability. Although diagnosis of depression is beyond the scope of practice of musculoskeletal clinicians, some studies have shown that depressive symptoms and high fear-avoidance scores can improve during some areas of musculoskeletal management and result in positive changes in patient outcomes of pain and disability (Fritz and George, 2002; Brox et al., 2003; Whitman et al., 2006). In addition, research has demonstrated that using an enhanced or multimodal team approach to treatment results in improved patient outcomes for musculoskeletal conditions such as low back pain (Sunderland et al., 1992; Whitman et al., 2006). Even though some physical, cognitive and psychological factors contributing to higher pre-treatment pain and disability and post-treatment outcomes have been identified in many musculoskeletal conditions, identifying all the behavioural factors that influence individuals with musculoskeletal disorders continues to be incomplete.

Similar to other health conditions, the daily lives of individuals with musculoskeletal disorders likely involve unanticipated challenges. Patients with musculoskeletal disorders must learn to navigate life with the stress of either acute or chronic pain, cope with reduced functioning, experience limitations to their physical and social abilities, manage through decreased activities, and face fears about recurrence or worsening of their condition. Previous research on arthritis and other health conditions has identified that persistent psychosocial needs can decrease the effectiveness of medical treatment, general health status and quality of life while increasing healthcare costs (Sullivan et al., 2005; Brooks, 2002; Steiner et al., 2002). Although unidentified in many areas of musculoskeletal literature, unaddressed personal and social needs may contribute to reduced participation with treatment and follow-up recommendations, diminished self-care and reduced overall health management (Marinelli and Orto, 1999). Therefore, we recommend that clinicians have a good understanding of the patient's experience of stressors, understand coping behaviours and identify patient resources that may contribute to an improved outcome.

Stress and Coping Model

Pain and disability have been identified as primary stressors in previous musculoskeletal literature. Differing experiences with musculoskeletal disorders result in different appraisals of the stressors of pain and disability. Moreover, individuals with musculoskeletal disorders can have different outcomes related to the experience of pain and disability even with the same treatment approaches. To better understand these main stressors, this chapter uses the underlying theoretical concepts in the stress and coping model (Lazarus and Folkman, 1984b) to define both stress and coping as well as identify the relationship of these concepts in musculoskeletal disorders. Within the stress and coping model (Lazarus and Folkman, 1984b), stress involves the relationship between an individual and his or her environment. This relationship or transaction between individuals and their environment indicates that stress is more than an internal stimulation or specific pattern of physiological, behavioural or subjective reactions (see Fig. 3.1). Two key mediators within the person–environment transaction are cognitive appraisal and coping effort. Cognitive appraisals and coping efforts are influenced by moderators such as personal and situational factors that result in individual adaptations that impact health on many levels. An understanding of stress and coping constructs underpins musculoskeletal clinicians' assessment of individual patients' stressors and coping behaviours that then informs how these may be addressed within clinical management.

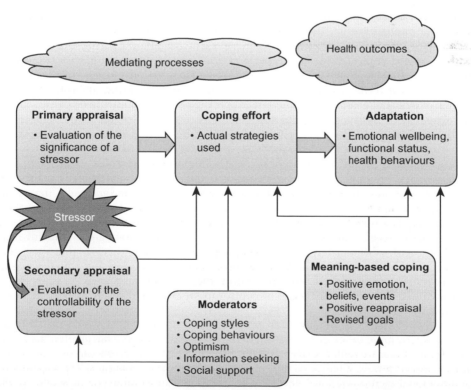

Fig. 3.1   Stress and coping model and stressful health conditions *(Adapted with permission from Glanz et al. [2008].)*

Cognitive Appraisal

The cognitive appraisal or evaluation by the individual is paramount to determining if the stress is threatening to his or her well-being or surpassing his or her resources. Upon appraising a stressor, the theory asserts that people engage in coping, defined as fluctuating behavioural exertions, in an effort to manage that stressor. The cognitive appraisal process helps an individual determine both the controllability and availability of coping resources identified as necessary to manage the stressor(s) (Lazarus and Folkman, 1984b).

Cognitive appraisal is a necessary component of dealing with a stressor. It accounts for the different ways in which individuals react to similar events. Health conditions such as those resulting in pain provocation and disability, as in many musculoskeletal disorders, can cause stress in nearly every person, yet people vary in their reactions and interpretations of the same event and condition (Lazarus and Folkman, 1984b). This variability in cognitive appraisals can change a person's level of vulnerability during a stressful health condition. Vulnerability is closely related to appraisal because vulnerability increases as a person appraises that he or she has reduced coping resources available. Vulnerability reflects the inability of individuals to withstand adverse impacts from a single stressor or multiple stressors to which they are exposed. It can be associated with a pattern of thought that is believed to predispose the individual to psychological problems and feelings of hopelessness. In addition, the variability of individual appraisals, as well as the individual's responses, helps to explain why some individuals experience similar health conditions but have differing quality, intensity and duration of physical, social and emotional outcomes.

Personal and Situational Factors

Two types of factors influence the cognitive appraisal process: personal factors and situational factors (Lazarus and Folkman, 1984a, 1984b). Personal factors consist of the personal values that motivate individuals to make certain decisions and beliefs that give the individual a personal sense of control. Therefore, at the individual level, commitments and beliefs are part of an individual's process of appraisal. Commitments are expressions of what is important to a person and can be related to vulnerability. For example, where a participation restriction may be an inconvenience to one patient that does not unduly add to the patient's stress, for another patient, the value and even self-identity he or she attaches to reduced or lost participation (e.g. work, sport) can represent a significant personal loss associated with increased vulnerability. The deeper a person's commitment, the greater potential for threat, but also the greater the push toward ameliorative action and hope. Beliefs are also important in determining how a person evaluates a stressful event or health condition. Beliefs of personal control over situations can relate to how an individual believes internal self-responses to situations (e.g. emotions) can be controlled. General control beliefs relate to the extent that the person believes the health-related outcomes can be controlled. For example, two patients may experience the same musculoskeletal injury, such as an anterior cruciate ligament rupture of the knee. One patient has had previous experience with an acute injury and rehabilitation and is confident he can emotionally manage this situation. The other patient is going through a difficult divorce and just went through the death of her mother. Her internal self-responses are exaggerated compared with normal and are highly emotional, so she does not believe that she can handle this additional life event. These beliefs will greatly impact each patient's evaluation of the stressful health condition and will ultimately affect the coping responses and strategies that they use to manage their knee rehabilitation. When working with the second patient who has negative health beliefs and a reduced sense of control, the clinician must work to address these beliefs and help improve her sense of control in order to help augment positive coping behaviours.

Another influence to the appraisal process is situational factors, which play a critical role in determining the external controllability of the stressor and what ameliorative action can be taken (Lazarus and Folkman, 1984a, 1984b). Situational factors can include predictability and uncertainty, temporal and life course factors and ambiguity. The modifiability of situational factors will vary, and as such, the potential to influence how and to what extent the stressor can be managed also varies. Although factors such as socio-economic status (SES) – recognized as a strong predictor of poor outcomes across a variety of health conditions – are less modifiable (although resources for financial assistance can still be explored), adverse workplace relations may be a situational factor amenable to change. For example, adverse workplace relations are a common situational factor and can be a source of stress for patients. Musculoskeletal clinicians can contribute to addressing workplace factors such as alternative work tasks and performance modifications that may improve workplace relations as a management strategy. In addition, patients with musculoskeletal disorders often vary in their stages of life and have aging-related concerns related to their potential for healing, recovery and future work or recreation opportunities. These age-related concerns are another example of a situational factor that could be a component of what a patient experiences, and they should be addressed by a clinician.

Maximum uncertainty is often extremely stressful for an individual experiencing a health condition such as an acute musculoskeletal injury or a chronic musculoskeletal disorder. Uncertainty is particularly common with persistent pain conditions that cannot be explained within the traditional biomedical framework or when patients encounter conflicting explanations and advice from different health professionals. The uncertainty can have immobilizing effects on anticipatory and actual coping processes and can cause mental confusion in the individual. Helping patients recognize the many personal and situational factors that may contribute to the stressors or improve coping behaviours can assist in reducing some of the uncertainty that comes with musculoskeletal disorders. Overall, it is important to assess both situational factors and personal factors in order for clinicians and patients to understand and recognize factors that ultimately influence the level of stress related to pain and disability in musculoskeletal disorders.

Different Appraisals

Although differences between individuals under similar circumstances are inevitable due to various personal and situational factors, the stress and coping model emphasizes that all individuals evaluating a stressor undergo a cognitive appraisal process involving primary appraisal, secondary appraisal and/or reappraisal (Lazarus and Folkman, 1984a). Primary appraisals involve assessment of the magnitude and significance of a stressor or traumatic event. During primary appraisal, the individual will assess the actual harm, loss, threat or challenge that must be encountered with a stressful health condition. When an individual first experiences a musculoskeletal condition or a reoccurrence of a musculoskeletal condition, primary appraisal takes place. Individuals with musculoskeletal conditions are often in the process of primary appraisal when they seek out medical care and treatment.

Secondary appraisal refers to an individual's assessment of the degree to which the stressor or traumatic event can be controlled and the available coping resources (Lazarus and Folkman, 1984a, 1984b). Secondary appraisals are a judgment about what might and can be done in the situation (Lazarus and Folkman, 1984b). Secondary appraisals include an evaluation about whether a coping option (e.g. rest, medication, therapy) will accomplish what it is supposed to do as well as the consequences in the context of other internal and/ or external demands and constraints. Appraisals of controllability of a health condition can be stress-reducing if one believes that the outcome is controllable or that one has the coping resources to manage the outcomes. However, appraisals of controllability can also heighten threat and give rise to negative emotions and beliefs about coping if perceptions of control and resources are diminished. For example, individuals with low back pain (LBP) will use secondary appraisals when their chronic LBP has reoccurred and their activities have been limited. This in turn motivates some to seek treatment to control their pain and disability as part of the coping process if they have the necessary access and resources. For others, their LBP reoccurrence may heighten negative emotions and beliefs about the seriousness of their condition and its underlying cause and diminish their ability to manage the condition.

Reappraisal is the final feature of the appraisal process and entails an altered or revised version of a previous appraisal. Reappraisals can occur multiple times for reasons such as changes in the environment or the health condition (Lazarus and Folkman, 1984a, 1984b). Reappraisals can also occur when an individual has gone through the cognitive coping process and has altered his or her assessment of the available coping resources. Because the complete process of appraisal is dynamic, a patient with a chronic disease or persistent pain state, such as with many musculoskeletal conditions, is likely to appraise and reappraise the stressors of pain and disability and respective coping resources before, during and after treatment multiple times and with each successive episode. Ultimately, reappraisal of previous unhelpful appraisals is the aim of educative, behavioural and activity/exercise management for patients with persistent musculoskeletal pain and disability associated with a nociplastic dominant pain type and unhelpful cognitions and coping behaviours.

Coping

Coping is intimately related to the concept of cognitive appraisal and the person–environment relationship. Coping involves the cognitive and behavioural efforts to address external and internal demands on the person experiencing a stressful encounter. Coping can either be focused on changing the person–environment problem behind the stress or be directed toward changing the appraisal of the situation. Moreover, coping can be focused toward trying to reduce a negative emotional state of the situation. Early identification of patients who have reduced coping behaviours could help target certain factors and resources needed to improve coping behaviours. For example, in patients with a musculoskeletal disorder, early identification of individuals who have negative appraisals and reduced coping resources can help direct clinicians to increase cognitive-behavioural management to improve patient beliefs, motivation and participation in treatment. Ultimately, understanding coping behaviours in relationship to health outcomes can be important in the big picture to identify and prioritize healthcare resources for individuals with a musculoskeletal condition.

Key Points

> Most musculoskeletal health conditions require an individual to make changes, either short or long term, to their activities and expectations. Patients will evaluate the situation (called appraisal) and interpret the magnitude of the effect this condition will have on their lives. Patients will respond to the situation differently, depending on how manageable they perceive the situation to be. Patients with stronger coping skills tend to feel more positive about being able to manage their health condition. A clinician who can identify which patients feel negative about their condition can work to provide extra support and/or refer patients to appropriate caregivers to assist in improving coping skills and behaviours to manage their condition.

Managing Stressors: Coping With the Stressor of Pain

The experience of pain is often described as stressful by an individual and identified as a source of stress for individuals (Jensen and Karoly, 1991). In recognizing the role of pain as a stressor, it is necessary to explore and expand upon an understanding of the factors contributing to an individual's experience of pain. The traditional biomedical model of pain dates back hundreds of years to an era when pain was understood to be a primarily sensory experience resulting from the stimulation of noxious sensory receptors, usually from physical damage or injury (Descartes, 1985). This theory of pain describes primarily nociceptive pain, defined as pain elicited when sensory receptors specialized to sense mechanical, thermal or chemical pain react when stimulated past a sensory threshold. This simplistic view suggests that pain only comes from specific physical pathology and is often called the biomedical model of pain. It does not take into account how pain is experienced by the individual, involving additional psychological, social and behavioural mechanisms of injury and illness. Chapter 2 goes into further depth about our current understanding of pain and its effects on the individual. In this chapter, a broader understanding of pain and its influences beyond the individual level that ultimately impact the individual's pain experience during a health condition will be explored. There are many potential avenues that can heighten or alter the pain experience. In the musculoskeletal condition of LBP, for example, patients with LBP often experience pain that is unrelated or only partly related to their radiographic severity or lumbar pathology (Boden, 1996; Pahl et al., 2006), illustrating that their pain experience is greater than the pure pathophysiological processes involved. Due to the narrow scope of the biomedical model of pain, it is often criticized for being reductionist and exclusionary, and broader concepts need to be explored (Turk and Flor, 1999).

Biopsychosocial Models of Pain

To encompass a broader view of pain, Turk and Flor (1999) described a biopsychosocial approach to pain which addresses many of the shortfalls found in traditional biomedical models. In this approach, it is recognized that the experience of pain is the reciprocal and dynamic interaction of biological, psychological and social factors. It is based on the concept that the experience of pain arises from illness behaviour, although it is typically initiated by and/or has contributions from nociceptive and/or neuropathic pain. Illness behaviour is a term used to describe the ways in which given symptoms may be differently perceived, evaluated and acted or not acted upon by different individuals (Mechanic, 1962). Illness behaviour is believed to be a dynamic process that allows for the role of the biological, psychological and social factors to change in health conditions and as the condition evolves (Engel, 1980).

In the 1980s, Waddell (1987) applied the construct of illness behaviour to LBP (see Fig. 3.2). Their view was that persons with chronic LBP experienced illness behaviours and not just nociceptive pain. This view represented a broader biopsychosocial model of pain stemming from physiological impairment but with broader cognition, affective and social factors resulting in the experience of pain perceived and reported by individuals with chronic LBP (Waddell, 1987). Since this work, the construct of illness behaviour has been recognized as an important construct in many health conditions but continues to be absent in evaluative and management strategies for most musculoskeletal conditions other than LBP.

Stress-Diathesis Model of Pain

Asmundson and Wright (2004) expanded on the biopsychosocial framework by describing pain behaviours and the additional factors that contribute to disability in patients with chronic pain. In their stress-diathesis model (see Fig. 3.3), the impact (stress) of a painful

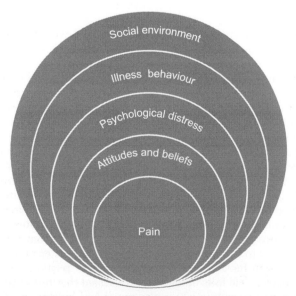

Fig. 3.2 Biopsychosocial model of pain. Cross-sectional representation of the Glasgow model representing the role of fear-avoidance beliefs in chronic low back pain and disability *(Adapted with permission from Waddell et al. [1987, 1993].)*

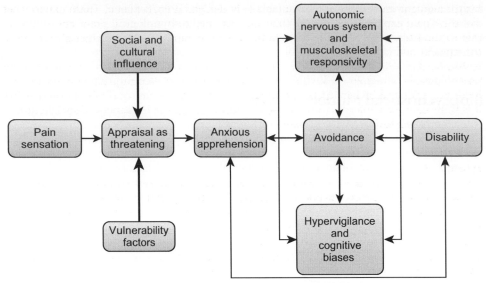

Fig. 3.3 The stress-diathesis model of pain and disability. An integrated stress-diathesis model of chronic pain *(Adapted with permission from Asmundson and Wright [2004].)*

condition is described in terms of the effects on the person and his or her social activities, and the model considers if the individual is vulnerable (diathesis) to additional comorbidities. A key part of the stress-diathesis model is the issue of pain appraisal. Pain appraisal refers to the meaning ascribed to pain by an individual (Sharp and Harvey, 2001). As already discussed with the stress and coping model (Lazarus and Folkman, 1984c), a distinction can be made between primary appraisal of pain in terms of it being threatening, benign or irrelevant and secondary appraisal, which evaluates the controllability of pain and one's coping resources. Primary appraisal of a threat or harm/loss is an indication of a stressor. Therefore, pain described as threatening by the stress-diathesis model is inherently stressful. The degree of the stress depends on the other factors of vulnerability, social and cultural influence and assessment of coping resources.

Let's use an example of a middle-aged male patient with sciatica. He rates his pain as 8/10 when sitting and 4/10 when walking or standing. He has tried multiple interventions, including physical therapy and injections, following surgery several years ago, with modest results. Although this is distressing to him, he has found ways to manage his pain and continue in activities that are important to him, including his spending time with his grandchildren and working. His work environment is flexible in that he is able to choose when he needs to move around and can control his schedule and activities. He has cut back on his activities with the grandchildren but enjoys his family time. By all accounts, this gentleman has low fear and avoidance behaviours and a good narrative in the aspects of the biopsychosocial model described by Waddell.

In the stress-diathesis framework, this gentleman does not perceive (appraise) his pain as a significant distress and has a social-cultural context which accommodates his level of pain, thus contributing to a low level of disability. But the stress-diathesis framework can help explain situations that are more complex. Let's take another patient, also male and middle-aged, with low back pain of the same intensity. This patient, too, has tried many interventions, including physiotherapy, injections and surgery. This patient works in an office which requires him to spend most of the time at the computer or phone, with few breaks. His home/active life is focused on his wife's recovery from breast cancer surgery and his son, who wants to hike and bike in the mountainous environment. He perceives his pain to interfere with his ability to focus at work, his relationship with his wife and the activities with his son. He feels limited and frustrated that he cannot be the person he wants to be. These are examples of how the social and cultural contexts influence the patient's perception of pain and contribute to disability. In addition, this patient has experienced feelings of helplessness before – after his first back surgery 15 years ago, after his discharge from the military and after his father had a heart attack. These experiences make him vulnerable to perceiving his LBP as very disabling and likely contribute to maintaining his persistent pain condition. This vulnerability is the 'diathesis' portion of the model.

In the stress-diathesis model, we can expect that patients with high vulnerability, psychological distress, low self-efficacy and/or complex social/cultural situations will have increased pain and higher levels of disability. In order to minimize disability (and pain), it is important for clinicians to understand and recognize the influences of social/cultural experiences and vulnerability as they impact outcomes.

Key Points

Pain is one of the key stressors of patients with both acute and chronic musculoskeletal conditions. In patients who have other psychological stressors, such as depression, or with complex social and cultural situations, a pain condition can lead to a significant level of disability. In order to improve patients' outcomes and quality of life, clinicians need to understand the patient's story, including psychological, social and cultural factors, along with their interpretation and appraisal of the situation.

Managing Stressors: Coping With the Stressor of Disability

As we see in the stress-diathesis model, pain is only one factor in a more complex set of factors contributing to disability. Coping behaviours can therefore ultimately differ when addressing the stressor of pain as compared with the stressor of disability. Understanding disability has been an evolving process in health and the healthcare literature. It is the role of musculoskeletal clinicians to reduce or limit the level of disability and improve function in patients, which requires the complex understanding we have today about disability and the factors that contribute to function.

Disability and Functioning

Over the years, multiple frameworks have been developed to explain a broader concept of disability. One of the earliest frameworks for disability, proposed in the 1960s by sociologist Saad Nagi, is the 'disablement model' that illustrates a disease pathway that is still used by healthcare professionals. The disablement model describes a pathway comprised of four inter-related but separate constructs that contribute in a linear fashion to disability (Nagi, 1965). The model starts with pathology as the underlying disease condition that eventually leads to impairments, functional limitations and disability. Much of current practice continues to describe the links between these constructs with the underlying implication that treating impairments will improve function and limit disability.

ICF Framework

In many ways, the disablement model describes a simplistic approach to treatment that does not address factors seen in other biopsychosocial models. Chapter 1 introduced the ICF model developed by the World Health Organization (WHO) and the Committee on a US National Agenda for the Prevention of Disabilities that combines previous research contributions to the concept of disability into a universal classification system to define and measure health and function by means of two domains: functioning and contextual factors. The domains characterize different factors that interact with the individual to facilitate or hinder functioning and/or disability (Bichkenbach et al., 1999). Changes to different factors often result in a decrement of health and thereby can be used to describe disability in the individual.

Functioning

Similar to the original disablement model, the ICF has components that encompass pathology, impairment and functioning. Problems in both body function and structure are together usually termed impairments by health professionals and defined as deviations or loss of structure or function. The other two components of activity and participation encompass a larger concept of functioning. Activity and participation are similar concepts, although each has a slightly different definition. Activity is defined as the action or task performance by an individual. Participation represents the involvement in life activities. Problems in an individual's ability to participate in activities will result in participation restrictions and limit actual activity. For example, individuals with LBP or knee pain may be limited in activities such as walking, climbing steps, or lifting objects. When a person with knee pain cannot perform activities such as walking or climbing stairs, it often precludes his or her participation in many social, recreational and daily chores that require both the functional ability and the psychological confidence to execute these activities, as well as the social supports to navigate these activities in a modified or assisted manner.

Contextual Factors

Contextual factors in the ICF are classified as either personal or environmental factors that influence disability. Contextual factors are similar to the two types of factors that influence the cognitive appraisal process during stress and coping: personal factors and situational factors (Lazarus and Folkman, 1984b). Environmental factors, similar to situational factors, refer to all aspects of the external or extrinsic world that form the context of an individual's personal life that have an impact on a person's functioning. Environmental factors can be both facilitators that can assist a person's functioning or barriers that hinder or limit a person's functioning. Our understanding of disability as a function of the interaction of individuals with the influence of social and physical environments has grown over the years. As a result, the environment has been seen to influence disability via the natural environment, the built environment, culture, the economic system, the political system and social systems. Previous literature has added increased emphasis that persons with disabilities have reduced access in the environment that restricts full participation in life and society (Oliver, 1996). Ultimately, the less supportive the environment is to an individual from both a physical and social perspective, the greater the resulting disability.

The other type of contextual factor, personal factors, can include anything that is an internal influence on a person's functioning and disability. Personal factors include individual markers such as age, sex and social status (Stucki and Ewert, 2005) and personal characteristics such as coping styles, lifestyle, habits, social background, past experiences, self-efficacy, self-advocacy and other psychosocial assets that, at least initially, are not directly related to the health condition. This overlaps with the concepts in the stress and coping model where personal factors consist of the personal values that motivate individuals to make certain decisions and beliefs that give the individual a personal sense of control (Lazarus and Folkman, 1984a, 1984b). These personality traits can influence how a person responds to possible limitations secondary to disability. Some individuals may have difficulty with assertiveness or have a negative outlook, regardless of the health condition and corresponding disability. Others may have a sense of positive optimism or self-determination that persists regardless of the disability. The individual's outlook or sense of self can be directly influenced by his or her larger social context. Overall, personal factors are attributes within the person that influence an individual's level of disability and in turn can be positively or negatively influenced by the pain or disability experienced. The recognition of personal factors in the ICF framework illustrates that a person is more than simply the sum of his or her physical functioning. The ICF framework and its components are displayed in Fig. 3.4.

Application of Functioning and Disability in LBP

The ICF model of function illustrates the complex and multifactorial nature of disability as currently understood by clinicians, researchers and the public health community. One

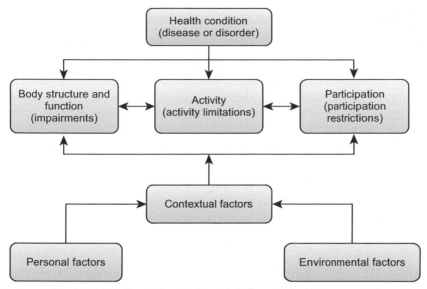

Fig. 3.4   International Classification of Functioning, Disability and Health framework. Representation of the different factors that interact and contribute to disruption of function and increase overall disablement *(Adapted with permission from the WHO ICF framework [WHO, 2001].)*

musculoskeletal area, LBP, has received a lot of attention by all of these groups because it is recognized as a significant cause of musculoskeletal-related disability in our society. In 1980, Waddell revolutionized the clinical perspective of LBP by illustrating that there were many nonorganic and behavioural components to an individual's experience of LBP (Waddell et al., 1980, 1989). The work to revise the concept of disablement along with continued research in LBP has resulted in a more complex understanding of the typical spectrum of musculoskeletal problems of functioning in patients with LBP. Various studies have used the ICF framework to assist in understanding the complexity of LBP (Krismer and Van Tulder, 2007; Sigl et al., 2006; Cieza et al., 2004). Psychosocial and environmental risk factors have been identified in the development and management of LBP (Gatchel et al., 1995; Waddell, 1987, 1991; Waddell et al., 1989, 1993). These studies show the complexity of LBP beyond somatic symptoms and support the multifactorial disablement models in musculoskeletal disorders such as LBP. Using the stress and coping model in combination with the ICF framework and the stress-diathesis model, respective coping processes and resources can be better identified that describe the experience of pain and disablement in patients with musculoskeletal disorders. Ultimately, these theoretical contributions serve to support the larger goal of improving clinicians' understanding of psychosocial factors contributing to musculoskeletal disorders and improving the allocation of resources to reduce the consequences of disability.

Resource Theories of Stress and Coping

To further understand how personal and environmental factors contribute to disablement in musculoskeletal disorders, theoretical constructs have been identified in a number of resource theories of stress and coping. In some health conditions, such as diabetes mellitus and cancer, social and personal constructs have been proposed to serve as coping resources that address stressful person–environmental transactions. More needs to be known about what personal and social constructs are important in coping by patients with musculoskeletal disorders. Specific constructs are explored in this chapter, including the constructs of self-rated health, self-efficacy and social support. Each construct reflects both the individual-level coping behaviours and the interpersonal role of society on influencing health and health behaviours.

Self-Rated Health as a Psychosocial Construct

Self-rated health is a commonly used measurement that identifies a patient's perspective of his or her health condition. It is believed that self-rated health may contribute to both poor coping behaviours as well as improvement in health outcomes. Self-ratings of health are used frequently in the health literature and have been shown to be predictors of morbidity and mortality (Ware and Sherbourne, 1992). Self-rated health has also been proven sensitive to improvements and declines in many health-related outcomes (Garrity et al., 1978; Rodin and McAvay, 1992). A 5-year study by Gold et al. (1996) of health outcomes in the community determined that both functional ability and self-rated health were independent predictors of health outcomes.

Self-rated health measures assess subjective well-being related to physical and mental domains of health. These measures are used extensively in clinical trials and in health services research, where they have shown evidence of reliability, validity and responsiveness (Stewart et al., 1988). These studies support the use of a health status measure as part of an initial intake for patients in musculoskeletal clinics. Even though most medical treatment still focuses on a person's actual physical state as it relates to pain and illness, perceived health may largely contribute to a person's well-being and function.

Appraisal of Health

Self-rated health, both physical and mental health, is likely to be part of a larger appraisal process when faced with a stressful health condition. The perception of health status during a negative health experience is believed to be just as relevant to health outcomes as the actual somatic state of the individual. When an individual has a better perception of his or her overall health, there is a greater potential for these health beliefs to bolster positive coping behaviours during illness experiences. For example, it has been shown that older adults' overall perception of health can be predictive of their use of active coping strategies to deal with age-related health challenges (Menec et al., 1999). Research has also shown that those who don't have a positive health perception may engage in sick-role behaviours that can lead to self-destructive behaviours during illness (Mechanic, 1962). One reason for this is that self-rated health is believed to be a reflection of an enduring self-concept of a healthy or unhealthy person (Bailis et al., 2003). There are many factors at and beyond the individual level that may influence and contribute to an individual's self-health concept. Therefore, this self-concept of health may act as a moderator when engaging in positive or negative illness behaviours.

Variance in physical measures and outcomes have also been shown to be related to respondents' previous self-rated health (Bailis et al., 2003). Longitudinal studies have illustrated that those with initial lower self-rated health predict poor functional ability and increased healthcare utilization over time (Rodin and McAvay, 1992; Ferraro et al., 1997). Negative self-rated health has been found to predict long-term disability and health decline in the general population (Ferraro et al., 1997). Change in self-rated health has been shown to coincide with long-term changes in physical health, mental health, perceived social support and performance-related behaviours (Bailis et al., 2003). Moreover, self-rated health has been shown to vary according to whether respondents intended to improve specific health-related behaviours in the future (Bailis et al., 2003). These findings suggest that self-rated health is both a current assessment of one's health status, similar to a self-concept, and a reflection of efforts to achieve relatively important health-related goals.

Application of Self-Rated Health

Measurement of perceived physical and mental health has been performed routinely in the health literature by several standardized tools (Brooks et al., 1990; Gold et al., 1996; Hicks and Manal, 2009; Ware and Sherbourne, 1992). A common tool used in the health literature is the Medical Outcomes Survey Short Form 36 Questionnaire or the SF-36. Other tools include the General Psychological Well Being Inventory (Dupuy, 1984), Health Perceptions Questionnaire (Davies and Ware, 1981), EuroQol (Group, 1990) and various other measures that assess physical and role functioning (Reynolds et al., 1974). General health surveys have been designed to measure overall self-rated health with a broad range of questions covering a variety of aspects of physical and mental health. It is commonly felt that the usefulness of general measures is in their ability to allow comparisons among patients with the same condition as well as between patients with different conditions. In some cases, general health measures may be able to identify unsuspected issues from a diagnostic group that would be highlighted as scores deviating from population- or disease-specific norms. These self-rated indicators likely take into account the patient's physical sensations (e.g. bodily pain), the patient's comparison of what he or she can perform in his or her daily life as compared with previously or as compared with his or her peers, his or her psychological status and his or her social perception of functioning and social role. Overall, understanding how an individual with a musculoskeletal disorder perceives his or her general physical and mental health may add to the larger role of personal and environmental-level influences on outcomes of pain and disability.

Looking closer at the SF-36 as an example, it is a general health survey which yields psychometrically based physical and mental health summary measures. In numerous previous studies, the SF-36 has been used for general and specific populations in evaluating health outcomes, comparing the relative burden of diseases and differentiating the perceived health benefits produced by a wide range of different treatments. The content validity of the SF-36 has been compared with that of other widely used generic health surveys (McHorney et al., 1993; Ware et al., 1995). The SF-36 was judged to be the most widely evaluated generic patient assessed health outcome measure in a study published in the *British Medical Journal* (Garratt et al., 2002). The SF-36 has proven useful in estimating disease burden and comparing disease-specific benchmarks with general population norms in more than 200 diseases and conditions. Among the most frequently studied diseases and conditions, with 50 or more SF-36 publications, are the following: arthritis, cancer, cardiovascular disease, chronic obstructive pulmonary disease, depression, diabetes, gastrointestinal disease, migraine headache, HIV/AIDS, hypertension, irritable bowel syndrome, kidney disease, LBP, multiple sclerosis, various musculoskeletal conditions, neuromuscular conditions, osteoarthritis, psychiatric diagnoses, rheumatoid arthritis, sleep disorders, spinal injuries, stroke, substance abuse, surgical procedures, transplantation and trauma (Turner-Bowker et al., 2008).

The SF-36 is 36-item, generic self-report measure of general health status covering eight domains: physical functioning, role limitations as a result of physical health problems, role limitations as a result of emotional health problems, energy/fatigue, emotional well-being, social functioning, pain and general health perceptions (McHorney et al., 1993; Ware and Sherbourne, 1992). LBP is a key area of musculoskeletal practice where the evidence for self-rated health and health behaviours has been explored. Psychosocial factors and emotional distress have been found to be stronger predictors of LBP outcomes compared with physical examination findings or severity of pain alone (Pincus et al., 2002). Psychosocial factors that predict poorer LBP outcomes include the presence of depression, passive coping strategies, higher disability levels or somatization (Fayad et al., 2004; Pincus et al., 2002). Chapter 4 discusses issues related to psychological factors in greater detail. However, it is important to remember that a general health status measure can give insight into which aspects of the patient's life are most affected, including the ability to participate in social activities or social roles.

In the general LBP literature, Fanuele et al. (2000) investigated the Medical Outcomes Survey SF-36 physical component scores (PCSs) in a prospective sample of 17,774 patients with spinal disorders. They found that individuals with LBP had a mean PCS of 30.4 ± 9.95 (standard deviation [SD]) compared with 50.0 ± 10.00 for the general U.S. population. This indicates that the PCS is greatly reduced in individuals with spinal disorders in general and is similar to the PCS in other patient populations, such as chronic heart failure (31.0), chronic obstructive pulmonary disorder (33.9), systemic lupus erythematosus (37.1), cancer (38.4) and other musculoskeletal disorders such as primary total hip arthroplasty (29.0), primary total knee arthroplasty (32.6) and glenohumeral degenerative joint disease (35.2) (Fanuele et al., 2000). Because LBP and other musculoskeletal disorders greatly impact an individual's perceived self-health, it is important to include a health status measure to guide further questioning and assessment, collaborative goal setting and outcome reassessment. Beyond the total score, clinicians can determine which of the domains are most influenced by the patient's condition and can target interventions or identify referrals to address these issues.

Key Points

Self-rated health is an indicator of how patients perceive their health. Patients with both acute and chronic musculoskeletal conditions may still rate their overall health as good; this can indicate that the patient also has good coping skills in dealing with health conditions. The converse is also true: patients who rate their overall health as poor may have lower abilities to manage their condition(s). Therefore, we recommend that an examination of patients with either acute or chronic pain condition(s) include a measure of health status. This measure can be used for patient outcomes as well as guidance for selecting interventions and as an indicator for adding and/or augmenting additional coping resources.

Social Cognitive Theory and the Psychosocial Construct of Self-Efficacy

Health status measures attempt to make a link between personal characteristics and social factors that together lead to the ability to function in both physical and social environments. Some frequently cited work by Bandura (1977a) views individuals both as products and as producers of their own environments and social systems. In this view, called social cognitive theory (SCT) (Bandura, 1977a, 1986), individuals possess a self-system that enables them to exert control over their thoughts, feelings, motivations and actions (Bandura, 2001). SCT hypothesizes that people's beliefs in their capabilities mediate how they behave in situations such as participating in treatment for a musculoskeletal disorder. Treatment provides an environment in which there are opportunities for physical and psychosocial support by health professionals, family or friends which can in turn affect beliefs about their capabilities. Both external social supports and individual physical actions during treatment may help to improve an individual's beliefs about his or her capacity to perform functional tasks.

Self-Efficacy

The construct of self-efficacy is a key concept within the SCT framework. Perceived self-efficacy is defined as a person's belief in his or her capacity to both organize and execute the necessary actions and behaviors needed to produce specific performance attainments (Bandura, 1997). It is a context-specific assessment of one's competence to perform a specific task or range of tasks in a given domain. Bandura (1997) describes self-efficacy as influencing four areas: (1) the choices that are made, (2) the effort put forth in task-specific roles, (3) the time one persists when there are obstacles and (4) one's feelings of confidence in performing specific tasks in specific situations.

Depending on what is being managed, the tasks over which personal influence is exercised may entail regulation of one's motivation, thought processes, affective states and actions, or changing environmental conditions. Self-efficacy beliefs are sensitive to these contextual factors. Therefore, they differ from other expectancy beliefs in that self-efficacy judgments are more task and situation specific, and individuals make use of these judgments in reference to the type of goal (Bandura, 1986; Bandura et al., 1989; Pintrich and Schunk, 1996). Self-efficacy can refer to sub-skills required to organize actions that are governed by broader self-regulatory skills, such as perceiving the practical needs for certain task demands or constructing and evaluating alternative strategies. Possessing these self-regulatory sub-skills can permit individuals to improve their performance across varied activities. This is particularly relevant to the patient who is experiencing a musculoskeletal or other health disorder. Individuals who have self-regulatory skills could theoretically participate in treatments and develop alternative strategies for task performance even when faced with sensations of pain during activities. Self-efficacy can also generalize across skills when commonalities are cognitively structured across activities. For example, confidence in physical exercises and motor skills practiced in musculoskeletal treatments may transfer to confidence in other activities performed in daily living if the tasks have generalizable features.

Theoretically, people make and shape self-efficacy beliefs in the context of performing a specific goal or task. Self-efficacy beliefs might influence a patient's experiences of pain, functional limitations and disability with a musculoskeletal disorder. Self-efficacy beliefs have the potential to be modifiable with the right support and reinforcement. A patient practicing functional activities like walking could increase his or her task-specific self-efficacy for walking through successful practice with a reconstructed understanding of pain provocation and pacing to avoid flare-up and, as a result, increase his or her confidence and activity participation outside of the clinic. Moreover, a patient who enters treatment with high self-efficacy for functional tasks might have even greater belief that he or she can organize and execute all of the actions needed to successfully complete tasks required in treatment. Theoretically, a patient with higher self-efficacy could have heightened beliefs about accomplishing tasks, including positive health behaviours such as attending regularly scheduled clinical appointments, following medical instructions, executing a series of home and clinic exercises and performing adaptive avoidance behaviours to minimize pain and discomfort. Overall, high self-efficacy beliefs can lead to setting challenging individual goals and maintaining a strong commitment to these goals, which ultimately could affect outcomes related to a musculoskeletal disorder.

Researchers think self-efficacy beliefs not only influence behaviours but in part determine outcome expectations (Bandura, 1997; Davis and Yates, 1982). Individuals who expect success in a particular task often produce successful outcomes in that task. The opposite is also true of those who lack such confidence in task performance; those who doubt their success will produce failed outcomes. Patients undertaking tasks such as those found in musculoskeletal treatment would have similar anticipatory outcome expectations about performing the specific tasks required for the process of treatment and transfer these beliefs to similar skills outside of treatment.

Issues of self-efficacy found in those with chronic conditions and in older adults often center on reappraisals and misappraisals of their capabilities. Because physical conceptions in chronicity and aging focus extensively on declining abilities, many physical functions can decrease as people regularly avoid activity due to chronic pain or general aging concerns. This process requires reappraisal of self-efficacy for activities in which physical functions have been significantly affected. However, evidence has shown that when older adults are taught to use their intellectual and physical capabilities, their improvement in cognitive and physical functioning more than offsets the average decrement in performance over two decades (Bandura, 1997). Similar situations arise from chronic health conditions. As a health condition becomes chronic, individuals can often reappraise their ability to perform tasks at much lower levels. However, intervention that targets both cognitive and physical capabilities can often mitigate some of this decline. Therefore, it is possible that perceived self-efficacy may affect the level of involvement in activities and theoretically mitigate the decline from musculoskeletal disorders seen in older adults or those with chronic conditions.

Application of Self-Efficacy

In many musculoskeletal disorders, it is unknown if self-efficacy for specific tasks can maintain or improve in the presence of the pain and disability perceived by many patients. It is known that pain can impede or prevent patients from participating in an activity because of the actual experience of pain, the fear and/or avoidance behaviours that pre-empt participation and the cognitive appraisals or reappraisals that are made after activities have repeatedly resulted in painful experiences. Reductions in function can also lower an individual's self-confidence and, as a result, continue to lower the levels of activity in which an individual participates in daily life.

In laboratory experiments, self-efficacy beliefs were found to predict tolerance levels to pain (Keefe et al., 2005). From a biological perspective of pain, perceived self-efficacy has been shown to affect the body's opioid and immune systems (Weisenberg et al., 1998). In patients with pain disorders related to LBP, self-efficacy positively affects physical and psychological functioning (Woby et al., 2007). Evidence shows that self-efficacy influences pain and function after acute physical interventions like surgery (Bastone and Kerns, 1995; Allen et al., 1990). Prospective studies in patients who underwent orthopedic surgery demonstrated that high self-efficacy before the start of treatment and larger increases over the course of treatment speed recovery and predict better long-term outcomes (Waldrop et al., 2001; Dohnke et al., 2005; Orbell et al., 2001). It is possible that individuals with high self-efficacy may be more motivated to engage in health-promoting behaviours and adhere better to treatment recommendations because they have higher performance success expectancies. In addition, it is believed that people with high self-efficacy are less likely to give up an activity when faced with barriers such as pain or weakness and are therefore less likely to become trapped in the negative spiral of activity avoidance, physical deconditioning, loss of social supports and depression.

Application of Self-Efficacy During Treatment

In rehabilitation literature, self-efficacy is measured by using task-specific constructs relevant to the chronic disease process and specific rehabilitation treatments being studied. Research indicates that task-specific self-efficacy can improve during the treatment process. Scherer and Schmieder (1997) demonstrated improved task-specific self-efficacy with patients who participated in treatment for dyspnoea due to chronic obstructive pulmonary disease. Patients who completed educational and exercise training had significant increases in their self-efficacy scores to manage or avoid breathing difficulty. In addition, patients increased their self-efficacy expectations for exercise endurance (Scherer and Schmieder, 1997). Carlson et al. (2001) showed that cardiac rehabilitation treatment involving physical exercise improved patients' post-treatment self-efficacy beliefs for independent exercise. Another study by Jeng and Braun (1997) found that greater success in functional outcomes from cardiac rehabilitation treatment correlated with higher exercise-specific self-efficacy scores. Finally, Rejeski et al. (1998) found that when patients engaged in aerobic and strength-training exercises for knee osteoarthritis (OA), those who actively engaged in physical exercises had increased self-efficacy outcomes for stair climbing, a task-specific limitation for patients with knee OA, compared with controls.

Research has demonstrated that self-efficacy is also an important factor in improved coping and psychological outcomes (Tinetti et al., 1994; Salbach et al., 2006; Lackner and Carosella, 1999b). Taal et al. (1993) surveyed patients with rheumatoid arthritis (RA) to determine their level of self-efficacy in relation to function, pain and disability when coping with RA. Higher self-efficacy scores correlated with improved coping abilities independent of pain, disease status and functional abilities. Moreover, Strahl et al. (2000) found that higher self-efficacy levels in patients with arthritis were predictive of better outcomes related to psychological functioning.

An investigation of self-efficacy for patients with chronic LBP found that initial self-efficacy beliefs predicted functional abilities. In a study by Lackner and Carosella (1999a) that included patients with chronic LBP, 100 patients rated their confidence to perform load-lifting tasks before any examination or treatment. Next, these patients underwent a subsequent physical examination and physical performance test for lifting loads. The results indicated a significant association between self-efficacy beliefs and lifting higher loads and higher physical performance. Lackner and Carosella did not find an association between pain perceptions or measures of psychological distress and the physical performance measures.

Overall, these studies indicate that self-efficacy is an important construct in healthcare management and should be recognized in musculoskeletal-related disorders. Two of the studies (Jeng and Braun, 1997; Lackner and Carosella, 1999a) found significant relationships demonstrating that self-efficacy beliefs have an impact on the outcomes of pain and disability for patients with chronic disease processes. Although the role of self-efficacy in the treatment process warrants more investigation, these studies indicate that heightened patient beliefs regarding the ability to perform specific tasks might also raise the functional, psychological and overall coping behaviours of patients during and post-treatment and therefore help to decrease overall perceptions of pain and disability. Although the role of self-efficacy is unknown in many musculoskeletal disorders, it is important for clinicians and researchers to appreciate the possible impact of self-efficacy in the appraisal of the pain, disability and coping behaviours of patients with musculoskeletal disorders.

Key Points

Self-efficacy plays a significant role in positive patient outcomes. Self-efficacy should be assessed as part of an initial examination as well as ongoing progression in rehabilitation for any musculoskeletal health condition. Clinicians can select interventions that lead to patient success and improve self-efficacy or note that additional efforts to increase confidence using graded exposures may be warranted to reduce fears resulting in poor self-efficacy and avoidance of certain tasks. This may involve the treating clinician and/or may necessitate additional referral to other care providers.

Social Relationships and Health

Although many of the models we have described in this chapter support the complex role of biology and physiology, personal characteristics and social factors (e.g. biopsychosocial model), less is known about the direct role of social factors in the health and management of patients with musculoskeletal disorders. In general, researchers have determined that people with social support and social ties, regardless of their source, live longer than people who are isolated (Putnam, 2000). People with a close network of ties with other people maintain better health, resist disease and deal more successfully with problems they encounter (Putnam, 2000; Guidi et al., 1998). People who are socially isolated and have fewer social relationships have been found to have mortality rates two to five times higher than those with good social relationships, regardless of gender, race, ethnic background and socioeconomic status (Berkman, 1985; Cohen et al., 2000).

As it relates to health and outcomes, assessment of a patient's social contacts and resources could lead to newer treatments and improved outcomes. Social integration and social networks are terms used to describe the existence and quantity of social connections that an individual has available as resources. Social integration is used to establish the existence of social ties (Berkman, 1985) and refers to having open and honest relationships with others. Families or work colleagues who engage in open communication about current and personal issues would be seen as having social integration. Social network is another social construct that describes the interconnectedness of social relationships that surround an individual (Cohen et al., 2000). Researchers investigating social networks describe the types and numbers of other individuals that someone interacts with. People who engage with neighbours, attend church, or participate in interest or civic engagement groups are examples of individuals who have strong and varied social networks. Together, social integration and social networks describe the existence and quantity of social connections that an individual has available.

Social support is another social-level concept that illustrates not only the existence of a social relationship but also the positive function of that social connection and its potential to play a supportive role specifically in an individual's health (Heaney and Israel, 2002; Schwarzer and Leppin, 1991). Social support is defined as the degree to which a person's basic social needs are met through interaction with other people (Cohen, 1992). It includes tangible and intangible resources, emotional support and informational and instructional support, as well as a person's perception of assistance in times of need. When assessing supportive social influences in health, assessment should include what support is available if needed (i.e. patient's perceived support availability) and functions that are currently being supported (i.e. patient's received support) (Schwarzer and Leppin, 1991; Cohen et al., 2000).

Social Support

The role of social support has evolved in health research and is believed to be a social construct that protects and preserves the well-being of an individual in the face of a

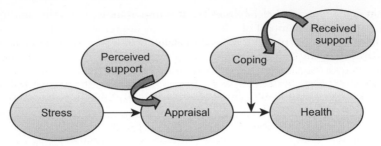

Fig. 3.5 Social support interactions with the stress and coping model. Interactions between perceived support with appraisals as well as received support with coping to modify the effect of a stressor on health.

stressful encounter such as a negative health condition (Cohen et al., 2000). Social support is believed to contribute to global self-evaluations of health (Krause and Borawski-Clark, 1994). In addition, social support serves as a social resource that can assist an individual in his or her capability to cope with stress (Lazarus and Folkman, 1984b). Even though social support comes from an external source, this external support is believed to be able to help protect people from the adverse effects of stress (Fig. 3.5). In the stress and coping literature, social support is a coping resource that can alter beliefs and commitments that can in turn alter how one appraises a stressful situation (Lazarus and Folkman, 1984b).

When considering the role of social support, stressors are believed to act on two different pathways. One pathway is through appraisals of available social support (see Fig. 3.5). The perception that social support is available may protect people from the adverse effects of stressors by leading them to appraise or interpret stressful situations less negatively. For example, a patient with a musculoskeletal disorder with high perceived social support might interpret his or her pain and disability less negatively than a person with low perceived social support and therefore approach the process of treatment and self-management more proactively. Patients' interpretations and reinterpretations of support may moderate their experience of pain and disability before, during and after the treatment process.

The other pathway social support is believed to assist in coping is by actual supportive actions, or received support. Received social support is the actual assistance of others during stress (Cohen and Lichtenstein, 1990; Coriell and Cohen, 1995). Received support is believed to interact with and alter a person's coping abilities in times of stress. This improved coping due to increased received support is theorized to reduce the impact of stress on a person's health (Cohen et al., 2000). When a person can reduce the impact of stress on his or her health, it is theorized that this could be measured through improved health outcomes such as reduced pain and/or disability. Therefore, social support can indirectly influence routine physical measures of pain and disability that are evaluated in patients with musculoskeletal disorders.

Social support can be measured in several ways. One way clinicians and researchers have measured social support is by quantifying the frequency or number of supportive actions a person reports as well as his or her perception of the quality of that received support (Masters et al., 2007). Retrospectively identifying the patient-reported frequency and quality of support received during a specific time period of treatment is an easy way to evaluate the social support beliefs of a patient. In addition, more information can be gained if the patient is asked to identify and report the actual supportive actions that were experienced. Finally, a further step is to investigate how the patient perceived the supportive action and how it interacted with his or her health by rating how the support was helpful or unhelpful. This brings up the key point that not all supportive actions are perceived by patients as helpful. In fact, some supportive actions performed by a healthcare professional, friend or family member may actually hinder the coping process by the individual with the health disorder. It is important to remember that the existence of social supports does not always result in positive coping behaviours by individuals with health conditions. Careful consideration and direct interpretation by a patient are always important to determine if social support plays a positive or negative role in managing stressors related to health.

Application of Social Support in Treatment

Evidence exists on the importance of overall social support in the treatment of chronic diseases, particularly in the treatment of cardiovascular disease (André-Petersson et al., 2007; Amick and Ockene, 1994) and stroke (Glass et al., 1993; Evans et al., 1987; Friedland and McColl, 1987; McLeroy et al., 1984). These studies have shown that improvements in physical functioning and psychological adjustment in cardiovascular and stroke recovery were greater among those with higher sources of social support (Amick and Ockene, 1994; Evans et al., 1987; Friedland and McColl, 1987; Glass et al., 1993; McLeroy et al., 1984; Morris et al., 1991; Stephens et al., 1987). Other studies have shown that social support from all sources positively correlated with increased perceived general health and quality of life after stroke (Angeleri et al., 1993; King, 1996; Handen, 1991). Researchers have also shown lack of social support in general to be associated with negative health consequences, including suicidal thoughts (Kishi et al., 2001), depression (Andersen, 2002), length of hospital stay (Rao et al., 2001), discharge to rehabilitation and nursing home facilities (Marottoli, 1994) and reduced physical functioning (Kawachi et al., 1996; LaCasse et al., 2001).

There is additional evidence that patients with a variety of disease processes benefit from social support from all sources. In one study, Littlefield et al. (1990) found that patients with type II diabetes mellitus had improved function associated with higher total social support scores but worse function associated with higher depression scores. In another study, Yates (1995) surveyed patients with cardiovascular disease who reported that both emotional support and tangible aid from healthcare providers and the patients' spouses were important sources of support for coping with their disease process and improving overall physical recovery. Additionally, Gulick (2001) conducted research involving patients with multiple sclerosis and found that higher total social support scores correlated positively with ADL function scores and inversely with depression scores.

Research investigating arthritis found that social support does mediate the response to the treatment process and function of the patient. In patients with rheumatoid arthritis (RA), Taal et al. (1993) found that tangible or instrumental support by caregivers corresponded positively with improved patient-reported health status and participation in daily physical activities. However, emotional support did not relate to patients' reported health status for this sub-group of patients with RA. Weinberger et al. (1990) illustrated that in research involving patients with osteoarthritis (OA) with concurrent functional limitations, both older age and lower levels of tangible support from caregivers, friends or family were directly associated with greater physical disability. Moreover, in patients with OA, greater psychological disability was associated with lower levels of emotional support from all sources.

Little research has directly examined the association between treatment for many musculoskeletal disorders and the quality or benefit of social support. Masters et al. (2007) investigated whether patients received social support in the treatment process for LBP. Retrospectively, the researchers asked patients who participated in treatment for LBP to indicate which sources of social support they received and whether this support was helpful or unhelpful. Out of the 50 patients surveyed, 43% indicated that they received tangible support from a physiotherapist and physician that was helpful. Thirty-three percent of the patients indicated they received helpful emotional support from physiotherapists, family and friends. Twenty-three percent of the patients additionally reported that they received helpful informational support from physiotherapists. However, 50% of the patients also reported that they received unhelpful emotional support from their family and friends during the treatment process. Additionally, 37% reported receiving unhelpful informational support, and 10% reported receiving unhelpful tangible support from their physicians during the treatment process. Unfortunately, the researchers did not evaluate the relationship of support to other general health, physical function or psychosocial measures. In addition, the researchers did not evaluate the relationship of social support to the outcomes of pain and disability in treatment for LBP. Overall, this study illustrates that social support sources are available and are identified as both helpful and unhelpful in treatment for LBP. Additional research needs to be conducted to understand how social support and other social factors can impact the experience of pain and disability in LBP and other musculoskeletal disorders and identify ways to best intervene to assist our patients to achieve more optimal outcomes.

Key Points

> The presence or lack of social support can influence the experience of pain and disability and affect coping behaviours. Although we don't know enough about which social support interventions are more likely to improve outcomes, clinicians should address the social situation of patients with musculoskeletal conditions. Clinicians should attempt to identify those social supports that play a positive role in the patient's life in order to identify additional resources for management strategies. Additionally, clinicians should attempt to identify support that is interpreted as negative and determine if alternative sources of support could improve coping behaviors. Minimally, positive support from the patient's family, friends and other caregivers can be involved in therapeutic activities, or related social activities could be included in the plan of care for rehabilitation.

Conclusion

A theoretical framework can assist clinicians in understanding psychosocial contributions to musculoskeletal conditions. Table 3.1 summarizes the theoretical framework described in this chapter. It is important for clinicians to understand the complex personal, social and environmental factors that influence health and functioning. Often, coping beliefs and behaviours due to health-related stressors are multifactorial. Early identification and assessment of these complex issues can assist clinicians in identifying resources and treatment approaches that enhance function and outcomes.

TABLE 3.1

FACTORS TO INCLUDE IN ASSESSMENT OF PATIENTS WITH MUSCULOSKELETAL CONDITIONS

Stressors
1. Pain and disability
   a. Biopsychosocial model
   b. Stress-diathesis model
   c. ICF framework

Coping
1. Perception/appraisal of the condition and how much control the patient feels
2. External/environmental factors influencing activity participation (contextual)
3. Personal factors influencing activity participation (contextual)
4. Coping beliefs and behaviours
   a. Self-rated health
   b. Self-efficacy
   c. Positive application of social support

REFERENCES

Allegrante, J.P., Marks, R., 2003. Self-efficacy in management of osteoarthritis. Rheum. Dis. Clin. North Am. 29, 747–768.

Allen, J.K., Becker, D.M., Swank, R.T., 1990. Factors related to functional status after coronary artery bypass surgery. Heart Lung 19, 337–343.

Amick, T., Ockene, J., 1994. The role of social support in the modification of risk factors for cardiovascular disease. In: Amick, T.L., Ockene, J.K. (Eds.), Social Support and Cardiovascular Disease. Springer, New York, pp. 259–278.

Andersen, B., 2002. Biobehavioral outcomes following psychological interventions for cancer patients. J. Consult. Clin. Psychol. 70, 590–610.

André-Petersson, L., Engström, G., Hedblad, B., Janzon, L., Rosvall, M., 2007. Social support at work and the risk of myocardial infarction and stroke in women and men. Soc. Sci. Med. 64, 830–841.

Angeleri, F., Angeleri, V., Foschi, N., Giaquinto, S., Nolfe, G., 1993. The influence of depression, social activity, and family stress on functional outcome after stroke. Stroke 24, 1478–1483.

Asmundson, G.J.G., Wright, K.D., 2004. Biopsychosocial approaches to pain. In: Hadjistavropoulos, T., Craig, K.D. (Eds.), Pain: Psychological Perspectives. Lawrence Erlbaum Associates, Mahwah, NJ, pp. 35–57.

Bailis, D.S., Segall, A., Chipperfield, J.G., 2003. Two views of self-rated general health status. Soc. Sci. Med. 56, 203–217.

Bandura, A. (Ed.), 1977a. Social Learning Theory. Prentice-Hall, Englewood, NJ.

Bandura, A., 1977b. Toward a unifying theory of behavioral change. Psychol. Rev. 84, 191–215.

Bandura, A. (Ed.), 1986. Social Foundations of Thought and Action: Social Cognitive Theory. Prentice-Hall, Englewood, NJ.

Bandura, A. (Ed.), 1997. Self-Efficacy: The Exercise of Control. W. H. Freeman, New York.

Bandura, A., 2001. Social cognitive theory: an agentive perspective. Annu. Rev. Psychol. 52, 1–26.

Bandura, A., O'Leary, A., Barr-Taylor, C., Gauthier, J., Gossard, D., 1989. Perceived self-efficacy and pain control: opioid and nonopioid mechanisms. J. Pers. Soc. Psychol. 53, 563–571.

Bastone, E.C., Kerns, R.D., 1995. Effects of self-efficacy and perceived social support on recovery-related behaviors after coronary artery bypass graft surgery. Anns Behav. Med. 17, 324–330.

Berkman, L.F., 1985. The relationship of social networks and social support to morbidity and mortality. In: Cohen, S., Syme, S.L. (Eds.), Social Support and Health. Academic Press, San Diego, CA, US, pp. 241–262.

Bickenbach, J., Chatterji, S., Badley, E., Üstün, T., 1999. Models of disablement, universalism and the international classification of impairments, disabilities and handicaps. Soc. Sci. Med. 48, 1173–1187.

Black, E.K., White, C.A., 2005. Fear of recurrence, sense of coherence and posttraumatic stress disorder in haematological cancer survivors. Psychooncology 14, 510–515.

Blank, T.O., Bellizzi, K.M., 2008. A gerontologic perspective on cancer and aging. Cancer 112, 2569–2576.

Boden, S., 1996. The use of radiographic imaging studies in the evaluation of patients who have degenerative disorders of the lumbar spine. J. Bone Joint Surg. Am. 78-A (1), 114–125.

Brooks, P.M., 2002. Impact of osteoarthritis on individuals and society: how much disability? Social consequences and health economic implications. Curr. Opin. Rheumatol. 14, 573–577.

Brooks, W.B., Jordan, J.S., Divine, G.W., Smith, K.S., Neelon, F.A., 1990. The impact of psychologic factors on measurement of functional status: assessment of the sickness impact profile. Med. Care 793–804.

Brox, I., Jens, M., Sorensen, R., Friis, A., Nygaard, O., Indahl, A., et al., 2003. Randomized clinical trial of lumbar instrumented fusion and cognitive intervention and exercises in patients with chronic low back pain and disc degeneration. Spine 28, 1913.

Buer, N., Linton, S., 2002. Fear-avoidance beliefs and catastrophizing: occurrence and risk factor in back pain and ADL in the general population. Pain 99, 485–491.

Carlson, J., Norman, G., Feltz, D., Franklin, B., Johnson, J., Locke, S., 2001. Self-efficacy, psychosocial factors, and exercise behavior in traditional versus modified cardiac rehabilitation. J. Cardiopulm. Rehabil. Prev. 21, 363.

Cieza, A., Stucki, G., Weigl, M., Disler, P., Jackel, W., van der Linden, S., et al., 2004. ICF Core Sets for low back pain. J. Rehabil. Med. 36, 69–74.

Cohen, S., 1992. Stress, social support, and disorder. In: Veiel, H.O.F., Baumann, U. (Eds.), The Meaning and Measurement of Social Support. Hemisphere Press, New York, pp. 109–124.

Cohen, S., Gottlieb, B., Underwood, L., 2000. Social relationships and health. In: Cohen, S., Underwood, L.G., Gottlieb, B.H. (Eds.), Social Support Measurement and Intervention: A Guide for Health and Social Scientists. Oxford University Press, New York, pp. 3–25.

Cohen, S., Lichtenstein, E., 1990. Perceived stress, quitting smoking, and smoking relapse. Health Psychol. 9, 466–478.

Coriell, M., Cohen, S., 1995. Concordance in the face of a stressful event: when do members of a dyad agree that one person supported the other? J. Pers. Soc. Psychol. 69, 289–299.

Davies, A.R., Ware, J.E., 1981. Measuring health perceptions in the health insurance experiment. Rand Corporation, Santa Monica, CA.

Davis, F., Yates, B., 1982. Self-efficacy expectancies versus outcome expectancies as determinants of performance deficits and depressive affect. Cognit. Ther. Res. 6, 23–35.

Descartes, R., 1985. The Philosophical Writings of Descartes. Cambridge University Press.

Dohnke, B., Knauper, B., Mallerae-Fahrnow, W., 2005. Perceived self-efficacy gained from, and health effects of, a rehabilitation program after hip joint replacement. Arthritis Care Res. 53, 585–592.

Dupuy, H.J., 1984. The psychological general well-being (PGWB) index. In: Wenger, N.S. (Ed.), Assessment of Quality of Life in Clinical Trials of Cardiovascular Therapies. Le Jacq, Darien, CT, pp. 170–183.

Elder, G.H., Jr., 1994. Time, human agency, and social change: perspectives on the life course. Soc. Psychol. Q. 57, 4–15.

Engel, G.L., 1980. The clinical application of the biopsychosocial model. Am. J. Psychiatry 137, 535–544.

Evans, R., Bishop, D., Matlock, A., Stranahan, S., Smith, G., Halar, E., 1987. Family interaction and treatment adherence after stroke. Arch. Phys. Med. Rehabil. 68, 513–517.

Fanuele, J., Birkmeyer, N., Abdu, W., Tosteson, T., Weinstein, J., 2000. The impact of spinal problems on the health status of patients: have we underestimated the effect? Spine 25, 1509–1514.

Fayad, F., Lefevre-colau, M.M., Poiraudeau, S., Fermanian, J., Rannou, F., Benyahya, R., et al., 2004. Chronicity, recurrence, and return to work in low back pain: common prognostic factors. Ann. Readapt. Med. Phys.

Ferraro, K.F., Farmer, M.M., Wybraniec, J.A., 1997. Health trajectories: long-term dynamics among black and white adults. J. Health Soc. Behav. 38–54.

Flynn, T., Fritz, J., Whitman, J., Wainner, R., Magel, J., Rendeiro, D., et al., 2002. A clinical prediction rule for classifying patients with low back pain who demonstrate short-term improvement with spinal manipulation. Spine 27, 2835–2843.

Friedland, J., McColl, M., 1987. Social support and psychosocial dysfunction after stroke: buffering effects in a community sample. Arch. Phys. Med. Rehabil. 68, 475–480.

Fritz, J., Delitto, A., Welch, W., Erhard, R., 1998. Lumbar spinal stenosis: a review of current concepts in evaluation, management, and outcome measurements. Arch. Phys. Med. Rehabil. 79, 700–708.

Fritz, J., George, S., 2002. Identifying psychosocial variables in patients with acute work-related low back pain: the importance of fear-avoidance beliefs. Phys. Ther. 82, 973.

Garratt, A., Schmidt, L., Mackintosh, A., Fitzpatrick, R., 2002. Quality of life measurement: bibliographic study of patient assessed health outcome measures. BMJ 324, 1417.

Garrity, T.F., Somes, G.W., Marx, M.B., 1978. Factors influencing self-assessment of health. Soc. Sci. Med. 12, 77–81. Part A: Medical Psychology and Medical Sociology.

Gatchel, R.J., Polatin, P.B., Mayer, T.G., 1995. The dominant role of psychosocial risk factors in the development of chronic low back pain disability. Spine 20, 2702–2709.

Glanz, K., Rimer, B.K., Viswanath, K., 2008. Health Behavior and Health Education: Theory, Research, and Practice. John Wiley and Sons, San Francisco.

Glass, T., Matchar, D., Belyea, M., Feussner, J., 1993. Impact of social support on outcome in first stroke. Stroke 24, 64–70.

Gold, M., Franks, P., Erickson, P., 1996. Assessing the health of the nation: the predictive validity of a preference-based measure and self-rated health. Med. Care 34, 163–177.

Group, T.E., 1990. EuroQol – a new facility for the measurement of health-related quality of life. Health Policy 16, 199–208.

Guidi, L., Tricerri, A., Frasca, D., Vangeli, M., Errani, A., Bartoloni, C., 1998. Psychoneuroimmunology and Aging. Logo 44.

Gulick, E., 2001. Emotional distress and activities of daily living functioning in persons with multiple sclerosis. Nurs. Res. 50, 147.

Handen, B., 1991. The influence of social support factors on the well-being of the elderly. In: Wisocki, P.A. (Ed.), Handbook of Clinical Behavior Therapy With the Elderly Client. Springer, New York, pp. 121–139.

Heaney, C., Israel, B., 2002. Social networks and social support. In: Glanz, K., Rimer, B.K., Lewis, F.M. (Eds.), Health Behavior and Health Education: Theory, Research, and Practice. Jossey-Bass, San Fransisco, pp. 185–209.

Hicks, G.E., Manal, T.J., 2009. Psychometric properties of commonly used low back disability questionnaires: are they useful for older adults with low back pain? Pain Med. 10, 85–94.

Hirsch, M.S., Liebert, R.M., 1998. The physical and psychological experience of pain: the effects of labeling and cold pressor temperature on three pain measures in college women. Pain 77, 41–48.

Jeng, C., Braun, L., 1997. The influence of self-efficacy on exercise intensity, compliance rate and cardiac rehabilitation outcomes among coronary artery disease patients. Prog. Cardiovasc. Nurs. 12, 13–24.

Jensen, M.P., Karoly, P., 1991. Control beliefs, coping efforts, and adjustment to chronic pain. J. Consult. Clin. Psychol. 59, 431.

Kawachi, I., Colditz, G., Ascherio, A., Rimm, E., Giovannucci, E., Stampfer, M., et al., 1996. A prospective study of social networks in relation to total mortality and cardiovascular disease in men in the USA. J. Epidemiol. Community Health 50, 245–251.

Keefe, F.J., Lefebvre, J.C., Maixner, W., Salley, A.N., Caldwell, D.S., 2005. Self-efficacy for arthritis pain: relationship to perception of thermal laboratory pain stimuli. Arthritis Rheum. 10, 177–184.

King, R., 1996. Quality of life after stroke. Stroke 27, 1467–1472.

Kirkaldy-Willis, W., Bernard, T. (Eds.), 1999. Managing Low Back Pain. Churchill Livingstone, Edinburgh.

Kishi, Y., Robinson, R., Kosier, J., 2001. Suicidal ideation among patients with acute life-threatening physical illness. Psychosomatics 42, 382–390.

Krause, N., Borawski-Clark, E., 1994. Clarifying the functions of social support in later life. Res. Aging 16, 251–279.

Krismer, M., Van Tulder, M., 2007. Low back pain (non-specific). Best Pract. Res. Clin. Rheumatol. 21, 77–91.

LaCasse, Y., Rousseau, L., Maltais, F., 2001. Prevalence of depressive symptoms and depression in patients with severe oxygen-dependent chronic obstructive pulmonary disease. J. Cardiopulm. Rehabil. Prev. 21, 80.

Lackner, J., Carosella, A., 1999a. The relative influence of perceived pain control, anxiety, and functional self efficacy on spinal function among patients with chronic low back pain. Spine 24, 2254.

Lackner, J.M., Carosella, A.M., 1999b. The relative influence of perceived pain control, anxiety, and functional self efficacy on spinal function among patients with chronic low back pain. Spine 24, 2254–2260, discussion 2260–2261.

Lazarus, R., Folkman, S., 1984a. Coping and adaptation. In: Gentry, W.D. (Ed.), The Handbook of Behavioral Medicine. Guildford, New York, pp. 282–325.

Lazarus, R.S., Folkman, S., 1984b. Stress, Appraisal, and Coping. Springer, New York.

Lazarus, R.S., Folkman, S., 1984c. Stress, Appraisal, and Coping. Springer, New York.

Littlefield, C., Rodin, G., Murray, M., Craven, J., 1990. Influence of functional impairment and social support on depressive symptoms in persons with diabetes. Health Psychol. 9, 737–749.

Marinelli, R.P., Orto, A.E.D., 1999. The Psychological and Social Impact of Disability. Springer, New York.

Marottoli, R., 1994. Predictors of mortality and institutionalization after hip fracture: the New Haven EPESE cohort. Established Populations for Epidemiologic Studies of the Elderly. Am. J. Pub. Health 84 (11), 1807–1812.

Masters, K., Stillman, A., Spielmans, G., 2007. Specificity of support for back pain patients: do patients care who provides what? J. Behav. Med. 30, 11–20.

McHorney, C.A., Ware, J.E., Jr., Raczek, A.E., 1993. The MOS 36-Item Short-Form Health Survey (SF-36): II. Psychometric and clinical tests of validity in measuring physical and mental health constructs. Med. Care 31 (3), 247–263.

McLeroy, K., Devellis, R., Devellis, B., Kaplan, B., Toole, J., 1984. Social support and physical recovery in a stroke population. J. Soc. Pers. Relat. 1, 395.

Mechanic, D., 1962. The concept of illness behavior. J. Chronic Dis. 15, 189.

Menec, V.H., Chipperfield, J.G., Perry, R.P., 1999. Self-perceptions of health: a prospective analysis of mortality, control, and health. J. Gerontol. B Psychol. Sci. Soc. Sci. 54, P85–P93.

Morris, P., Robinson, R., Raphael, B., Bishop, D., 1991. The relationship between the perception of social support and post-stroke depression in hospitalized patients. Psychiatry 54, 306–316.

Nagi, S., 1965. Some conceptual issues in disability and rehabilitation. In: Sussman, M.B. (Ed.), Sociology and Rehabilitation. American Sociological Association, Washington, DC, pp. 100–113.

Oliver, M., 1996. Defining impairment and disability: issues at stake. In: Barnes, C., Mercer, G. (Eds.), Exploring the Divide: Illness and Disability. The Disability Press, Leeds, UK, pp. 39–54.

Orbell, S., Johnston, M., Rowley, D., Davey, P., Espley, A., 2001. Self-efficacy and goal importance in the prediction of physical disability in people following hospitalization: a prospective study. Br. J. Health Psychol. 6, 25–40.

Pahl, M.A., Brislin, B., Boden, S., Hilibrand, A.S., Vaccaro, A., Hanscom, B., et al., 2006. The impact of four common lumbar spine diagnoses upon overall health status. Thomas Jefferson University, Department of Orthopaedic Surgery Faculty Papers. http://jdc.jefferson.edu/cgi/viewcontent.cgi?article=1001&context=orthofp.

Painter, J.E., Borba, C.P.C., Hynes, M., Mays, D., Glanz, K., 2008. The use of theory in health behavior research from 2000 to 2005: a systematic review. Anns Behav. Med. 35, 358–362.

Pincus, T., Burton, A.K., Vogel, S., Field, A.P., 2002. A systematic review of psychological factors as predictors of chronicity/disability in prospective cohorts of low back pain. Spine 27, E109–E120.

Pinsky, J.L., Jette, A.M., Branch, L.G., Kannel, W.B., Feinleib, M., 1990. The Framingham Disability Study: relationship of various coronary heart disease manifestations to disability in older persons living in the community. Am. J. Public Health 80, 1363–1367.

Pintrich, P., Schunk, D. (Eds.), 1996. Motivation in Education: Theory, Research, and Applications. Prentice-Hall, Englewood Cliffs, NJ.

Putnam, R., 2000. Bowling Alone: The Collapse and Revival of American Community. Simon & Schuster, New York.

Rao, R., Jackson, S., Howard, R., 2001. Depression in older people with mild stroke, carotid stenosis and peripheral vascular disease: a comparison with healthy controls. Int. J. Geriatr. Psychiatry 16, 175–183.

Rejeski, W., Ettinger, W., Jr., Martin, K., Morgan, T., 1998. Treating disability in knee osteoarthritis with exercise therapy: a central role for self-efficacy and pain. Arthritis Care Res. 11, 94–101.

Reynolds, W.J., Rushing, W.A., Miles, D.L., 1974. The validation of a function status index. J. Health Soc. Behav. 271–288.

Rodin, J., McAvay, G., 1992. Determinants of change in perceived health in a longitudinal study of older adults. J. Gerontol. 47, P373–P384.

Rowland, J.H., 1989. Developmental Stage and Adaptation: Adult Model. In: Holland, J.C., Rowland, J.H. (Eds.), Handbook of Psychooncology: Psychological Care of the Patient With Cancer. Oxford University Press, New York.

Salbach, N.M., Mayo, N.E., Robichaud-Ekstrand, S., Hanley, J.A., Richards, C.L., Wood-Dauphinee, S., 2006. Balance self-efficacy and its relevance to physical function and perceived health status after stroke. Arch. Phys. Med. Rehabil. 87, 364–370.

Scherer, Y., Schmieder, L., 1997. The effect of a pulmonary rehabilitation program on self-efficacy, perception of dyspnea, and physical endurance. Heart Lung 26, 15.

Schwarzer, R., Leppin, A., 1991. Social support and health: a theoretical and empirical overview. J. Soc. Pers. Relat. 8, 99–127.

Shakil, M., Vaccaro, A., Albert, T., Klein, G., 1999. Efficacy of conservative treatment of lumbar spinal stenosis. Spine 11, 229–233.

Shanahan, M.J., Macmillan, R., 2008. Biography and the Sociological Imagination: Contexts and Contingencies. W.W. Norton, New York.

Sharp, T.J., Harvey, A.G., 2001. Chronic pain and posttraumatic stress disorder: mutual maintenance? Clin. Psychol. Rev. 21 (6), 857–877.

Sigl, T., Cieza, A., Brockow, T., Chatterji, S., Kostanjsek, N., Stucki, G., 2006. Content comparison of low back pain-specific measures based on the International Classification of Functioning, Disability and Health (ICF). Clin. J. Pain 22, 147–153.

Steiner, W.A., Ryser, L., Huber, E., Uebelhart, D., Aeschlimann, A., Stucki, G., 2002. Use of the ICF model as a clinical problem-solving tool in physical therapy and rehabilitation medicine. Phys. Ther. 82, 1098–1107.

Stephens, M., Kinney, J.M., Norris, V.K., Ritchie, S.W., 1987. Social networks as assets and liabilities in recovery from stroke by geriatric patients. Psychol. Aging 2 (2), 125–129.

Stewart, A.L., Hays, R.D., Ware, J.E., 1988. The MOS short-form general health survey: reliability and validity in a patient population. Med. Care 26, 724–735.

Strahl, C., Kleinknecht, R.A., Dinnel, D.L., 2000. The role of pain anxiety, coping, and pain self-efficacy in rheumatoid arthritis patient functioning. Behav. Res. Ther. 38, 863–873.

Stucki, G., Ewert, T., 2005. How to assess the impact of arthritis on the individual patient: the WHO ICF. Ann. Rheum. Dis. 64, 664–668.

Sullivan, M.J.L., Feuerstein, M., Gatchel, R., Linton, S.J., Pransky, G., 2005. Integrating psychosocial and behavioral interventions to achieve optimal rehabilitation outcomes. J. Occup. Rehabil. 15, 475–489.

Sunderland, A., Tinson, D., Bradley, E., Fletcher, D., Langton Hewer, R., Wade, D., 1992. Enhanced physical therapy improves recovery of arm function after stroke. A randomised controlled trial. Br. Med. J. 55, 530–535.

Taal, E., Rasker, J., Seydel, E., Wiegman, O., 1993. Health status, adherence with health recommendations, self-efficacy and social support in patients with rheumatoid arthritis. Patient Educ. Couns. 20, 63–76.

Tinetti, M.E., Mendes de Leon, C.F., Doucette, J.T., Baker, D.I., 1994. Fear of falling and fall-related efficacy in relationship to functioning among community-living elders. J. Gerontol. 49, M140–M147.

Turk, D.C., Flor, H., 1999. Chronic pain: a biobehavioral perspective. Psychosocial Factors in Pain: Critical Perspectives 1, 18.

Turner-Bowker, D.M., Derosa, M.A., Ware, J.E., Jr., 2008. SF-36 Health Survey. In: Boslaugh, S. (Ed.), Encyclopedia of Epidemiology, vol. 2. Sage Publications, Thousand Oaks, CA.

Waddell, G., 1987. A new clinical model for the treatment of low back pain. Spine 12, 632–644.

Waddell, G., 1991. Occupational low-back pain, illness behavior, and disability. Spine 16, 683–685.

Waddell, G., McCulloch, J.A., Kummel, E., Venner, R.M., 1980. Nonorganic physical signs in low-back pain. Spine 5, 117–125.

Waddell, G., Newton, M., Henderson, I., Somerville, D., Main, C.J., 1993. A Fear-Avoidance Beliefs Questionnaire (FABQ) and the role of fear-avoidance beliefs in chronic low back pain and disability. Pain 52, 157–168.

Waddell, G., Pilowsky, I., Bond, M.R., 1989. Clinical assessment and interpretation of abnormal illness behaviour in low back pain. Pain 39, 41–53.

Waldrop, D., Lightsey, O.R., Jr., Ethington, C.A., Woemmel, C.A., Coke, A.L., 2001. Self-efficacy, optimism, health competence, and recovery from orthopedic surgery. J. Couns. Psychol. 48, 233.

Ware, J.E., Jr., Kosinski, M., Bayliss, M.S., McHorney, C.A., Rogers, W.H., Raczek, A., 1995. Comparison of methods for the scoring and statistical analysis of SF-36 health profile and summary measures: summary of results from the Medical Outcomes Study. Med. Care 33 (Suppl. 4), AS264–AS279.

Ware, J.E., Jr., Sherbourne, C.D., 1992. The MOS 36-item short-form health survey (SF-36): I. Conceptual framework and item selection. Med. Care 30 (6), 473–483.

Weinberger, M., Terney, W., Booher, P., Hiner, S., 1990. Social support, stress and functional status in patients with osteoarthritis. Soc. Sci. Med. 30 (4), 503–508.

Weinstein, J.N., Tosteson, T.D., Lurie, J.D., Tosteson, A.N., Blood, E., Hanscom, B., et al., 2008. Surgical versus nonsurgical therapy for lumbar spinal stenosis. N. Engl. J. Med. 358, 794–810.

Weisenberg, M., Raz, T., Hener, T., 1998. The influence of film-induced mood on pain perception. Pain 76, 365–375.

Whitman, J., Flynn, T., Fritz, J., 2003. Nonsurgical management of patients with lumbar spinal stenosis: a literature review and case series of three patients managed with physical therapy. Phys. Med. Rehabil. Clin. N. Am. 14, 77–101.

Whitman, J.M., Flynn, T.W., Childs, J.D., Wainner, R.S., Gill, H.E., Ryder, M.G., et al., 2006. A comparison between two physical therapy treatment programs for patients with lumbar spinal stenosis: a randomized clinical trial. Spine 31, 2541–2549.

Woby, S.R., Roach, N.K., Urmston, M., Watson, P.J., 2007. The relation between cognitive factors and levels of pain and disability in chronic low back pain patients presenting for physiotherapy. Eur. J. Pain 11, 869–877.

World Health Organization, 2001. ICIDH-2: International Classification of Functioning, Disability and Health: Final Draft, Full Version. Classification, Assessment, Surveys and Terminology Team. World Health Organization, Geneva.

Yates, B., 1995. The relationships among social support and short- and long-term recovery outcomes in men with coronary heart disease. Res. Nurs. Health 18 (3), 193–203.

4

Assessment, Reasoning and Management of Psychological Factors in Musculoskeletal Practice

Jason M. Beneciuk • Steven Z. George • Mark A. Jones

Pain and associated disability are an overall experience and not simply isolated sensory, emotional or physiological responses (Institute of Medicine, 2011; Sim and Smith, 2004). Pain and disability occur in both a psychological and sociocultural context. As reflected in the International Classification of Functioning, Disability and Health (ICF) of the World Health Organization (2001) biopsychosocial framework depicted in Chapters 1 and 3, biological and psychosocial factors interact reciprocally in determining patients' pain and disability experiences that are both individual and complex (Borrell-Carrio et al., 2004). Within the literature, the term 'psychosocial' is commonly used as a single construct capturing both psychological and social influences. However, although psychological and social factors are intimately associated with each other, and in turn with pain and disability, they are individually comprised of specific characteristics that need to be understood and considered in musculoskeletal clinicians' patient assessment and management. Although the 'psychosocial' construct is used within this chapter because it is more broadly linked to the literature, this chapter focuses on psychological factors, with Chapter 3 focussing more explicitly on the influences of stress, coping and the interaction of social factors.

An important point to establish at the outset of this chapter is that psychological factors should not all be construed as negative. As an example, as discussed in Chapter 3, high self-efficacy related to pain-provoking tasks has been identified as a positive prognostic indicator for musculoskeletal pain clinical outcomes (Foster et al., 2010; Sarda et al., 2009). Building on the clinical reasoning theory in Chapter 1 and the theoretical foundations for the interaction between psychological and social factors covered in Chapter 3, this chapter discusses clinical reasoning associated with the identification and management of psychological factors that have been described as complications associated with recovery because they provide modifiable treatment targets.

There is increasing evidence that negative psychosocial factors are adversely influential in the transition from acute to chronic pain conditions (Burton et al., 1995; Linton, 2000; Linton, 2005; Nicholas et al., 2011; Chou et al., 2007; Chou and Shekelle, 2010). For example, a systematic review involving psychological factors as prognostic indicators for persistent pain and disability suggests there can be consistent relationships between depression, pain catastrophizing, pain intensity and beliefs about pain with future clinical or occupational outcomes in patients with acute or subacute low back pain (LBP) (Nicholas et al., 2011). A similar, yet separate systematic review involving predictors of poor clinical outcomes indicated that nonorganic signs, elevated maladaptive pain coping behaviors, elevated baseline LBP-related disability, the presence of psychiatric comorbidities and low general health status were the strongest predictors of poor clinical outcomes at 1-year follow-up (Chou and Shekelle, 2010). The theoretical foundations of coping beliefs and behaviours, pain, disability and general health status are covered in Chapter 3. Although most of the previous research in this area has explored the influence negative psychological factors have on LBP outcomes, it seems plausible (from a theoretical perspective) that similar relationships may be relevant for musculoskeletal pain complaints in other body regions (Nicholas et al., 2008; Hunt et al., 2013; Sullivan et al., 2006, 2009; George et al., 2007, 2011; Hartigan et al., 2013). Similarly, although not the focus of research, psychological factors can impact positively and negatively on any patient, and negative factors can contribute to attitudes, beliefs and behaviours that underpin the slow recovery and recurrence of any problem, thus supporting their screening in all patients.

Key Points

- Pain and associated disability occur in both a psychological and sociocultural context which creates an overall experience and not simply isolated sensory, emotional or physiological responses.
- Psychological factors are an important component within the biopsychosocial framework.
- Considering the wide spectrum of psychological factors, their influence on musculoskeletal pain clinical outcomes can be either positive or negative.
- There is increasing evidence that negative psychosocial factors are adversely influential in the transition from acute to chronic pain conditions.

Musculoskeletal Clinicians' Lack of Knowledge and Ability to Assess and Manage Psychological Factors

Although musculoskeletal clinicians are generally well educated to assess and manage the physical and many environmental dimensions of the patient's health condition, formal education and experience assessing, evaluating and managing psychological and social factors contributing to both acute and chronic pain are often less developed and less structured (Barlow, 2012; Bishop and Foster, 2005; Foster and Delitto, 2011; Main and George, 2011; Overmeer et al., 2005; Sanders et al., 2013; Singla et al., 2015). This was evident in survey responses from Australian primary care clinicians ($n = 651$), including musculoskeletal specialists ($n = 255$; 39.2%), that indicated formal psychosocial screening is not common (Kent et al., 2009). These results are alarming when one considers that formal screening has been shown to be more accurate than informal judgement (Spitzer et al., 1994; Haggman et al., 2004). Therefore, it seems apparent that embedding attention to psychological factors into musculoskeletal clinicians' management strategies is faced with several challenges, including inconsistency in breadth and depth of psychosocial education during entry-level study, competency in application of theory to practice (which is difficult to measure) and clinician culture (Foster and Delitto, 2011; Main and George, 2011). Most notably, biomedical or impairment-based perspectives are predominantly emphasized during the formal education and ongoing professional development of many musculoskeletal clinicians, with little, if any, content being provided from a biopsychosocial perspective (Foster and Delitto, 2011; Main and George, 2011; Smart and Doody, 2007; Daykin and Richardson, 2004; Bishop and Foster, 2005; Simmonds et al., 2012). Further complicating this issue is that collectively and traditionally, there has been a lack of clear knowledge regarding musculoskeletal clinicians' psychosocial assessment, reasoning and management best practice (Linton and Shaw, 2011; Nicholas et al., 2011; Foster and Delitto, 2011). However, suggestions have been put forward (Jones and Edwards, 2008), and a growing body of literature is now available informing musculoskeletal clinicians' psychosocial assessment and management, as well as underpinning reasoning (French and Sim, 2004; Hasenbring et al., 2012; Jones and Edwards, 2008; Keefe et al., 2006; Main et al., 2008).

Key Points

- Traditionally, musculoskeletal clinicians do not receive adequate training in biopsychosocial perspectives of patient management.
- Clinical reasoning has strong potential to be enhanced through standardized screening of psychological factors.

The 'Flag' System of Screening for Psychosocial-Related Risk Factors

The 'flag' system has been suggested as a framework to classify patients and assist in clinical decision-making processes based on colours representing different types of risk factors (Nicholas et al., 2011; Main and George, 2011):

- Red flags – serious pathology (e.g. fracture)
- Orange flags – psychopathology (e.g. clinical depression)
- Yellow flags – psychological reactions to symptoms (e.g. fear-avoidance beliefs about physical activity)
- Blue flags – perceptions about work and health relationships (e.g. belief that increased work will lead to further injury)
- Black flags – healthcare system influence on clinical decisions and contextual factors (e.g. insurance restrictions, socioeconomic status)

Although sociocultural influences outside the workplace and healthcare system (e.g. family, community, government, etc.) are not represented in the flag classifications, they are equally important to consider, as discussed in Chapter 3.

An important component to incorporating the flag system into musculoskeletal practice is the ability to distinguish between different types of clinical decisions (Nicholas et al., 2011). 'Psychologically informed practice' has been presented as a secondary prevention approach for chronic musculoskeletal pain that integrates both biomedical (focused on pathology or physical impairments) and cognitive-behavioural (focused on psychological distress or behaviour) principles (Main and George, 2011). Psychologically informed practice also underpins cognitive-behavioural approaches used for patients who may be experiencing recurrent symptoms or have already progressed to chronicity. The primary goal of psychologically informed musculoskeletal practice is minimization of current and future disability related to musculoskeletal pain by emphasizing (1) identification of individuals who are at high risk for developing chronic or recurrent symptoms based on the presence of psychological factors and (2) targeted treatment aimed at psychological factors in conjunction with traditional, impairment-based therapy (Main and George, 2011). Therefore, although screening for 'red flags' as indicators of serious pathology is an important component of routine clinical practice, psychologically informed practice is predominantly characterized by screening for elevated and functionally maladaptive 'yellow flags' to identify patients at risk for poor outcomes primarily based on psychological factors that potentially can be targeted through direct therapeutic intervention.

It is also important to distinguish between modifiable and non-modifiable psychosocial risk factors from a musculoskeletal intervention perspective because both may be strong predictors of future outcomes and can be identified through screening. Some psychosocial risk factors are non-modifiable through musculoskeletal clinical intervention. For example, social class has been identified as a predictor of poor outcome in patients with neck pain treated by physical therapists (Hill et al., 2007); however, it is non-modifiable through musculoskeletal clinical intervention. From a psychological perspective, Main and George (2011) have suggested that the ability to distinguish between modifiable and non-modifiable risk factors based on the flag system is a critical component of psychologically informed practice because musculoskeletal clinicians are not trained to address all psychological risk factors. For instance, properly trained musculoskeletal clinicians are equipped to identify and provide interventions tailored to addressing yellow flags (e.g. maladaptive pain coping), which are considered modifiable psychological risk factors. However, it is not within the scope of musculoskeletal practice to provide direct treatment interventions that target orange flags (e.g. clinical depression), which are considered non-modifiable psychological risk factors, through direct musculoskeletal treatment interventions alone. Therefore, orange flag screening combined with frequent and early re-assessment is a vitally important role for musculoskeletal clinicians during the ongoing clinical reasoning process to determine if referral to other healthcare professionals (e.g. clinical psychologist) is warranted. Similar to screening for visceral disease masquerading as a musculoskeletal disorder, the appropriately trained musculoskeletal clinician's role in orange flag screening is, for example, to screen for symptoms of clinical depression and other psychological disorders (e.g. anxiety) and not to diagnose psychological or psychiatric disorders. Just as every clinical feature listed as a potential red flag does not necessitate immediate referral, not every patient with elevated depressive symptoms will need to be referred to a psychologist or back to the referring practitioner. This is an area requiring more attention in musculoskeletal education to assist clinicians to be able to recognize indicators warranting immediate referral or consultation (e.g. suicidal tendencies, features of post-traumatic stress syndrome). Musculoskeletal clinicians are advised to add this screening to their current patient assessment, to monitor any overt symptoms linked to orange flags and to consult with the referring practitioner or a psychologist when uncertain about the significance of such symptoms.

Psychosocial yellow flags are probably the most manageable from a musculoskeletal clinical perspective; therefore, increased emphasis should be placed on clinical reasoning associated with information obtained from yellow flag assessments to identify individuals who may benefit from psychologically based interventions (Nicholas and George, 2011). Expert musculoskeletal clinicians have been shown to employ a range of 'clinical reasoning strategies' incorporating different foci of reasoning, including psychosocially oriented reasoning (i.e. 'narrative reasoning') (Edwards et al., 2004) as discussed in Chapter 1. Expanding your knowledge of theoretical constructs that characterize pain coping behaviours, as covered in Chapter 3, combined with an understanding of narrative reasoning, will facilitate clinical assessment, analysis and management of yellow flags for patients experiencing musculoskeletal pain.

Key Points

- The flag system is a framework to classify different types of risk factors by colour to assist clinicians' recognition, reasoning and management of such factors in their patients.
- Psychologically informed practice is a secondary prevention approach for chronic musculoskeletal pain that integrates both biomedical and cognitive-behavioural principles.
- Psychologically informed practice is also used for patients who are experiencing recurrent symptoms or have already progressed to chronicity. Psychologically informed practice emphasizes (1) identification of individuals who may be at high risk for poor clinical outcomes and (2) targeted treatment aimed at psychological factors in conjunction with traditional, impairment-based therapy.
- Clinical reasoning can be enhanced when clinicians are able to distinguish between modifiable and non-modifiable psychosocial risk factors.

Psychosocial 'Yellow Flag' Screening and Assessment Process

The intent of primary prevention is the protection of health by personal and community-wide efforts. As a potential component of primary prevention, screening can provide valuable information regarding risk factors for future disease among healthy individuals in the general population (e.g. demographics or lifestyle) (Straus et al., 2005). However, screening is also commonly associated with secondary prevention processes where the intent is early identification of individuals with the potential for poor future outcomes (e.g. disability related to musculoskeletal pain). Early risk factor screening has been advocated as one strategy to identify patients who may be at risk of poor clinical outcomes and as a potential method to improve the efficiency and effectiveness of care (Pransky et al., 2011; Hill and Fritz, 2011; Chou et al., 2007). Risk factor screening can be achieved by questionnaire and by patient interview. Validated questionnaires provide quantitative measurement of psychological factors while also opening the door to important areas of assessment patients may not spontaneously volunteer. Information provided via questionnaire can then be explored further through the patient interview for a fuller understanding of the patient and psychological factors that may be contributing to the patient's pain and disability.

Although psychosocial factor screening to inform psychologically informed management has mostly been investigated and discussed in the area of LBP, the overarching premise of routine screening may have applicability to many if not all musculoskeletal conditions (Nicholas et al., 2008, 2011).

Psychological Factor Screening by Questionnaire

Self-report psychological factor screening questionnaires are commonly used by clinicians as a component of the assessment process. The design of these questionnaires can range from unidimensional measures that provide an assessment of a specific psychological construct to multidimensional measures that provide an assessment of overall psychological distress. Each of these approaches is associated with strengths and weaknesses. For example, a potential weakness in using unidimensional questionnaires is that they do not provide information beyond the targeted psychological factor(s) of interest. In addition, it has been suggested that many commonly used unidimensional psychological screening instruments (e.g. Tampa Scale of Kinesiophobia) may be better suited for patients with persistent pain, rather than acute or sub-acute pain (Nicholas et al., 2011). On the other hand, there are potential benefits of using multidimensional instruments with a small number of items (e.g. STarT Back screening tool) for estimating patient risk of a poor outcome (based on assessment of modifiable risk factors), for example, with respect to disability, return to work and, to a lesser extent, pain (Nicholas et al., 2011; Hill and Fritz, 2011; Chou et al., 2007; Chou and Shekelle, 2010; Karran et al. 2017). Considering time is commonly indicated as a barrier to administering and interpreting questionnaires with patients in clinical settings, the use of brief multidimensional measures that have prognostic value while also highlighting for the clinician areas to explore further through the patient interview is potentially advantageous. However, although a potential strength of multidimensional questionnaires is their broader screening of psychological distress, they do not provide detailed information on specific psychological factors that may serve as behavioural treatment targets. Therefore, in later sections of this chapter, we describe a two-step screening approach that consists of using multidimensional measures to identify those patients at high risk for poor outcomes and then further screening those high-risk patients using unidimensional measures and the patient interview.

Disability and health screening questionnaires are often completed as part of an intake process. We suggest these include an initial multidimensional psychosocial screening tool. Although unidimensional psychosocial screening questionnaires can also be completed at that time, this would require prior review of the multidimensional screening scores and a judgment on which unidimensional measures to use. Also, the administering of excessive questionnaires at the one time can be overwhelming to patients. Therefore, completion of a multidimensional screening measure followed by the patient interview may be more feasible for clinical practice, and together both will assist in identifying the need for and selection of the more focused unidimensional psychosocial questionnaires to subsequently administer.

Key Points

- Multidimensional measures are capable of providing a general assessment of overall psychological distress.
- Unidimensional measures are capable of providing a more comprehensive assessment of a specific psychological construct.
- Both multidimensional and unidimensional measures are associated with individual strengths and limitations.
- We suggest clinicians attempt to incorporate both multidimensional and unidimensional measures (if appropriate), in conjunction with a thorough patient interview, to enhance the assessment of psychological distress and associated clinical reasoning.

Examples of Multidimensional Measures

STarT Back Screening Tool (SBT)

The SBT is a nine-item measure used to identify subgroups of patients associated with different levels of risk for persistent LBP-related disability based on the presence of modifiable prognostic factors which may be useful in matching patients with targeted interventions (Hill et al., 2008). The SBT contains items related to physical and psychosocial factors that have been identified as strong independent predictors for persistent, disabling LBP. The SBT overall score (ranging from 0 to 9) is determined by summing all positive responses, and the SBT psychosocial subscale score (ranging from 0 to 5) is determined by summing items related to bothersomeness, fear, catastrophizing, anxiety and depression. Based on the patient's responses, the SBT categorizes the patient as either 'high risk' (psychosocial subscale score ≥4), in which high levels of psychosocial prognostic factors are present with or without physical factors being present; 'medium risk' (overall score >3, psychosocial subscale score <4), in which physical and psychosocial factors are present, but not a high level of psychosocial factors; or 'low risk' (overall score 0–3), in which few prognostic factors are present (Hill et al., 2008). Other studies on the horizon should (and will) further evaluate the capabilities of these multidimensional tools and do so in different capacities (i.e. purely prognostic capabilities versus treatment that is provided based on stratification strategies) while also evaluating different screening instruments' prognostic accuracy for specific outcome parameters. For example, Karran et al. (2016) demonstrated that the accuracy of the risk assessment classification via a range of prognostic screening instruments administered within the first 3 months of an episode of LBP is best for predicting return to work (>80% probability), somewhat less accurate for predicting persistent disability (70%–80% probability), and least accurate for predicting persistent pain (60%–70% probability), highlighting the importance of considering different outcome dimensions when seeking prognostic information. As with any new and evolving area of research, clinicians need caution in relying on a single measure, and hence the three-dimensional approach to psychosocial factor assessment recommended in this chapter incorporates multidimensional questionnaires, unidimensional questionnaires and the patient interview.

Örebro Musculoskeletal Pain Screening Questionnaire (OMPSQ)

The OMPSQ was originally developed to assist primary care practitioners in identifying psychosocial 'yellow flags' and patients at risk for future work disability due to pain. The OMPSQ is a 25-item screening questionnaire (of which 21 are scored) that consists of items involving pain location (item 4), work absence due to pain (item 5), pain duration (item 6), pain intensity (items 8 and 9), control over pain (item 11), frequency of pain episodes (item 10), functional ability (items 20–24), mood (items 12 and 13), perceptions of work (items 7 and 16), patient's estimate of prognosis (items 14 and 15) and fear avoidance (items 17–19) (Linton and Hallden, 1997). The scored items are summed to provide a total score potentially ranging from 0 to 210, with higher scores indicating a higher risk of poor outcome. The ability of the OMPSQ to predict long-term pain, disability and sick leave has been supported in previous studies (Maher and Grotle, 2009), including a notable systematic review (Hockings et al., 2008). Karran et al. (2016) similarly found the OMPSQ was 'excellent' for discriminating workers at risk of prolonged absenteeism, and they reported that this was regardless of country and across varied clinical settings, supporting its wider utility for return-to-work risk assessment. A 10-item short-form OMPSQ (Linton et al., 2012) has been shown to have similar properties to the long version.

Examples of Unidimensional Measures

Fear Avoidance Beliefs Questionnaire (FABQ)

The FABQ assesses the degree of fear-avoidance beliefs specific to LBP (Waddell et al., 1993); however, modified versions have been used for other body regions (Piva et al., 2009; Hart et al., 2009; Cleland et al., 2008; Simon et al., 2011). The FABQ consists of a 4-item FABQ physical activity scale (FABQ-PA; score potentially ranging from 0 to 24) and a 7-item FABQ work scale (FABQ-W; score potentially ranging from 0 to 42), with higher scores indicating higher levels of fear avoidance for both FABQ scales.

Pain Catastrophizing Scale (PCS)

The PCS assesses the degree of exaggerated negative orientation toward actual or anticipated pain experiences and catastrophic cognitions due to musculoskeletal pain (Sullivan et al., 1995). The PCS consists of 13 items with a potential score range from 0 to 52, with higher scores indicating higher levels of pain catastrophizing (Sullivan et al., 1995).

Tampa Scale of Kinesiophobia (TSK-11)

The TSK-11 assesses the degree of fear of movement and injury or re-injury (Woby et al., 2005). The TSK-11 consists of 11 items with a potential score range from 11 to 44, with higher scores indicating greater fear of movement and increased injury or re-injury due to painful symptoms.

Pain Anxiety Symptoms Scale (PASS-20)

The PASS-20 assesses the degree of pain-related anxiety symptoms for individuals with pain disorders (McCracken and Dhingra, 2002). The PASS-20 consists of 20 items with a potential score range from 0 to 100, with higher scores indicating elevated symptoms of pain-related anxiety.

Patient Health Questionnaire (PHQ-9)

The PHQ-9 assesses the degree of depressive symptoms (Kroenke et al., 2001). The PHQ-9 consists of nine items with a potential score range from 0 to 27, with higher scores indicating elevated depressive symptoms.

Pain Self-Efficacy Questionnaire (PSEQ)

The PSEQ assesses the degree of self-efficacy beliefs in the context of pain that can be either low or high (Nicholas, 2007). The PSEQ consists of 10 items with a potential score range from 0 to 60, with higher scores indicating elevated levels of pain-related self-efficacy, which is a positive prognostic indicator.

Chronic Pain Acceptance Questionnaire (CPAQ)

The CPAQ assesses the degree of pain acceptance from a functional perspective by focusing on behavioural aspects (McCracken et al., 2004). The CPAQ consists of 20 items with a potential score range from 0 to 120, with higher scores indicating an increased level of pain acceptance, also a positive prognostic indicator.

Brief Illness Perception Questionnaire (Brief IPQ)

The Brief IPQ assesses cognitive and emotional representations of illness (Broadbent et al., 2006). The Brief IPQ consists of nine items rated using a 0–10 scale, except for the causal question. Five of the items assess cognitive illness representations: consequences (item 1), timeline (item 2), personal control (item 3), treatment control (item 4) and identity (item 5). Two of the items assess emotional representations: concern (item 6) and emotions (item 8). One item assesses illness comprehensibility (item 7). An open-ended response is provided so that patients are able to list the three most important causal factors of their illness (item 9).

Psychological Factor Screening by Patient Interview

The patient interview is an essential component of a musculoskeletal clinical examination, with respect to both information gathering and associated clinical reasoning and establishment of the patient–therapist therapeutic alliance. It provides the framework for psychological factor screening by questionnaire in an iterative process, with questionnaires providing standardized, measurable assessments supplemented by more in-depth exploration and qualification through the initial patient interview and ongoing discussions. Assessing for psychological factors by interview and questionnaire interconnects to the 'patient's perspective on his or her experience' hypothesis category discussed in Chapter 1. Formulation of unique patient perspectives associated with pain and disability experiences was discussed in greater detail in Chapter 3. Assessment of patient perspectives incorporates aspects such as the following:

- Patients' understanding of their problem (including attributions about the cause, beliefs about pain and associated cognitions)
- Patients' responses to stressors in their lives and any relationship these have with their clinical presentation
- Effects the problem and any stressors appear to have on patients' thoughts, feelings, coping, motivation and self-efficacy to actively participate in management and the recovery process
- Effects the problem and any stressors appear to have on patients' work or social participation
- Patients' goals and expectations for management

When assessing patients' perceptions of their problem (e.g. diagnosis, pain), it is important to question sufficiently to discover their unique perspectives with respect to the potential nature of cause, management and likely recovery trajectory – that is, their 'illness (problem) schema' (Leventhal et al., 1980). As Chapter 3 describes, research into patients' health and disability perspectives highlights important components that make up patients' understanding/beliefs and concerns about their problem. Greater understanding of the components that comprise patients' perceptions of their problems assists in knowing what to listen for and what to more overtly screen for, as psychosocially oriented information often emerges spontaneously during patient and clinician interactions. The 'self-regulation model' proposes that internal (e.g. experience of symptoms) and external (e.g. medical, family, media warnings) experiences that patients perceive as threats (e.g. to body/health, self, life, etc.) lead patients to develop individual illness perceptions or schemas that determine how they respond to those threats (Leventhal et al., 1998). Illness perceptions represent individuals' implicit theories of their health problem(s) that they use in order to interpret and respond to health threats (see also the discussion of the stress and coping model in Chapter 3). Illness perceptions across different musculoskeletal pain conditions have been shown to be related to the severity of pain, affective distress, muscle and joint tenderness, pain-related disability and poor treatment outcome (van Wilgen et al., 2014). These schemas are learned (consciously or unconsciously) through social and personal experiences and are comprised of the following elements:

- A label that identifies the problem (e.g. 'disc prolapse')
- Beliefs regarding how long they expect the problem to last
- Beliefs regarding what caused the problem
- Beliefs regarding the problem's likely effects (immediate and long-term consequences or prognosis)
- Beliefs regarding management and potential for change or coping strategies

There are also a range of dimensions that people use in evaluating their health problem, including their perception of its seriousness (e.g. self-limiting versus can't be helped), extent of impact on their life (work, family, sport, social), self-concept and self-worth (e.g. embarrassed, shame, guilt) and changeability or controllability. Therefore, it is not only patients' existing beliefs and assumptions that make up their illness perceptions and contribute to determining their coping strategies, but, as discussed in Chapter 3, it is also their 'primary appraisal' of the threat their health condition/problem poses and their 'secondary appraisal' of its controllability. This highlights the importance of assessing, and if necessary addressing through education and cognition-targeted activities and exercise (Nijs et al., 2011, 2014), the patient's threat appraisal (Jones and Edwards, 2006; Louw and Puentedura, 2018; Moseley, 2004; Moseley and Butler, 2017).

While questioning to understand the patient's activity and participation restrictions and capabilities, areas to listen for and explicitly screen as part of a psychological factor assessment by clinical interview can include the following:

- What are the patient's perspectives of his or her pain/disability experience with respect to the following:
  - Their understanding of the diagnosis/problem?
  - Their understanding of pain (e.g. acute versus chronic)?
  - Excessively negative cognitions (e.g. catastrophizing) associated with the problem?

- Their emotions (e.g. depressive symptoms, feelings of vulnerability) associated with the problem?
  - Their goals and future predictions?
  - Their expectations and beliefs about management and their role in management?
- What is the basis of the patient's beliefs and expectations?
- How does the patient think he or she is perceived by partner, workmates and employer, and how does this affect how the patient feels about him- or herself with respect to:
  - What they can and cannot do?
  - Their perceptions of their contributions?
  - Their self-concept and conception of self-worth?
- Does the patient perceive they have social support from family, friends, work mates, employers?
- How is the patient coping, emotionally (e.g., anger, depressive symptoms, feelings of vulnerability, etc.) and behaviorally? Do they have any specific coping strategies (e.g. medication, rest, alcohol, medication, exercise, avoidance), and if so, are they effective?
- Is change important to the patient? If so, to what extent and in regard to what domain? Does the patient display self-efficacy to positively contribute to change? What tasks does the patient currently believe he or she can perform? What tasks does the patient believe he or she will be able to return to following management?
- What is the patient's threat appraisal with respect to:
  - Seriousness?
  - Vulnerability?
  - Extent of impact on their life, on activity and participation (work, home, sport, social), and on their relationships?
  - Changeability and controllability?

These areas should be considered as a suggested framework only, and not as a prescribed list or set sequence of questions that must be followed. Realistically, there will be some degree of overlap in regard to patient perspectives and threat appraisal because they are both capable of influencing one another to a certain extent, particularly for individuals experiencing chronic musculoskeletal pain. Whereas patient interview questions directed at understanding the patient's problem(s) and associated musculoskeletal 'diagnostic reasoning' typically follow a routine structure, question timing and structure to assess psychosocial status will vary according to a patient's readiness for this line of enquiry and the rapport established. Although some patients will spontaneously offer much of this information (hence the importance of knowing what to listen for), for others, it will take longer for them to feel comfortable discussing non-physical issues related to their problem. This point emphasizes the importance of establishing a therapeutic alliance with an effective collaborative relationship between the patient and clinician very early during an episode of care. When assessing patient perspectives by interview, commencing with a question regarding the patient's understanding of the problem followed by clarification of why the patient has that understanding is less intrusive and hence generally accepted. Moreover, acknowledging patient efforts to change (i.e. improve) whenever possible is recommended because this strategy will potentially help foster a collaborative relationship and enhance patient motivation. If clues in the patient interview regarding, for example, patient fears, repeated negative statements, stress, adverse coping or depression do emerge, then further assessment through the use of unidimensional questionnaires can still be conducted.

Three Avenues for Psychological Factor Screening and Monitoring

Thus, as the reader might have gleaned, three avenues exist for psychological factor screening: direct communication with the patient in the form of formal interview and ongoing discussions, and both multidimensional and unidimensional questionnaires (Beneciuk et al., 2014; Mirkhil and Kent, 2009; Nicholas et al., 2011; Bergbom et al., 2014). Traditionally, screening for pathological disease (e.g. cardiovascular disease) should occur prior to the onset of symptoms, with one rationale being that the risk of poor outcome is decreased if certain diseases are detected early and managed accordingly. This rationale for early screening can also be applied to psychological factors which have the potential to adversely influence musculoskeletal pain outcomes (e.g. transition to chronicity) if not identified and addressed early during the episode of care.

A concrete example of the three-avenue screening process would consist of (1) the patient interview to understand, in conjunction with diagnostically oriented inquiries, the patient's context (e.g. living, work, social and economic circumstances, activity/fitness/exercise behaviours) and the patient's 'perspectives on the pain/disability experience'; (2) a multidimensional measure (e.g. STarT Back screening tool for patients with LBP) to identify those at high risk of persistent disability primarily based on the influence of psychological factors; and (3) unidimensional measures to specifically identify psychological factors to target with treatment (e.g. pain-related fear) that should be administered close to initiating treatment and can be used to monitor responses to psychologically informed interventions. Although we are suggesting that unidimensional measures be used specifically for patients identified as being at high risk for persistent disability, we also acknowledge that they may similarly enhance clinical reasoning for other patients when, in certain cases, the adverse influence of a particular psychological construct may become apparent during the patient interview, thus requiring more objective assessment. Ongoing discussions with the patient are then iteratively used to clarify select responses from multidimensional and unidimensional screening questionnaires and to provide further depth of understanding regarding the patient's perspectives on his or her experiences (Fig. 4.1).

Utilization of multidimensional and unidimensional (if appropriate) questionnaires will ensure a standardized screening and assessment process for all patients that will provide information to enhance clinical reasoning regarding psychological (yellow flag) factors. On the other hand, lack of a standardized assessment process can lead to self-selecting which patients are best suited for psychological factor screening, which has the potential to bias clinical decision-making. The patient interview provides further screening and allows for open-ended responses which may provide additional insight related to the patient's perspective. Ongoing follow-up communication to clarify responses from unidimensional measures and continued exploration of the patient's pain and disability experiences that often emerge as the therapeutic relationship develops are both important and should continue during the entire episode of care. That is, understanding a patient's psychosocial status takes time, and clinicians should be cognisant that initial findings may change rapidly for better or worse following communication with a healthcare provider and initiation of treatment. Facilitation of self-disclosure is a specific strategy that can be used to encourage patients to discuss their concerns about their problems and may serve as a method to collaboratively engage patients in clinical decision-making. For example, item responses on unidimensional

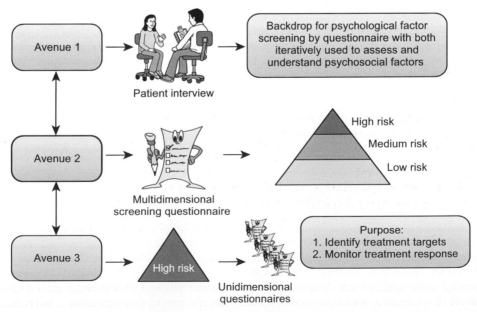

Fig. 4.1   Iterative three-avenue psychological factor screening.

questionnaires (e.g. TSK-11) can be more fully understood by having patients elaborate as to why they feel they may become injured with exercise (as a specific example). It is essential that patients understand that the purpose of discussion regarding the completed questionnaire is to better understand their perspectives on their responses. Following this explanation, it is best to employ open questions regarding completed questionnaires, such as, 'After reviewing your responses, I realize that you may be fearful of certain activities because you think they will make your problem worse – can you tell me more about that?'

Collectively, responses from multidimensional measures and information gathered during the patient interview can guide whether unidimensional psychosocial measures need to be administered, and if so, which constructs require further exploration that can subsequently be targeted with psychologically informed interventions and monitored accordingly. In the event that the patient is not identified as being at high risk for a poor outcome using multidimensional measures, and the interview also does not suggest further screening is necessary, then the administration of unidimensional measures is arguably not required. However, as previously discussed, further questioning regarding the patient's perspectives on his or her experiences is still warranted to fully understand the 'person behind the problem'.

An additional consideration is that information obtained during psychological assessment has the potential to vary based on the timing (e.g. pre-treatment, over an episode of care, post-treatment) and number of repeated assessments (Wand et al., 2009; Dunn and Croft, 2006; Sieben et al., 2002; Turner et al., 2007; Hart et al., 2011; Werneke et al., 2011), with some studies indicating that changes in psychological risk factors may improve the prediction of clinical outcomes when compared with pre-treatment assessments (Sieben et al., 2002; Turner et al., 2007; Hart et al., 2011; Werneke et al., 2011). The clinical relevance of these findings is that changes in psychological risk factors have potential not only for use as prognostic indicators administered at the initial patient encounter but also for treatment monitoring (i.e. re-assessment) during a patient encounter, particularly for psychologically oriented interventions (van der Windt et al., 2008; Nicholas et al., 2011; Bergbom et al., 2014). Although potentially appealing, using a single measure for multiple purposes (e.g. prognostic screening and treatment monitoring) is not always appropriate because many screening measures were developed to be used only as brief triage instruments and are not capable of providing specific information or being responsive to change. Nevertheless, if, for example, a patient's beliefs regarding the problem were judged to be unhelpful and possibly contributing to the patient's pain and disability, those beliefs would not only be targeted within both the education and physical activity or exercise management provided, they would also need to be reassessed to determine if those negative beliefs had changed for better or worse throughout the course of management (see the research on social support and LBP discussed in Chapter 3 for a further perspective). Therefore, we advocate for early re-assessments during an episode of care so that the clinician is provided with important clinical decision-making information that can be used to determine whether treatment modifications are required, sooner as opposed to later.

Key Points

- The patient interview provides an avenue to understand the patient's context and perspectives on his or her pain and disability experience, and related categories of information regarding patient perspectives to listen for and screen are proposed.
- A multidimensional measure provides an avenue to identify patients at high risk for poor clinical outcomes primarily based on the influence of psychological factors.
- Utilization of unidimensional measures (if appropriate) provides an avenue to enhance clinical reasoning regarding psychological (yellow flag) factors.

Psychological Factor Management

Several opportunities exist for musculoskeletal clinicians to provide interventions that target psychological factors that may influence the development and maintenance of chronic musculoskeletal pain and therefore enhance musculoskeletal management generally. We fully acknowledge that in extreme cases, psychological distress could require referral to another provider. However, more commonly, psychological distress is a precursor of delayed recovery or an indication for psychologically informed interventions that could provide better outcomes than standard treatment approaches alone (Nicholas and George, 2011; Nicholas et al., 2011).

It is important to appreciate that stress in a person's life can be minor or more significant; that is, it occurs along a continuum. Similarly, the psychological response to stress (distress) also occurs along a continuum. Pincus and colleagues (Pincus and Morley, 2001; Pincus, 2004; Rusu and Pincus, 2012) discuss continuums of stress and distress associated with pain and disability. Some patients present with selective attention to sensory information, low levels of fear avoidance of movement perceived as dangerous and frustration with their activity and participation restrictions. Many of these patients will either adjust to this themselves over time or will respond well to education and activation strategies, such as graded activity. Generally, the greater the pain- and disability-associated stress, the greater the distress, with the emergence of catastrophizing cognitions, hypervigilance and broader fear avoidance being common in chronic pain presentations. Higher levels of distress where the person's negative cognitions and emotions regarding his or her pain and disability become integrated with the person's self-concept and self-worth (see schema enmeshment theory [Pincus and Morley, 2001]) can lead to emotions of helplessness, hopelessness, guilt and despair associated with depression. Musculoskeletal clinicians with training in the provision of pain education and cognitive-behavioural application of activity promotion and exercise are well placed to manage patients' unhelpful/maladaptive cognitions and behaviours at the lower end of these continuums. However, at the higher end, as with clinical depression, and when stressors include issues outside of clinicians' scope of practice, such as a relationship breakdown, clinicians need to facilitate referral to other, more qualified mental health professionals. Importantly, referral to a psychologist (for example) does not necessarily equate to discharge from musculoskeletal therapy, as pain education, activity promotion and exercise are still important, and optimal management will likely involve the integration of musculoskeletal therapy and psychology (Johnson and Moores, 2006).

As previously described, psychologically informed musculoskeletal practice emphasizes (1) identification of individuals who are at high risk of developing chronic pain based on the presence of psychological distress and (2) targeted treatment aimed at psychological factors in conjunction with traditional, impairment-based musculoskeletal therapy (Main and George, 2011). From a clinical reasoning perspective and specifically related to musculoskeletal pain, this approach to management is consistent with prognostic stratified care that has been investigated for LBP and which has been described as targeting treatment to subgroups of patients based on key characteristics (e.g. psychological factors) (Foster et al., 2013).

What follows is an example of the three-avenue psychological factor screening and assessment process and one particular yellow flag management approach for LBP that consists of a sensitive initial screening using a multidimensional measure followed by the patient interview, then a more comprehensive third-order assessment using a battery of unidimensional measures. Realistically, administering a multidimensional measure prior to the patient interview may not always be feasible in the clinical setting; however, we strongly suggest that both are incorporated early during an episode of care. The STarT Back screening tool is being used to illustrate a patient scenario related to LBP. We acknowledge that further research is needed to establish the clinical utility of the STarT Back screening tool (and other screening tools) to determine if similar targeted treatment approaches based on responses to these tools are generalizable to other musculoskeletal conditions. Nonetheless, we support the general principle of the three-avenue screening and assessment process as described here as a strategy to further enhance clinical reasoning.

The STarT Back screening tool (SBT) is used as the first-order screening to categorize patients into one of three subgroups (low, medium or high risk) for persistent LBP-related disability. For patients categorized as high risk on the SBT, clinical reasoning can be enhanced by the patient interview to both clarify issues highlighted in the SBT screening and to gain further understanding of the patient, including the context of the patient's problems and his or her perspectives on the experience. Together, the SBT and the patient interview can guide the selection of appropriate unidimensional psychological measures. Information obtained through the unidimensional measure screening can then be used to identify specific psychological factors that may be negatively impacting the patient's pain and disability experience (and can potentially be targeted by musculoskeletal clinicians through direct treatment). Because two patients can provide the same response for quite different reasons, clarification of select interview and unidimensional measure responses is used to better understand the meaning and basis of those responses (refer to the previous discussion of facilitation of self-disclosure), thus providing explicit targets for psychosocially oriented treatment strategies such as pain belief education and cognition-targeted exercise.

Brief Case Example

A 38-year-old female presents with LBP following an afternoon of gardening at home 2 weeks prior. The patient was administered the SBT, and based on her responses, she was categorized as 'high risk' for persistent disability. During the patient interview, she was asked to elaborate on her perception of the current pain experience and indicated she felt hopeless and was very concerned that her condition would never improve because a friend experienced similar symptoms several years ago and ultimately received surgical intervention. Additional information collectively obtained during the patient interview and supported by careful clarification of responses to the SBT also indicated that (1) she was avoiding any physical activity due to concerns her symptoms would become worse, and (2) this was the worst experience she had ever had.

Based on the information obtained, the patient was subsequently administered the Fear-Avoidance Beliefs Questionnaire (FABQ) and Pain Catastrophizing Scale (PCS) to enhance clinical reasoning regarding fear of physical activity (via the FABQ – physical activity scale) and catastrophic cognitions (via the PCS). Over the course of treatment, the clinician was then able to compare these early scores to later scores (e.g. 1–2 weeks) to monitor for change and progress (or lack thereof). This information was then used to determine if modification of the treatment plan was necessary.

It is beyond the scope of this chapter to present the details of the psychologically informed management for this patient. Instead, key principles and general strategies for psychologically informed musculoskeletal therapy management are presented. Examples of specific strategies for psychologically informed musculoskeletal therapy management through education and activity are covered in several chronic pain case studies later in this book.

Management

In the case of LBP, suggested targeted treatment pathways are matched to each SBT subgroup such that patients categorized as low risk receive minimal care, primarily consisting of reassurance, education and self-management, with the potential to benefit from minimal therapy based on physical examination findings. Patients categorized as medium risk also receive reassurance and education, but their treatment is supplemented with therapy focused on restoring function and targeting physical signs identified from the physical examination. For patients categorized as high risk, therapy is focused on restoring function using a combination of physical and psychological approaches (described in greater detail later in this case study).

Prior to providing descriptions of how communication style, education and activity-based interventions can be implemented to target previously identified psychological factors, it is important to acknowledge that skilled communication strategies can (and should) be used to enhance other interventions. Importantly, skilled communication can enhance clinical reasoning by providing clinicians with information that otherwise may not be detected.

Communication Style

Musculoskeletal clinicians should incorporate effective communication skills, including active listening, facilitation of self-disclosure, empathy and collaborative decision-making, in order to optimize the patient–clinician therapeutic alliance (as discussed in Chapter 1). Active listening skills are important for picking up potentially relevant information spontaneously offered by patients, for example, regarding their expectations, beliefs and behaviours related to pain and physical activity (as discussed in Chapter 3). Previous studies have indicated relationships between patient expectations and musculoskeletal therapy outcomes (Bishop et al., 2011, 2013), with findings from an experimental study suggesting the potential role that clinicians may have in influencing patient expectations (Bialosky et al., 2008). Facilitation of self-disclosure is enhanced when rapport is good and when the patient perceives genuine interest from their clinician. Skilled communication through the psychosocial screening not only elicits more relevant information important to making a judgment regarding the patient's perspectives on his or her experiences and in identifying negative psychological factors to address in management, but it also enriches the therapeutic relationship and is

Continued on following page

Brief Case Example (Continued)

important for optimizing outcomes (Ferreira et al., 2013; Hall et al., 2010).

Education-Based Approaches

Musculoskeletal clinicians should consider incorporating a combination of educational approaches where psychosocial factors are judged to be contributing to patients' pain and disability. Education-based approaches commonly include 'pain neuroscience' and 'activation philosophy' as two broad components. A systematic review of available randomized controlled trials supports the use of pain neuroscience education for changing pain beliefs and improving health status in patients with chronic musculoskeletal pain (Louw et al., 2011), and guidelines for application of pain neuroscience education are readily available (Nijs et al., 2011; van Wilgen and Keizer, 2012). Content related to pain neuroscience can be used to provide a general overview about the nature of pain, neurophysiological processes associated with pain perception, mechanisms of pain associated with the development of disability, and the role of psychosocial factors in transitioning from acute to chronic pain. Ideally, information is contextualized to the patient's unique presentation, for example, by referring to specific unhelpful beliefs, behaviours and social factors uncovered in the overall psychosocial factor screening when discussing different pain neuroscience constructs. Importantly, pain neuroscience education should not unduly focus on biomedical constructs such as pathology, biomechanics and anatomical structures. Although we acknowledge that there is the potential for a direct link between musculoskeletal pain symptoms, anatomical structures, pathology (e.g. disc bulge) and biomechanics, when the intent is to target psychological obstacles, the language of physical impairments (mobility, control/strength, fitness, etc.) rather than that of pathology is advised, particularly for those patients who already overly focus on pathology and demonstrate maladaptive fears, hypervigilance and catastrophization. When pathology is raised, skill is needed to acknowledge confirmed pathology, explain that pathology can be asymptomatic and reassure the patient that any exercises and graded activity recommended will not cause them harm. Two excellent resources to assist clinicians understanding and application of pain neuroscience education are the texts Explain Pain Supercharged by Moseley and Butler (2017) and Pain Neuroscience Education. Vol 2. by Louw, Puentedura, Schmidt & Zimney (2018).

In general, activation philosophies involve encouraging patients to be active participants in the recovery process (Nicholas and George, 2011). Activation philosophy strategies can be used to provide patients with reassurance (e.g. there is no permanent damage) and encouragement to resume normal activities (if appropriate), as well as to emphasize positive attitudes and coping styles. However, providing passive reassurance in the form of pamphlets or booklets alone is not sufficient. Previous review studies (Nicholas and George, 2011; Linton et al., 2008) have indicated the vital importance of addressing specific patient concerns or misapprehensions during educational approaches that incorporate an activation philosophy component. Moreover, the importance of incorporating an education-based approach involving activation philosophy content within an activity-based approach (described later in this case study) has been previously highlighted (Nicholas and George, 2011). This requires clinical judgments (i.e. 'reasoning about teaching'; see Chapter 1) regarding when to address patient concerns and misapprehensions, how best to challenge existing beliefs and present alternatives, when to initiate activation philosophy discussions, how much to cover at a single time, and re-assessment to determine understanding, acceptance and integration of new perspectives. Pain neuroscience education and activation philosophy are important precursors to promote adaptive pain and activity beliefs prior to commencing activity-based interventions, and education needs to continue throughout any cognition-targeted activities and prescribed exercise (Nijs et al., 2011, 2014). Equally, education and interventions specifically tailored to address pain coping strategies are vitally important for successful management, as discussed in some of this book's patient cases (for example, see Chapters 9, 13, 14, 24 and 25).

Activity-Based Approaches

Information obtained through psychological (and social) factor screening assessments can also be utilized to enhance clinical reasoning during the planning of activity-based interventions. Two common activity-based approaches are graded exercise or activity and graded exposure, which are described in greater detail elsewhere (Nicholas and George, 2011). Graded exercise or activity encourages continued activity despite the presence of pain and utilizes a quota-based system (Nicholas and George, 2011). For example, baseline levels (i.e. initial quotas) are first determined by having the patient perform an activity (e.g. treadmill walking) until limited by pain tolerance. Initial quotas serve as the basis for subsequent treatment sessions and should be set relatively low (e.g. 60%) to optimize success because successful completion of prescribed exercise and activity is in itself usually reinforcing. An important component of this treatment strategy is patient participation in goal setting because this contributes to guiding subsequent quota increases. The activities and exercises utilized should not only be

Brief Case Example (Continued)

time-contingent, but they should also be 'cognition targeted', that is, reinforcing of previous pain education by addressing the patient's unhelpful cognitions regarding the problem during the activity and exercise instruction, and they should be practiced with progression from more simple (including motor imagery) to more complex activities and exercise (Nijs et al., 2014).

Alternatively, graded exposure is primarily for patients presenting with high levels of fear and avoidance behaviours and utilizes a hierarchical exposure approach (Nicholas and George, 2011). For example, fearful activities (e.g. forward bending to retrieve objects from ground level) are specifically identified, and low levels of those activities are initially incorporated into the treatment plan. As the level of fear decreases, the level of activity subsequently increases. The Fear of Daily Activities Questionnaire (FDAQ) provides an example of a self-report measure that can be utilized to specifically

identify fearful activities and levels of fear associated with those activities that can then be used to monitor treatment responses (George et al., 2009). George and Zeppieri (2009) have previously described how the FDAQ can be used to positively impact clinical reasoning during the management of patients with LBP. The principle underpinning both graded activity/exercise and graded exposure is 'exposure without danger' to reduce maladaptive pain memories associated with maintained pain and pain behaviours (Zusman, 2004, 2008). The combination of pain neuroscience education assisting patients to reconceptualize their perceptions of danger followed by cognition-targeted graded activity/exercise or graded exposure (as required) facilitates increased activity and participation capability. More specific details for implementation of cognition-targeted interventions are provided elsewhere (Nijs et al., 2014, 2015), with examples also presented in some case studies in this book.

Key Points

- Skilled communication (including active listening, facilitation of self-disclosure, empathy and collaborative decision-making) is essential to optimize the patient–clinician therapeutic alliance, the extent to which the patient shares his or her full story (i.e. the patient's perspectives), the clinician's reasoning and, ultimately, the success of management.
- Education-based interventions, including 'pain neuroscience' and 'activation philosophy', are important in the management of psychosocial factors and should be supplemented with pain coping strategies.
- Activity-based interventions (e.g. graded exercise/activity and graded exposure), along with ongoing education, should be implemented collaboratively with the patient to help facilitate increased activity and participation capabilities.

Summary

Musculoskeletal pain experiences are unique to each individual patient and can be strongly influenced by psychological factors. An increased understanding of these relationships will enhance clinical reasoning, which in turn has strong potential to improve patient outcomes. In this chapter we have described a three-avenue psychological factor screening and assessment process consisting of (1) direct communication with the patient in the form of formal interview and ongoing discussions, (2) a multidimensional screening measure to identify those patients at risk of persistent disability and (3) unidimensional measures (where appropriate) to identify specific psychological factors to target and monitor through psychologically informed interventions. The overall intent of this chapter is to provide musculoskeletal clinicians with strategies and understandings to enhance their clinical reasoning by embracing a biopsychosocial framework with special emphasis placed on psychological factors.

REFERENCES

Barlow, S., 2012. The barriers to implementation of evidence-based chronic pain management in rural and regional physiotherapy outpatients: realising the potential [Online]. NSW Ministry of Health. Available: www.aci.health.nsw.gov.au 2015].

Beneciuk, J.M., Fritz, J.M., George, S.Z., 2014. The STarT Back Screening Tool for prediction of 6-month clinical outcomes: relevance of change patterns in outpatient physical therapy settings. J. Orthop. Sports Phys. Ther. 44, 656–664.

Bergbom, S., Boersma, K., Linton, S.J., 2014. When matching fails: understanding the process of matching pain-disability treatment to risk profile. J. Occup. Rehabil. 25 (3), 518–526.

Bialosky, J.E., Bishop, M.D., Robinson, M.E., Barabas, J.A., George, S.Z., 2008. The influence of expectation on spinal manipulation induced hypoalgesia: an experimental study in normal subjects. BMC Musculoskelet. Disord. 9, 19.

Bishop, M.D., Bialosky, J.E., Cleland, J.A., 2011. Patient expectations of benefit from common interventions for low back pain and effects on outcome: secondary analysis of a clinical trial of manual therapy interventions. J. Man. Manip. Ther. 19, 20–25.

Bishop, A., Foster, N.E., 2005. Do physical therapists in the United Kingdom recognize psychosocial factors in patients with acute low back pain? Spine 30, 1316–1322.

Bishop, M.D., Mintken, P.E., Bialosky, J.E., Cleland, J.A., 2013. Patient expectations of benefit from interventions for neck pain and resulting influence on outcomes. J. Orthop. Sports Phys. Ther. 43, 457–465.

Borrell-Carrio, F., Suchman, A.L., Epstein, R.M., 2004. The biopsychosocial model 25 years later: principles, practice, and scientific inquiry. Ann. Fam. Med. 2, 576–582.

Broadbent, E., Petrie, K.J., Main, J., Weinman, J., 2006. The brief illness perception questionnaire. J. Psychosom. Res. 60, 631–637.

Burton, A.K., Tillotson, K.M., Main, C.J., Hollis, S., 1995. Psychosocial predictors of outcome in acute and subchronic low back trouble. Spine 20, 722–728.

Chou, R., Qaseem, A., Snow, V., Casey, D., Cross, J.T., Jr., Shekelle, P., et al., 2007. Diagnosis and treatment of low back pain: a joint clinical practice guideline from the American College of Physicians and the American Pain Society. Ann. Intern. Med. 147, 478–491.

Chou, R., Shekelle, P., 2010. Will this patient develop persistent disabling low back pain? JAMA 303, 1295–1302.

Cleland, J.A., Fritz, J.M., Childs, J.D., 2008. Psychometric properties of the Fear-Avoidance Beliefs Questionnaire and Tampa Scale of Kinesiophobia in patients with neck pain. Am. J. Phys. Med. Rehabil. 87, 109–117.

Daykin, A.R., Richardson, B., 2004. Physiotherapists' pain beliefs and their influence on the management of patients with chronic low back pain. Spine 29, 783–795.

Dunn, K.M., Croft, P.R., 2006. Repeat assessment improves the prediction of prognosis in patients with low back pain in primary care. Pain 126, 10–15.

Edwards, I., Jones, M., Carr, J., Braunack-Mayer, A., Jensen, G.M., 2004. Clinical reasoning strategies in physical therapy. Phys. Ther. 84, 312–330, discussion 331–335.

Ferreira, P.H., Ferreira, M.L., Maher, C.G., Refshauge, K.M., Latimer, J., Adams, R.D., 2013. The therapeutic alliance between clinicians and patients predicts outcome in chronic low back pain. Phys. Ther. 93, 470–478.

Foster, N.E., Delitto, A., 2011. Embedding psychosocial perspectives within clinical management of low back pain: integration of psychosocially informed management principles into physical therapist practice–challenges and opportunities. Phys. Ther. 91, 790–803.

Foster, N.E., Hill, J.C., O'Sullivan, P., Hancock, M., 2013. Stratified models of care. Best Pract. Res. Clin. Rheumatol. 27, 649–661.

Foster, N.E., Thomas, E., Bishop, A., Dunn, K.M., Main, C.J., 2010. Distinctiveness of psychological obstacles to recovery in low back pain patients in primary care. Pain 148, 398–406.

French, S., Sim, J., 2004. Physiotherapy: A Psychosocial Approach. Elsevier, Edinburgh.

George, S.Z., Coronado, R.A., Beneciuk, J.M., Valencia, C., Werneke, M.W., Hart, D.L., 2011. Depressive symptoms, anatomical region, and clinical outcomes for patients seeking outpatient physical therapy for musculoskeletal pain. Phys. Ther. 91, 358–372.

George, S.Z., Dover, G.C., Fillingim, R.B., 2007. Fear of pain influences outcomes after exercise-induced delayed onset muscle soreness at the shoulder. Clin. J. Pain 23, 76–84.

George, S.Z., Valencia, C., Zeppieri, G., Jr., Robinson, M.E., 2009. Development of a self-report measure of fearful activities for patients with low back pain: the fear of daily activities questionnaire. Phys. Ther. 89, 969–979.

George, S.Z., Zeppieri, G., 2009. Physical therapy utilization of graded exposure for patients with low back pain. J. Orthop. Sports Phys. Ther. 39, 496–505.

Haggman, S., Maher, C.G., Refshauge, K.M., 2004. Screening for symptoms of depression by physical therapists managing low back pain. Phys. Ther. 84, 1157–1166.

Hall, A.M., Ferreira, P.H., Maher, C.G., Latimer, J., Ferreira, M.L., 2010. The influence of the therapist–patient relationship on treatment outcome in physical rehabilitation: a systematic review. Phys. Ther. 90, 1099–1110.

Hart, D.L., Werneke, M.W., Deutscher, D., George, S.Z., Stratford, P.W., Mioduski, J.E., 2011. Using intake and change in multiple psychosocial measures to predict functional status outcomes in people with lumbar spine syndromes: a preliminary analysis. Phys. Ther. 91, 1812–1825.

Hart, D.L., Werneke, M.W., George, S.Z., Matheson, J.W., Wang, Y.C., Cook, K.F., et al., 2009. Screening for elevated levels of fear-avoidance beliefs regarding work or physical activities in people receiving outpatient therapy. Phys. Ther. 89, 770–785.

Hartigan, E.H., Lynch, A.D., Logerstedt, D.S., Chmielewski, T.L., Snyder-Mackler, L., 2013. Kinesiophobia after anterior cruciate ligament rupture and reconstruction: noncopers versus potential copers. J. Orthop. Sports Phys. Ther. 43, 821–832.

Hasenbring, M., Rusu, A., Turk, D., 2012. From Acute to Chronic Back Pain: Risk Factors, Mechanisms, and Clinical Implications. Oxford University Press, Oxford.

Hill, J.C., Dunn, K.M., Lewis, M., Mullis, R., Main, C.J., Foster, N.E., et al., 2008. A primary care back pain screening tool: identifying patient subgroups for initial treatment. Arthritis Rheum. 59, 632–641.

Hill, J.C., Fritz, J.M., 2011. Psychosocial influences on low back pain, disability, and response to treatment. Phys. Ther. 91, 712–721.

Hill, J.C., Lewis, M., Sim, J., Hay, E.M., Dziedzic, K., 2007. Predictors of poor outcome in patients with neck pain treated by physical therapy. Clin. J. Pain 23, 683–690.

Hockings, R.L., McAuley, J.H., Maher, C.G., 2008. A systematic review of the predictive ability of the Örebro Musculoskeletal Pain Questionnaire. Spine 33, E494–E500.

Hunt, M.A., Keefe, F.J., Bryant, C., Metcalf, B.R., Ahamed, Y., Nicholas, M.K., et al., 2013. A physiotherapist-delivered, combined exercise and pain coping skills training intervention for individuals with knee osteoarthritis: a pilot study. Knee 20, 106–112.

Institute of Medicine, 2011. Relieving Pain in America: A Blueprint for Transforming Prevention, Care, Education, and Research. The National Academies Press, Washington, DC.

Johnson, R., Moores, L., 2006. Pain management: integrating physiotherapy and clinical psychology in practice. In: Gifford, L. (Ed.), Topical Issues in Pain 5. CNS Press, Falmouth.

Jones, M., Edwards, I., 2006. Learning to facilitate change in cognition and behaviour. In: Gifford, L. (Ed.), Topical issues in pain 5. CNS Press, Falmouth.

Jones, M., Edwards, I., 2008. Clinical reasoning to facilitate cognitive-experiential change. In: Higgs, J., Jones, M., Loftus, S., Christensen, N. (Eds.), Clinical Reasoning in the Health Professions, third ed. Butterworth Heinemann Elsevier, Amsterdam.

Karran, E.L., McAuley, J.H., Traeger, A.C., Hillier, S.L., Grabherr, L., Russek, L.N., et al., 2017. Can screening instruments accurately determine poor outcome risk in adults with recent onset low back pain? A systematic review and meta-analysis. BMC Med. 15 (13), 1–15.

Karran, E., McAuley, J., Traeger, A., Hillier, S., Moseley, L., 2016. How accurate are low back pain screening instruments at determining chronic pain risk? A systematic review and meta-analysis. International Low Back and Neck Pain Forum, Buxton, United Kingdom.

Keefe, F., Scipio, C., Perri, L., 2006. Psychosocial approaches to managing pain: current status and future directions. In: Gifford, L. (Ed.), Topical Issues in Pain 5. CNS Press, Falmouth.

Kent, P.M., Keating, J.L., Taylor, N.F., 2009. Primary care clinicians use variable methods to assess acute nonspecific low back pain and usually focus on impairments. Man. Ther. 14, 88–100.

Kroenke, K., Spitzer, R.L., Williams, J.B., 2001. The PHQ-9: validity of a brief depression severity measure. J. Gen. Intern. Med. 16, 606–613.

Leventhal, H., Leventhal, E., Contrada, R., 1998. Self-regulation, health, and behavior: a perceptual-cognitive approach. Psychology & Health 3, 717–733.

Leventhal, H., Meyer, D., Nerenz, D., 1980. The common sense representation of illness danger. In: Rachman, S. (Ed.), Contributions to Medical Psychology. Pergamon Press, New York.

Linton, S.J., 2000. A review of psychological risk factors in back and neck pain. Spine 25, 1148–1156.

Linton, S.J., 2005. Do psychological factors increase the risk for back pain in the general population in both a cross-sectional and prospective analysis? Eur. J. Pain 9, 355–361.

Linton, S.J., Hallden, K., 1997. Risk factors and the natural course of acute and recurrent musculoskeletal pain: developing a screening instrument. In: Jensen, T.S., Turner, J.A., Wiesenfeld-Hallin, Z. (Eds.), Proceedings of the 8th World Congress on Pain. IASP Press, Seattle, pp. 527–536.

Linton, S.J., McCracken, L.M., Vlaeyen, J.W., 2008. Reassurance: help or hinder in the treatment of pain. Pain 134, 5–8.

Linton, S.L., Nicholas, M.K., MacDonald, S., 2012. Development of a short form of the Örebro Musculoskeletal Pain Screening Questionnaire. Spine 36 (22), 1891–1895.

Linton, S.J., Shaw, W.S., 2011. Impact of psychological factors in the experience of pain. Phys. Ther. 91, 700–711.

Louw, A., Diener, I., Butler, D.S., Puentedura, E.J., 2011. The effect of neuroscience education on pain, disability, anxiety, and stress in chronic musculoskeletal pain. Arch. Phys. Med. Rehabil. 92, 2041–2056.

Louw, A., Puentedura, E., Schmidt, S., Zimney, K., 2018. Pain Neuroscience Education, vol. 2. OPTP, Minneapolis, MN.

Maher, C.G., Grotle, M., 2009. Evaluation of the predictive validity of the Örebro Musculoskeletal Pain Screening Questionnaire. Clin. J. Pain 25, 666–670.

Main, C.J., George, S.Z., 2011. Psychologically informed practice for management of low back pain: future directions in practice and research. Phys. Ther. 91, 820–824.

Main, C., Sullivan, M., Watson, P., 2008. Pain Management: Practical Applications of the Biopsychosocial Perspective in Clinical and Occupational Settings. Churchill Livingstone Elsevier, Edinburgh.

McCracken, L.M., Dhingra, L., 2002. A short version of the Pain Anxiety Symptoms Scale (PASS-20): preliminary development and validity. Pain Res. Manag. 7, 45–50.

McCracken, L.M., Vowles, K.E., Eccleston, C., 2004. Acceptance of chronic pain: component analysis and a revised assessment method. Pain 107, 159–166.

Mirkhil, S., Kent, P.M., 2009. The diagnostic accuracy of brief screening questions for psychosocial risk factors of poor outcome from an episode of pain: a systematic review. Clin. J. Pain 25, 340–348.

Moseley, G.L., 2004. Evidence for a direct relationship between cognitive and physical change during an education intervention in people with chronic low back pain. Eur. J. Pain 8, 39–45.

Moseley, G.L., Butler, D.S., 2017. Explain Pain Supercharged. Noigroup Publications, Adelaide.

Nicholas, M.K., 2007. The pain self-efficacy questionnaire: taking pain into account. Eur. J. Pain 11, 153–163.

Nicholas, M.K., Asghari, A., Blyth, F.M., 2008. What do the numbers mean? Normative data in chronic pain measures. Pain 134, 158–173.

Nicholas, M.K., George, S.Z., 2011. Psychologically informed interventions for low back pain: an update for physical therapists. Phys. Ther. 91, 765–776.

Nicholas, M.K., Linton, S.J., Watson, P.J., Main, C.J., Decade of the Flags Working Group, 2011. Early identification and management of psychological risk factors ("yellow flags") in patients with low back pain: a reappraisal. Phys. Ther. 91, 737–753.

Nijs, J., Lluch Girbes, E., Lundberg, M., Malfliet, A., Sterling, M., 2015. Exercise therapy for chronic musculoskeletal pain: innovation by altering pain memories. Man. Ther. 20, 216–220.

Nijs, J., Meeus, M., Cagnie, B., Roussel, N.A., Dolphens, M., Van Oosterwijck, J., et al., 2014. A modern neuroscience approach to chronic spinal pain: combining pain neuroscience education with cognition-targeted motor control training. Phys. Ther. 94, 730–738.

Nijs, J., Paul Van Wilgen, C., Van Oosterwijck, J., Van Ittersum, M., Meeus, M., 2011. How to explain central sensitization to patients with 'unexplained' chronic musculoskeletal pain: practice guidelines. Man. Ther. 16, 413–418.

Overmeer, T., Linton, S.J., Holmquist, L., Eriksson, M., Engfeldt, P., 2005. Do evidence-based guidelines have an impact in primary care? A cross-sectional study of Swedish physicians and physiotherapists. Spine 30, 146–151.

Pincus, T., 2004. The psychology of pain. In: French, S., Sim, K. (Eds.), Physiotherapy: A Psychosocial Approach. Elsevier, Edinburgh.

Pincus, T., Morley, S., 2001. Cognitive-processing bias in chronic pain: a review and integration. Psychol. Bull. 127, 599–617.

Piva, S.R., Fitzgerald, G.K., Wisniewski, S., Delitto, A., 2009. Predictors of pain and function outcome after rehabilitation in patients with patellofemoral pain syndrome. J. Rehabil. Med. 41, 604–612.

Pransky, G., Borkan, J.M., Young, A.E., Cherkin, D.C., 2011. Are we making progress?: the tenth international forum for primary care research on low back pain. Spine 36, 1608–1614.

Rusu, A., Pincus, T., 2012. Cognitive processing and self-pain enmeshment in chronic back pain. In: Hasenbring, M., Rusu, A., Turk, D. (Eds.), From Acute to Chronic Back Pain. Risk Factors, Mechanisms, and Clinical Implications. Oxford University Press, Oxford.

Sanders, T., Foster, N.E., Bishop, A., Ong, B.N., 2013. Biopsychosocial care and the physiotherapy encounter: physiotherapists' accounts of back pain consultations. BMC Musculoskelet. Disord. 14, 65.

Sarda, J., Jr., Nicholas, M.K., Asghari, A., Pimenta, C.A., 2009. The contribution of self-efficacy and depression to disability and work status in chronic pain patients: a comparison between Australian and Brazilian samples. Eur. J. Pain 13, 189–195.

Sieben, J.M., Vlaeyen, J.W., Tuerlinckx, S., Portegijs, P.J., 2002. Pain-related fear in acute low back pain: the first two weeks of a new episode. Eur. J. Pain 6, 229–237.

Sim, J., Smith, M., 2004. The sociology of pain. In: French, S., Sim, J. (Eds.), Physiotherapy: A Psychosocial Approach. Elsevier, Edinburgh.

Simmonds, M.J., Derghazarian, T., Vlaeyen, J.W., 2012. Physiotherapists' knowledge, attitudes, and intolerance of uncertainty influence decision making in low back pain. Clin. J. Pain 28, 467–474.

Simon, C.B., Stryker, S.E., George, S.Z., 2011. Comparison of work-related fear-avoidance beliefs across different anatomical locations with musculoskeletal pain. J. Pain Res. 4, 253–262.

Singla, M., Jones, M., Edwards, I., Kumar, S., 2015. Physiotherapists' assessment of patients' psychosocial status: Are we standing on thin ice? A qualitative descriptive study. Man. Ther. 20, 328–334.

Smart, K., Doody, C., 2007. The clinical reasoning of pain by experienced musculoskeletal physiotherapists. Man. Ther. 12, 40–49.

Spitzer, R.L., Williams, J.B., Kroenke, K., Linzer, M., Degruy, F.V., 3rd, Hahn, S.R., et al., 1994. Utility of a new procedure for diagnosing mental disorders in primary care. The PRIME-MD 1000 study. JAMA 272, 1749–1756.

Straus, S.E., Richardson, W.S., Glasziou, P., Haynes, R.B., 2005. Evidence-Based Medicine: How to Practice and Teach EBM. Elsevier, Churchill Livingstone, New York.

Sullivan, M.J., Adams, H., Rhodenizer, T., Stanish, W.D., 2006. A psychosocial risk factor–targeted intervention for the prevention of chronic pain and disability following whiplash injury. Phys. Ther. 86, 8–18.

Sullivan, M., Bishop, S., Pivik, J., 1995. The Pain Catastrophizing Scale: development and validation. Psychol. Assess. 7, 524–532.

Sullivan, M., Tanzer, M., Stanish, W., Fallaha, M., Keefe, F.J., Simmonds, M., et al., 2009. Psychological determinants of problematic outcomes following Total Knee Arthroplasty. Pain 143, 123–129.

Turner, J.A., Holtzman, S., Mancl, L., 2007. Mediators, moderators, and predictors of therapeutic change in cognitive-behavioral therapy for chronic pain. Pain 127, 276–286.

van der Windt, D., Hay, E., Jellema, P., Main, C., 2008. Psychosocial interventions for low back pain in primary care: lessons learned from recent trials. Spine 33, 81–89.

van Wilgen, P., Beetsma, A., Neels, H., Roussel, N., Nijs, J., 2014. Physical therapists should integrate illness perceptions in their assessment in patients with chronic musculoskeletal pain; a qualitative analysis. Man. Ther. 19, 229–234.

van Wilgen, C.P., Keizer, D., 2012. The sensitization model to explain how chronic pain exists without tissue damage. Pain Manag. Nurs. 13, 60–65.

Waddell, G., Newton, M., Henderson, I., Somerville, D., Main, C.J., 1993. A Fear-Avoidance Beliefs Questionnaire (FABQ) and the role of fear-avoidance beliefs in chronic low back pain and disability. Pain 52, 157–168.

Wand, B.M., McAuley, J.H., Marston, L., De Souza, L.H., 2009. Predicting outcome in acute low back pain using different models of patient profiling. Spine 34, 1970–1975.

Werneke, M.W., Hart, D.L., George, S.Z., Deutscher, D., Stratford, P.W., 2011. Change in psychosocial distress associated with pain and functional status outcomes in patients with lumbar impairments referred to physical therapy services. J. Orthop. Sports Phys. Ther. 41, 969–980.

Woby, S.R., Roach, N.K., Urmston, M., Watson, P.J., 2005. Psychometric properties of the TSK-11: a shortened version of the Tampa Scale for Kinesiophobia. Pain 117, 137–144.

World Health Organization, 2001. International Classification of Functioning, Disability and Health. World Health Organization, Geneva.

Zusman, M., 2004. Mechanisms of musculoskeletal physiotherapy. Phys. Ther. Rev. 9, 39–49.

Zusman, M., 2008. Associative memory for movement-evoked chronic back pain and its extinction with musculoskeletal physiotherapy. Phys. Ther. Rev. 13, 57–68.

Clinical Prediction Rules: Their Benefits and Limitations in Clinical Reasoning

Robin Haskins • Chad E. Cook • Peter G. Osmotherly • Darren A. Rivett

An Overview of Statistics in Healthcare Clinical Reasoning

Decision-making in the healthcare context has undergone a long and complex evolution. Perhaps surprisingly, the explicit integration of statistics to inform certain types of clinical decisions is a relatively more recent adjunct. A key driver of this more recent focus and conscientious employment of statistics in the clinical setting has been the evidence-based movement. Statistical data regarding disease and outcome prevalence (Laupacis et al., 1994; Richardson et al., 1999), diagnostic test accuracy (Jaeschke et al., 1994) and the quantification of treatment effect (Guyatt et al., 1994), among many others, have been increasingly used to help inform clinical decision-making.

In contemporary healthcare practice, the application of statistics facilitates the transformation of data into evidence-based diagnostic, prognostic and treatment decisions (Horvitz, 2010). Several different types of statistical prediction tools have been developed for use in the clinical setting, ranging from simple actuarial tables to more computationally complex approaches, such as artificial neural networks (Baxt, 1995; Meehl, 1954). Irrespective of the type, all statistical prediction tools use statistical analysis of prior cases with known outcomes to identify the quantified relationship between predictor variables and a particular diagnosis or outcome, such that they may be used to make future predictions (Swets et al., 2000b). This is simultaneously their strength and limitation.

A notable advantage of statistical prediction tools over unassisted clinician judgement is the control of human cognitive biases that are a common contributor to decision-making errors (Grove et al., 2000; Graber et al., 2005). Such errors in clinical problem solving are thought, at least in part, to be a consequence of limitations in the human cognitive capacity (Elstein and Schwarz, 2002). Simon (1990) described this as the principle of 'bounded rationality' – decision-making is limited by human behaviour being only partly rational, thereby causing limitations in information processing and complex problem solving, thus requiring the use of suboptimal approximation methods and heuristics. The need for fast and efficient decision-making 'shortcuts' and the resulting cognitive biases are believed, at least in part, to have arisen adaptively through our evolutionary history as a result of their intrinsic advantages for survival (Johnson et al., 2013). Such adaptive cognitive processes may, however, be suboptimal in many modern decision-making contexts, and their identification is frequently cited as central to reducing errors in medical practice (Croskerry, 2009; Ely et al., 2011; Graber et al., 2005, 2002; Hicks and Kluemper, 2011).

A critical limitation, however, of statistical prediction tools is their inherent inflexibility and fragility. That is, their predictions are limited to the specific outcome/diagnosis for which they were designed and are generated based on the limited subset of information considered within the tool. They are consequently not able to inform all categories of clinical judgements and are not able to integrate all of the available information that may be pertinent to a decision. The use of statistical procedures to inform decisions is therefore crucially reliant on a skilled individual's ability to judge the appropriateness of its application, an awareness of its limitations and assumptions, and the accurate interpretation of its results (Dawes et al., 1989; Swets et al., 2000a, 2000b).

P. E. Meehl (1954) first highlighted the crucial role of the skilled individual in the application of statistical prediction models in what is known as the 'broken leg countervailing'. This is where a prediction model may normally perform well under usual circumstances (e.g. a model that predicts someone's attendance at the movies given the day of the week) but will require human adjustment in the light of additional information not accounted for in the model that will influence the predicted outcome (e.g. in the rare case that someone has broken his or her leg, he or she is much less likely to attend the movies) (Grove and Meehl, 1996).

Importantly, statistics are not always available to inform all categories of clinical judgement, limiting the applicability of statistical prediction tools. Greater awareness of common cognitive errors and strategies to reduce some errors may assist in minimizing errors of clinical judgment (see Chapter 1 for further discussion). Rather than being a slave to a mathematical formula, it is suggested that clinicians using statistical prediction models integrate the objective data produced from such tools with all other existing information to facilitate their decision-making (Swets et al., 2000a). That is, statistical predictions do not form a clinical decision but, instead, inform a clinical decision.

The remainder of this chapter focuses specifically on a type of statistical prediction tool most commonly referred to as a 'clinical prediction rule'.

Clinical Prediction Rules

A clinical prediction rule (CPR) has been defined as a 'a clinical tool that quantifies the individual contributions that various components of the history, physical examination and basic laboratory results make towards the diagnosis, prognosis, or likely response to treatment in an individual patient' (McGinn et al., 2008, p. 493). Common synonyms include 'clinical prediction guides' (McGinn et al., 2008; US National Library of Medicine, 2009), 'clinical prediction tools' (Randolph et al., 1998), 'clinical decision rules' (Osmond et al., 2010), 'clinical decision guides' (Schneider et al., 2014) and 'clinical decision tools' (Thiruganasambandamoorthy et al., 2014).

CPRs may be conceptualized as a method of incorporating research evidence into clinical decision-making (Beattie and Nelson, 2006). They are clinical tools composed of the most *parsimonious* set of variables that have been empirically identified to predict a meaningful diagnosis or outcome (Childs and Cleland, 2006). Variables are commonly components of the history, physical examination and/or other tests or investigations that may be reliably collected within a standard clinical encounter (Laupacis et al., 1997). Some forms of CPRs enable the calculation of the probability of a given outcome or diagnosis, whilst others function to directly inform a specific course of action (Reilly and Evans, 2006). It is generally considered that CPRs may be of greatest utility when developed to assist in complex clinical decisions (McGinn et al., 2000).

Three major types of CPRs have been identified in the medical literature: diagnostic, prognostic and prescriptive (C. Cook, 2008).

Diagnostic Clinical Prediction Rules

Diagnostic CPRs function to inform clinical decisions regarding an individual patient's diagnosis or present classification/status. An example of a diagnostic CPR is the Ottawa Knee Rule (Stiell, Greenberg, et al., 1995). This five-item tool is designed to help inform decisions regarding which patients presenting to an emergency department following an acute knee injury require an x-ray. A patient's status on this CPR is determined by considering the presence or absence of five clinical variables (Table 5.1). In the absence of all five clinical variables, the likelihood of a knee fracture is remote (Bachmann et al., 2004), and consequently, an x-ray of the knee is unlikely to yield valuable clinical information.

TABLE 5.1

EXAMPLE OF A DIAGNOSTIC CLINICAL PREDICTION RULE: THE OTTAWA KNEE RULE

1. Age ≥55 years
2. Tenderness at head of fibula
3. Isolated tenderness of patella
4. Inability to flex knee to 90 degrees
5. Inability to bear weight (twice on each limb regardless of limping), both immediately and in the emergency department

(Stiell, Greenberg, et al., 1995)

Prognostic Clinical Prediction Rules

Prognostic CPRs differ from their diagnostic counterparts with respect to their dependence on the dimension of time. Prognostic CPRs function to inform clinical judgements regarding future outcomes or events, such as an individual's pain severity or likelihood of returning to work in 6 months' time. An example of a prognostic CPR is the 'Cassandra rule' (Dionne, 2005; Dionne et al., 1997, 2011). This CPR was derived in a population of patients with back pain presenting to primary care physicians and aims to identify individuals with differing degrees of risk of developing long-term significant functional limitations. The CPR uses a measure of depression and a measure of somatization from selected items of the Symptoms Checklist 90 Revised (Derogatis, 1977) questionnaire to stratify patients by their degree of risk of having 50% or greater disability on the Roland-Morris Disability Questionnaire (Roland and Morris, 1983) at 2 years.

Prescriptive Clinical Prediction Rules

Prescriptive CPRs are the third major type of these tools and function to sub-classify patient populations by matching patients to treatments based on their predicted responsiveness to that treatment, independent of a diagnostic classification (Foster et al., 2013). As such, prescriptive CPRs inform clinical decisions regarding treatment selection (C. Cook, 2008) and can be conceptualized as a special form of prognostic CPR that specifically relates to treatment effects. The treatment effect is the difference in outcome that is achieved by one intervention in comparison to that achieved by an alternative or control intervention (Kamper et al., 2010). Prescriptive CPRs are thus comprised of treatment effect modifiers (also known as effect moderators) – these are the baseline variables that differentiate patient subgroups which experience differing magnitudes of treatment effect (Kraemer et al., 2006). Such variables are subsequently distinct from prognostic variables, which predict outcomes independent of treatment (Hill and Fritz, 2011).

A patient's status on a treatment effect modifier predicts the relative benefit the patient will likely achieve from one intervention compared with another. Fig. 5.1 illustrates this relationship. Treatment effect modifiers are identified in randomized clinical trials by exploring interaction effects between candidate baseline variables and treatment groups (Hancock et al., 2009; Sun et al., 2010). The sample sizes required for such trials are, however, very large. To adequately power a study to detect an interaction effect, the sample size needs to be approximately four times that required to detect an overall treatment effect of the same magnitude (Brookes et al., 2004).

Development of Clinical Prediction Rules

The development a CPR occurs across three main stages: derivation, validation and impact analysis (Fig. 5.2) (Childs and Cleland, 2006; McGinn et al., 2000, 2008). Each stage functions to develop and investigate a specific aspect of a CPR and has crucial implications for its ability to be applied in clinical practice. The following subsections describe the processes involved in each of the main stages of a CPR's development.

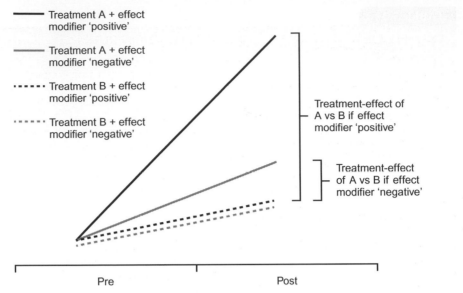

Fig. 5.1 Illustration of a treatment effect that is modified by a patient's status on a baseline variable.

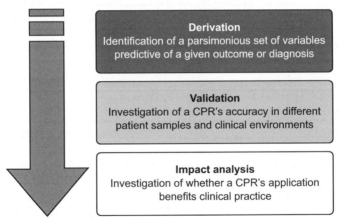

Fig. 5.2 Stages in the development of a clinical prediction rule (CPR) *(Adapted with permission from Childs and Cleland [2006]).*

Derivation

The first step in the development of a CPR is derivation. This process commences with the identification of a meaningful problem for which the development of a CPR may be perceived as clinically useful. Considerations that help inform the need for a CPR include the complexity of clinical decision-making, the accuracy of unassisted clinician judgement, clinician attitudes, variations in practices and the hypothesized potential for a tool to beneficially impact practice by improving patient outcomes or improving resource efficiencies (Fritz, 2009; Stiell and Wells, 1999).

The study design required to derive a CPR is dependent on the type of CPR under development. Diagnostic CPRs are derived in cross-sectional studies, prognostic CPRs are derived in longitudinal cohort studies and prescriptive CPRs require randomized controlled trials (Hancock et al., 2009; Hill and Fritz, 2011). In all instances, a meaningful, valid and clearly defined dependent outcome that is able to be reliably measured requires selection (Stiell and Wells, 1999). A small number of candidate predictor variables also need to be selected *a priori* and considered within the context of their hypothesized predictive performance, validity and reliability, as well as their practicality and availability within the

TABLE 5.2		
TECHNIQUES USED TO DEVELOP CLINICAL PREDICTION RULES		
Technique	**Advantages**	**Disadvantages**
Univariate analysis	Simple to develop. Easy to use.	Predictors may not be independent. Weightings are arbitrary. Less accurate.
Multivariable analysis	Improved accuracy.	Slightly more complicated to develop.
Nomograms	Improved accuracy. Easy to use.	More complicated to develop.
Classification and regression trees (recursive partitioning)	Easy to use. Enables development of rules that are optimized for sensitivity or specificity.	Can often be less accurate than other techniques. Does not work well for continuous variables. Prone to overfitting.
Artificial neural network	Improved accuracy over time with new data. Identifies complex non-linear relationships and interactions.	More complicated to develop. Prone to overfitting. Hard to apply in most clinical settings.

(Adapted from Grobman and Stamilio [2006] and Adams and Leveson [2012])

clinical environment (C. Cook et al., 2010; Lubetzky-Vilnai et al., 2014; Seel et al., 2012). Clinical judgement, literature reviews, focus groups and questionnaires have been used to select candidate predictor variables in some CPR derivation studies (Dionne et al., 2005; Hewitt et al., 2007; Heymans et al., 2007, 2009).

The patient population sampled in CPR derivation studies needs to represent the spectrum of patients to which the tool is likely to be applied (Stiell and Wells, 1999). Generally, large sample sizes are required to satisfy the assumptions of the statistical techniques that are used and to also generate greater precision of the findings (Childs and Cleland, 2006). Larger sample sizes are particularly required when investigating an outcome with a very low prevalence (e.g. cancer in patients with low back pain), when testing large numbers of candidate predictors and when investigating treatment effect modifiers (Babyak, 2004; Brookes et al., 2004).

Once data collection is complete, statistical analysis is used to identify the candidate variables that have a significant predictive relationship with the dependent outcome. There are several different techniques that have been used to derive CPRs in the medical literature. Table 5.2, adapted from Grobman and Stamilio (2006) and Adams and Leveson (2012), provides an overview of these techniques and their relative advantages and disadvantages.

Univariate analysis, whereby the relationships between each predictor variable and the dependent outcome are examined separately, is the simplest technique but has several limitations. Most notably, it does not account for the relationship among candidate predictor variables. Multivariable analysis overcomes this limitation by examining the independent relationship of each predictor variable with the target outcome, and it also enables the assignment of variable weightings based on the interpretation of the regression coefficients (Laupacis et al., 1997). Various forms of multivariable analysis have been commonly used to derive CPRs (Bouwmeester et al., 2012), and in some cases, automated methods of variable selection (e.g. forward stepwise, backward deletion, best subset) are applied. However, given the increased chance of identifying spurious associations using automated procedures, these approaches may not be well suited for CPR development and may best be reserved for exploratory analysis (Babyak, 2004; Katz, 2003). Multivariable models are generally well suited to construct nomograms, which are graphical calculating tools that facilitate the application of otherwise-complicated mathematical equations (Grobman and Stamilio, 2006).

Classification and regression trees are another approach used to derive CPRs. This analysis uses non-parametric statistical procedures to identify mutually exclusive and exhaustive subgroups based on the variables that predict the dependent outcome (Lemon et al., 2003). Recursive partitioning accounts for interactions between predictor variables

(E. F. Cook and Goldman, 1984; Dionne et al., 1997) and is subsequently better suited for deriving CPRs from datasets with interacting variables than logistic regression (Katz, 2006). This approach is also considered to be well suited in instances where a CPR requires optimization of either sensitivity or specificity (Stiell and Wells, 1999).

Artificial neural networks require advanced computational resources and are another approach used to develop CPRs. Artificial neural networks are inherently statistically more flexible than regression approaches and, all else being equal, provide models that better fit the study data (Kattan, 2002). However, as a consequence, they are also more vulnerable to overfitting, thus potentially reducing the likelihood that these approaches will perform well outside of the derivation study data (Tu, 1996).

To illustrate the development of a CPR, the Ottawa Knee Rule (Table 5.1) will be used as an example (Stiell, Greenberg, et al., 1995). A need for a tool to help decide which patients require an x-ray was based on the finding that whilst almost three-quarters of patients presenting with acute knee injury to an emergency department were referred for radiology, only 5% were identified to have a fracture (Stiell, Wells, et al., 1995). This contributes to increased costs of care, increased waiting times and unnecessary radiation exposure. It was also identified that experienced clinicians believed that the probability of a fracture was less than 10% in the majority of patients sent for radiology (Stiell, Wells, et al., 1995).

Consequently, a prospective study was conducted involving 1047 adult patients with acute knee injuries presenting to one of two university hospital emergency departments in Ottawa, Canada. The dependent outcome was any fracture of the knee seen on plain x-ray and was determined blinded to knowledge of the candidate predictor variables. For ethical reasons, patients thought not to require a knee x-ray were not sent for radiology, but follow-up was conducted via a telephone questionnaire with the aim of detecting any missed fractures. Twenty-three candidate predictor variables were selected based on clinician judgement, literature review and pilot study data. Explicit definitions of each variable were provided to clinicians in a handout.

Following data collection, recursive partitioning was used to derive the CPR. The tool was developed to optimize sensitivity, given that a missed fracture would be of greater consequence than an unnecessary x-ray. Many different models were identified to fit the data, and the research team decided to select the model that gave the greatest specificity and used the fewest number of variables whilst maintaining 100% sensitivity. The accuracy of the Ottawa Knee Rule in the derivation study was a sensitivity of 100% (95% confidence interval [CI] 95%–100%) and a specificity of 54% (95% CI 51%–57%).

Validation

A CPR models the study dataset from which it was derived (Beattie and Nelson, 2006). Consequently, it may not always perform well when applied outside of this original context (Justice et al., 1999). Validation is the second stage of a CPR's development and functions to examine the internal validity and generalizability of the derived tool in new patient populations and clinical environments (McGinn et al., 2008). Validation of a CPR is therefore not something achievable within a single study but, rather, an attribute that arises across multiple investigations (Hancock et al., 2009).

Methodological issues within a derivation study that challenge the internal validity of a CPR will have consequences for the tool's ability to perform well in other studies (C. Cook, 2008). However, there are at least three reasons why even a robustly derived CPR may not necessarily perform well outside of the original study (McGinn et al., 2000). These are as follows:

- Chance associations. It is possible that some statistically significant relationships identified in the derivation study are purely due to chance. Consequently, it is unlikely that such associations will hold true in new datasets, thus reducing the predictive performance of a CPR.
- Differences related to the patient population or clinical environment. It is possible that some of the predictive relationships identified in the derivation study are unique to the patient sample or clinician group under investigation. As such, derivation study findings may not generalize to other patient and clinician populations.

- Differences related to the implementation of a CPR. Inconsistencies may arise with regard to the operational definitions of predictor and dependent variables, as well as the accurate application and interpretation of the rule. These will influence a CPR's predictive performance.

Statistical validation (e.g. split samples, bootstrapping) will only account for the first of these threats (McGinn et al., 2000). As such, prospective studies involving different patients, clinicians and clinical settings are required to validate a CPR. 'Narrow validation' refers to the process by which a CPR is tested for its ability to replicate its predictive performance in patients and settings similar to those of the original derivation study (Kamper et al., 2010; Keogh et al., 2014; McGinn et al., 2000). The findings of such studies give insight into the variability of the predictive accuracy of a CPR in a specific patient population (Kent et al., 2010). 'Broad validation', by contrast, examines the generalizability of a CPR to different settings and patient populations unlike those in used in the derivation study (Kamper et al., 2010; Keogh et al., 2014; McGinn et al., 2000).

Toll et al. (2008) further delineate between the temporal, geographic and domain validation of a CPR. Temporal validation refers to the replication of a CPR's performance over time, with little change to the patient population sampled or other elements of the clinical setting. Geographic validation refers to the investigation of a CPR's performance in similar patient populations but in different clinical environments. Finally, domain validation, which is considered to provide the strongest evidence of generalizability, refers to the assessment of a CPR's performance in different clinical environments and in different patient populations that differ non-randomly from that of the derivation sample.

Several studies have contributed to the validation of the Ottawa Knee Rule (Bachmann et al., 2004). Ketelslegers et al. (2002) investigated the performance of this tool when applied by clinicians with differing levels of training in an emergency teaching centre in Brussels, Belgium. Medical students and surgical residents were trained in the accurate implementation of the CPR by the research team. The 261 patients recruited in this study were assessed with regard to their status on the Ottawa Knee Rule. Blinded outcome assessment for the presence of a fracture was determined by x-ray (84%) or by telephone or face-to-face follow-up. The results of this study demonstrated that the Ottawa Knee Rule had a sensitivity of 100% (95% CI 99%–100%) and a specificity of 32% (95% CI 26%–38%). No difference in the predictive accuracy of the CPR was identified between medical students and surgical residents, thus providing evidence of generalizability of the tool to different clinician populations of varying experience. The finding of the 100% sensitivity of the tool is also consistent with that of the derivation study and provides further evidence of the predictive performance of the CPR in identifying patients presenting with acute knee injury who are unlikely to benefit from radiological assessment.

Impact Analysis

The final stage of a CPR's development is called 'impact analysis' and is the investigation of whether a tool's application in clinical practice results in meaningful beneficial consequences, such as improved outcomes or resource efficiencies (Childs and Cleland, 2006). This step is important because even a well-validated CPR may not necessarily outperform unassisted clinician judgement. Further, if a CPR is difficult to use or if there are other factors that impede its implementation, it may not necessarily be successfully adopted in clinical practice (McGinn et al., 2000). Despite the growing volume of CPRs relevant to musculoskeletal practitioners that have been derived at this time, very few have undergone any form of impact analysis (Georgopoulos and Taylor, 2016; Haskins et al., 2015a, 2015b, 2012; Kelly et al., 2017; May and Rosedale, 2009; Stanton et al., 2010; van Oort et al., 2012; Wallace et al., 2016).

The best study design to conduct an impact analysis is a randomized controlled trial, whereby the outcomes produced from the use of a CPR are able to be rigorously evaluated (Toll et al., 2008). Randomization may be at the level of the patient, the clinician or the facility, with the latter helping to minimize potential contamination (Wallace et al., 2011). Before-and-after designs are often a more feasible approach to assessing the impact of the use of a CPR; however, the evidence from such designs is weaker than that produced from a randomized control trial due to the greater potential for bias (Childs and Cleland, 2006; Reilly and Evans, 2006).

In addition to exploring the effectiveness of a CPR on patient outcomes and resource consumption, it may also be useful to investigate changes in clinician practice behaviours, clinicians' acceptance of the tool and patient satisfaction (Beattie and Nelson, 2006; Childs and Cleland, 2006; McGinn et al., 2000; Stiell and Wells, 1999). Clinician acceptance of a CPR may be assessed using the 12-item Ottawa Acceptability of Decision Rules Instrument (Brehaut et al., 2010). Qualitative assessment of the perspectives of study participants may also be advantageous to gain greater understanding regarding the modifiable aspects of a CPR's implementation that may facilitate its successful clinical application (Wallace et al., 2011).

Continuing the Ottawa Knee Rule example, Stiell et al. (1997) used a before-and-after non-randomized controlled trial to evaluate the impact of the clinical application of this CPR. Two control and two intervention hospitals were used in this 2-year study, with the intervention hospitals applying the Ottawa Knee Rule in the last year of the study period. Following the implementation of the CPR in the intervention hospitals, there was a 20.5% absolute reduction in the use of knee x-rays (77.6%–57.1%). Over the same period, the use of knee x-rays in the control hospitals decreased by just 1% (76.9%–75.9%). Those patients not receiving knee radiography spent an average of 33 minutes less time in the emergency department, and their overall costs of care were US$103 less. During the period of use of the Ottawa Knee Rule in the intervention hospitals, clinicians overruled the CPR in 6.9% of cases. The main reasons for this related to patient preferences (either wanting or not wanting an x-ray) and clinician judgement. Almost all patients (95.7%) who did not receive a knee x-ray during the period of Ottawa Knee Rule application reported being satisfied with their episode of care. The sensitivity of the CPR in this study was 100% (95% CI 94%–100%), and the specificity was 48% (95% CI 45%–51%).

Methodological Considerations

The development of a CPR, irrespective of its type, requires consideration of a number of methodological standards specific to its stage of development. Such standards are an extension to the various methodological requisites that are specific to the underlying study design. A 23-item quality checklist has been developed to help guide the derivation of prescriptive CPRs (C. Cook et al., 2010); however, no universally accepted validated tool exists to help inform the development of all other forms of CPRs at their respective stages of development. Nevertheless, many publications within the medical literature provide commentary regarding the appropriate methodological considerations relevant to the development of CPRs. Tables 5.3, 5.4 and 5.5 provide an overview of the relevant methodological considerations highlighted within five well-cited publications on the derivation, validation and impact assessment of CPRs, respectively (Beattie and Nelson, 2006; Childs and Cleland, 2006; Laupacis et al., 1997; McGinn et al., 2000; Stiell and Wells, 1999).

Readiness for Application in Clinical Practice

The stage of a CPR's development has direct implications for its readiness to be applied in clinical practice (Fig. 5.3). This is due to the structured process of a CPR's development enabling progressively greater confidence in the tool's accuracy and generalizability (Childs and Cleland, 2006). McGinn et al. (2000) proposed a hierarchical framework to determine the degree to which a CPR may be used to confidently inform clinical decisions based on its stage of development:

- CPRs that have been derived, but have not yet undergone validation, are not considered within this framework to be ready to be applied in clinical practice. There are many reasons why even a rigorously derived CPR may not perform well outside of the original study data. McGinn et al. (2000) suggest that clinicians may wish to consider which variables were and were not identified to have a significant predictive relationship with the target outcome or diagnosis within a derivation study to cautiously inform their clinical practice. Clinicians need to be wary, however, that such relationships may simply

TABLE 5.3

METHODOLOGICAL CONSIDERATIONS COMMON TO THE DERIVATION OF ALL FORMS OF CLINICAL PREDICTION RULES

	Laupacis et al. (1997)	Stiell and Wells (1999)	McGinn et al. (2000)	Beattie and Nelson (2006)	Childs and Cleland (2006)
Prospective design	■	■		■	■
Outcomes defined	■		■	■	■
Outcome clinically important	■		■	■	■
Blinded outcome assessment	■		■		
All important predictors included	■		■	■	■
Predictive variables clearly defined	■	■	■		■
Blinded predictor assessment	■	■	■		■
Assessment of the reliability of the predictive variables	■	■			■
Important patient characteristics described	■			■	■
Inclusion criteria explicitly stated	■			■	■
Representative sample		■		■	■
Complete follow-up	■			■	■
Study site described	■			■	■
Justification for the number of study subjects		■	■	■	■
At least 10 outcome events per independent variable in the rule		■	■	■	■
Important predictors present in a significant proportion of the study population		■	■		■
Mathematical techniques described	■	■		■	■
Multivariate analysis	■	■	■	■	■
Results of the rule described	■	■	■	■	■
Clinically sensible/reasonable	■	■	■	■	■
Easy to use	■	■		■	■
Probability of diagnosis or outcome described	■			■	■
Course of action described	■				■
Estimation of potential impact of use	■				

reflect chance associations or may be specific to the unique characteristics of the derivation study's patient sample, clinicians or setting.

- CPRs that have undergone 'narrow validation' (examination of the tool's performance in a population and setting very similar to that in which the CPR was derived) may be cautiously applied with some confidence in their predictive accuracy in the limited instances where a clinician's caseload closely approximates that of the validation and derivation studies. This stage of a CPR's development does not, however, provide evidence that it may accurately perform outside of this limited context. Additionally, the application of a CPR at this stage of development, even within this limited context, may not necessarily result in improved patient outcomes or other improvements in clinical care.
- CPRs that have undergone 'broad validation' (examination of the tool's performance in heterogeneous patient populations and settings different from that used in the derivation

TABLE 5.4

METHODOLOGICAL CONSIDERATIONS COMMON TO THE VALIDATION OF ALL FORMS OF CLINICAL PREDICTION RULES

	Laupacis et al. (1997)	Stiell and Wells (1999)	McGinn et al. (2000)	Beattie and Nelson (2006)	Childs and Cleland (2006)
Prospective validation in new patient population	■				
Different clinical setting to derivation study		■			
Different clinicians to derivation study		■			
Representative sample				■	
The rule is applied accurately					■
Complete follow-up		■			
Blinded outcome assessment			■		
Blinded predictor assessment			■		
Accuracy of the rule in the validation study sample described			■		
Justification of the validation study sample size		■			
Assessment of the inter-observer reliability of the rule	■	■			
Assessment of clinicians' perceived ease of use of the rule		■			
Rule is refined when indicated		■			
Estimation of potential impact of use		■			

TABLE 5.5

METHODOLOGICAL CONSIDERATIONS COMMON TO THE IMPACT ASSESSMENT OF ALL FORMS OF CLINICAL PREDICTION RULES

	Laupacis et al. (1997)	Stiell and Wells (1999)	McGinn et al. (2000)	Beattie and Nelson (2006)	Childs and Cleland (2006)
Effects of clinical use prospectively measured	■				■
Assessment of changes to clinician behaviour/practice		■	■	■	■
Assessment of rules' ability to improve outcomes			■	■	■
Effect on efficiency assessed		■			
Accuracy of the rule is described				■	
Clinician acceptance is assessed				■	
Patient satisfaction is assessed		■			■

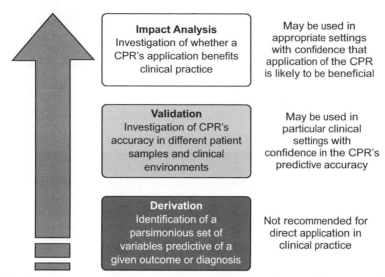

Fig. 5.3   Relationship between a clinical prediction rule (CPR) development phase and readiness to be applied in clinical practice.

study) may be applied with some confidence in their predictive accuracy across various clinical settings. This stage of CPR development does not, however, provide evidence that the use of a CPR will have beneficial clinical consequences.

- CPRs that have undergone impact analysis may be applied with confidence that their application in clinical practice is likely to result in improved patient outcomes and/or resource efficiencies while maintaining quality of care and patient satisfaction. At the present time, however, very few CPRs relevant to musculoskeletal practice have undergone this necessary phase of development (Georgopoulos and Taylor, 2016; Haskins et al., 2012, 2015a, 2015b; Kelly et al., 2017; May and Rosedale, 2009; Stanton et al., 2010; van Oort et al., 2012; Wallace et al., 2016).

Clinical Application of CPRs in Musculoskeletal Practice

It is our interpretation that there is potential value in the use of CPRs in musculoskeletal clinical practice; however, that value is presently limited to well-developed diagnostic and prognostic forms of CPRs. Diagnostic and prognostic CPRs have fewer assumptions relative to their prescriptive counterparts, and in the case of diagnostic CPRs, they have more definitive outcomes. Although prognostic CPRs use outcomes similar to those of prescriptive CPRs, these tools look primarily at baseline measures and their relationships with general outcomes findings. Prognostic CPRs do not require the discrimination of outcomes based on a treatment provided, as prescriptive CPRs assume.

We feel that diagnostic CPRs can provide value in clinical decision-making by helping clinicians reason through the potential underlying element supplying the diagnosis. Diagnostic CPRs will use an outcome variable of disease or no disease (or disorder/syndrome, no disorder/syndrome), thus improving the likelihood of discriminating the given situation at hand. Diagnostic CPRs are developed by combining clinical findings that are the closest component to a reference standard (the best mechanism for determining the diagnosis), and in some cases, they actually make up the reference standard (e.g. patellofemoral pain syndrome).

Prescriptive CPRs suffer from many challenges that may actually erode the clinical reasoning processes used by clinicians. By their nature, prescriptive CPRs (1) assume the validity of an outcome value, (2) assume that the treatment interventions have distinguishing effects (effects that are different for dissimilar populations) and (3) assume that the treatment effects are strong enough to distinguish from the given prognostic influence of the baseline characteristics of the patient. These are lofty assumptions that, to date, have not been verified in most mechanically oriented musculoskeletal conditions.

Past work has shown that altering one's threshold of 'success' within an outcome measure can lead to different CPRs (Haskins and Cook, 2016). Simply put, if one adjusts what he or she considers to be the threshold measure, commonly referred to as a minimal clinically important difference score, one will find multiple different prescriptive CPRs within the same group of patients receiving the same treatment. This suggests that the modelling is fragile and will differ across studies, populations and definitions of success/non-success in outcome measures. Further, when different outcome measures are used, different CPRs are also created – within the same population (Haskins and Cook, 2016).

Let us consider the assumption that treatment interventions have distinguishing effects. In the psychological literature, the *shared mechanisms theory* suggests that there is similarity in outcomes across presumably different treatment approaches. There are many examples in the psychological literature that demonstrate, comparatively, that there are no differences among the many forms of interventions for major depression (Cuijpers et al., 2008), pain (Wampold et al., 1997) and panic disorder and obsessive-compulsive disorder (Ougrin and Latif, 2011).

Consequently, for musculoskeletal clinical practice, we support the use of well-developed prognostic and diagnostic CPRs but do not support the use of nearly all musculoskeletal-based prescriptive CPRs derived to date. Regardless of your strategy for using CPRs, we advocate for the use of clinical reasoning as the 'trump card' over any CPR presently available. For multiple reasons, CPRs will not always be available for the particular clinical decision at hand or be appropriate for all categories of clinical judgement. Further, CPRs by design are limited to a subset of information, which, importantly, may omit critical aspects of an individual's presentation pertinent to decision-making. Statistical modelling methods such as CPRs assist in informing clinical reasoning, not replacing it.

Future Directions

CPRs represent one branch of an evolving approach to clinical practice that conscientiously incorporates quantified research evidence into clinical decision-making. Many clinical presentations encountered by musculoskeletal practitioners are probable ideal targets for such tools given the complexity of clinical judgements and the numerous assessment and management alternatives. It is widely hypothesized that the development of CPRs for musculoskeletal presentations has the potential to lead to substantial patient and system-level gains, particularly those tools that are explicitly developed to address a currently unmet need identified by clinicians.

REFERENCES

Adams, S.T., Leveson, S.H., 2012. Clinical prediction rules. Br. Med. J. 344, d8312.

Babyak, M.A., 2004. What you see may not be what you get: a brief, nontechnical introduction to overfitting in regression-type models. Psychosom. Med. 66 (3), 411–421.

Bachmann, L.M., Haberzeth, S., Steurer, J., ter Riet, G., 2004. The accuracy of the Ottawa knee rule to rule out knee fractures: a systematic review. Ann. Intern. Med. 140 (2), 121–124.

Baxt, W.G., 1995. Application of artificial neural networks to clinical medicine. The Lancet 346 (8983), 1135–1138.

Beattie, P., Nelson, R., 2006. Clinical prediction rules: what are they and what do they tell us? Aust J. Physiother. 52 (3), 157–163.

Bouwmeester, W., Zuithoff, N.P.A., Mallett, S., Geerlings, M.I., Vergouwe, Y., Steyerberg, E.W., et al., 2012. Reporting and methods in clinical prediction research: a systematic review. PLoS Med. 9 (5), e1001221.

Brehaut, J.C., Graham, I.D., Wood, T.J., Taljaard, M., Eagles, D., Lott, A., et al., 2010. Measuring acceptability of clinical decision rules: validation of the Ottawa acceptability of decision rules instrument (OADRI) in four countries. Med. Decis. Making 30 (3), 398–408.

Brookes, S.T., Whitely, E., Egger, M., Smith, G.D., Mulheran, P.A., Peters, T.J., 2004. Subgroup analyses in randomized trials: risks of subgroup-specific analyses; power and sample size for the interaction test. J. Clin. Epidemiol. 57 (3), 229–236. http://dx.doi.org/10.1016/j.jclinepi.2003.08.009. doi.

Childs, J.D., Cleland, J.A., 2006. Development and application of clinical prediction rules to improve decision making in physical therapist practice. Phys. Ther. 86 (1), 122–131.

Cook, C., 2008. Potential pitfalls of clinical prediction rules. J. Man. Manip. Ther. 16 (2), 69–71.

Cook, C., Brismee, J.M., Pietrobon, R., Sizer, P., Jr., Hegedus, E., Riddle, D.L., 2010. Development of a quality checklist using delphi methods for prescriptive clinical prediction rules: the QUADCPR. J. Manipulative Physiol. Ther. 33 (1), 29–41. Doi:http://dx.doi.org/10.1016/j.jmpt.2009.11.010.

Cook, E.F., Goldman, L., 1984. Empiric comparison of multivariate analytic techniques: advantages and disadvantages of recursive partitioning analysis. J. Chronic Dis. 37 (9–10), 721–731. Doi:http://dx.doi.org/10.1016/0021-9681(84)90041-9.

Croskerry, P., 2009. Clinical cognition and diagnostic error: applications of a dual process model of reasoning. Adv. Health Sci. Educ.Theory Pract 14 (1), 27–35.

Cuijpers, P., Brannmark, J.G., van Straten, A., 2008. Psychological treatment of postpartum depression: a meta-analysis. J. Clin. Psychol. 64 (1), 103–118. doi:10.1002/jclp.20432.

Dawes, R.M., Faust, D., Meehl, P.E., 1989. Clinical versus actuarial judgement. Science 243, 1668–1674.

Derogatis, L.R., 1977. Symptoms Checklist-90. Administration, scoring and procedures manual for the revised version. Baltimore: Clinical Psychometric Research.

Dionne, C.E., 2005. Psychological distress confirmed as predictor of long-term back-related functional limitations in primary care settings. J. Clin. Epidemiol. 58 (7), 714–718.

Dionne, C.E., Bourbonnais, R., Frémont, P., Rossignol, M., Stock, S.R., Larocque, I., 2005. A clinical return-to-work rule for patients with back pain. Can. Med. Assoc. J. 172 (12), 1559–1567.

Dionne, C.E., Koepsell, T.D., Von Korff, M., Deyo, R.A., Barlow, W.E., Checkoway, H., 1997. Predicting long-term functional limitations among back pain patients in primary care settings. J. Clin. Epidemiol. 50 (1), 31–43.

Dionne, C.E., Le Sage, N., Franche, R.-L., Dorval, M., Bombardier, C., Deyo, R.A., 2011. Five questions predicted long-term, severe, back-related functional limitations: evidence from three large prospective studies. J. Clin. Epidemiol. 64 (1), 54–66. doi: http://dx.doi.org/10.1016/j.jclinepi.2010.02.004.

Elstein, A.S., Schwarz, A., 2002. Clinical problem solving and diagnostic decision making: selective review of the cognitive literature. Br. Med. J. 324 (7339), 729–732.

Ely, J.W., Graber, M.L., Croskerry, P., 2011. Checklists to reduce diagnostic errors. Acad. Med. 86 (3), 307–313. doi:10.1097/ACM.0b013e31820824cd.

Foster, N.E., Hill, J.C., O'Sullivan, P., Hancock, M., 2013. Stratified models of care. Best Pract. Res. Clin. Rheumatol. 27 (5), 649–661.

Fritz, J.M., 2009. Clinical prediction rules in physical therapy: coming of age? J. Orthop. Sports Phys. Ther. 39 (3), 159–161.

Georgopoulos, V., Taylor, A., 2016. Clinical prediction rules in the prognosis of Whiplash Associated Disorder (WAD): a systematic review. Pain and Rehabilitation - the Journal of Physiotherapy Pain Association 41, 5–16.

Graber, M.L., Franklin, N., Gordon, R., 2005. Diagnostic error in internal medicine. Arch. Intern. Med. 165 (13), 1493–1499.

Graber, M.L., Gordon, R., Franklin, N., 2002. Reducing diagnostic errors in medicine: what's the goal? Acad. Med. 77 (10), 981–992.

Grobman, W.A., Stamilio, D.M., 2006. Methods of clinical prediction. Am. J. Obstet. Gynecol. 194 (3), 888–894.

Grove, W.M., Meehl, P.E., 1996. Comparative efficiency of informal (subjective, impressionistic) and formal (mechanical, algorithmic) prediction procedures: the clinical–statistical controversy. Psychol. Public Policy Law 2 (2), 293–323.

Grove, W.M., Zald, D.H., Lebow, B.S., Snitz, B.E., Nelson, C., 2000. Clinical versus mechanical prediction: a meta-analysis. Psychol. Assess. 12 (1), 19–30.

Guyatt, G.H., Sackett, D., Cook, D.J., Evidence Based Medicine Working Group, 1994. Users' guides to the medical literature. II. How to use an article about therapy or prevention. B. What were the results and how will they help me in caring for my patients? J. Am. Med. Assoc. 271, 59–63.

Hancock, M.J., Herbert, R.D., Maher, C.G., 2009. A guide to interpretation of studies investigating subgroups of responders to physical therapy interventions. Phys. Ther. 89 (7), 698–704.

Haskins, R., Cook, C., 2016. Enthusiasm for prescriptive clinical prediction rules (eg, back pain and more): a quick word of caution. Br. J. Sports Med. 50 (16), 960–961. doi:10.1136/bjsports-2015-095688.

Haskins, R., Osmotherly, P.G., Rivett, D.A., 2015a. Diagnostic clinical prediction rules for specific subtypes of low back pain: a systematic review. J. Orthop. Sports Phys. Ther. 45 (2), 61–76.

Haskins, R., Osmotherly, P.G., Rivett, D.A., 2015b. Validation and impact analysis of prognostic clinical prediction rules for low back pain is needed: a systematic review. J. Clin. Epidemiol. 68 (7), 821–832.

Haskins, R., Rivett, D.A., Osmotherly, P.G., 2012. Clinical prediction rules in the physiotherapy management of low back pain: a systematic review. Man. Ther. 17 (1), 9–21.

Hewitt, J.A., Hush, J.M., Martin, M.H., Herbert, R.D., Latimer, J., 2007. Clinical prediction rules can be derived and validated for injured Australian workers with persistent musculoskeletal pain: an observational study. Aust J. Physiother. 53 (4), 269–276.

Heymans, M.W., Anema, J.R., van Buuren, S., Knol, D.L., van Mechelen, W., De Vet, H.C.W., 2009. Return to work in a cohort of low back pain patients: development and validation of a clinical prediction rule. J. Occup. Rehabil. 19 (2), 155–165.

Heymans, M.W., Ford, J.J., McMeeken, J.M., Chan, A., de Vet, H.C.W., van Mechelen, W., 2007. Exploring the contribution of patient-reported and clinician based variables for the prediction of low back work status. J. Occup. Rehabil. 17 (3), 383–397.

Hicks, E.P., Kluemper, G.T., 2011. Heuristic reasoning and cognitive biases: are they hindrances to judgments and decision making in orthodontics? Am. J. Orthod. Dentofacial Orthop. 139 (3), 297–304. doi:10.1016/j.ajodo.2010.05.018.

Hill, J.C., Fritz, J.M., 2011. Psychosocial influences on low back pain, disability, and response to treatment. Phys. Ther. 91 (5), 712–721. doi:10.2522/ptj.20100280.

Horvitz, E., 2010. From Data to Predictions and Decisions: Enabling Evidence-Based Healthcare. Computing Community Consortium. https://cra.org/ccc/wp-content/uploads/sites/2/2015/05/Healthcare.pdf.

Jaeschke, R., Guyatt, G.H., Sackett, D., Evidence-Based Medicine Working Group, 1994. Users' guides to the medical literature: III. How to use an article about a diagnostic test b. What are the results and will they help me in caring for my patients? J. Am. Med. Assoc. 271 (9), 703–707.

Johnson, D.D.P., Blumstein, D.T., Fowler, J.H., Haselton, M.G., 2013. The evolution of error: error management, cognitive constraints, and adaptive decision-making biases. Trends Ecol. Evol. (Amst.) 28 (8), 474–481.

Justice, A.C., Covinsky, K.E., Berlin, J.A., 1999. Assessing the generalizability of prognostic information. Ann. Intern. Med. 130 (6), 515–524.

Kamper, S.J., Maher, C.G., Hancock, M.J., Koes, B.W., Croft, P.R., Hay, E., 2010. Treatment-based subgroups of low back pain: a guide to appraisal of research studies and a summary of current evidence. Best Pract. Res. Clin. Rheumatol. 24 (2), 181–191.

Kattan, M., 2002. Statistical prediction models, artificial neural networks, and the sophism "I am a patient, not a statistic." J. Clin. Oncol. 20 (4), 885–887.

Katz, M.H., 2003. Multivariable analysis: a primer for readers of medical research. Ann. Intern. Med. 138 (8), 644–650.

Katz, M.H., 2006. Multivariable Analysis. A Practical Guide for Clinicians, second ed. Cambridge University Press, New York.

Kelly, J., Ritchie, C., Sterling, M., 2017. Clinical prediction rules for prognosis and treatment prescription in neck pain: a systematic review. Musculoskeletal Sci. Pract. 27, 155–164. Doi:https://doi.org/10.1016/j.math.2016.10.066.

Kent, P.M., Keating, J.L., Leboeuf-Yde, C., 2010. Research methods for subgrouping low back pain. BMC Med. Res. Methodol. 10 (1), 62.

Keogh, C., Wallace, E., O'Brien, K.K., Galvin, R., Smith, S.M., Lewis, C., et al., 2014. Developing an international register of clinical prediction rules for use in primary care: a descriptive analysis. Ann. Fam. Med. 12 (4), 359–366. doi:10.1370/afm.1640.

Ketelslegers, E., Collard, X., Vande Berg, B., Danse, E., El-Gariani, A., Poilvache, P., et al., 2002. Validation of the Ottawa knee rules in an emergency teaching centre. Eur. Radiol. 12 (5), 1218–1220. doi:10.1007/s00330-001-1198-9.

Kraemer, H.C., Frank, E., Kupfer, D.J., 2006. Moderators of treatment outcomes: clinical, research, and policy importance. J. Am. Med. Assoc. 296 (10), 1286–1289. Doi: http://dx.doi.org/10.1001/jama.296.10.1286.

Laupacis, A., Sekar, N., Stiell, I.G., 1997. Clinical prediction rules: a review and suggested modifications of methodological standards. J. Am. Med. Assoc. 277 (6), 488–494.

Laupacis, A., Wells, G., Richardson, W.S., Tugwell, P., Guyatt, G.H., Browman, G., et al., 1994. Users' guides to the medical literature: V. How to use an article about prognosis. J. Am. Med. Assoc. 272 (3), 234–237.

Lemon, S.C., Roy, J., Clark, M.A., Friedmann, P.D., Rakowski, W., 2003. Classification and regression tree analysis in public health: methodological review and comparison with logistic regression. Anns Behav. Med. 26 (3), 172–181.

Lubetzky-Vilnai, A., Ciol, M., McCoy, S.W., 2014. Statistical analysis of clinical prediction rules for rehabilitation interventions: current state of the literature. Arch. Phys. Med. Rehabil. 95 (1), 188–196.

May, S., Rosedale, R., 2009. Prescriptive clinical prediction rules in back pain research: a systematic review. J. Man. Manip. Ther. 17 (1), 36–45.

McGinn, T.G., Guyatt, G.H., Wyer, P.C., Naylor, C.D., Stiell, I.G., Richardson, W.S., 2000. Users' guides to the medical literature: XXII: how to use articles about clinical decision rules. Evidence-Based Medicine Working Group. JAMA 284 (1), 79–84.

McGinn, T.G., Wyer, P., Wisnivesky, J., Devereaux, P.J., Stiell, I., Richardson, S., et al., 2008. Advanced topics in diagnosis: clinical prediction rules. In: Guyatt, G., Rennie, D., Meade, M.O., Cook, D.J. (Eds.), Users' Guides to the Medical Literature. A Manual for Evidence-Based Clinical Practice, second ed. McGraw Hill Medical, New York, pp. 491–505.

Meehl, P.E., 1954. Clinical Versus Statistical Prediction: A Theoretical Analysis and a Review of the Evidence. University of Minnesota Press.

Osmond, M.H., Klassen, T.P., Wells, G.A., Correll, R., Jarvis, A., Joubert, G., et al., 2010. CATCH: a clinical decision rule for the use of computed tomography in children with minor head injury. Can. Med. Assoc. J. 182 (4), 341–348. doi:10.1503/cmaj.091421.

Ougrin, D., Latif, S., 2011. Specific psychological treatment versus treatment as usual in adolescents with self-harm. Crisis 32 (2), 74–80.

Randolph, A.G., Guyatt, G.H., Calvin, J.E., Doig, G., Richardson, W.S., Cook, D.J., 1998. Understanding articles describing clinical prediction tools. Crit. Care Med. 26 (9), 1603–1612.

Reilly, B.M., Evans, A.T., 2006. Translating clinical research into clinical practice: impact of using prediction rules to make decisions. Ann. Intern. Med. 144 (3), 201–209.

Richardson, W.S., Wilson, M.C., Guyatt, G.H., Cook, D.J., Nishikawa, J., Evidence-Based Medicine Working Group, 1999. Users' guides to the medical literature: XV. How to use an article about disease probability for differential diagnosis. J. Am. Med. Assoc. 281 (13), 1214–1219.

Roland, M., Morris, R., 1983. A study of the natural history of back pain: part I: development of a reliable and sensitive measure of disability in low-back pain. Spine 8 (2), 141–144.

Schneider, G.M., Jull, G.A., Thomas, K., Smith, A., Emery, C., Faris, P., et al., 2014. Derivation of a Clinical Decision Guide in the Diagnosis of Cervical Facet Joint Pain. Arch. Phys. Med. Rehabil. 95 (9), 1695–1701. doi:10.1016/j.apmr.2014.02.026.

Seel, R.T., Steyerberg, E.W., Malec, J.F., Sherer, M., Macciocchi, S.N., 2012. Developing and evaluating prediction models in rehabilitation populations. Arch. Phys. Med. Rehabil. 93 (8), S138–S153.

Simon, H.A., 1990. Invariants of human behavior. Annu. Rev. Psychol. 41 (1), 1–20.

Stanton, T.R., Hancock, M.J., Maher, C.G., Koes, B.W., 2010. Critical appraisal of clinical prediction rules that aim to optimize treatment selection for musculoskeletal conditions. Phys. Ther. 90 (6), 843–854.

Stiell, I.G., Greenberg, G.H., Wells, G.A., McKnight, R.D., Cwinn, A.A., Cacciotti, T., et al., 1995. Derivation of a decision rule for the use of radiography in acute knee injuries. Ann. Emerg. Med. 26 (4), 405–413.

Stiell, I.G., Wells, G.A., 1999. Methodologic standards for the development of clinical decision rules in emergency medicine. Ann. Emerg. Med. 33 (4), 437–447.

Stiell, I.G., Wells, G.A., Hoag, R.H., Sivilotti, M.L.A., Cacciotti, T.F., Verbeek, P.R., et al., 1997. Implementation of the Ottawa Knee Rule for the use of radiography in acute knee injuries. J. Am. Med. Assoc. 278 (23), 2075–2079.

Stiell, I.G., Wells, G.A., McDowell, I., Greenberg, G.H., McKnight, R.D., Cwinn, A.A., et al., 1995. Use of radiography in acute knee injuries: need for clinical decision rules. Acad. Emerg. Med. 2 (11), 966–973.

Sun, X., Briel, M., Walter, S.D., Guyatt, G.H., 2010. Is a subgroup effect believable? Updating criteria to evaluate the credibility of subgroup analyses. Br. Med. J. 340, c117. doi:10.1136/bmj.c117.

Swets, J.A., Dawes, R.M., Monahan, J., 2000a. Better decisions through science. Sci. Am. 283 (4), 82–87.

Swets, J.A., Dawes, R.M., Monahan, J., 2000b. Psychological science can improve diagnostic decisions. Psychol. Sci. Public Interest 1 (1), 1–26.

Thiruganasambandamoorthy, V., Stiell, I.G., Sivilotti, M.L.A., Murray, H., Rowe, B.H., Lang, E., et al., 2014. Risk stratification of adult emergency department syncope patients to predict short-term serious outcomes after discharge (RiSEDS) study. BMC Emerg. Med. 14, 8–doi. http://dx.doi.org/10.1186/1471-227X-14-8.

Toll, D.B., Janssen, K.J.M., Vergouwe, Y., Moons, K.G.M., 2008. Validation, updating and impact of clinical prediction rules: a review. J. Clin. Epidemiol. 61 (11), 1085–1094. Doi:http://dx.doi.org/10.1016/j.jclinepi.2008.04.008.

Tu, J.V., 1996. Advantages and disadvantages of using artificial neural networks versus logistic regression for predicting medical outcomes. J. Clin. Epidemiol. 49 (11), 1225–1231.

US National Library of Medicine, 2009. PubMed Clinical Queries. From http://www.ncbi.nlm.nih.gov/pubmed/clinical/. (Retrieved December 2014.)

van Oort, L., van den Berg, T., Koes, B.W., de Vet, R.H.C.W., Anema, H.J.R., Heymans, M.W., et al., 2012. Preliminary state of development of prediction models for primary care physical therapy: a systematic review. J. Clin. Epidemiol. 65 (12), 1257–1266. Doi:http://dx.doi.org/10.1016/j.jclinepi.2012.05.007.

Wallace, E., Smith, S.M., Perera-Salazar, R., Vaucher, P., McCowan, C., Collins, G.A., et al., 2011. Framework for the impact analysis and implementation of Clinical Prediction Rules (CPRs). BMC Med. Inform. Decis. Mak. 11 (1), 62.

Wallace, E., Uijen, M.J.M., Clyne, B., Zarabzadeh, A., Keogh, C., Galvin, R., et al., 2016. Impact analysis studies of clinical prediction rules relevant to primary care: a systematic review. BMJ Open 6 (3), doi:10.1136/bmjopen-2015-009957.

Wampold, B.E., Mondin, G.W., Moody, M., Stich, F., Benson, K., Ahn, H., 1997. A meta-analysis of outcome studies comparing bona fide psychotherapies: Empirically, "all must have prizes." Psychol. Bull. 122 (3), 203–215.

SECTION 2

Clinical Reasoning in Action: Case Studies From Expert Musculoskeletal Practitioners

A Multifaceted Presentation of Knee Pain in a 40-Year-Old Woman

Jenny McConnell • Darren A. Rivett

Subjective History

Karina, a 40-year-old female patient, presented for treatment of bilateral knee pain (Fig. 6.1). The pain started in her left knee 3 years earlier after a period of intensive running.

Past History of Complaint

Three months after her pain had commenced, she consulted a sports physician, who prescribed Mobic (a non-steroidal anti-inflammatory drug [NSAID]) and referred her for physiotherapy after obtaining a magnetic resonance imaging (MRI) scan of her left knee. The MRI scan showed that Karina had changes, including chondromalacia patellae in the lateral patellar articular facet and mild Hoffa's fat-pad change, suggesting patellar mal tracking or fat-pad impingement, as well as a 5-mm undisplaced, chondral flap of the posterior inner medial femoral condyle. Because there was inflammation in the fat pad, the sports physician administered a corticosteroid injection into the fat pad of her left knee, which initially provided some relief.

The previous physiotherapy program undertaken by Karina consisted of soft tissue massage, taping her knee across the patella and gluteal and quadriceps exercises involving clam exercises, squats and lunges, as well as hamstrings stretches. Three months after commencing physiotherapy, she returned to the sports physician because her right knee was now painful. The sports physician instructed her to cease taking the Mobic because it did not seem to be helping. The physiotherapist had informed the sports physician that Karina was now able to descend stairs without pain and that there was improvement as measured on biofeedback, with the medial quadriceps almost equal to the lateral quadriceps. However, the physiotherapist also noted that Karina was feeling frustrated at her lack of progress because she was still not back to running, so she was getting quite depressed.

The sports physician suggested Karina stop physiotherapy, increase her walking, start swimming but avoid breaststroke and participate in gym activities, as long as there was no bent-knee work. He also suggested that she purchase the *Explain Pain* (Butler and Moseley, 2003) book online, feeling that she was developing a degree of 'pain syndrome around her knees', and this approach might help direct her attention away from her knees. He emphasized to her that the MRI scan did not show any significant pathology and that her present discomfort did not mean that she was further damaging her knee.

Twelve months after her left knee pain commenced, Karina experienced left-sided back pain, with intermittent non-specific referral of pain into the left thigh (Fig. 6.1). She believed that she had ruptured a disc, although she did not have a scan. She received physiotherapy involving back and sacro-iliac joint mobilization, as well as transversus abdominis exercises for the back problem, but she was unsure whether physiotherapy helped her back or whether the 'disc problem' resolved itself with time because the symptoms gradually became more manageable. Her back was still intermittently problematic depending on what she was doing.

Present History of Complaint

Before her initial examination at our clinic, Karina was sent for a new MRI scan of her left knee (Figs 6.2 and 6.3), which again showed low-grade Hoffa's fat-pad oedema, in keeping with changes resulting in patellar mal-tracking, patellar alta with a mildly flattened trochlear groove (interestingly enough, this was not commented upon in the first MRI report), and

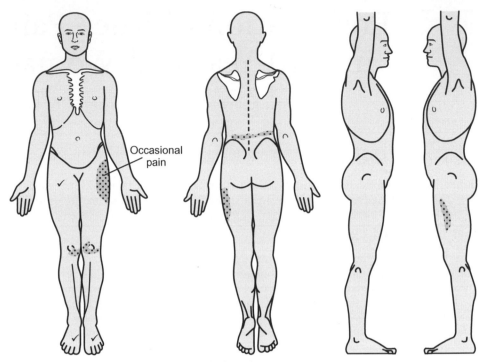

Fig. 6.1   Body chart depicting symptoms.

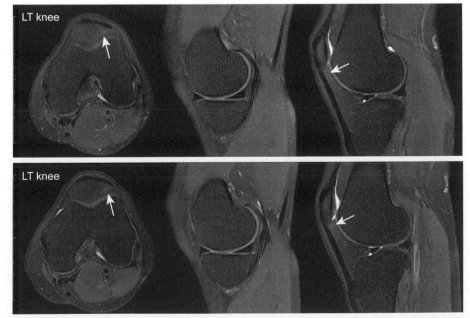

Fig. 6.2   MRI scans of the left knee. The axial view (left) demonstrates chondromalacia, and the sagittal view, medial side (middle) and lateral side (right), demonstrates inflammation of the infrapatellar fat pad and patellar alta.

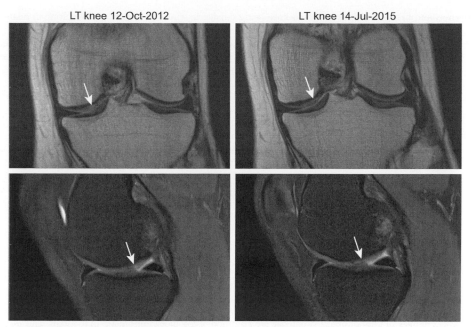

Fig. 6.3 MRI scans of the left knee demonstrating a 5-mm undisplaced chondral flap of the posterior inner medial femoral condyle (unchanged from previous scans).

increased signal in the patellar articular cartilage. When asked during the history why she had come for physiotherapy this time, she stated that she had complex regional pain syndrome (CRPS). She had been attending the pain clinic at the nearby hospital for the last 2 years, where the psychiatrist had prescribed Pristiq (desvenlafaxine), which is a selective serotonin and norepinephrine reuptake inhibitor designed to rebalance the brain's chemicals in people with major depressive disorders.

Karina also volunteered that her 3-year-old nephew had been diagnosed with leukaemia but was now in remission. This diagnosis had caused significant distress and upheaval in her family. Her stress release was running, which she was no longer able to do because of her knee pain. She felt that her inability to run and the strain of her nephew's diagnosis might have contributed to her emotional state of not being able to cope with her knee problems.

Reasoning Question:

1. Karina presented to you with a previous history of unilateral knee pain, which had become bilateral by the time of your first consultation. She also reported a prior episode of low back pain, and she still had some intermittent back pain at presentation. What were your early thoughts about the mechanisms involved in these symptomatic presentations?

Answer to Reasoning Question:

Karina initially experienced unilateral knee pain because she had either increased the frequency of her running with not enough time for recovery or because she had increased the intensity of her running and was running steeper gradients. She was therefore outside her envelope of function, so she had breached the threshold of what her knee could cope with, as her quadriceps muscle had either fatigued or was not strong enough eccentrically for descending steep hills. Her inner-range quadriceps control was likely compromised, so she hyperextended her knee, which inflamed the infrapatellar (Hoffa's) fat pad.

The infrapatellar fat pad is highly innervated and when inflamed causes quadriceps inhibition (Dragoo et al., 2012; Bennell et al., 2004). During walking, 0.5× body weight goes through the knee, but with stairs, this increases to 3–4× body weight (Reilly and Martens, 1972), so if the quadriceps is inhibited, and the demand through the joint increases, the patient will offload the painful knee by solely using the other knee for stair ascent and descent. This can cause an overloading of the other

Continued on following page

knee, and hence it will result in that knee being outside its envelope of function, resulting in bilateral knee pain.

When a patient has bilateral knee pain, she will be more reluctant to flex her knees when she is lifting objects or picking things off the floor, so she will bend her back more, which will put increased pressure on her lumbar spine and hence predispose her to back strain or injury. Interestingly, it has been established in feline spines that a 20-minute bout of sustained flexion or 20-minute bout of intermittent flexion and extension causes a hundred-fold increase in neutrophil density in the supraspinous ligament 7 hours later, indicative of an acute soft tissue inflammation. This is accompanied by a reflexive increase in multifidus activity (Solomonow et al., 2003a, 2003b, 2008).

When the quadriceps is weak, a patient may compensate by using the hamstrings and gastrocnemius muscles to stabilize the knee (Besier et al., 2009; Henriksen et al., 2007). With the hamstrings stabilizing the knee, the hamstrings become tighter, and a tight hamstrings muscle is associated with an increased incidence of low back pain (Feldman et al., 2001). Patients with low back pain also often have a decrease in gluteus maximus and medius activity (Nadler et al., 2001; Nelson Wong et al., 2008). Pain and the accompanying muscle activation changes can contribute greatly to an alteration in the patient's gait pattern and therefore loading through her joints. She will likely continue to experience low back pain and knee pain unless these muscle imbalances are addressed.

Reasoning Question:

2. The sports physician initially administered Mobic and a cortisone injection into the fat pad of the patient's left knee, which gave some short-term relief. What were your thoughts about this, and how relevant did you think the MRI findings were in this case?

Answer to Reasoning Question:

MRI changes of chondromalacia patellae are common, even in asymptomatic individuals, and do not cause pain. The 5-mm chondral flap of the posterior inner medial femoral condyle could cause symptoms of locking if it were displaced, but it would not cause pain, and because the flap was undisplaced, there was no need for any surgical intervention.

The sports physician addressed the inflammatory changes in the infrapatellar fat pad evident on the MRI scan by performing a cortisone injection. A targeted ultrasound-guided cortisone injection into the fat pad can provide pain relief; however, the outcome from the injection is not always consistent, particularly if the cortisone does not reach the area of inflammation in the fat pad. Mobic, an NSAID, is effective if there is a knee joint effusion but is generally not effective for an inflamed fat pad.

The MRI finding of an inflamed fat pad is very significant to the case because it informs us that the quadriceps will continue to be inhibited while the fat pad is inflamed. The knowledge that the fat pad is inflamed should guide our rehabilitation so that we do not give exercises or advice that will further compromise the fat pad. For example, straight leg raises and freestyle kicking in swimming are both activities that will further aggravate the fat pad.

Reasoning Question:

3. If you had been the treating physiotherapist at the initial presentation, what would have been the direction of your treatment?

Answer to Reasoning Question:

It is crucial as a treating clinician, once you have listened to the patient's history, to give the patient some knowledge about why he or she has pain, where the pain is coming from, and the expected length of time it may take for recovery. Knowledge is power, and it is our responsibility to empower patients to manage their problems and to emphasize that musculoskeletal problems are managed, not cured.

Explaining Dye's (1996) model of homeostasis and envelope of function (Fig. 6.4) helps the patient to have an idea as to why her knee pain started. Informing the patient about the loading through the

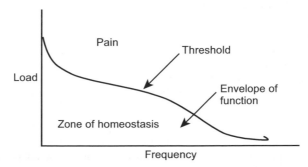

Fig. 6.4 Dye's (1996) model of homeostasis and envelope of function illustrating the effect of intensity and frequency of load on joints. *(Reproduced with permission from Springer Healthcare Ltd.)*

knee with activities is important, as is discussing with the patient the effect of pain and fear of pain on quadriceps muscle activity.

Initially, the patient would have been asked to stand in front of the mirror to observe her lower limb alignment – for example, does she have pronated feet or hyperextending knees or internally rotated femurs? While still in front of the mirror, the patient would then be asked to watch her knee as she steps down from a step to see if she has a dynamic knee valgus (or medial knee collapse), and the implications of this abnormal loading of her knee would be discussed with her. Once on the plinth, she would be asked to palpate her infrapatellar fat pad to determine its size and compare it with the opposite leg. She would be able to see that it is enlarged compared with the other leg. It would be explained to the patient that the infrapatellar fat pad has a large number of nerve fibres, so when it is inflamed, it causes a great deal of pain. This pain turns the quadriceps muscle off, and if the quadriceps is turned off, she will feel more pain, which in turn causes fear of pain, which then results in an inhibition of the medial quadriceps causing a mal-tracking of the kneecap, causing more knee pain and so forth. It can be summarized for the patient as follows:

Increased loading through the knee (0.5× body weight through knee when walking; 3–4× body weight on stairs; 7–8× body weight during squatting; 8–10× body weight when running on a level surface) or rapid straightening of the knee ⇨ inflamed fat pad ⇨ knee pain ⇨ ⇩ quadriceps activity ⇨ more knee pain ⇨ fear of pain ⇨ ⇩ inside quadriceps activity ⇨ mal-tracking of the kneecap ⇨ more knee pain ⇨ further ⇩ quadriceps activity ⇨ ⇧ hamstring and calf muscle activity ⇨ ⇩ gluteal muscle activity ⇨ ⇧ limping which may ⇨ low back pain(⇨, leads to; ⇩, decrease in; ⇧, increase in; ×, times).

Initially, the need for improved recruitment of the lower limb muscles is emphasized because strengthening for activities such as running takes a while. So until she is able to do the activity pain-free, it is advisable for the patient not to participate in that activity.

In summary, the more knowledge patients have after the initial examination, the more empowered they are and more on board they are with your treatment.

Clinical Reasoning Commentary:

An understanding of the importance of the strategy of 'reasoning about teaching' (see Chapter 1) is evident in this response – that is, reasoning associated with the planning, execution and evaluation of individualized and context-sensitive teaching. In this case, the importance of education for conceptual understanding (e.g. musculoskeletal diagnosis, pain), for physical performance (e.g. rehabilitative exercise, postural correction) and for behavioural change (e.g. running) in patient management is discussed. By enhancing the patient's knowledge about her problem and how to 'self-manage' it, she is empowered to increasingly take control of her situation and minimize the impact on her lifestyle. Education to improve understanding can lead to a decrease in patient fear, greater compliance and a concurrent improvement in pain experienced and movement impairments. Musculoskeletal clinicians require significant skills in teaching patients, an aspect of their formal education which is often only minimally addressed.

Physical Examination

Karina was shown in front of a full-length mirror what was being looked for in the examination (flat feet, puffy looking knees, knees that looked at each other when she put her legs together and straightened out when she squeezed her gluteals) and informed that she had inherited her less-than-ideal anatomy from her parents. She presented with internally rotated femurs (Fig. 6.5), pronated feet and enlarged infrapatellar fat pads, with the left worse than the right. She locked her knees back into extension during walking, and although she had an enlarged fat pad on the left, walking was pain-free. Slight pain (measured on a visual analogue scale [VAS] 3/10) was reproduced going down stairs.

Further examination revealed that her entire left leg was smaller than her right, including the calf, gluteals and particularly the quadriceps, with the girth of her left quadriceps being 1 cm smaller than the right. This finding suggested muscle atrophy, consistent with long-term disuse of her leg. In supine lying, Karina's pain was reproduced with an isometric quadriceps contraction (VAS 5/10 left, 3/10 right). Because she was very apprehensive about her knee being touched, the examination was modified to light touch to determine if there was any temperature difference along the legs and between the legs (Goubert et al., 2017; Lazaro, 2016). An 8-cm area above and below the left knee was markedly colder than the surrounding area, with the area over the patella being particularly cold. There was a slight

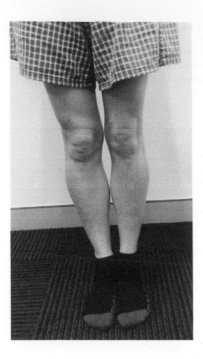

Fig. 6.5 With the patient standing with her legs together, note the internal rotation of the femurs, slight genu varum and quadriceps wasting of the left leg.

change in skin colour associated with the temperature change. Karina then palpated her own knee to feel the temperature difference herself. Her hamstrings flexibility was measured by flexing her hip to 90 degrees and then straightening the left knee, which could only straighten to 40 degrees of knee flexion. This is a good method of assessing hamstrings flexibility without putting too much stress and strain on the knee.

The anterior hip structures were assessed in a figure-of-four position, first in supine lying, which caused no pain, then in prone lying to determine the flexibility of her hip flexors, adductors and internal rotators. This is because if these structures are tight, it will cause an increase in the dynamic valgus vector force (medial knee collapse) when descending stairs. Karina's anterior superior iliac spine (ASIS) was four fingers away from the plinth in the prone position (L>R).

Reasoning Question:

4. Can you please discuss why you didn't perform a more comprehensive assessment of lower limb biomechanics, muscle strength, length and so forth in your physical examination?

Answer to Reasoning Question:

At the initial presentation, Karina was extremely apprehensive about her knee and whether physiotherapy would make her worse, particularly because she knew she had been diagnosed with CRPS, so a modified examination was deemed necessary until she was more comfortable with how she would fare with the treatment. Passive knee movement and muscle strength tests were therefore not performed on the knees at this time because, from experience, this only aggravates the symptoms in someone who has all the hallmarks of what we used to call 'reflex sympathetic dystrophy' (now complex regional pain syndrome, CRPS), as evidenced by the colour and temperature changes around her knee. The immediate concern was to get this patient on board with treatment and to have her feel that physiotherapy would be able to help her navigate her knee problems.

Reasoning Question:

5. What was your hypothesis regarding the pain type (nociceptive, neuropathic, nociplastic) involved? What was your interpretation of the area of the left knee that had temperature changes?

Answer to Reasoning Question:

Karina's pain was multi-faceted. She had an inflamed fat pad (nociceptive pain). She also had an increased sensitivity to touch, and there was decreased temperature and slight skin discolouration from about four fingers above the knee to four fingers below, with the greatest difference being at the knee (particularly the medial aspect). Interestingly, Karina had no pain on walking and did not experience a great deal of pain when stepping off just one step, but she was extremely anxious about movement causing pain. This suggests there was an element of central sensitization, but she had been to a pain clinic as well as having seen a psychiatrist to help with this aspect. Temperature and colour changes are very common around the knee if a patient has central sensitization.

Reasoning Question:

6. How did you explain Karina's pain to her?

Answer to Reasoning Question:

Musculoskeletal clinical practice is a journey toward self-management for a patient. This involves the clinician getting 'buy-in' from the patient, so it is imperative that at the first consultation, you explain to the patient what has happened, why it has happened and what you and the patient can do to improve the symptoms. This means the patient must be aware from the outset that musculoskeletal conditions are not cured but can be self-managed very successfully. It also means that you should intermittently check how the patient is doing every 6–12 months, even after the patient has been 'discharged' from treatment.

During the initial examination, the effect of the intensity and frequency of loads on joints and what happens when their threshold is exceeded should be discussed (see Fig. 6.4). It should be explained to the patient that during walking, 0.5× body weight goes through the knee, 3–4× body weight on stair ascent and descent, 7–8× body weight in squatting and 8–10× body weight with running (Chen et al., 2010). It should be further explained that once she has pain, her function decreases because pain decreases quadriceps activity, which in turn increases the load through the joint because the muscle is no longer supporting the joint. This in turn causes more knee pain, which then results in fear of pain, which causes a decrease in medial (not lateral) quadriceps activity, which will cause lateral tracking of the patella and, of course, more knee pain.

Clinical Reasoning Commentary:

An overlap in pain type mechanisms (e.g. nociceptive with sensitization) requires prioritization of interventions. In this case, sensitization is hypothesised as a consequence of cognitive and emotional input (e.g. unhelpful thoughts, fears about physiotherapy treatment, incorrect beliefs about the cause of her pain, anxiety about movement) with nociception from pathological, inflamed or overloaded tissues (e.g. inflamed fat pad, overloaded patellofemoral joint). The clinician has deemed that the immediate priority is to address the cognitive and emotional factors, through education and other strategies to decrease pain and sensitisation through better understanding, decreased fear and better load management.

Treatment 1

In Karina's case, any treatment directed to the knee would have exacerbated her symptoms, so the concept of why minimal mechanical stimuli are interpreted by the brain as being painful was explained. This was achieved by using the analogy of an electric stove, which keeps cooking the food even when the stove is turned off; the patient's system is similarly tuned so that it responds to all stimuli as if they were painful. The only way the patient can diminish this is to consciously 'turn off' the input by desensitizing the area.

To decrease the hypersensitivity around her knee, Karina was shown a desensitizing regime, which involved rubbing the knee with different textures in a circular fashion, then a stroking fashion. She was instructed to perform the procedure for up to 5 minutes every day. These textures are commonly found in the clinic and consisted of, among others, cotton wool, a pot-scouring pad, a piece of elasticated tubular support bandage and a piece of elastic resistance exercise band; these were given to Karina to take home so that she could maintain the daily regime.

Because Karina needed to have the focus of rehabilitation shifted away from her knee, she was given some strategies to improve limb loading for daily activities. For example, she was instructed that when sitting down and standing up from a chair, she should not use her hands and should keep her knees over her feet; she was also instructed to stand in a modified ballet third position when she had to stand for long periods.

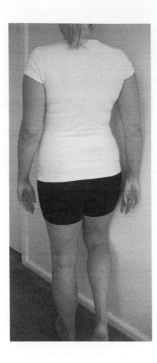

Fig. 6.6 Lower limb weight-bearing training to simulate walking and running. The patient stands as tall as possible at 45–60 degrees to a wall, with all the weight on the outside leg. The pelvis is tucked under slightly, the weight is back through the heel and the knee is very slightly flexed. The knee of the other leg rests against the wall for balance, and the toes remain on the ground, simulating the push-off phase of gait. The patient is instructed to very slightly externally rotate the top of the standing leg thigh, without moving the hip or the foot. The patient maintains this position for 15 seconds and repeats the training often throughout the day.

She was also given a weight-bearing gluteal activity that simulated weight transference from double to single support during gait. This is quite challenging mentally for a patient because it involves a very subtle shifting of weight. The object is to train the brain so that a slightly different muscle pattern is activated to shift the patient out of the end of range, changing the loading through the lower extremity for weight-bearing activities. The gluteal exercise involves training the symptomatic leg (in Karina's case, both legs were symptomatic) to cope with accepting weight, so she was instructed to stand at 45–60 degrees to the wall, with most of her weight through the leg furthest from the wall. The knee of the leg closest to the wall is bent onto the wall for balance, and the heel of that leg is off the floor to simulate the heel-off phase in gait (Fig. 6.6). Karina was then asked to stand tall, with a slight posterior tilt of the pelvis, weight back through the heel and then to very slightly externally rotate the standing thigh.

The instructions to Karina for this gluteal exercise were as follows: (1) stand close enough to the wall so that you can imagine you are about to take a step; (2) turn into the wall so that you are not quite facing the wall; (3) stand on your outside leg; (4) stand tall by keeping the distance from your belly button to the bottom of your ribs as long as possible; (5) tuck your bottom underneath a tiny bit; (6) shift your weight back through your heel; (7) bend your other knee up against the wall for balance, but don't put pressure through it; (8) lift the heel of that leg up off the ground, keeping the toes on the ground; (8) slightly turn the standing (outside) leg thigh without moving the hip or the foot; (9) hold the position for 5 seconds. The patient should feel the contraction in the gluteals; no pain should be felt in the knee, lateral thigh, calf, anterior hip or other leg. If the contraction is felt anywhere else, the position has to be modified. Karina was instructed to practice the exercise often, holding for only 5 seconds initially but building up to 15 seconds.

Karina was also asked to actively stretch her anterior hip structures in a figure-of-four position to help decrease the soft tissue adaptation to her femoral anteversion and to facilitate a gluteal contraction (Fig. 6.7). She was asked to hold the adductors to decrease the tightness and allow a distinct separation of hip and spine movement. This stretch was to be held for 5 seconds, repeated five times and performed twice a day.

Treatment 2 (1 Week Later)

Karina returned a week later to ensure that she was able to do the prescribed training (body management strategies) without any problems and to check that her desensitizing

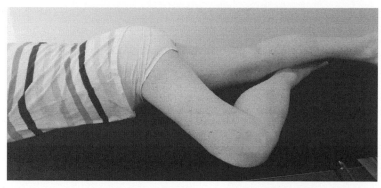

Fig. 6.7   The patient lies prone with the foot of the bent leg positioned under the straight leg just below the tibial tubercle. Ideally, in this position, the anterior superior iliac spine should almost be flat on the table. To perform the exercise, the patient is instructed to elongate the thigh along the plinth without moving the spine, which will result in a stretching of the anterior hip structures.

regime was helping re-establish her connection with her left knee. The gluteal exercise was able to be progressed at this time, such that when she was standing on her left leg, she was able to lift the right leg off the floor. If she felt any pain in her knee, she had to put her toes back on the floor. Again, this was practiced to start with for 5 seconds and performed often, particularly when she stood up after prolonged sitting or if she was about to go for a walk or had just returned from a walk.

Treatment 3 (4 Weeks Later)

As Karina was going on holidays, her next treatment was 4 weeks later. Her pain was improving, and she wanted to return to the gym. She had tried doing a 'dodgy' knee class focussing on people with knee problems and had tried lunging, but this increased her pain. She had returned for her regular checkup with the psychiatrist, who reported that the patient had found that 'physiotherapy had been helpful, particularly the desensitization exercises which seem to be helping reduce the central sensitization', and so the psychiatrist suggested that she 'explore some of the approaches in Norman Doidge's recent book' (Doidge, 2015). The temperature around her knee was now the same as the rest of the leg and the same as the other leg. The discolouration was also gone.

On examination, it was apparent that Karina's ability to descend stairs in a controlled fashion was poor because:

1. The quadriceps were weak, so eccentric control of the knee was poor; and
2. Talocrural joint movement was restricted, as was evidenced by the mid-foot pronating early, causing a dynamic knee valgus collapse.

The restriction of talocrural joint movement was confirmed by evaluating the knee-to-wall test, which showed the left leg was restricted compared with the right. Karina was also unable to walk on her toes on the left, which indicated that the gastrocnemius had been stabilizing her knee because the quadriceps were weak.

At this treatment, we were able to start focussing more on the knee, and the effect of pain and fear of pain on quadriceps activity was reiterated. It was explained that every time she went to the gym or did an exercise class, the strong muscle (vastus lateralis) would get stronger, and the weak muscle (vastus medialis) would stay weak, further increasing the quadriceps imbalance and creating more knee pain. Karina was shown how to inhibit her lateral quadriceps by using firm tape across the muscle belly, which she was to put on every time she was exercising (Fig. 6.8).

Karina commenced doing sets of five small knee bends, four times/day, bending to as far as being able to just see her toes, coming up to 'soft' knees with no locking of the knees, and squeezing her gluteals at the same time. Because she demonstrated a valgus knee collapse during stair descent and because this poor alignment was contributing to her pain, her left talocrural joint was mobilized in weight bearing using a seat belt (in

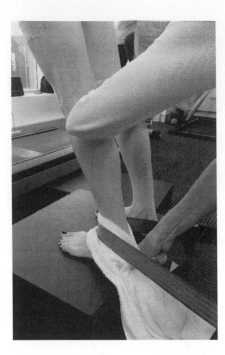

Fig. 6.8 The patient stands on a box and holds on to an immovable object (treadmill). The therapist places a seat belt and towel around the distal end of the tibia and pulls posteriorly while the patient leans forward into the treadmill. Using one hand, the therapist pushes the proximal end of the tibia anteriorly. This position simulates the stance phase of gait and will help increase dorsiflexion range at the talocrural joint. This will then decrease the need for the patient to pronate and internally rotate the femur when descending stairs, which will decrease the stress through the patellofemoral joint.

knee extension to simulate mid-stance phase of gait and also stretch the gastrocnemius muscle) (Fig. 6.8). This is because decreased talocrural joint range when descending stairs causes increased mid-foot pronation, contributing to valgus knee collapse. To help maintain improved foot loading, she was also asked to practice lifting the arch of her foot (activating the tibialis posterior muscle), keeping the base of her big toe on the floor, whenever she stood up from sitting.

Treatment 4 (1 Month Later)

Karina's fourth treatment was 1 month later, where her body management strategies (exercises) – stretching her anterior hip structures, weight-bearing gluteal training, arch lifting and small knee bends – were all reviewed. She had started using an exercise bike at the gym, which she found quite helpful. She was still intermittently desensitizing her knee when she felt she needed to do so.

Her left talocrural joint was mobilized again, and footwear options were discussed. Karina already knew that high-heeled shoes exacerbated her symptoms, but she was confused about why her knees felt worse in ballet flats. It was explained to her that when she came down steps, the ballet flat decreased the available range in her ankle joint, so the foot had to roll more, increasing the loading through the knee joint. Second, ballet flats tend to tip the wearer backward, which causes the knee to lock back, further irritating the fat pad. Because Karina's hamstrings were tight, which adversely affects the quadriceps and gluteal activation, not only loading the knee more but also increasing the strain on the lumbar spine, it was important to indirectly improve hamstrings flexibility. This was achieved by mobilizing her thoracic spine in sitting with the arms supported on the plinth, as this indirect approach would not irritate her inflamed fat pad or increase any CRPS symptoms. The effect of the mobilization was reviewed after 2 weeks, and because it had a positive effect, it was repeated.

Treatment 5 (2 Months Later)

Because the holiday season was approaching and because Karina was now better at managing her symptoms, she returned for further treatment 2 months later. Again, what she had been doing in her home programme was reviewed, and she reported she was able to do most things without much pain. However, whenever she tried to do too much, she had recurrences of her symptoms. On being asked what she expected/wanted to do with her knees, she replied she didn't want to run a marathon, but she would like to be able to do activities with her kids without suffering for days afterward. It was discussed with her how this could be possible and the glacial speed at which muscle recovery occurs. In this treatment, her talocrural joint was mobilized, which had improved in range, and her thoracic spine was again mobilized.

Treatment 6 (2 Months Later)

Before seeing me for her next treatment, Karina had once again seen the psychiatrist, who in his letter to me stated that 'overall she had done very well with her bilateral knee pain. She continues to exercise and live a full life and has been assisted by her physiotherapy treatment. As her mood and anxiety symptoms are stable, she would like to wean off Pristiq (desvenlafaxine), and I have suggested she do this slowly by taking one tablet on alternate days.'

Karina's interpretation of the visit to the psychiatrist was quite different. She told the psychiatrist that she was managing well and having no trouble exercising, particularly when she put two pieces of firm horizontal tape across her lateral quadriceps. She claimed that the psychiatrist told her that putting firm tape across her lateral thigh was 'OCD [obsessive-compulsive disorder] behaviour' and that there was nothing physiologically wrong with her knees and that the pain was all in her mind. At this appointment, she was again shown that there was a considerable difference in size between her right and left quadriceps (when measured, there was a 2-cm decrease in girth of the left thigh at a distance of both 5 cm and 10 cm from the patella). It was reiterated that knee pain causes quadriceps atrophy and that her knee pain was worse, and had been more longstanding in her left knee than the right, because of the decrease in girth of the left thigh relative to the right.

Because Karina could now touch her left knee and cope with others touching her knee, she was able to be shown that her patella was tilted laterally and posteriorly. She could palpate her patella and see that it was tilted, and when she contracted her quadriceps, she could feel the patella glide laterally. Stretching of the tight deep lateral retinacular tissues was undertaken, and she was taught how she could stretch these structures herself. We discussed how she could get a more sustained stretch of the lateral retinacular tissues by taping the patella. Karina was then shown how to tape her own patella, sitting on the edge of a chair with her leg straight but relaxed so that the patella could be moved. She was to start the tape one-third up from the distal pole, in the middle of the patella. This tape lifted the lateral border up and tilted the inferior pole out of the fat pad. She was to place a second piece of tape just past the lateral border, again one-third up from the distal pole of the patella. She was instructed to tape like this as often as she could to improve the seating of the patella in the trochlea, which in turn would improve the activity of the vastus medialis oblique.

Treatment 7 (2 Weeks Later)

Because the management was now being more interventionist at the knee, it was decided to see Karina after just 2 weeks to ascertain the effect of the more directed treatment to the knee. At this next session, it was found that she had managed taping her own knees quite well, and she reported that her knees felt much better. This session involved mobilizing her lateral retinacular tissues, her anterior hip structures and her thoracic spine with the left leg extended, as well as checking her taping and gluteal exercise. Karina was given a sitting hamstrings stretch (Fig. 6.9), where she had to sit on a kitchen bench with the trunk at 90 degrees to the hips and the lumbar spine in a neutral position while the lower leg was extended (she could get her lower leg to 45 degrees in this position) and the foot was dorsiflexed and plantarflexed five times. The stretch was to last 15 seconds and be repeated twice for each leg.

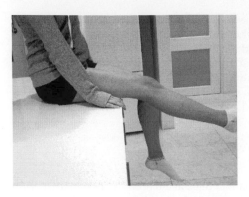

Fig. 6.9 The patient sits tall (in a neutral spine position) with the trunk at 90 degrees to the hips on a kitchen bench so that the legs can dangle. The patient then extends one leg as much as possible without allowing the spine to slump or flex or the trunk to move back. The stretch is held for 15 seconds, repeated twice and performed twice a day.

Treatment 8 (3 Months Later)

Karina was still doing her body management strategies – anterior hip stretches, weight-bearing gluteal training, hamstrings stretches and standing in modified ballet third position. She was progressing well and reported intermittently taping her knee for strenuous activity and going to the gym. She had progressed the weight-bearing gluteal training and now two to three times per week undertook the exercise standing on a pillow, which simulated an unstable surface. Karina was also strengthening her quadriceps by stepping down slowly from a step in front of a mirror, ensuring that her knee was over the middle of her foot and that her pelvis was kept parallel to the floor, as well as by cycling for 30 minutes three times every week.

No further intervention was deemed necessary, but it was agreed Karina would be reviewed every 6 months or so.

Review Note (6 Months Later)

Karina was still going to the gym and doing her body management strategies. She reported being able to do some running, enjoying playing tennis and exercising with her children. She had accepted that she has a condition she has to manage and that it will never be cured.

Reasoning Question:

7. In a nutshell, what were the 'key' learnings you would stress to readers of this case?

Answer to Reasoning Question:

Once Karina's sensitization signs had settled (i.e. the skin was the same temperature as the other leg, and there was no longer any skin-colour change in the area), then the focus was able to be shifted to very slowly increasing quadriceps activity. Karina would have continued to have had marked knee problems unless she was able to improve the strength of her quadriceps muscle, as it is impossible to go up and down stairs without a functioning quadriceps. This must begin with small movements and gradually progress further into range, but for effective strengthening (as opposed to graded activity for desensitization), any training you give a patient must be pain-free. If Karina continues to ensure her quadriceps and gluteals are strong, this will decrease the chances of her condition progressing and may even reverse some of the chondral changes.

Finally, it became apparent that the psychiatrist's reported comments were potentially detrimental to Karina's recovery, as she initially felt that her problem was all in her head. Once the mechanism behind her pain was explained – in particular that it would be difficult for her to improve when her quadriceps were not working effectively – she was able to overcome these unhelpful beliefs and engage in her body management strategies.

Clinical Reasoning Commentary:

An understanding of the patient's problems must include consideration of the patient's attributions about the cause, beliefs about pain and associated cognitions (see Chapter 1). In Karina's case, the identified sensitization likely occurred in response to both internal and external inputs, including cognitive and emotional input, such as her unhelpful thoughts, erroneous beliefs, fears and anxiety that may have resulted from the psychiatrist's comments. Clarifying relationships between beliefs, cognitions and emotions within the history and behaviour of the patient's symptoms assists in the recognition of such unhelpful beliefs and stressors that are contributing to the patient's pain and disability experience. By initially clarifying Karina's thoughts and beliefs regarding the cause of her pain, management could address these misconceptions and associated emotions, first through education, and then gradually through her active engagement in her own rehabilitation.

REFERENCES

Bennell, K., Hodges, P., Mellor, R., et al., 2004. The nature of anterior knee pain following injection of hypertonic saline into the infrapatellar fat pad. J. Orthop. Res. 22 (1), 116–121.

Besier, T.F., Fredericson, M., Gold, G.E., Beaupré, G.S., Delp, S.L., 2009. Knee muscle forces during walking and running in patellofemoral pain patients and pain-free controls. J. Biomech. 42 (7), 898–905.

Butler, D., Moseley, L. 2003. Explain Pain. NOI Group, Adelaide.

Chen, Y.J., Scher, I., Powers, C.M., 2010. Quantification of patellofemoral joint reaction forces during functional activities using a subject-specific three-dimensional model. J. Appl. Biomech. 26 (4), 415–423.

Doidge, N., 2015. The Brain's Way of Healing. Penguin, New York.

Dragoo, J.L., Johnson, C., McConnell, J., 2012. Evaluation and treatment of disorders of the infrapatellar fat pad. Sports Med. 42 (1), 51–67.

Dye, S.F., 1996. The knee as a biologic transmission with an envelope of function: a theory. Clin. Orthop. Relat. Res. 325, 10–18.

Feldman, D., Shrier, I., Rossignol Abenhaim, L., 2001. Risk factors for the development of low back pain in adolescence. M. Am. J. Epidemiol. 154, 30–36.

Goubert, D., Danneels, L., Graven-Nielsen, T., Descheemaeker, F., Meeus, M., 2017. Differences in pain processing between patients with chronic low back pain, recurrent low back pain, and fibromyalgia. Pain Physician 20 (4), 307–318.

Henriksen, M., Alkjaer, T., Lund, H., Simonsen, E.B., Graven-Nielsen, T., Danneskiold-Samsøe, B., et al., 2007. Experimental quadriceps muscle pain impairs knee joint control during walking. J. Appl. Physiol. 103 (1), 132–139.

Lazaro, R.P., 2016. Complex regional pain syndrome: medical and legal ramifications of clinical variability and experience and perspective of a practicing clinician. J. Pain Res. 19 (10), 9–14.

Nadler, S.F., Malanga, G.A., Feinberg, J.H., Prybicien, M., Stitik, T.P., DePrince, M., 2001. Relationship between hip muscle imbalance and occurrence of low back pain in collegiate athletes: a prospective study. Am. J. Phys. Med. Rehabil. 80 (8), 572–577.

Nelson-Wong, E., Gregory, D., Winter, D.A., Callaghan, J.P., 2008. Gluteus medius muscle activation patterns as a predictor of low back pain during standing. Clin. Biomech. 23 (5), 45–553.

Reilly, D., Martens, M., 1972. Experimental analyses of the quadriceps muscle force and patellofemoral joint reaction force for various activities. Acta Orthopaedica Scandinavia 43, 126–137.

Solomonow, D., Davidson, B., Zhou, B.H., Lu, Y., Patel, V., Solomonow, M., 2008. Neuromuscular neutral zones response to cyclic lumbar flexion. J. Biomech. 41 (13), 2821–2828.

Solomonow, M., Baratta, R.V., Zhou, B.H., Burger, E., Zieske, A., Gedalia, A., 2003a. Muscular dysfunction elicited by creep of lumbar viscoelastic tissue. J. Electromyogr. Kinesiol. 13 (4), 381–396.

Solomonow, M., Hatipkarasulu, S., Zhou, B.H., Baratta, R.V., Aghazadeh, F., 2003b. Biomechanics and electromyography of a common idiopathic low back disorder. Spine 28 (12), 1235–1248.

7

Lateral Elbow Pain With Cervical and Nerve-Related Components

Robert J. Nee • Michel W. Coppieters • Mark A. Jones

Initial Examination

Patient Profile and Reported Symptoms

Henry (age 46) reported to physical therapy with a physician diagnosis of 'tennis elbow'. He worked as a safety engineer consultant for the navy. His job involved computer and desk work interspersed with on-site ship inspections at the naval base. He enjoyed golf, gardening and home improvement projects.

Henry's main problem was right (dominant-limb) lateral elbow pain that limited his ability to perform computer work (keyboard and mouse) and power-grip activities (Fig. 7.1). He took frequent breaks from the computer to complete his work duties. He had no ship inspections at the time of the initial examination, but he thought that pain with gripping handrails would make it difficult to negotiate steep stairwells to reach the different levels of a ship. Henry also took frequent breaks to complete weekly gardening activities and did not start any new gardening or home improvement projects because of his symptoms. Although he liked to golf two or three times a week, he could not play because his elbow pain did not allow him to grip and swing a golf club.

Henry also reported having right-sided headaches, right low cervical and upper trapezius area symptoms and a 'falling asleep' feeling in his right arm since a motor vehicle accident (MVA) 25 years ago (Fig. 7.1). He stated these symptoms had not changed since his lateral elbow pain started approximately 1 year ago.

Behaviour of Symptoms

Henry's computer work was limited to 20 minutes because of achiness in his lateral elbow and forearm. Symptoms settled in 10 minutes with resting the arm by his side, and he could then repeat another 20 minutes of computer work. The lateral elbow and forearm did not get more sensitive with repeated 20-minute sessions of computer work throughout the day.

Power-grip activities (e.g. gardening tools, other tools) also aggravated the lateral elbow and forearm symptoms. The 'ache' increased to a 'sharp pain' when objects were heavier or required a larger grip. Henry was able to continue the activity as long as the object was not too heavy (i.e. <5 kg). The 'sharp pain' always settled immediately, but the time required for the 'ache' to settle varied from a few minutes to as long as 60 minutes depending on how hard he pushed the activity. Power-grip activities in elbow extension or in greater degrees of forearm pronation or supination were more painful and took closer to 60 minutes for the 'ache' to settle. The issues with elbow extension and forearm pronation/supination prevented Henry from gripping and swinging a golf club. The 'sharp pain' created by the impact of hitting the golf ball was also problematic. Henry modified power-grip activities to make sure that the 'ache' settled within 60 minutes.

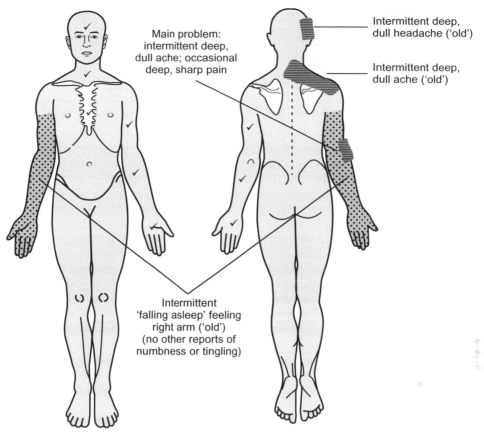

Fig. 7.1 Body chart showing Henry's symptoms at the initial examination. Check marks indicate areas where Henry denied the presence of any symptoms.

In addition to taking more frequent breaks and modifying activities, Henry used an over-the-counter non-steroidal anti-inflammatory drug (NSAID) that helped keep the lateral elbow and forearm 'ache' intermittent, rather than constant. He also occasionally iced his lateral elbow and forearm to help ease his symptoms.

Henry reported no problems sleeping, but his right elbow was generally stiff (lateral side > medial side) when waking in the morning. Gentle flexion and extension movements helped reduce the stiffness in 20 minutes, but if he did not move the elbow, the stiffness lingered for 60 minutes. Even with pacing activities during the day, the lateral elbow and forearm felt more 'tired' and 'achy' at the end of the day, but these feelings were gone by the next morning.

Henry also stated that using his right arm to brush his teeth or reach overhead caused his arm to 'fall asleep'. This feeling settled immediately after stopping the activity. He considered this to be more of a nuisance than a real problem because it had been present since his MVA 25 years ago. As noted previously, the feeling of his arm 'falling asleep' had not changed since his lateral elbow pain started about 1 year ago.

The impact that Henry's symptoms had on his daily function was quantified with the Patient-Specific Functional Scale (PSFS) (Hefford et al., 2012; Stratford et al., 1995). Computer work, gardening and swinging a golf club were the activities Henry nominated for the PSFS at the initial examination (Table 7.1).

History

Approximately 1 year ago, Henry was pulling a heavy bookcase across the floor and felt a 'twinge' in his right lateral elbow. He thought nothing of it at the time and continued his activities without problems. One week later he performed a ship inspection that required

TABLE 7.1	
PATIENT-SPECIFIC FUNCTIONAL SCALE (PSFS) SCORES AT THE INITIAL EXAMINATION*	
Activity	**Initial Exam**
Computer	4
Gardening	4
Swing golf club	0
Average	**2.7**

*Each activity nominated by the patient is rated from 0 (unable to perform the activity) to 10 (able to perform activity at 'pre-injury' level).

a lot of power-grip activities to use the handrails to ascend and descend steep stairwells to reach different levels of the ship. He also had to lift thick and heavy safety manuals to look at information required for the inspection. The inspection lasted 1 week, and during this time, he noticed a gradual onset of the lateral elbow ache. At the end of the week, the lateral elbow ache had increased to the point that he could no longer perform power-grip activities, and he also noticed the sharp pain.

Henry saw his physician 2 months later (10 months ago) because the symptoms had not improved. He received a cortisone injection to his lateral elbow that provided some relief. However, 4 months after the cortisone injection (6 months ago), he was still having symptoms and was referred to physical therapy. Henry reported that physical therapy treatment focused on stretching and strengthening exercises for the common wrist extensors. After 2 months of treatment with no change in his symptoms, he received a second cortisone injection (4 months ago). The second injection led to some additional improvement, but his symptoms had plateaued at his current level of function for the past 2 months.

Henry had no significant medical history, no medical 'red flags' and no symptoms suggestive of potential cervical arterial dysfunction. He was involved in a 'head-on' MVA 25 years ago. He did not lose consciousness and drove his vehicle from the scene. The right-sided headaches and right low cervical and upper trapezius area symptoms started a few days later. He saw a physician shortly after the MVA. Radiographs of his neck were negative, and the physician prescribed pain medication for his symptoms, but it did not help very much. He did not recall how soon after the MVA that the 'falling asleep' feeling started in his right arm. Henry had not pursued any other treatment for these symptoms.

During the patient interview, Henry expressed some frustration with the lack of improvement in his lateral elbow symptoms and not being able to golf. He also wondered whether his neck and arm symptoms from the MVA might partly explain why his elbow symptoms had not responded to previous treatment. A more formal assessment of psychosocial status was not pursued because, other than this frustration, Henry did not convey any overt yellow flags during the patient interview.

Reasoning Question:

1. What were your hypotheses and reasoning at the end of your patient interview regarding dominant 'pain type' (nociceptive, neuropathic, nociplastic), possible 'sources of symptoms' and specific 'pathology'?

Answer to Reasoning Question:

The findings from the patient interview related to Henry's main problem of lateral elbow pain were consistent with lateral epicondylalgia (Coombes et al., 2015). Signs of central sensitization have been documented in lateral epicondylalgia (Coombes et al., 2015) and after MVAs (Sterling, 2014). However, peripheral sensitization of non-neural and neural tissues at the lateral elbow was thought to be the primary contributor to Henry's pain experience. This hypothesis would be consistent with a combination of nociceptive and peripheral neuropathic pain types. Peripheral sensitization of non-neural tissues was likely because the lateral elbow symptoms were relatively localized and consistently aggravated by activities that apply mechanical forces to the common extensor origin and the humero-ulnar, humero-radial and proximal radio-ulnar joints (Coombes et al., 2015; Gifford & Butler, 1997; Smart et al., 2010). Peripheral sensitization of neural tissues was likely because studies show that neurodynamic tests often reproduce symptoms in patients who have lateral epicondylalgia (Berglund et al., 2008; Coombes et al., 2014; Waugh et al., 2004; Yaxley & Jull, 1993). Furthermore, sensitization of upper limb neural tissues can be relatively common in patients who have experienced an MVA (Sterling et al., 2002). Although the 'falling asleep' feeling in the right arm had not changed with the onset of lateral elbow pain, it suggested that neural tissues may have already been sensitized. Impairments in the middle and lower cervical spine were also likely contributing to peripheral sensitization of nociceptive and non-nociceptive pathways associated with lateral elbow and neural structures (Berglund et al., 2008; Cleland et al., 2005; Coombes et al., 2014; Waugh et al., 2004).

Tendinopathy at the common extensor origin was the tissue pathology most likely related to Henry's lateral elbow symptoms (Coombes et al., 2015). Despite recent debate about the nature and amount of any inflammatory process (Rees et al., 2014), tendinopathy is characterized by a dysfunctional healing response to repetitive microtrauma that reduces the load-bearing capabilities of the tendon complex (Coombes et al., 2015; Scott et al., 2013). However, there is no direct relationship between pathology and reports of pain or other symptoms (Chourasia et al., 2013; Coombes et al., 2015; Scott et al., 2013). We therefore thought that treatment should focus on reducing signs of sensitivity in lateral elbow and neural structures, rather than trying to change tendon pathology (Coombes et al., 2015).

Clinical Reasoning Commentary:

Deductive reasoning, based on recognition of accepted criteria, has elicited a diagnostic hypothesis of lateral epicondylalgia, potentially involving multiple local non-neural and neural tissues, with tendinopathy considered the most likely pathology. As discussed in Chapter 1, clinical patterns incorporate enabling or predisposing factors, pathobiological and psychosocial processes and the resulting consequences or disability:

- Enabling conditions: conditions or constraints under which a disease or problem occurs, such as personal, social, medical, hereditary and environmental (e.g. load and ergonomics) factors
- Fault: the pathobiological and psychosocial processes associated with any given disease or disability
- Consequences of the fault: signs and symptoms of the particular problem, as well as its functional impact on the patient's life

Although pattern recognition has been shown to be the dominant mode of reasoning of expert clinicians confronted with familiar, straightforward presentations, musculoskeletal clinicians are frequently presented with more complex presentations requiring more thorough assessment and deductive analysis (i.e. 'slow thinking' discussed in Chapter 1). Musculoskeletal diagnostic reasoning has been made more challenging with the increasing knowledge of pain science highlighting the influence that 'pain type' and mechanisms of peripheral and central sensitisation can have on local tissues.

Tendinopathy is hypothesized as the most likely 'pathology,' and research demonstrating the lack of relationship between pathology and symptoms has guided the proposed plan of management. The limitations of pathology-focused reasoning are discussed in Chapter 1, with the suggestion for a balance between pathology- and impairment-oriented reasoning being needed.

Reasoning Question:

2. What were your hypotheses and reasoning regarding potential 'contributing factors' to the development and onset of his pain and disability and 'precautions to your physical examination and management'?

Answer to Reasoning Question:

The onset of Henry's lateral elbow pain appeared to be related to a gripping and traction injury when pulling the heavy bookcase, followed by a large amount of power-grip activity during the ship inspection 1 week later. As mentioned previously, pre-existing cervical and neural tissue sensitivity from the MVA might have contributed to the development of the lateral elbow symptoms. However, pulling a heavy bookcase and a substantial power-grip activity could lead to similar lateral elbow symptoms in an individual who has no history of neck pain or injury. The relationship between pulling the heavy bookcase and the onset of symptoms suggested that ergonomic issues for computer work, gardening and golf were not likely to be related to the development of Henry's lateral elbow pain. Any ergonomic advice for these activities during treatment would aim to provide relative rest for sensitive tissues, rather than trying to change movement patterns that might have contributed to the initial onset of symptoms.

There were no specific precautions for the physical examination or management. Henry's lateral elbow symptoms were low on the irritability scale (Maitland, 1991), there were no medical 'red flags' and there were no concerns about cervical arterial dysfunction. Despite Henry's previous MVA, upper

Continued on following page

cervical stability testing was not planned for the physical examination because the middle and lower cervical spine would be the target for testing and any initial treatment. Furthermore, initial cervical spine treatment was not likely to involve high-velocity thrust techniques.

It was also important to examine Henry's cervical spine from a psychosocial and management perspective. First, he wondered whether his neck and arm symptoms might partly explain why his lateral elbow pain had not responded to previous treatment. Examining the cervical spine was necessary to help answer his question. Second, previous physical therapy treatment had apparently focused on musculotendinous tissues at the elbow and was not successful, and Henry was frustrated by the lack of improvement in his symptoms. Examining factors not addressed during previous treatment, such as the cervical spine and upper-quarter neural tissues, could reveal different treatment options that might lead to better outcomes. Even if the result of examining these other factors indicated that treatment should still target the musculotendinous tissues at the elbow, the examination process and subsequent explanation of the results might strengthen the therapeutic alliance with Henry and change the context surrounding any local elbow treatment (O'Keefe et al., 2016; Pinto et al., 2012; Stenner et al., 2018). A stronger therapeutic alliance between the patient and clinician is associated with better outcomes (Hall et al., 2010).

Clinical Reasoning Commentary:

Judging the relevance of potential intrinsic and extrinsic contributing factors to the development and maintenance of a patient's problem(s) is challenging given that these, like pathology, do not correlate well with symptoms and signs (or pathology). Because extrinsic factors, such as excessive tissue load and poor ergonomics, and intrinsic factors, such as impaired muscle length and motor control/strength, do not necessarily result in symptoms, skilled clinical reasoning is needed to identify historical and other relationships between potential factors and patient symptoms to generate hypotheses regarding which factors are likely relevant in the individual patient's clinical presentation. Ultimately, all such hypotheses must then be 'tested' in the management phase through targeted interventions and outcome re-assessment.

Information regarding irritability of symptoms and screening for red flags has contributed to the reasoning concerning precautions for physical examination and treatment. See Chapter 1 for further discussion of this important hypothesis category and examples within the range of information that can inform these clinical decisions.

A biopsychosocial approach is evident in the consideration of Henry's queries regarding the possible relevance of his neck and arm symptoms and his frustration with the failure of previous treatments to the physical examination planned, despite no significant psychosocial yellow flags being present.

Physical Examination

Henry showed no relevant postural deviations. Active right elbow extension with the forearm supinated was limited by lateral elbow stiffness at 25 degrees from full extension (full extension on left). Active right elbow flexion with the forearm supinated was limited by lateral elbow stiffness at 115 degrees (130 degrees on left). With the elbow in 90 degrees of flexion, active right forearm supination was limited by lateral elbow stiffness at 65 degrees (85 degrees on left). Active right forearm pronation was full range with no symptoms.

Passive physiological movements were consistent with active movements. Passive right elbow extension (forearm supinated) was much stiffer than other movements and reproduced Henry's lateral elbow pain. Passive elbow flexion was stiff and provoked lateral elbow pain that was not as intense as with elbow extension. Passive forearm supination (elbow flexed 90 degrees) was stiff and provoked stiffness in the lateral elbow region but not pain. Restrictions in passive forearm supination were greater when the elbow was near full extension. Passive forearm pronation was unremarkable.

Passive accessory movement testing focused on the head of the radius with the elbow extended and forearm supinated (Kaltenborn et al., 1980). Anterior-posterior (A-P) and posterior-anterior (P-A) glides of the radial head were very stiff and provoked lateral elbow pain. However, A-P glides were stiffer and more painful.

A dynamometer was not available for measuring grip strength. Therefore, large power grip was tested by having Henry squeeze the distal portion of the examiner's forearm. When tested in 90 degrees of elbow flexion, grip pressure was moderately decreased on the right compared to the left and provoked lateral elbow pain. When tested in elbow extension, there were greater reductions in grip pressure on the right with provocation of more intense lateral elbow pain (De Smet & Fabry, 1996; Dorf et al., 2007).

Resisted isometric wrist extension (Coombes et al., 2015; Cyriax, 1982) showed findings similar to large power grip. Weakness and provocation of lateral elbow pain were more evident during testing in elbow extension than during testing in 90 degrees of elbow flexion.

The shoulder complex was screened with a combination of active movements and resisted isometric tests (Maitland, 1991). Active abduction and hand-behind-back had full range of movement and were pain-free with passive overpressure. Resisted isometric abduction with the shoulder abducted to 30 degrees was full strength and pain-free (Cyriax, 1982).

Deep tendon reflexes and sensory testing of dermatomes were normal. Myotomal testing was negative except for C6. Resisted isometric elbow flexion was weak and provoked lateral elbow pain. As noted previously, resisted isometric wrist extension was also weak and painful. Testing for the C6 myotome was therefore considered inconclusive because it was unclear whether the weakness reflected a neurological impairment or pain inhibition from sensitive structures in the elbow complex (Cyriax, 1982).

The median nerve upper limb neurodynamic test ($ULNT_{MEDIAN}$) on the right provoked lateral elbow and forearm pain at 40 degrees from full elbow extension ($ULNT_{MEDIAN}$ range of motion on left to 20 degrees from full elbow extension and pain-free) (Fig. 7.2). Side-bending the neck away from the tested limb increased the lateral elbow pain (structural differentiation) (Butler, 2000; Elvey, 1997; Nee et al., 2012). The radial nerve test ($ULNT_{RADIAL}$) on the right was modified to accommodate Henry's lack of full elbow extension (Butler, 2000; Elvey, 1997; Nee et al., 2012) (Fig. 7.3). Passive wrist/finger flexion during $ULNT_{RADIAL}$ provoked lateral elbow and forearm pain. However, structural differentiation by altering the amount of shoulder girdle depression or side-bending the neck away from the tested limb did not change these symptoms.

Active cervical flexion had full range of movement and was pain-free with passive overpressure. Extension was limited by stiffness at 55 degrees (measured with inclinometer) with poor segmental motion in the low cervical spine. Passive overpressure provoked right low cervical discomfort. Right rotation was limited by stiffness at 55 degrees (measured with goniometer) and passive overpressure provoked right low cervical discomfort similar to extension. Left rotation was significantly less stiff at 75 degrees (measured with goniometer),

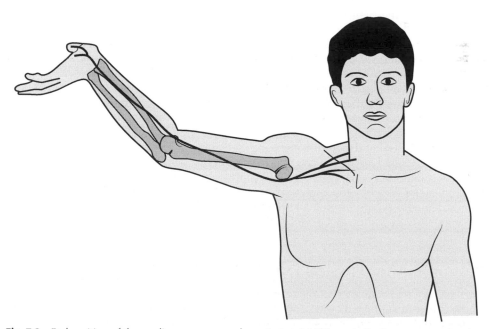

Fig. 7.2 End position of the median nerve neurodynamic test ($ULNT_{MEDIAN}$). Testing sequence involves the following: shoulder girdle stabilization, shoulder abduction, wrist/finger extension, forearm supination, shoulder lateral rotation and elbow extension. Side-bending the neck away from the tested limb or releasing wrist extension can be used for structural differentiation *(Butler, 2000; Elvey, 1997; Nee et al., 2012.)*

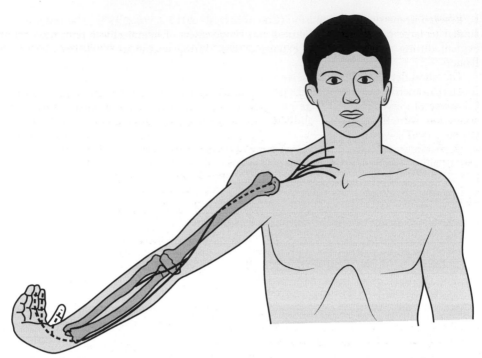

Fig. 7.3 End position of the radial nerve neurodynamic test (ULNT$_{RADIAL}$). Testing sequence involves the following: shoulder girdle depression, elbow extension, shoulder internal rotation and forearm pronation, wrist/finger flexion and shoulder abduction as needed. Side-bending the neck away from the tested limb, releasing shoulder girdle depression, or releasing wrist/finger flexion can be used for structural differentiation (*Butler, 2000; Elvey, 1997; Nee et al., 2012.*)

and passive overpressure did not provoke any discomfort. Combined extension, side-bending and rotation to the right (low cervical quadrant) (Maitland, 1986) had 50% less motion than to the left and provoked right low cervical discomfort. Cervical movements and passive overpressures did not provoke lateral elbow or forearm symptoms.

Palpation examination of the cervical spine involved unilateral A-P pressures and caudal pressures on the first rib in supine as well as central and unilateral P-A pressures in prone (Hengeveld & Banks, 2014; Maitland, 1982). Unilateral A-P pressures from C5 to C7 were significantly stiffer on the right and provoked Henry's symptoms in the right low cervical and upper trapezius area but no elbow symptoms (C6 stiffest and most sensitive). Caudal pressures on the first rib were also significantly stiffer on the right but only provoked local discomfort. Central and right unilateral P-A pressures from C5 to C7 were also very stiff and provoked right low cervical and upper trapezius area symptoms but no elbow symptoms (C6 stiffest and most sensitive). Central P-A pressures were stiffer and more sensitive than right unilateral P-A pressures. Overall, unilateral A-P pressures were stiffest and provoked the most intense symptoms in the low cervical and upper trapezius area. Central and right unilateral P-A pressures at C1 and C2 were also significantly stiff and provoked local discomfort.

Response After Physical Examination

After palpation examination of the cervical spine, active and passive extension of the right elbow (forearm supinated) were only 15 degrees from full extension with noticeably less stiffness, and Henry reported significantly less lateral elbow pain. A-P and P-A glides of the radial head were less stiff and less painful. Large power-grip pressure (elbow extended) was noticeably improved and significantly less painful. ULNT$_{MEDIAN}$ still provoked lateral elbow pain, but symptoms were not provoked until the elbow was 30 degrees from full extension.

Reasoning Question:

3. Please discuss your interpretation of these physical examination findings with respect to whether they supported or did not support your previous hypotheses regarding 'pain type', 'sources of symptoms' and 'pathology'.

Answer to Reasoning Question:

The physical examination findings supported earlier hypotheses that Henry had lateral epicondylalgia with cervical and nerve-related components. Painful decreases in force production during grip testing and resisted isometric wrist extension were consistent with lateral epicondylalgia, especially because these impairments were worse in elbow extension (Coombes et al., 2015; Cyriax, 1982; De Smet & Fabry, 1996; Dorf et al., 2007). Passive stretching of the common extensor origin was incorporated into the ULNT$_{RADIAL}$. Passive wrist/finger flexion with the elbow extended at the end of the ULNT$_{RADIAL}$ provoked Henry's lateral elbow and forearm pain, but structural differentiation did not change these symptoms. This response to the ULNT$_{RADIAL}$ suggested that the provocation of lateral elbow and forearm pain was related to stretching sensitized musculotendinous tissues at the common extensor origin, another finding that was consistent with lateral epicondylalgia (Cyriax, 1982; Waugh et al., 2004). Limited motion and provocation of lateral elbow pain/stiffness with passive elbow extension, passive forearm supination and radial head glides were relevant 'articular' signs that are present in many individuals who have lateral epicondylalgia (Waugh et al., 2004). The humero-radial joint was likely involved because symptoms were at the lateral elbow, deficits in forearm supination were worse when tested in elbow extension and radial head glides were restricted when tested in elbow extension and forearm supination (Kaltenborn et al., 1980; Maitland, 1991).

The cervical and nerve-related components of Henry's problem were supported by the physical examination and re-assessment immediately after cervical palpation examination. Provocation of lateral elbow pain during the ULNT$_{MEDIAN}$ and changing this pain with structural differentiation suggested that Henry's elbow symptoms were at least partly related to increased nerve sensitivity (Nee et al., 2012). The fact that the lateral elbow pain provoked during the ULNT$_{RADIAL}$ did not change with structural differentiation was unexpected because the ULNT$_{RADIAL}$ is the neurodynamic test that typically provokes symptoms in patients who have lateral epicondylalgia (Berglund et al., 2008; Coombes et al., 2014; Waugh et al., 2004; Yaxley & Jull, 1993). The inability to achieve full elbow extension during testing was thought to be the likely reason for the 'negative' response to the ULNT$_{RADIAL}$. Impairments in motion from C5 to C7 during cervical palpation examination were consistent with data showing that many patients who have lateral epicondylalgia also have cervical spine findings (Berglund et al., 2008; Coombes et al., 2014; Waugh et al., 2004). The cervical spine findings were thought to be relevant to Henry's lateral elbow pain because re-assessment showed immediate improvements in passive elbow extension, radial head A-P and P-A glides, grip pressure and ULNT$_{MEDIAN}$ range of motion.

The proportional responses to mechanical testing of tissues supported the hypothesis from the patient interview that peripheral sensitization of lateral elbow and neural structures was the main contributor to Henry's pain experience (Gifford & Butler, 1997; Smart et al., 2010). However, categorizing the peripheral sensitization of these structures into specific pain types can be challenging. The impairments in grip pressure, resisted isometric wrist extension and physiological and accessory movements at the elbow supported the previous hypothesis of a nociceptive pain type (Gifford & Butler, 1997; Smart et al., 2010). The physical examination did not definitively support the previous hypothesis of peripheral neuropathic pain because Henry did not exhibit signs of hyperesthesia or hypoesthesia that are needed to diagnose this type of pain clinically (Finnerup et al., 2016; Treede et al., 2008). Although clinicians feel that positive responses to the ULNTs can help diagnose peripheral neuropathic pain (Smart et al., 2010), we are not aware of any data showing that the ULNTs can diagnose this type of pain in patients who have lateral epicondylalgia (Nee et al., 2012). Even though we could not apply a definitive label of peripheral neuropathic pain to Henry's symptoms, we thought that the increased nerve sensitivity identified during the ULNT$_{MEDIAN}$ needed to improve during treatment because it was associated with the provocation of his lateral elbow pain.

Clinical Reasoning Commentary:

A hypothesis-oriented approach to clinical reasoning, as evident here, is important to reduce the risk of bias from medical diagnosis ('priming' influence discussed in Chapter 1) and initial impressions formulated through the patient interview. It is essential that clinical reasoning is an evolving process of data gathering, analysis, 'testing' of hypotheses and hypothesis revision when supported by a synthesis of information. Here initial hypotheses from the patient interview regarding pain type, sources of symptoms and pathology are all supported by the physical examination. Although specific pathology associated with lateral epicondylalgia cannot be confirmed with the clinical examination, specific physical impairments can, and these are highlighted here with supporting research, thus providing options for impairment-targeted treatments and the ongoing re-assessment necessary for management progression. Re-assessment between key aspects of the physical examination (e.g. cervical palpation

Continued on following page

and elbow 'articular', isometric contraction and neurodynamic assessments) has provided support to hypothesized relationships between these different impairments and the patient's symptoms. Although time consuming, these brief re-assessments enable evaluation of the influence of movement and/or adding load to one impairment on another that can assist treatment decisions while also ensuring that the progressive physical assessment is not worsening the patient's signs and symptoms.

Reasoning Question:

4. Please also discuss the implications of the physical examination findings with respect to overall management plans and specific treatments considered.

Answer to Reasoning Question:

The cervical, neurodynamic and elbow 'articular' findings provided different options for management that might lead to better outcomes than Henry's previous treatments. Clinical trial data support mobilizing the cervical spine in patients who have lateral epicondylalgia (Cleland et al., 2005; Hoogvliet et al., 2013). Evidence for mobilizing the elbow is variable, with less support for simply mobilizing the radial head and more support for a mobilization with movement (MWM) technique where a lateral glide of the proximal ulna is combined with repetitive pain-free gripping (Hoogvliet et al., 2013; Lucado et al., 2018; Mulligan, 1999). Prospective case series data support using radial nerve gliding techniques for patients who have lateral epicondylalgia (Arumugam et al., 2014; Ekstrom & Holden, 2002). Despite its lack of effect during previous treatment, evidence also suggests that therapeutic exercise for the common extensor origin should be part of the overall management of lateral epicondylalgia (Cullinane et al., 2014; Hoogvliet et al., 2013). Exercise for the common extensor origin might be more effective if cervical, neurodynamic and elbow 'articular' signs are also addressed during treatment (Hoogvliet et al., 2013; Lucado et al., 2018). The immediate improvements following cervical palpation examination suggested that it would be a good option to start treatment by mobilizing the cervical spine. The progression of treatment at future visits would be dictated by the results of re-assessment of physical examination findings and Henry's report of changes in symptoms and function (Maitland, 1991). As stated previously, intervention needed to focus on techniques that reduced signs of sensitivity in the lateral elbow and neural structures and allowed Henry to perform computer work, gardening, golf and other power-grip activities without limitations (Coombes et al., 2015).

Clinical Reasoning Commentary:

Evidence-informed practice requires awareness of critically appraised research relevant to your patient's clinical presentation that is then used as a guide to assessment and management. Here, the research-supported identified physical impairments commonly associated with lateral epicondylalgia and research-supported management strategies are highlighted. In the absence of definitive evidence for best management, significant improvement in signs and symptoms following cervical palpation examination is used to support initial treatment directed to the cervical spine. Most clinical problems present with a range of potentially relevant symptomatic and asymptomatic physical impairments and some mix of physical, environmental and/or psychosocial potential contributing factors, almost all of which can be linked to some level of research evidence supporting their attention in management. Although Henry's treatment may have been differently commenced by some clinicians, what is essential is that the treatment options considered are evidence-informed, tailored to the patient's particular presentation, and guided by ongoing re-assessment.

Treatment (Appointment 1, Day 1)

Three main points were discussed with Henry: (1) examination findings were consistent with a diagnosis of 'tennis elbow', (2) lack of long-term improvement from cortisone injections was consistent with published data (Coombes et al., 2013) and (3) sensitivity and stiffness in his right low cervical spine (Berglund et al., 2008; Cleland et al., 2005; Coombes et al., 2014; Waugh et al., 2004) and neurodynamic test findings (Berglund et al., 2008; Coombes et al., 2014; Waugh et al., 2004; Yaxley & Jull, 1993) could be contributing his elbow symptoms.

Reasoning Question:

5. Please discuss your rationale for the discussion with Henry prior to commencing treatment and what you hoped to achieve. Was there anything specific from your assessment of his 'perspectives' (e.g. understanding, beliefs, emotions, etc.) that prompted this discussion?

Answer to Reasoning Question:

Patients expect previous treatment to be changed if it has not been helpful (Peersman et al., 2013; Pinto et al., 2012). The lack of improvement with repeated cortisone injections and previous physical therapy meant that we needed to find alternate treatment strategies. Patients also want accurate and understandable information about their problem so that they can participate in decision-making with the clinician (O'Keefe et al., 2016; Peersman et al., 2013; Pinto et al., 2012; Stenner et al., 2018). The rationale for discussing these three items with Henry was to give him an accurate picture of our interpretation of his pain experience so that he could help make and understand treatment decisions. Henry's question about the role his pre-existing neck and arm symptoms might have in the lack of improvement from previous treatment, and his clear frustration with the overall lack of improvement, made discussing these items even more important. Given his expressed frustration, another aim of this discussion was to reassure him that his experience was not unusual for patients who have lateral epicondylalgia. Although no formal assessments were performed, Henry's frustration appeared to be the only psychosocial factor that was present at the initial examination, so it needed to be acknowledged and addressed. Discussing these three items reflects the type of patient-centred communication that, as mentioned previously, enhances the therapeutic alliance between the patient and clinician and can lead to improved outcomes (Hall et al., 2010; Peersman et al., 2013; Pinto et al., 2012). We believe that these types of individually tailored discussions should be routine clinical practice for all patients.

Clinical Reasoning Commentary:

Psychosocial factors evident in 'patients' perspectives on their experience' (see Chapter 1 for discussion of this hypothesis category) can be present in all patient presentations, from acute to chronic. Even when informal or formal screening for psychosocial factors suggests there are no significant maladaptive factors driving the patient's pain experience, addressing these is still important to optimize the therapeutic alliance, as highlighted with the example of Henry's expressed frustration. The therapeutic alliance is one of a number of factors influencing clinical reasoning discussed in Chapter 1.

Because of improvements in physiological and accessory movements of the elbow, grip pressure and $ULNT_{MEDIAN}$ range-of-motion after palpation examination of the cervical spine, initial treatment focused on mobilizing right unilateral A-P pressures from C5 to C7. Grade III and IV mobilizations that provoked symptoms in the right low cervical and upper trapezius area in rhythm with each oscillation were used to address stiffness (Maitland, 1986). After cervical mobilization, active and passive elbow extension remained 15 degrees from full extension, but Henry reported a further reduction in lateral elbow pain. A-P and P-A glides of the radial head were unchanged. Large-grip pressure was slightly increased with a further reduction in lateral elbow pain. $ULNT_{MEDIAN}$ did not provoke lateral elbow pain until 25 degrees from full extension. Henry was instructed to perform active craniocervical flexion while supine or against a wall for 10–15 repetitions three times each day, with an emphasis on elongating the posterior cervical spine to facilitate low cervical extension. Provocation of symptoms in the right low cervical and upper trapezius area at the end range of the movement was permitted.

Appointment 2, Day 4 (3 Days Later)

Henry reported no soreness after the initial examination and treatment and no problems with the active craniocervical flexion exercise. He stated that his elbow felt generally less sensitive, but he had not noticed any significant increases in the amount of computer work or power-grip activities that he could perform. The feeling of his right arm 'falling asleep' had not been aggravated by the active craniocervical flexion exercise.

Active and passive extension of the right elbow were limited by stiffness at 20 degrees from full extension (25 degrees from full extension at initial examination). Passive extension still provoked lateral elbow pain. A-P and P-A glides of the radial head were slightly less stiff than at the initial examination. Large-grip pressure (elbow extended) was improved but still provoked lateral elbow pain. $ULNT_{MEDIAN}$ provoked lateral elbow pain at 30 degrees from full elbow extension (40 degrees from full elbow extension at initial examination). Right unilateral A-P pressures at C5 to C7 were still stiff and provoked right low cervical discomfort.

Treatment continued with Grade III and IV right unilateral A-P pressures from C5 to C7. However, the technique was progressed by placing the right arm in 60 degrees of shoulder abduction (elbow extended) to preload the upper-quarter neural tissues (Coppieters, 2006; Elvey, 1986; Nee & Butler, 2006) (Fig. 7.4). After treatment, active and passive elbow extension improved to 10 degrees from full extension with significantly less stiffness

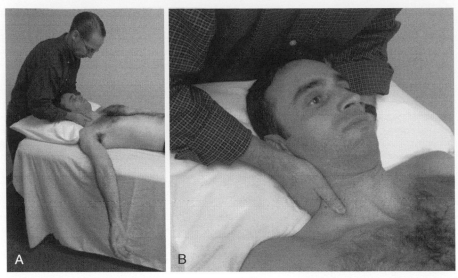

Fig. 7.4 Unilateral anterior-posterior (A-P) pressures at C5–C7 with the upper extremity in shoulder abduction and elbow extension to preload the upper-quarter neural tissues. (A) Patient and therapist positions. (B) Close-up view of the therapist's hand contacts.

and pain. A-P and P-A glides of the radial head were much less stiff. Large-grip pressure was significantly improved and much less painful. ULNT$_{MEDIAN}$ did not provoke lateral elbow pain until 20 degrees from full elbow extension. Henry was instructed to continue performing the active craniocervical flexion exercise but place his arm in 60 degrees of shoulder abduction to preload the upper-quarter neural tissues as during treatment.

Reasoning Question:

6. Please discuss your rationale for the grades of cervical mobilization used (III and IV). Also, what do you hypothesize underlies the treatment responses occurring – for example, how does treating the cervical spine affect radial head glide stiffness/pain and grip strength/pain?

Answer to Reasoning Question:

The perceived restrictions in mobility during the examination using unilateral A-P pressures suggested that stiffness from C5 to C7 contributed to the peripheral sensitisation of lateral elbow and neural structures. Additionally, Henry's symptoms were low on the irritability scale (Maitland, 1991). It was therefore considered appropriate to use grades of mobilization that are thought to be able to address both 'through-range' (Grade III) and 'end-range' (Grade IV) stiffness (Maitland, 1986, 1991). Lastly, Grade III and IV mobilizations might also provide a more appropriate stimulus to elicit the neurophysiological responses described next (Bialosky et al., 2009; Bialosky et al., 2018).

Neurophysiological mechanisms most likely explain why cervical mobilization appeared to make relatively rapid changes in impairments at the elbow. Cervical mobilization provides a mechanical stimulus that activates analgesic responses from higher centres in the central nervous system (e.g. periaqueductal gray area of the midbrain) and spinal cord (Bialosky et al., 2009; Bialosky et al., 2018; Chu et al., 2014; Schmid et al., 2008; Wright, 1995). This type of neurophysiological response to cervical mobilization has been documented in patients who have lateral epicondylalgia (Vicenzino et al., 1998, 1996). The end result clinically is that cervical mobilization can be associated with immediate improvements in passive elbow extension range/pain, radial head glide stiffness/pain, grip strength/pain and neurodynamic testing range/pain. The reduction in signs of sensitivity in lateral elbow and neural structures after cervical mobilization might also allow subsequent treatment directed to the elbow itself to be more effective (Hoogvliet et al., 2013).

Clinical Reasoning Commentary:

As discussed in this answer, the neurophysiological effects of manual therapy are now well documented as the likely mechanism underpinning short-term improvements in musculoskeletal signs and symptoms. Although use of manual therapy has been criticized by some for its lack of efficacy in producing long-term improvements, this fails to appreciate that contemporary musculoskeletal practice generally promotes selective use of manual therapy as a component of management, whereby short-term improvements in pain and function enable inclusion of additional (or progression of existing) management strategies. Skilled clinical reasoning following a comprehensive examination enables identification of where manual therapy may be adventitious as part of a differential diagnosis and, as discussed in this answer, as a means to decreasing sensitivity that may optimize other management strategies.

TABLE 7.2

PATIENT-SPECIFIC FUNCTIONAL SCALE (PSFS) SCORES AT THE THIRD APPOINTMENT*

Activity	Initial Exam (Day 1)	Appointment 3 (Day 8)
Computer	4	6
Gardening	4	5
Swing golf club	0	1
Average	**2.7**	**4.0**

*Each activity nominated by the patient is rated from 0 (unable to perform the activity) to 10 (able to perform activity at 'pre-injury' level).

Appointment 3, Day 8 (4 Days Later)

Henry reported no problems after the second appointment and no problems with progression of the active craniocervical flexion exercise. He noticed improvements in computer work and power-grip activities as reflected by his PSFS ratings (Table 7.2).

Active and passive extension of the right elbow were limited by stiffness at 10 degrees from full extension (20 degrees from full extension at appointment 2). Passive extension still provoked lateral elbow pain. A-P and P-A glides of the radial head continued to be stiff and painful. Large-grip pressure (elbow extended) continued to improve but still provoked lateral elbow pain. ULNT$_{MEDIAN}$ did not provoke lateral elbow pain until 20 degrees from full elbow extension (30 degrees from full elbow extension at appointment 2). Right unilateral A-P pressures at C5 to C7 were less stiff and did not provoke as much right low cervical discomfort.

Treatment continued with mobilization of right unilateral A-P pressures from C5 to C7 with the arm abducted to preload the neural tissues. Although cervical mobilization continued to reduce end-range pain with elbow extension, improve grip pressure and reduce lateral elbow pain provoked by ULNT$_{MEDIAN}$, it had less impact on stiffness with end-range passive elbow extension and with A-P and P-A glides of the radial head. Treatment was progressed by adding Grade III and IV A-P glides of the radial head with the elbow extended and forearm supinated. Lateral elbow pain was provoked in rhythm with each oscillation. Radial head mobilization decreased end-range stiffness and pain with active and passive elbow extension and further improved grip pressure. However, it did not change ULNT$_{MEDIAN}$. Henry continued the active craniocervical flexion exercise with the arm in abduction and was instructed in self-mobilization of elbow extension in a partial weight-bearing position (Fig. 7.5). Provocation of lateral elbow pain at the end range of the self-mobilization technique was permitted.

Appointment 4, Day 11 (3 Days Later)

Henry reported no problems from adding radial head mobilization and self-mobilization into elbow extension. His bouts of computer work had increased to 30 minutes, and symptoms after power-grip activities were consistently settling in less than 45 minutes. He also reported that his morning stiffness lasted less than 10 minutes with elbow flexion and extension movements.

Treatment continued with right unilateral A-P mobilization of C5–C7 with preloading of the upper-quarter neural tissues (now 90 degrees of shoulder abduction with elbow extended) and A-P glides of the radial head in elbow extension and forearm supination. The active craniocervical flexion exercise was progressed by placing the arm in 90 degrees

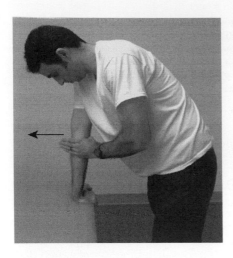

Fig. 7.5 Patient position and hand placement to self-mobilize elbow extension in partial weight bearing of the upper extremity. Arrow shows direction of force to self-mobilize elbow extension.

TABLE 7.3		
PATIENT-SPECIFIC FUNCTIONAL SCALE (PSFS) SCORES AT THE FIFTH APPOINTMENT*		
Activity	**Initial Exam (Day 1)**	**Appointment 5 (Day 15)**
Computer	4	7
Gardening	4	6
Swing golf club	0	2
Average	**2.7**	**5.0**

*Each activity nominated by the patient is rated from 0 (unable to perform the activity) to 10 (able to perform activity at 'pre-injury' level).

of shoulder abduction. Henry also continued with self-mobilization of elbow extension in a partial weight-bearing position.

Appointment 5, Day 15 (4 Days Later)

Henry continued to have no problems with treatments or home exercises. PSFS ratings indicated a clinically important improvement in function compared with the initial examination (Abbott and Schmitt, 2014; Hefford et al., 2012) (Table 7.3).

Active and passive extension of the right elbow had improved to 5 degrees from full extension. Passive elbow extension still provoked lateral elbow pain at the end range of movement. Active and passive forearm supination (elbow in 90 degrees flexion) had improved to 75 degrees (85 degrees on left) but still provoked lateral elbow stiffness at end range. A-P and P-A glides of the radial head were much less stiff and less painful. Large-grip pressure (elbow extended) was still reduced, but Henry stated that lateral elbow pain provoked during this test was 50% less intense than at the initial examination. ULNT$_{\text{MEDIAN}}$ no longer provoked lateral elbow pain at 20 degrees from full elbow extension. Right unilateral A-P pressures at C5–C7 continued to be less stiff and provoked less discomfort in the right low cervical area.

Improvements in elbow extension and ULNT$_{\text{MEDIAN}}$ necessitated progression of the physical examination to continue to identify comparable findings for monitoring Henry's condition (Maitland, 1986, 1991). The passive elbow extension-adduction test (Hyland et al., 1990; Maitland, 1991) was very stiff on the right and provoked more intense lateral elbow pain than passive extension. ULNT$_{\text{RADIAL}}$ was rechecked with Henry's improved amount of elbow extension. Passive wrist/finger flexion during the test still provoked lateral elbow and forearm pain. However, in contrast to the initial examination, structural differentiation by decreasing the amount of shoulder girdle depression reduced these symptoms. Resisted

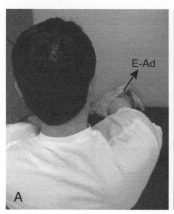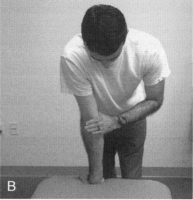

Fig. 7.6 Self-mobilization of elbow extension-adduction in partial weight bearing of the upper extremity. Patient position and hand placement are the same as for self-mobilizing elbow extension (Fig. 7.5). (A) Arrow in overhead view shows the direction of force to self-mobilize elbow extension-adduction (E-Ad). (B) Anterior view shows that with the hand fixed in the partial weight-bearing position, the force applied to the elbow simultaneously extends and adducts the distal forearm relative to the upper arm.

isometric elbow flexion for the C6 myotome was also rechecked and was now full strength and pain-free.

Treatment continued with right unilateral A-P mobilization of C5–C7, but the arm position for preloading the neural tissues was changed to mimic ULNT$_{RADIAL}$ (20 degrees shoulder abduction, shoulder internal rotation, elbow extension and forearm pronation) (Vicenzino et al., 1996). After cervical mobilization, passive elbow extension remained 5 degrees from full extension but was less painful. Passive elbow extension-adduction and A-P and P-A glides of the radial head were unchanged. Large-grip pressure had increased and was less painful. ULNT$_{RADIAL}$ had improved so that lateral elbow pain was not provoked until 20 degrees of shoulder abduction (45 degrees shoulder abduction on left). Treatment was progressed by substituting Grade III and IV right elbow extension-adduction for A-P mobilization of the radial head. Lateral elbow pain was provoked in rhythm with each oscillation. After elbow extension-adduction mobilization, active and passive elbow extension were near full range with less lateral elbow pain. A-P and P-A glides of the radial head were much less stiff and no longer painful. Large-grip pressure was again improved and less painful. ULNT$_{RADIAL}$ was unchanged. Henry continued with the active craniocervical flexion exercise with the arm in abduction. However, self-mobilization of elbow extension in partial weight bearing was modified so that Henry mobilized into elbow extension-adduction (Fig. 7.6). Provocation of lateral elbow pain at the end range of the self-mobilization technique was permitted.

Reasoning Question:

7. Selection and progression of treatment is a largely unresearched area of clinical practice. Would you discuss the general reasoning guiding your approach to 'treatment selection and progression'? Please also comment on your decision to mobilize articular structures (cervical, elbow) rather than the ULNT movements themselves.

Answer to Reasoning Question:

As mentioned previously, treatment focused on reducing signs of sensitivity in lateral elbow and neural structures, rather than trying to change tendon pathology (Coombes et al., 2015). Additionally, we needed to find different treatment strategies because Henry had not responded to previous management. The principle of 'treat and re-assess' guided treatment selection and progression (Maitland 1986, 1991). Relevant impairments (i.e. 'comparable findings' (Maitland, 1991) were treated, and re-assessment determined whether treatment was effective and indicated when changes were needed. The relevance of each impairment was judged by whether it was (1) present in a structure that was within the area of elbow symptoms (e.g. grip force, radial head glides) or able to influence the area of elbow symptoms (e.g. right unilateral A-P pressures from C5 to C7); (2) significant enough to 'fit' with Henry's report

Continued on following page

of symptoms and limitations in function; (3) associated with provocation/reduction of elbow symptoms; (4) consistent with our clinical experience with other patients who had lateral epicondylalgia; and (5) in accordance with available evidence from the literature.

Although not studied specifically in patients who have lateral epicondylalgia, data on patients who have low back pain (Cook et al., 2012; Hahne et al., 2004), neck pain (Cook et al., 2014; Trott et al., 2014; Tuttle, 2005; Tuttle et al., 2006) and shoulder pain (Garrison et al., 2011) support using re-assessment to guide treatment selection and progression. Within-session and between-session improvements in impairments are consistently associated with future improvements in impairment-related outcomes such as pain intensity, range of motion and centralization of symptoms. However, associations with future improvements in self-reported function are less consistent. This means that re-assessment should include both impairment- and function-related outcomes so that treatment selection and progression are as effective and efficient as possible (Tuttle, 2009; Tuttle et al., 2006). The need for function-related outcomes was why the PSFS was an important part of our re-assessment process when treating Henry.

Mobilizing the cervical spine and elbow prior to mobilizing ULNT movements with nerve gliding techniques was based on the results of re-assessment at the initial examination and at follow-up visits. As stated previously, the immediate improvements following cervical palpation examination suggested that it would be a good option to start treatment by mobilizing the cervical spine. Continued improvement in reported symptoms, neurodynamic testing and other physical examination findings at subsequent visits supported this choice. However, we did try to more specifically address nerve sensitivity early in management (appointment 2) by mobilizing and self-mobilizing the cervical spine with the arm in a position that preloaded the upper quarter neural tissues. Re-assessment at appointment 3 showed that although cervical spine mobilization continued to improve neurodynamic test findings, it was having progressively less impact on 'articular' findings at the elbow. Therefore, we decided to start mobilizing the elbow. We are not aware of any data showing that this approach is superior to beginning treatment with nerve gliding techniques in patients who have signs of increased nerve sensitivity. It is conceivable that incorporating nerve gliding techniques earlier in treatment could have led to similar or better outcomes.

Clinical Reasoning Commentary:

This answer reflects the clinical reasoning principle discussed in Chapter 1 that management should not simply follow some predetermined recipe or protocol but instead should be guided by research evidence and clinical experience tailored to the patient's particular presentation and preferences, with re-assessments sufficient to adequately monitor meaningful change. It should be 'collaborative', as shown in this case with attending to Henry's concerns about lack of progress with prior treatments, which both strengthens the therapeutic alliance and optimizes outcomes, as discussed in Chapter 1 and highlighted in the Answer to Reasoning Question 2. Here an overarching aim to reduce signs of sensitivity in lateral elbow and neural structures has been combined with interventions targeting specific physical impairments supported by research related to this pattern of presentation. The rationale for judging the relevance (i.e. weighting) of physical impairment findings is outlined in detail, enabling the clinician to sort incidental impairments/findings from those directly related to the structural source(s) of the pain or contributing to the maintenance of the problem. Being able to articulate the rationale and criteria underpinning your clinical decisions in this way is an important aspect of the critical thinking incorporated in skilled clinical reasoning. Although future research may lead to some revision in our understanding and philosophy of practice (e.g. treatment selection and progression), for this to occur, it is essential that we first understand our own individual reasoning, including the assumptions on which it is based (Brookfield, 2008; Mezirow, 2012).

Appointment 6, Day 22 (1 Week Later)

Henry reported no problems with the progression of treatments or home exercises. His bouts of computer work had increased to nearly 45 minutes, and symptoms after power-grip activities were consistently settling in less than 30 minutes. He reported minimal to no morning stiffness. Henry also stated that the feeling of his arm 'falling asleep' did not come on as quickly with brushing teeth or reaching overhead and seemed to be less intense.

Active and passive elbow extension were near full range of movement. Passive elbow extension was still stiff at end range and provoked mild lateral elbow pain. Passive extension-adduction was still significantly stiff and provoked more intense lateral elbow pain. A-P glides of the radial head were mildly stiff but not painful, and P-A glides were unremarkable. Large-grip pressure (elbow extended) continued to increase and continued to be less painful. ULNT$_{RADIAL}$ provoked lateral elbow pain at 25 degrees shoulder abduction (45 degrees shoulder abduction on left). Although still stiff, cervical extension had increased

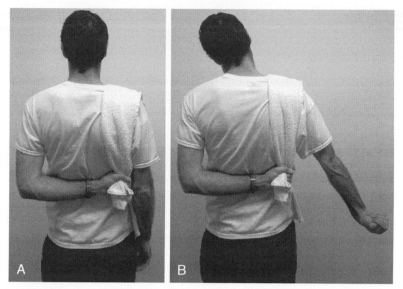

Fig. 7.7 Nerve gliding exercise for gentle, repetitive tensile loading of the radial nerve. (A) Start position. (B) Finish position that mimics the end position of the radial nerve neurodynamic test (ULNT$_{RADIAL}$). Towel prevents shoulder girdle elevation during active movements of the neck and upper extremity.

to 65 degrees (55 degrees at initial examination). Right rotation had increased to 70 degrees (55 degrees at initial examination), but passive overpressure was still stiff and provoked some right low cervical discomfort. Right unilateral A-P pressures from C5 to C7 were still mildly stiff and provoked a small amount of right low cervical discomfort.

Treatment continued with mobilizing right unilateral A-P pressures from C5 to C7 with the arm in a position that mimicked ULNT$_{RADIAL}$ and with mobilizing elbow extension-adduction. Each technique continued to make independent improvements in physical examination findings. At the end of treatment, active and passive elbow extension had full range of movement with no pain. Passive elbow extension-adduction was significantly less stiff and less painful. A-P glides of the radial head were unremarkable. Large-grip pressure was improved and no longer painful. ULNT$_{RADIAL}$ had improved so that lateral elbow pain was not provoked until 35 degrees shoulder abduction. Henry was instructed to continue with the active craniocervical flexion and elbow extension-adduction self-mobilization exercises. He was also asked to perform a radial nerve gliding exercise that focused on gentle, repetitive tensile loading (Coppieters & Butler, 2008; Wright et al., 2005) (Fig. 7.7). Provocation of lateral elbow pain was permitted during each repetition of the radial nerve gliding exercise but needed to settle immediately.

Appointment 7, Day 35 (2 Weeks Later)

Henry had no problems after the previous appointment or with the radial nerve gliding home exercise. PSFS ratings indicated a clinically important improvement in function compared with 3 weeks earlier at appointment 5 (Abbott & Schmitt, 2014; Hefford et al., 2012) (Table 7.4). Computer work was no longer a problem, and the lateral elbow would only feel tired (not painful) with gardening. Swinging shorter golf clubs (e.g. 9 iron) was fine, but swinging longer golf clubs (e.g. driver) provoked mild discomfort in the lateral elbow. Henry had not tried to actually hit a golf ball at this point.

Active and passive elbow extension were unremarkable. Passive elbow extension-adduction was slightly stiff and provoked mild discomfort in the lateral elbow. Large-grip pressure (elbow extended) was still mildly reduced but not painful. Resisted isometric wrist extension (elbow extended) was slightly weak and provoked mild discomfort in the lateral elbow. ULNT$_{RADIAL}$ did not provoke lateral elbow discomfort until 40 degrees shoulder abduction (45 degrees shoulder abduction on left).

Henry was instructed to continue his current home exercise program with the addition of wrist extensor strengthening using a large grip. Wrist extensor strengthening focused

TABLE 7.4

PATIENT-SPECIFIC FUNCTIONAL SCALE (PSFS) SCORES AT THE SEVENTH APPOINTMENT*

Activity	Initial Exam (Day 1)	Appointment 5 (Day 15)	Appointment 7 (Day 35)
Computer	4	7	10
Gardening	4	6	8
Swing golf club	0	2	6
Average	2.7	5.0	8.0

*Each activity nominated by the patient is rated from 0 (unable to perform the activity) to 10 (able to perform activity at 'pre-injury' level).

on eccentric training in positions of elbow flexion and extension (Cullinane et al., 2014). He was encouraged to gradually return to hitting golf balls once he was able to swing all clubs without discomfort. Henry was discharged from formal therapy but was asked to continue with his home exercise program for 2 months after he had returned to all activities without discomfort. He was encouraged to contact us with any questions or if he encountered any problems with his gradual return to all activities.

Reasoning Question:

8. What was your rationale for using eccentric strengthening with Henry?

Answer to Reasoning Question:

Despite being significantly less painful, large grip and resisted isometric wrist extension still had deficits in force production, so it was important to address this remaining impairment. Exercise has positive effects on force production and tendon remodeling (Coombes et al., 2015). In addition to any positive effects there might be on local structures, it is important to consider that exercise might also have positive effects on the neural circuitry involved in the patient's pain experience. Progressive mechanical loading through exercise and functional tasks helps the patient perform previously symptomatic activities with minimal to no pain. These experiences enable the conscious and non-conscious parts of the patient's nervous system to 'learn' that the previously painful area can be used without exacerbating symptoms (Littlewood et al., 2013; Moseley, 2003). This 'learning process' may further reduce the sensitivity of the neural circuitry involved in the patient's pain experience (Littlewood et al., 2013; Moseley, 2003). Regardless of the ultimate mechanisms, incorporating eccentric exercise into a multimodal treatment program improves outcomes for patients who have lateral epicondylalgia (Cullinane et al., 2014).

When reflecting on Henry's treatment, questions could be raised that the prescribed exercise focused on grip and wrist extension but did not address forearm pronation/supination. It would have been logical to assess force production with forearm pronation/supination in more detail because these movements had aggravated Henry's lateral elbow symptoms. We do not have a specific explanation for why this was not done. If Henry had not continued to improve with treatment, we would hopefully have thought about a more detailed assessment of force production with forearm pronation/supination and modified treatment accordingly. Fortunately, our omission did not appear to have a negative impact on Henry's overall outcome.

Clinical Reasoning Commentary:

A clear rationale for the inclusion of exercise in management is provided with critical awareness that both local and neuromodulatory mechanisms may underpin any improvements realized. What is particularly refreshing is the honest critical reflection that additional assessment of force production with forearm pronation/supination could have been undertaken and may have provided further treatment options. Key factors influencing the development of expertise, as discussed in Chapter 1, include critical thinking, metacognition, knowledge organization, data-collection and procedural skills and the patient–therapist therapeutic alliance. Inherent in critical thinking and metacognition is open-minded self-reflection. Although experts know a great deal, they also have sufficiently advanced metacognitive skills to recognize what they don't know and to frankly critique their own performance.

Follow-Up (1 Month Later)

Henry was contacted by phone 1 month after his last treatment. He was gardening, performing home improvement projects and playing 9 holes of golf two times a week without any limitations. The feeling of his arm 'falling asleep' was continuing to decrease. He wanted to increase to playing 18 holes of golf two times a week over the next month and intended to continue his home exercise program for 2 months after he had achieved this goal.

REFERENCES

Abbott, J., Schmitt, J., 2014. Minimum important differences for the Patient-Specific Functional Scale, 4 region-specific outcome measures, and the numeric pain rating scale. J. Orthop. Sports Phys. Ther. 44, 560–564.

Arumugam, V., Selvam, S., MacDermid, J., 2014. Radial nerve mobilization reduces lateral elbow pain and provides short-term relief in computer users. Open Orthop. J. 8, 368–371.

Berglund, K., Persson, B., Denison, E., 2008. Prevalence of pain and dysfunction in the cervical and thoracic spine in persons with and without lateral elbow pain. Man. Ther. 13, 295–299.

Bialosky, J., Bishop, M., Price, D., Robinson, M., George, S., 2009. The mechanisms of manual therapy in the treatment of musculoskeletal pain: a comprehensive model. Man. Ther. 14, 531–538.

Bialosky, J.E., Beneciuk, J.M., Bishop, M.D., Coronado, R.A., Penza, C.W., Simon, C.B., et al., 2018. Unraveling the mechanisms of manual therapy: modeling an approach. J. Orthop. Sports Phys. Ther. 48, 8–18.

Brookfield, S., 2008. Clinical reasoning and generic thinking skills. In: Higgs, J., Jones, M., Loftus, S., Christensen, N. (Eds.), Clinical Reasoning in the Health Professions, third ed. Butterworth Heinemann Elsevier., Amsterdam, pp. 65–75.

Butler, D., 2000. The Sensitive Nervous System. NOI Group Publications, Adelaide, Australia.

Chourasia, A., Buhr, K., Rabago, D., Kijowski, R., Lee, K., Ryan, M., et al., 2013. Relationships between biomechanics, tendon pathology, and function in individuals with lateral epicondylosis. J. Orthop. Sports Phys. Ther. 43, 368–378.

Chu, J., Allen, D., Pawlowsky, S., Smoot, B., 2014. Peripheral response to cervical or thoracic spinal manual therapy: an evidence-based review with meta-analysis. J. Man. Manip. Ther. 22, 220–229.

Cleland, J., Flynn, T., Palmer, J., 2005. Incorporation of manual therapy directed at the cervicothoracic spine in patients with lateral epicondylalgia: a pilot clinical trial. J. Man. Manip. Ther. 13, 143–151.

Cook, C., Lawrence, J., Michalak, K., Dhiraprasiddhi, S., Donaldson, M., Petersen, S., et al., 2014. Is there preliminary value to a within- and/or between-session change for determining short-term outcomes of manual therapy on mechanical neck pain? J. Man. Manip. Ther. 22, 173–180.

Cook, C., Showalter, C., Kabbaz, V., O'Halloran, B., 2012. Can a within/between-session change in pain during reassessment predict outcome using manual therapy intervention in patients with mechanical low back pain? Man. Ther. 17, 325–329.

Coombes, B., Bisset, L., Brooks, P., Khan, A., Vicenzino, B., 2013. Effect of corticosteroid injection, physiotherapy, or both on clinical outcomes in patients with unilateral lateral epicondylalgia: a randomized controlled trial. J. Am. Med. Assoc. 309, 461–469.

Coombes, B.K., Lissett, L., Vicenzino, B., 2015. Management of lateral elbow tendinopathy: one size does not fit all. J. Orthop. Sports Phys. Ther. 45, 938–949.

Coombes, B., Bisset, L., Vicenzino, B., 2014. Bilateral cervical dysfunction in patients with unilateral lateral epicondylalgia without concomitant cervical or upper limb symptoms: a cross-sectional case-control study. J. Manipulative Physiol. Ther. 37, 79–86.

Coppieters, M., 2006. Shoulder restraints as a potential cause for stretch neuropathies: biomechanical support for the impact of shoulder girdle depression and arm abduction on nerve strain. Anesthesiology 104, 1351–1352.

Coppieters, M., Butler, D., 2008. Do 'sliders' slide and 'tensioners' tension? An analysis of neurodynamic techniques and considerations regarding their application. Man. Ther. 13, 213–221.

Cullinane, F., Boocock, M., Trevelyan, F., 2014. Is eccentric exercise an effective treatment for lateral epicondylitis? A systematic review. Clin. Rehabil. 28, 3–19.

Cyriax, J., 1982. Textbook of Orthopaedic Medicine, vol. 1: Diagnosis of Soft Tissue Lesions. Bailliere Tindall, London.

De Smet, L., Fabry, G., 1996. Grip strength in patients with tennis elbow. Influence of elbow position. Acta Orthop. Belg. 62, 26–29.

Dorf, E., Chhabra, A., Golish, S., McGinty, J., Pannunzio, M., 2007. Effect of elbow position on grip strength in the evaluation of lateral epicondylitis. J. Hand Surg. Am. 32A, 882–886.

Ekstrom, R., Holden, K., 2002. Examination of and intervention for a patient with chronic lateral elbow pain with signs of nerve entrapment. Phys. Ther. 82, 1077–1086.

Elvey, R., 1986. Treatment of arm pain associated with abnormal brachial plexus tension. Aust. J. Physiother. 32, 225–230.

Elvey, R., 1997. Physical evaluation of the peripheral nervous system in disorders of pain and dysfunction. J. Hand Ther. 10, 122–129.

Finnerup, N.B., Haroutounian, S., Kamerman, P., Baron, R., Bennett, D.L., Bouhassira, D., et al., 2016. Neuropathic pain: an updated grading system for research and practice. Pain 157, 1599–1606.

Garrison, J., Shanley, E., Thigpen, C., Hegedus, E., Cook, C., 2011. Between-session changes predict overall perception of improvement but not functional improvement in patients with shoulder impingement syndrome seen for physical therapy: an observational study. Physiother. Theory Pract. 27, 137–145.

Gifford, L., Butler, D., 1997. The integration of pain sciences into clinical practice. J. Hand Ther. 10, 86–95.

Hahne, A., Keating, J., Wilson, S., 2004. Do within-session changes in pain intensity and range of motion predict between-session changes in patients with low back pain? Aust. J. Physiother. 50, 17–23.

Hall, A., Ferreira, P., Maher, C., Latimer, J., Ferreira, M., 2010. The influence of the therapist-patient relationship on treatment outcome in physical rehabilitation: a systematic review. Phys. Ther. 90, 1099–1110.

Hefford, C., Abbott, J., Arnold, R., Baxter, G., 2012. The Patient-Specific Functional Scale: validity, reliability, and responsiveness in patients with upper extremity musculoskeletal problems. J. Orthop. Sports Phys. Ther. 42, 56–65.

Hengeveld, E., Banks, K. (Eds.), 2014. Maitland's Vertebral Manipulation, eighth ed. Churchill Livingstone, Edinburgh.

Hoogvliet, P., Randsdorp, M., Dingemanse, R., Koes, B., Huisstede, B., 2013. Does effectiveness of exercise therapy and mobilisation techniques offer guidance for the treatment of lateral and medial epicondylitis? A systematic review. Br. J. Sports Med. 47, 1112–1119.

Hyland, S., Nitschke, J., Matyas, T., 1990. The extension-adduction test in chronic tennis elbow: soft tissue components and joint biomechanics. Aust. J. Physiother. 36, 147–153.

Kaltenborn, F., Evjenth, O., Hinsen, W., 1980. Mobilization of the Extremity Joints: Examination and Basic Treatment Techniques. Olaf Norlis Bokhandel, Oslo.

Littlewood, C., Malliaras, P., Bateman, M., Stace, R., May, S., Walters, S., 2013. The central nervous system - an additional consideration in 'rotator cuff tendinopathy' and a potential basis for understanding response to loaded therapeutic exercise. Man. Ther. 18, 468–472.

Lucado, A.M., Dale, R.B., Vincent, J., Day, J.M., 2018. Do joint mobilizations assist in the recovery of lateral elbow tendinopathy? A systematic review and meta-analysis. J. Hand Ther. In Press: doi:10.1016/j.jht.2018.01.010.

Maitland, G., 1982. Palpation examination of the posterior cervical spine: the ideal, average and abnormal. Aust. J. Physiother. 28, 3–12.

Maitland, G., 1986. Vertebral Manipulation. Butterworths, London.

Maitland, G., 1991. Peripheral Manipulation. Butterworth-Heinemann, London.

Mezirow, J., 2012. Learning to think like an adult. Core concepts in transformative theory. In: Taylor, E., Cranton, P. (Eds.), The Handbook of Transformative Learning, Theory, Research, and Practice. Jossey-Bass., San Francisco, pp. 73–95.

Moseley, G., 2003. A pain neuromatrix approach to patients with chronic pain. Man. Ther. 8, 130–140.

Mulligan, B., 1999. Manual Therapy: "NAGS", "SNAGS", "MWMS" etc. Plane View Services, Ltd, Wellington, New Zealand.

Nee, R., Butler, D., 2006. Management of peripheral neuropathic pain: integrating neurobiology, neurodynamics, and clinical evidence. Phys. Ther. Sport 7, 36–49.

Nee, R., Jull, G., Vicenzino, B., Coppieters, M., 2012. The validity of upper-limb neurodynamic tests for detecting peripheral neuropathic pain. J. Orthop. Sports Phys. Ther. 42, 413–424.

O'Keefe, M., Cullinane, P., Hurley, J., Leahy, I., Bunzli, S., O'Sullivan, P.B., et al., 2016. What influences patient-therapist interactions in musculoskeletal physical therapy? Qualitative systematic review and meta-synthesis. Phys. Ther. 96, 609–622.

Peersman, W., Rooms, T., Bracke, N., Van Waelvelde, H., De Maeseneer, J., Cambier, D., 2013. Patients' priorities regarding outpatient physiotherapy care: a qualitative and quantitative study. Man. Ther. 18, 155–164.

Pinto, R., Ferreira, M., Oliveira, V., Franco, M., Adams, R., Maher, C., et al., 2012. Patient-centred communication is associated with positive therapeutic alliance: a systematic review. J. Physiother. 58, 77–87.

Rees, J., Stride, M., Scott, A., 2014. Tendons - time to revisit inflammation. Br. J. Sports Med. 48, 1553–1557.

Schmid, A., Brunner, F., Wright, A., Bachmann, L., 2008. Paradigm shift in manual therapy? Evidence for a central nervous system component in the response to passive cervical joint mobilisation. Man. Ther. 13, 387–396.

Scott, A., Docking, S., Vicenzino, B., Alfredson, H., Murphy, R., Carr, A., et al., 2013. Sports and exercise-related tendinopathies: a review of selected topical issues by participants of the second International Scientific Tendinopathy Symposium (ISTS) Vancouver 2012. Br. J. Sports Med. 47, 536–544.

Smart, K., Blake, C., Staines, A., Doody, C., 2010. Clinical indicators of 'nociceptive', 'peripheral neuropathic' and 'central' mechanisms of musculoskeletal pain. A Delphi survey of expert clinicians. Man. Ther. 15, 80–87.

Stenner, R., Palmer, S., Hammond, R., 2018. What matters most to people in musculoskeletal physiotherapy consultations? A qualitative study. Musculoskelet Sci. Pract. 35, 84–89.

Sterling, M., 2014. Physiotherapy management of whiplash-associated disorders (WAD). Physiotherapy 60, 5–12.

Sterling, M., Treleaven, J., Jull, G., 2002. Responses to a clinical test of mechanical provocation of nerve tissue in whiplash associated disorder. Man. Ther. 7, 89–94.

Stratford, P., Gill, C., Westaway, M., Binkley, J., 1995. Assessing disability and change on individual patients: a report of a patient specific measure. Physiother. Can. 47, 258–263.

Treede, R., Jensen, T., Campbell, J., Cruccu, G., Dostrovsky, J., Griffin, J., et al., 2008. Neuropathic pain: redefinition and a grading system for clinical and research purposes. Neurology 70, 1630–1635.

Trott, C., Aguila, M., Leaver, A., 2014. The clinical significance of immediate symptom response to manual therapy treatment for neck pain: observational secondary data analysis of a randomized trial. Man. Ther. 19, 549–554.

Tuttle, N., 2005. Do changes within a manual therapy treatment session predict between-session changes for patients with cervical spine pain? Aust. J. Physiother. 51, 43–48.

Tuttle, N., 2009. Is it reasonable to use an individual patient's progress after treatment as a guide to ongoing clinical reasoning? J. Manipulative Physiol. Ther. 32, 396–403.

Tuttle, N., Laakso, L., Barrett, R., 2006. Change in impairments in the first two treatments predicts outcome in impairments, but not in activity limitations, in subacute neck pain: an observational study. Aust. J. Physiother. 52, 281–285.

Vicenzino, B., Collins, D., Benson, H., Wright, A., 1998. An investigation of the interrelationship between manipulative therapy-induced hypoalgesia and sympathoexcitation. J. Manipulative Physiol. Ther. 21, 448–453.

Vicenzino, B., Collins, D., Wright, A., 1996. The initial effects of a cervical spine manipulative physiotherapy treatment on the pain and dysfunction of lateral epicondylalgia. Pain 68, 69–74.

Waugh, E., Jaglal, S., Davis, A., Tomlinson, G., Verrier, M., 2004. Factors associated with prognosis of lateral epicondylitis after 8 weeks of physical therapy. Arch. Phys. Med. Rehabil. 85, 308–318.

Wright, A., 1995. Hypoalgesia post-manipulative therapy: a review of a potential neurophysiological mechanism. Man. Ther. 1, 11–16.

Wright, T., Glowczewskie, F., Cowin, D., Wheeler, D., 2005. Radial nerve excursion and strain at the elbow and wrist associated with upper-extremity motion. J. Hand Surg. Am. 30A, 990–996.

Yaxley, G., Jull, G., 1993. Adverse tension in the neural system: a preliminary study of tennis elbow. Aust. J. Physiother. 39, 15–22.

Nonspecific Low Back Pain: Manipulation as the Approach to Management

Timothy W. Flynn • Bill Egan • Darren A. Rivett • Mark A. Jones

Patient History

Dave is a 46-year-old male who is self-employed as a plumber. He referred himself to our private clinic seeking help for his low back pain. He reported an onset of pain 8 days prior to his initial evaluation. The symptoms had begun shortly after he had been working in his yard operating a chainsaw and lifting and hauling heavy branches and limbs to clear away brush and trees following a recent storm. Dave noticed lower back soreness and fatigue during this work, but he was not concerned because these symptoms were usual for him in his occupation as a plumber. However, the following day upon waking and getting out of bed, he experienced sharp lower back pain, muscle spasm and difficulty moving and Dave felt like he was standing 'crooked.' He subsequently did not work that day and began taking over-the-counter ibuprofen (400 mg three to four times a day). Since that time, his symptoms had remained stable, neither better nor worse.

Dave's current chief complaint was right-sided low back and buttock pain as shown in the body chart (Fig. 8.1). He rated his pain on a numerical rating of pain scale (NPRS) as 5/10 on average, 3/10 at best and 7/10 at worst (Childs et al., 2005). His symptoms were aggravated by the following activities: sitting for longer than 10 minutes; standing for longer than 15 minutes; sitting to stand when getting out of bed or his car; turning over in bed. He reported that when he had been sitting or driving for longer than 10 minutes or upon rising in the morning, it took him a minute or two to be able to stand upright. His back generally felt best when moving, and he frequently changed position to ease his symptoms. His symptoms eased if he lay on his back with his knees flexed (crook lying). Throughout a 24-hour-day, he stated that his back was generally stiff and sore for the first 30 minutes after rising and that his symptoms varied throughout the day depending on activity. His sleep was mildly disturbed due to the pain he experienced while rolling over in bed at night.

Dave denied radiating leg pain or numbness and tingling. On his medical screening form and during follow-up questioning, he denied recent weight loss, night pain, fever or chills, bowel or bladder dysfunction, abdominal pain or gastrointestinal symptoms, a history of cancer or shortness of breath. His medical history was unremarkable with the exception of elevated cholesterol, for which he took Lipitor (statin medication). He denied a family history of rheumatologic disease, but there was a history of heart disease, with his father suffering a myocardial infarction at age 55 requiring coronary artery bypass graft surgery. Dave had experienced intermittent episodes of low back pain occurring approximately twice per year for the past 10 years. The symptoms had typically settled on their own within a week or two, and he had not sought care for his back pain previously. For the current episode, his pain was more severe than any previous episode, and this was the first time he had experienced the postural deviation and a sense of feeling 'crooked'.

Dave lived in the suburbs of moderate-size metropolitan city area with his wife and two school-aged children. He had been employed as a plumber since completing trade

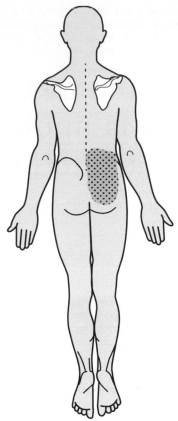

Fig. 8.1 Body chart.

school and currently owned and ran his own business doing residential plumbing work. His wife helped run the business. His job was physically demanding and stressful, at times, but he generally enjoyed his work. He started his work very early in the morning, and there were periods when he worked up to 12 hours/day. In his spare time, Dave enjoyed coaching youth football for his son's team. He did not exercise outside of work and reported that his job provided him with significant amounts of physical activity involving using hand tools, lifting, carrying, bending and working in awkward postures for prolonged periods. Dave did not smoke and drank socially on the weekends.

When asked about what he thought was the cause of his back pain, Dave reported that he thought he 'strained something' while working out in the yard. He expressed some concern that his years of plumbing might have created some 'wear and tear' in his back. He had several friends in his profession who had chronic back pain requiring various medical interventions, and he had some concerns about being able to return to work. Due to the nature of his job, Dave thought it would be very difficult to perform all of his job-related activities while he was experiencing his current level of back pain. He asked if he should get magnetic resonance imaging (MRI) to see 'what is going on and make sure he did not slip a disc'. Because Dave sought physical therapy services at our facility based on a friend's recommendation, he was not really sure what to expect. He had not had physical therapy previously but stated that perhaps 'some stretching exercises' might help his back pain. In general, he was optimistic that he would get better but was worried about continued injury in the future and the potential 'damage' to his back from his job. His goals were to return to all of his required work activities and to 'strengthen his back' in order to prevent further injury.

As part of his initial intake information, Dave completed the Modified Oswestry Disability Index (ODI) (Fritz and Irrgang, 2001) and the Fear Avoidance Beliefs Questionnaire (Waddell et al., 1993). He scored a 22/50, or 44%, on the ODI, indicating a moderate level of perceived disability. This score is typical of patients presenting to outpatient physical therapy for acute low back pain. The Fear Avoidance Beliefs Questionnaire (FAB-Q) is a measure of fear-avoidance beliefs related to work and physical activity and consists of two sub-scales: Work and Physical Activity. Dave scored 14/42 on the work subscale and 6/24 on the physical activity subscale, indicating a low level of fear-avoidance beliefs related to his back pain.

Reasoning Question:

1. Can you outline the range of hypotheses you had at this stage regarding the possible sources of symptoms? Did you recognize a pattern emerging following the subjective examination?

Answer to Reasoning Question:

For a patient such as Dave with acute back pain, the first hypotheses to consider and rule out are more sinister or serious causes of back pain. Recent research has questioned the validity of the so-called 'low-back-pain red flags' as being indicative of serious pathology such as cancer or fractures (Downie et al., 2013). As clinicians, informed by the research, we recommend and use a health history screening questionnaire with follow-up questioning to probe for the potential presence of serious pathology. Based on the totality of the information and clinical judgement, we determine the probability of serious pathology. In Dave's case, there was no indication of any potential serious pathology based on the following: (1) He was younger than 50. (2) He did not report significant personal or family health history making him more likely to have serious pathology as the cause of his back pain. (3) He denied symptoms that could indicate serious pathology, such as constant pain that does not change with position, prolonged morning stiffness, night pain, weight loss or changes to bowel or bladder function. Even though the possibility of serious pathology after the history/interview seemed remote, we would still be mindful to consider it throughout the physical examination and subsequent treatment. For example, if Dave's examination did not match up with what we might typically expect, if he did not respond to treatment as expected or if his status changed over the course of time, we would reconsider the possibility of more serious pathology. Once we have considered serious pathology, the next condition to consider is to assess for lumbar nerve root pathology. He denied any lower extremity symptoms at the time. It did not appear that he had a lumbar radiculopathy, but there was a chance that a radiculopathy could subsequently develop or be present without him overtly sensing or reporting typical radicular symptoms. Therefore, part of our physical examination for Dave consisted of a lower-quarter neurological examination and passive straight leg raise test to assess for the presence of a radiculopathy. Once serious pathology and specific nerve root disorders have been considered, the remaining back disorders have been described as non-specific, indicating there is no readily identifiable pathology for the patient's back pain. There are a variety of methods to sub-classify this group of patients, and as clinicians, we would consider the treatment-based classification (TBC) (Alrwaily et al., 2016) (Table 8.1) scheme for a patient such as Dave with acute back pain. Using the TBC, Dave would likely fit into the manipulation group given his recent onset of back pain (<16 days) and his denial of symptoms radiating below the knee. He could also fit into the specific exercise category if he demonstrated a directional preference.

Continued on following page

TABLE 8.1

DECISION MAKING USING THE LOW BACK PAIN (LBP) TREATMENT-BASED CLASSIFICATION

Consideration of LBP 'red flags' requiring medical management	Patient presents without red flags, significant comorbidities or signs of serious pathology.
Consideration of psychosocial risk profile	Patient presents with minimal psychosocial risk factors.
Staging of the back pain disorder	Patient presents with acute onset, moderate pain and disability, initially indicating Stage 1 management strategies which focus on symptom modulation.
Stage 1 interventions	Patient presents with indication for spinal manipulation. A clear directional preference is not present initially but emerges following manipulation.
Manipulation • Pain <16 days • No symptoms distal to the knee • Lumbar manipulative procedures and mobility exercise	Specific exercise: • Clear lumbar directional preference is present. • Extension, flexion or side-glide procedures matching the directional preference

Other possibilities of sources of symptoms from outside the low back include the hip joint and related soft tissues and the pelvic girdle. The sudden onset of his symptoms, the pattern and location of his symptoms and the aggravating and easing factors did not seem to implicate the hip as a source of symptoms. However, as part of the examination, we would examine Dave's hips to determine if symptoms arise with provocation of the hip joint or if there are relevant movement impairments, such as mobility, muscle length, strength or motor control impairments. Given his age and gender, pelvic girdle pain seemed a remote possibility for Dave. However, if assessment of the lumbar did not reproduce his symptoms, we would next consider pelvic girdle pain provocation tests to explore that region as a potential source of symptoms.

Reasoning Question:

2. What was your hypothesis regarding the 'pain type' (nociceptive, neuropathic, nociplastic)? Did the scores Dave achieved on the questionnaires influence your hypothesis?

Answer to Reasoning Question:

Dave seemed to present with a dominant peripheral nociceptive pain mechanism (Smart et al., 2011). He had acute, relatively localized pain, and the behavior of his symptoms, including the aggravating and easing factors, indicated a mechanical pattern. As described previously, there was a possibility of a potential lumbar radiculopathy developing, which in that case, the dominant mechanism would be peripheral neuropathic. A dominant nociplastic pain type was not present. His symptoms were not widespread, they followed a mechanical pattern and he did not report additional symptoms (sensitivity to pressure, temperature, light) or comorbid conditions (additional regions of pain, gastro-intestinal [GI] distress, headaches) that are suggestive of a dominant central pain pattern. His ODI score of 42 is typical of a patient with acute low back pain (LBP); a much higher score might have indicated significant psychosocial distress and/or a more dominant central pain mechanism. His FAB-Q scores indicated low fear avoidance for work and physical activities, supporting a more peripheral nociceptive pain pattern and suggesting that maladaptive beliefs are minimal.

Reasoning Question:

3. How did the previous lack of contact with a physical therapist, Dave's beliefs about his injury and his reference to friends who have developed chronic pain influence your clinical reasoning at this stage?

Answer to Reasoning Question:

Individual beliefs about back pain are shaped by friends, family, colleagues, media and previous contact with medical providers. In Dave's case, his beliefs were not uncommon for the typical patient presenting with LBP. Patients are often concerned about the seriousness of their current back pain as well as what the future might hold. As the owner and primary employee for his business, in an industry that requires manual work, Dave was concerned for his health and his financial livelihood. Our clinical reasoning at this point suggested that we should provide Dave with a thorough examination, taking time to explain the examination findings, and also spend time discussing with him his current condition and his prognosis. The goals were to provide reassurance that he would recover from his current episode, get him back into his activities as soon as possible and work out strategies with Dave to assist with reducing his risk of future recurrent episodes of acute back pain. It was also important to find a management strategy that would help to reduce his current symptoms rapidly to promote a positive outlook on his recovery.

Clinical Reasoning Commentary:

Clinical reasoning regarding 'sources of symptoms' follows a triage approach that initially considers sinister sources informed through a combination of broad health screening and follow-up questioning in the patient interview. As discussed in Chapter 1, screening for other symptoms, health comorbidities and other potential aggravating and easing factors is an important strategy to minimize the chance of missing relevant information the patient may not spontaneously provide. Although sinister pathology was not supported at this stage of the assessment, consistent with the hypothesis-oriented reasoning framework, this would be 'tested' further through an analysis of the physical examination findings and response to treatments. Similarly, a lumbar nerve root source for Dave's symptoms was not supported by the presenting features but would be tested further in the physical examination. Lastly, somatic low back, hip and pelvic girdle sources would be considered, with the clinical pattern thus far supporting a non-specific low lumbar source. The TBC scheme promotes classification of impairments as identified through the examination. This is consistent with the reasoning framework proposed in Chapter 1 that argues for a balance in pathology- and impairment-based reasoning. Although classification systems assist structured assessments and reasoning, patients do not always fit the designated boxes, and initial classification hypotheses may need to be revised, highlighting the importance of continued reappraisal (i.e. reasoning) over time.

A clinical pattern of a nociceptive dominant pain type was recognized. Although fear avoidance screened via the FAB-Q was judged as low, and Dave's beliefs are not considered maladaptive, the

Answer to Reasoning Question 3 illustrates the importance of analyzing patients' beliefs (component of 'patient perspectives' hypothesis category discussed in Chapter 1) within the broader context of their personal circumstances. That is, beliefs such as understanding of the problem and concerns regarding the future cannot be judged normatively (like range of movement or strength) on their own as adaptive versus maladaptive and need to be explored further, for example, with respect to their relationship to symptom behavior and patient behavior (e.g. coping strategies). As seen here, even when beliefs are judged as reasonable (i.e. not maladaptive), it is still important to address them through education and reassurance within management.

Physical Examination
Observations and Functional Examination

While standing from the chair and walking back from the waiting room, Dave displayed antalgic postures and movement patterns. He sat with his weight shifted to the left and stood with deviation of his weight to the left. His gait was guarded, with decreased rotation of his trunk and a decrease in his stride length bilaterally. Dave stood with a moderate left lateral shift with his shoulders deviated to the left with respect to his pelvis. While undressing, he displayed similar guarded movement patterns and sat down on a chair to remove his shoes quite slowly and carefully.

Standing Lumbar Active Range of Motion

On examination of the active range of lumbar movement, Dave reported his baseline symptoms at 3/10 and the location of his symptoms in the right lower lumbar and buttock region. Because his condition was considered moderately irritable, Dave was instructed to bend only to the first onset of his pain.

Lumbar motion was measured using a single inclinometer placed over T12.

- Standing flexion: 40 degrees forward flexion. Dave's trunk deviated slightly to the left, and he reported that the intensity of his symptoms increased to 6/10 without a change in location.
- Extension: 10 degrees, increased his pain to 6/10 without a change in location.
- Left side bend: 30 degrees, no change in symptoms.
- Right side bend: 5 degrees, pain increased to 6/10 without a change in location.
- Right side-glide: moderately limited, and pain increased to 6/10 without a change in location. Repeated side-glide to the right further increased his symptoms, and his motion did not improve.
- Left side-glide: full, no change in symptoms.

Sitting

A lower-quarter neurological examination was performed, including manual muscle testing, reflexes and sensation to light touch. This revealed no neurological deficits.

Supine

Supine passive straight leg testing was 70 degrees bilaterally with a report of a stretching sensation in the hamstrings muscles.

Passive hip mobility testing in supine revealed increased resistance bilaterally into flexion/adduction without pain. Passive flexion, abduction, external rotation (FABER) of the hips revealed full motion without pain bilaterally.

Prone

Prone passive mobility testing using central and unilateral posterior-to-anterior pressures (PAs) revealed concordant pain rated at 6/10 during central and right unilateral PAs over L4 and L5. Increased resistance was noted at these levels, and these segments were assessed as hypomobile.

Reasoning Question:

4. Did the findings of the physical examination support your earlier thoughts about the 'pain type' and the likely 'source of symptoms'?

Answer to Reasoning Question:

Yes, his examination was consistent with acute mechanical LBP without signs or symptoms of serious pathology or a lumbar radiculopathy. The dominant pain mechanism appeared to be peripheral nociceptive given the discrete location of his symptoms that could be reproduced with lumbar movement and palpation.

Reasoning Question:

5. You assessed straight leg raise. Can you explain what information you intended to gain from performing this test?

Answer to Reasoning Question:

We used the passive straight leg raise test for assessment of neural tissue sensitivity and as a means to 'rule out' a potential lumbar radiculopathy. This test is reported to be sensitive for a lumbar radiculopathy due to lumbar disc herniation, although some studies report that it is more specific than sensitive depending on the reference standard used in the study (Scaia et al., 2012). Going on the premise that the passive straight leg raise is a sensitive test for radiculopathy due to lumbar disc herniation, if the passive straight leg test is found to be 'negative,' the clinician can more confidently 'rule out' a radiculopathy. The negative passive straight leg raise, the absence of leg symptoms and the normal lower-quarter neurological exam together suggested that a lumbar radiculopathy was not currently present with Dave.

Reasoning Question:

6. Can you describe your reasoning process behind arriving at your final diagnosis and your thoughts on initial treatment selection?

Answer to Reasoning Question:

During the examination, we considered the possibility of hip joint pathology given Dave's limited weight bearing on the right side and the lateral shift to the left. Based on his history and age, hip pathology, such as osteoarthritis or non-arthritic intra-articular hip joint pathology, such as femoral acetabular impingement or labral pathology, did not seem likely. This was confirmed by the lack of symptom reproduction with passive hip mobility testing, including the FABER and flexion adduction internal rotation (FADIR) combined movement positions. Pelvic girdle or sacroiliac joint pain was also a consideration. However, in our opinion, if the patient's symptoms are reproduced by movement and provocation of the lumbar spine, pelvic girdle pain is much less likely, and conducting pelvic girdle pain provocation tests could potentially lead to false-positive tests given the common pain-referral patterns between the lumbar spine and pelvic girdle joints. Reflecting retrospectively, we could have considered the possibility of the lower thoracic spine or thoracolumbar junction as the source of symptoms. Although less prevalent than the more typical lower lumbar spine injuries, the lower thoracic spine and thoracolumbar junction region can be a source of mechanical nociception with pain referral into the iliac crest and gluteal region (Maigne, 1980).

Dave was assessed as having an acute, non-specific mechanical low back disorder. Serious pathology was ruled out given the absence of red flags, an unremarkable medical history and screening and a normal neurological examination. Although Dave did have some concerns about his back and how his job activities would relate to the long-term health of his back, he did not have significant yellow flags (psychosocial risk factors of chronicity) related to his back disorder. Furthermore, based on clinical research, Dave had several factors suggestive of a favourable prognosis if he was provided with lumbar manipulation (Table 8.2) (Flynn et al., 2002; Childs et al., 2004; Fritz et al., 2005). The two key factors were a recent onset of symptoms and no symptoms below the knee. He also had low fear-avoidance beliefs and had at least one lumbar segment judged to be hypomobile. Given these findings, Dave potentially had a greater-than-90% chance of success with lumbar manipulation. Success is defined as achieving a greater-than-50% reduction on the ODI score. According to the LBP TBC, Dave also appeared to fit the specific exercise category (Fig. 8.2) (Fritz et al., 2007; Stanton et al., 2011). Patients in this category display a directional preference for a specific lumbar motion. In Dave's case, with the acute lateral shift, side-gliding exercises are typically performed with an attempt to reduce the shift. Dave appeared to fit both the manipulation and specific exercise categories. Given the large benefit of manipulation in terms of pain reduction and functional improvement in appropriately matched patients, it was determined to start with manipulation. Addditionally, it has been demonstrated that provider preferences for treatment positively influence pain outcomes in patients with acute LBP, and joint-biased interventions resulted in a greater chance of meeting participants' expected outcomes. (Bishop et al., 2017). Given that we preferred manipulation in this population that supported our decision as well. Finally, manipulation could facilitate his right side-glide mobility in order to decrease the lateral shift. This would then be followed by directional preference exercises.

TABLE 8.2

THE LUMBAR SPINE MANIPULATION CLINICAL PREDICTION RULES

1. Onset of low back pain (LBP) occurred <16 days ago.*
2. Patient reports no symptoms distal to the knee.*
3. Clinician judges at least one lumbar vertebral level as hypomobile with central posterior-to-anterior (PA) testing.
4. Fear Avoidance Beliefs Questionnaire (physical activity subscale) score <19.
5. Patient has greater than 35 degrees of internal rotation of at least one hip.

If four to five factors are present, +LR of 13.2 for successful outcome with spinal manipulation and exercise.

*Two-factor rule: if the first two factors are present, +LR of 7.2 for successful outcome with spinal manipulation and exercise.

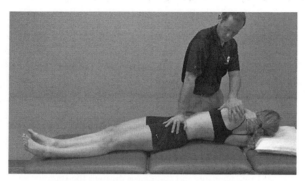

Fig. 8.2   Supine lumbopelvic manipulation.

Reasoning Question:

7. You don't mention any radiological investigations. Can you outline if any findings would have influenced your clinical reasoning and selection of management strategy?

Answer to Reasoning Question:

As physical therapists with the ability to examine and treat patients directly, we consider the potential need for imaging studies in all patients presenting with acute LBP. In Dave's case, there was no indication of a need for immediate imaging. The American College of Physicians Clinical Practice Guidelines (Chou et al., 2011) recommend against routine imaging for patients with acute back pain. The guidelines recommend immediate imaging only in cases where cancer or cauda equina syndrome are suspected. In Dave's case, he did not present with any signs, symptoms, or findings of these disorders. Had Dave presented with a previous history of cancer, lumbar spine radiographs would have been warranted to rule out potential bone metastases as a cause of his LBP. Had he presented with other red flags for cancer, such as night pain, recent weight loss and/or no positions of relief, but without a history of cancer, then clinical judgement might suggest to wait and see how he responds to treatment. If he was responding favourably to therapy, then no imaging would be necessary. If he was not responding as expected to treatment, or his symptoms were worsening, then imaging might be indicated at that time. The bottom line is that for the majority of patients with acute LBP, immediate imaging is not only unnecessary, but it could be potentially harmful, leading to an iatrogenic increase in the patient's self-perceived disability (Flynn et al., 2011). Dave's case is a good example of how physical therapists can effectively serve as first-contact providers for patients with musculoskeletal disorders and potentially reduce unnecessary imaging and other procedures, such as opioid medications, injections and surgery (Ojha et al., 2014).

Reasoning Question:

8. You have outlined your clinical reasoning for your selection of management strategies. Although the clinical prediction rule (CPR) suggested Dave would have a favourable outcome with these measures, did you also draw from any previous experience in determining your management plan?

Answer to Reasoning Question:

This is an important question because the application of CPRs has often been portrayed as akin to 'cookbook' physical therapy. The manipulation CPR serves as a useful guide in the initial clinical reasoning process of clinical pattern recognition. The clinical pattern of a patient with acute LBP without radiculopathy, low fear-avoidance beliefs and lumbar mobility deficits suggests that the patient may have a

Continued on following page

favourable prognosis when treated with spinal manipulation and exercise. However, it is not the authors' contention that manipulation *must* be provided in all cases of patients presenting with these criteria or, more importantly, that manipulation should be withheld from patients who do not fit the CPR. Clinical judgement, experience and the patient's values certainly come into play when considering the manipulation CPR, similar to all other treatment decisions within an evidence-informed clinical practice paradigm. It is interesting to note that during the lumbar manipulation derivation study (Flynn et al., 2002), several patients who were eligible and enrolled in the study presented with an acute lumbar lateral shift. These patients all received lumbar manipulation, and there were no adverse events reported. Prior to this study, many clinicians, including the authors, would have been less likely to provide manipulation as the initial intervention for a patient presenting with acute LBP and a lumbar lateral shift. Since that initial study, the authors have provided manipulation to patients with an acute lumbar lateral shift in clinical practice with varying success and without adverse events. In Dave's case, he met the CPR criteria and did not display contraindications to manipulation, and after a discussion about manipulation as a treatment option, he was very amenable to receiving it. Our clinical experience is that patients such as Dave often have an immediate reduction in symptoms and improvement in lumbar spine motion that can facilitate subsequent and complementary treatment interventions such as exercise. Furthermore, manipulation and other manual therapy procedures, despite being labeled as 'passive' treatments, can play a role in providing a 'cognitive' intervention. In other words, if manipulation is provided and the patient experiences an immediate reduction in symptoms, this can enhance the patient's expectation for recovery and create a positive shift in the patient's beliefs.

Clinical Reasoning Commentary:

The clinical reasoning discussed in these answers illustrates how errors of confirmation bias and premature conclusions are avoided by testing hypotheses formulated in the patient history (subjective examination) in the physical examination. Although it is hoped that this is standard practice for all musculoskeletal clinicians, the relatively newer hypothesis category of pain type (or pain mechanisms) similarly requires learning the typical (but not absolute) clinical patterns for different pain types (see Chapters 1 and 2). Hypotheses in all hypothesis categories (see Chapter 1) should then be tested through both the physical examination and then later through the ongoing re-assessments that occur as management is progressed.

Prognosis and Goals

Dave had a favourable prognosis given the recent onset of symptoms, his overall good health, the low level of psychosocial factors and the lack of symptoms or examination findings suggestive of serious pathology or nerve root involvement. The physical demands of Dave's job were a potential factor that could make returning to work in the short term more difficult while his symptoms were more acute and irritable. However, being self-employed gave Dave the ability to schedule his own work, to modify his job tasks as needed, and to have his employees assist him with more difficult tasks. Dave and I agreed that his short-term goal was to return to work with modified duties within 1 week. Long-term goals were to return to full work duties within 4 weeks in addition to learning self-management strategies and an exercise program to lessen the chances of further episodes of acute LBP.

Treatment 1 (Day 1)

After the initial evaluation, it was explained to Dave that he had an acute low back strain injury without signs of serious pathology or nerve root compromise. I reassured him that despite his pain and limitations, he had a very good chance of recovery. Our clinical experience has been that patients such as Dave who access physical therapy directly and early after an acute episode of LBP, do not have signs of a radiculopathy and have minimal psychosocial factors that would place them at risk for prolonged disability tend to make a rapid recovery. Fritz and colleagues (2015) reported that patients who met the manipulation CPR and received early physical therapy consisting of four sessions of manipulation and exercise experienced an average of a 30-point decrease on the ODI and a decrease of over 3 points on the NPRS from baseline to 4 weeks. We discussed that returning to work and remaining active as tolerated leads to a more rapid recovery and decreases the potential for deconditioning. I explained that although his job was physically demanding, the spine is a strong structure that is meant to be loaded and that his job activities do not necessarily place him at risk for prolonged pain and disability or future 'wear and tear' of his spine. I further emphasized that his active work lifestyle was actually positive in that he was using his back muscles and making them stronger more than if he worked at a desk. We discussed the main findings from his physical exam, including the normal neurological exam, the negative straight leg raise and the mobility impairments of his spine. I explained that spinal manipulation could enhance his recovery by helping to improve his motion and decrease his pain. We discussed that manipulation is a safe procedure when applied to the appropriate patient and that there were several indications from his examination that he would benefit from manipulation. Dave consented to the manipulation and was eager to receive treatment that might help.

I applied the supine lumbopelvic manipulation with right side bending and left rotation of the trunk on the pelvis, which creates tension at the right lumbopelvic region. The clinician applies a thrust to the right anterior pelvic region in a smooth, curvilinear fashion (Fig. 8.2). Care is taken during the setup to ensure maximum patient comfort and that the thrust is performed smoothly and quickly but with low force and amplitude. Afterward, Dave stood up, he reported a reduction in his baseline pain and there was a reduction in his lateral shift. Additionally, there was an improvement in the pain-free range into extension, right side-gliding and right side bending. We then applied repeated right side-glide in standing. As Dave repeated the side-glide, his motion improved, and his pain gradually reduced and centralized toward the central lumbar spine. After two sets of 10 repetitions of the right side-glide, his lateral shift was no longer present. He was then instructed to perform lumbar extension in standing, and after 10 repetitions, his range of motion increased to nearly full, and he had mild end-range pain located in the central low lumbar region. Dave was instructed to continue the side-glide exercise followed by the extension exercises at home every 1 to 2 hours. I explained that his lateral shift was likely to return and that the side-glide exercise should be performed first to address the shift, followed by lumbar extension. At the end of the session, Dave reported an overall decrease in baseline pain (1/10) and had decreased pain with end-range extension and right side-gliding (3/10). Furthermore, his symptoms were no longer present in the right buttock region; they were confined to the lower lumbar spine. I explained to Dave that during his recovery, his symptoms were likely to continue to fluctuate and that soreness or a temporary increase in symptoms following his initial treatment is normal.

Treatment 2 (3 Days Later)

Dave reported an overall reduction in pain (3/10) and noted that his lateral shift was no longer present. He had returned to work the previous day but had avoided heavier lifting and was taking frequent breaks throughout the day to perform his exercise program. He reported a baseline pain of 2/10 located in the right lower lumbar region and denied any pain below L5. Right side-glide and right side-bending range were mildly limited compared to the left, with moderate (5/10) end-range pain. The supine lumbopelvic manipulation was again performed with the thrust on the right anterior pelvic region. Afterward, his side-glide and side bending were full, with mild pain at the end range. After 10 repetitions of repeated right side-glide, this motion was pain-free. Dave was instructed to perform repeated extension every 1–2 hours and only to perform the side-glide exercise as needed if he felt like he was laterally shifted. We discussed continued modification of his work activities as necessary and tolerated and decided to follow up in physical therapy in 5 days. I also explained that his symptoms were likely to fluctuate over the next week but should continue to decrease overall. We also continued to provide pain neuroscience education to include positive messages that "hurt doesn't equal harm" and that his spine is robust and strong (Louw et al., 2017).

Treatment 3 (5 Days Later)

Dave reported that he did not have much pain except when sitting or standing for greater than 30 minutes, stooping over to perform manual work for greater than 5 minutes or when engaging in heavier lifting. He completed a follow-up ODI, which was scored at 18%, indicating a greater-than-50% reduction from his baseline score. His lumbar extension

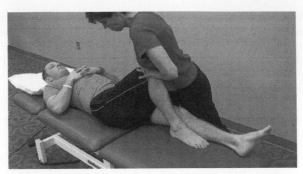

Fig. 8.3 Supine anterior-to-posterior hip mobilization.

and right side-gliding and right side bending were full and pain-free. His lumbar flexion was moderately limited, and he reported end-range pain in the right low lumbar region. It was noted that he did not anteriorly tilt his pelvis forward during forward bending; in other words, he appeared to be moving mostly from his lumbar spine during forward bending. During sitting, squatting and simulated stooping similar to a typical job-related position for Dave, he also displayed increased posterior pelvic tilt and flexion of his low lumbar spine. Based on these observations, in addition to Dave's report of LBP during these positions and activities, it was determined that Dave had a lumbar flexion motor control impairment (MCI) (O'Sullivan, 2005). From a regional interdependence standpoint, restricted hip mobility, particularly into hip flexion, could be related to the lumbar flexion MCI. In Dave's case, supine passive hip flexion with adduction was limited bilaterally. I spent several minutes performing graded hip mobilization in an AP direction (Fig. 8.3) on the right and left sides.

Afterward, there was an improvement in passive hip flexion range. Dave was instructed on how to perform passive hip flexion stretches in supine as part of his home exercise program. To retrain motor control of the lumbopelvic region, Dave was instructed on how to anteriorly rotate his pelvis in supine, quadruped (4-point kneeling) and sitting. In standing, Dave was then cued to bend his knee slightly and to anteriorly rotate his pelvis during forward bending. Tactile cueing was used to help Dave get a feel for how the pelvis should rotate forward with the spine during forward bending. After a few repetitions, Dave was able to bend to full range without pain. We then practiced squatting and stooping using the same principles of rotating the pelvis. We discussed sitting and how to anteriorly rotate his pelvis, and this was a position that felt most comfortable to Dave. An ergonomic setup in his truck was discussed, which helped to best facilitate this position, including tilting the front part of his seat down. Dave was instructed to continue the lumbar extension exercises as needed for pain relief. He was instructed to perform the hip self-stretching exercises, pelvic tilting in supine and sitting and quadruped and to practice squatting while moving through the hips and keeping the lumbar spine in neutral for his home exercise program. Furthermore, Dave was instructed to try using the new way of moving his back throughout his workday. We discussed with Dave that aerobic exercise would greatly benefit his overall health and could potentially decrease future recurrences of LBP. It has been reported that approximately one-half of patients who have recovered from an episode of acute LBP will experience another episode within 1 year (Steffens et al., 2016). Various mechanisms and interventions for a reduction in recurrence rates have been put forward, with little evidence to favour any one mechanism or method. A systematic review reported that programs combining education and exercise led to a 45% risk reduction in LBP episodes for up to a year (Steffens et al., 2016). In Dave's case, he was physically active at work but did not participate in a regular exercise program outside of work. Our thought was that an aerobic exercise program could increase his endurance capacity, provide stress relief and positive benefits to his mental health and decrease other health-related risk factors, such as those for cardiovascular disease. Aside from the general health benefits, the exercise program may potentially assist with reducing future episodes of LBP. Furthermore, Dave's job involved a significant amount of driving, bending and lifting and a program of walking could provide a beneficial variation in the load and stress on his back that he does not regularly receive throughout the day. However, these theories are speculative, and it must be recognized that preventing LBP is a difficult undertaking and that the evidence for low back injury prevention is not very robust. Dave reported that he enjoyed going for walks with his wife and thought that he could do this 3 to 4 days per week, with the goal of working up to 45–60 minutes. We discussed that the intensity of the walk is important and that he should strive to get his heart rate to 104–120 beats/minute. We incresed our pain neuroscience education to include a deeper discussion of pain as an alarm system that alerts us of potential danger and we are going to strengthen the system (Louw et al., 2017).

Treatment 4 (5 Days Later)

Dave reported minimal to no pain with work activities. On examination, he had full, pain-free lumbar range of motion. His lumbar flexion showed an improvement in motion quality with an increased anterior tilt of the pelvis. He demonstrated sitting, squatting and stooping over with improved motion quality. Dave reported that these activities seemed less stressful on his back since learning how to perform them in a different way. Dave had started to take walks with his wife and had worked up to 30 minutes. Dave was instructed to perform squatting using dumbbell weights for external resistance in addition to lunges, single-limb dead-lift exercises, push-ups and rows. These exercises were prescribed to build strength and endurance throughout his lumbopelvic and lower extremity regions in addition to reinforcing the previously learned motor patterns of enhancing hip and pelvic motion during bending and lifting activities to reduce the flexion stress on his lower back. We discussed that maintaining an exercise program involving both aerobic and strength-training exercises could help to decrease the occurrence of future episodes of LBP (Steffens et al., 2016). However, I also explained that recurrent back pain episodes are not unusual. We discussed 'first-aid' interventions should his back become painful again, including the lumbar side-glide and extension exercises. Dave was discharged from therapy with instructions to follow up or call as necessary.

Reasoning Question:

9. You cautioned Dave that he might experience future episodes of LBP. What are your thoughts regarding the long-term prognosis for Dave?

Answer to Reasoning Question:

This is a difficult question to answer with a degree of certainty. From both the literature and clinical experience, we know that back pain in general is highly prevalent and that recurrence rates are high. Dave works in a job involving heavy manual work that could put him at a higher risk for persistent disability related to back pain. However, Dave is the owner of his business and has control over his work tasks, work hours and other aspects of his job that could cause an individual who is an employee to have high work stress and job dissatisfaction. Work stress and job dissatisfaction combined with heavy manual work have been reported as risk factors for persistent work-related LBP and disability (Shaw et al., 2011). Dave is in overall good health, lives a generally healthy lifestyle, has financial stability and has a stable family life. Furthermore, he experienced a rapid recovery from this current episode of back pain and appeared to have a shift in positive beliefs about his back throughout the course of his care. Our hunch is that he will continue to experience minor back strains from time to time given his previous history and his job demands. We do not foresee that his back pain will be very disabling, nor is he likely to develop a persistent LBP disorder. Recent research has shed some light on the trajectory of back pain disorders (Kongsted et al., 2016). Back pain has typically been divided into acute and chronic disorders, with the thought that patients with acute LBP will either improve rapidly or develop chronic pain. However, studies monitoring back pain over time and employing a statistical process known as latent class analysis have reported that trajectories of back pain are more variable. This is observed when back pain trajectories are considered at the level of the individual as opposed to the average of the population. For example, individuals presenting with acute back pain may be experiencing a flare-up of a mild-moderate persistent back pain condition. In these cases, initial management is directed toward the flare-up, and long-term management strategies would then address the more persistent, mild back pain condition. We believe that Dave's case is an example of a mild, persistent back pain disorder accompanied by occasional acute flare-ups. The goal with Dave is that his exercise program and lifestyle modifications could decrease his persistent mild pain and reduce his recurrent flare-up episodes. Furthermore, improved knowledge of how pain works could potentially decrease fear and the over-medicalization of a future flare-up.

Continued on following page

Clinical Reasoning Commentary:

All patients understandably want to know if therapy will help them and how long it is likely to take. Clinicians often struggle with this question, partly because, as highlighted in this answer, research results focus on the average for a population rather than a specific individual. However, research allows the clinician to provide probabilities for the expected outcome of a specific patient for the clinical features (variables) that have been investigated. Sound clinical reasoning integrates these probabilities into a patient-centred discussion. Prognostic reasoning is also often challenging because it is a judgement category clinicians typically attend to with less overt reflection as compared with diagnosis and treatment selection.

Broadly, as discussed in Chapter 1, a patient's prognosis is determined by the nature and extent of the patient's problem(s) and the patient's ability and willingness to make the necessary changes (e.g. to lifestyle, psychosocial and physical contributing factors) to facilitate recovery or improved quality of life. In addition to research evidence of prognosis for different categorizations of patient presentations, at the level of the individual patient, clues will be available throughout the subjective and physical examination and the ongoing management, including the following:

- Patient's perspectives and expectations (including readiness, motivation and confidence to make changes);
- External incentives (e.g. return to work) and disincentives (e.g. litigation, lack of employer support);
- Extent of activity/participation restrictions;
- Nature of problem (e.g. systemic disorder such as rheumatoid arthritis versus local ligamentous problem such as ankle sprain);
- Extent of 'pathology' and physical impairments;
- Social, occupational and economic status;
- Dominant pain type present;
- Stage of tissue healing;
- Irritability of the disorder;
- Length of history and progression of disorder; and
- Patient's general health, age and pre-existing disorders.

Although prognostic decisions are not an exact science, as pointed out in this answer, it is helpful to consider a patient's prognosis by reflecting on the positives and negatives from the previous list or other sets of criteria. Importantly, to then get better at these prognostic judgements, clinicians need to critically reflect on their initial judgement after they have seen the patient for a limited number of sessions and reappraise the patient's prognosis. When that judgement has not been correct, the key is to learn from that by returning to the initial judgement and the basis for that judgement (research and individual patient presentation) to identify where particular features may have been under- or overweighted.

REFERENCES

Alrwaily, M., Timko, M., Schneider, M., et al., 2016. Treatment-based classification system for low back pain: revision and update. Phys. Ther. 96 (7), 1057–1066.

Bishop, M., Bialosky, J., Penza, C., et al., 2017. The influence of clinical equipoise and patient preferences on outcomes of conservative manual interventions for spinal pain: an experimental study. J. Pain Res. 10, 965–972.

Childs, J.D., Fritz, J.M., Flynn, T.W., et al., 2004. Validation of a clinical prediction rule to identify patients with low back pain likely to benefit from spinal manipulation. Ann. Intern. Med. 141, 920–928.

Childs, J.D., Piva, S.R., Fritz, J.M., 2005. Responsiveness of the numeric pain rating scale in patients with low back pain. Spine 30, 1331–1335.

Chou, R., Qaseem, A., Owens, D.K., et al., 2011. Diagnostic imaging for low back pain: advice for high-value health care from the American College of Physicians. Ann. Intern. Med. 154, 181–189.

Downie, A., Williams, C.M., Henschke, N., et al., 2013. Red flags to screen for malignancy and fracture in patients with low back pain: systematic review. BMJ 347, f7095.

Flynn, T., Fritz, J.M., Whitman, J., et al., 2002. A clinical prediction rule for classifying patients with low back pain who demonstrate short-term improvement with spinal manipulation. Spine 27, 2835–2843.

Flynn, T.W., Smith, B., Chou, R., 2011. Appropriate use of diagnostic imaging in low back pain: a reminder that unnecessary imaging may do as much harm as good. J. Orthop. Sports Phys. Ther. 41, 838–846.

Fritz, J.M., Irrgang, J.J., 2001. A comparison of a modified Oswestry disability questionnaire and the Quebec back pain disability scale. Phys. Ther. 81, 776–788.

Fritz, J.M., Childs, J.D., Flynn, T.W., 2005. Pragmatic application of a clinical prediction rule in primary care to identify patients with low back pain likely to respond quickly to spinal manipulation. BMC Fam. Pract. 6, 29.

Fritz, J.M., Cleland, J.A., Childs, J.D., 2007. Subgrouping patients with low back pain: evolution of a classification approach to physical therapy. J. Orthop. Sports Phys. Ther. 37, 290–302.

Fritz, J.M., Magel, J.S., McFadden, M., 2015. Early physical therapy vs usual care in patients with recent-onset low back pain: a randomized clinical trial. JAMA 13 (314), 1459–1467.

Kongsted, A., Kent, P., Axen, I., et al., 2016. What have we learned from ten years of trajectory research in low back pain? BMC Musculoskelet. Disord. 21 (17), 220.

Louw, A., Nijs, J., Puentedura, L., 2017. A clinical perspective on a pain neuroscience education approach to manual therapy. J. Man. Manip. Ther. 25 (3), 160–168.

Maigne, R., 1980. Low back pain of thoracolumbar origin. Arch. Phys. Med. Rehabil. 61, 389–395.

Ojha, H.A., Snyder, R.S., Davenport, T.E., 2014. Direct access compared with referred physical therapy episodes of care: a systematic review. Phys. Ther. 94, 14–30.

O'Sullivan, P., 2005. Diagnosis and classification of chronic low back pain disorders: maladaptive movement and motor control impairments as underlying mechanism. Man. Ther. 10, 242–255.

Scaia, V., Baxter, D., Cook, C., 2012. The pain provocation-based straight leg raise test for diagnosis of lumbar disc herniation, lumbar radiculopathy, and/or sciatica: a systematic review of clinical utility. J. Back Musculoskelet. Rehabil. 5, 215–223.

Shaw, W.S., Main, C.J., Johnston, V., 2011. Addressing occupational factors in the management of low back pain: implications for physical therapist practice. Phys. Ther. 91, 777–789.

Smart, K.M., Blake, C., Staines, A., Doody, C., 2011. The discriminative validity of 'nociceptive,' 'peripheral neuropathic,' and 'central sensitization' as mechanisms-based classifications of musculoskeletal pain. Clin. J. Pain 27, 655–663.

Stanton, T.R., Fritz, J.M., Hancock, M.J., et al., 2011. Evaluation of a treatment-based classification algorithm for low back pain: a cross-sectional study. Phys. Ther. 91, 496–509.

Steffens, D., Maher, C.G., Pereira, L.S., et al., 2016. Prevention of low back pain: a systematic review and meta-analysis. JAMA Intern. Med. 176, 199–208.

Waddell, G., Newton, M., Henderson, I., et al., 1993. A Fear-Avoidance Beliefs Questionnaire (FABQ) and the role of fear-avoidance beliefs in chronic low back pain and disability. Pain 52, 157–168.

9

Chronic Facial Pain in a 24-Year-Old University Student: Touch-Based Therapy Accessed via Auditory Pathways

G. Lorimer Moseley • Mark A. Jones

Interview

Tina was a 24-year-old right-handed female university student who presented along with her father. Tina reported a 9-year history of unilateral face pain, triggered by being hit on the side of the face with a softball. She presented for treatment of her face pain because it was greatly limiting her quality of life. She lived with her parents and a younger brother, who together provided substantial physical and emotional support. Her parents were both medical practitioners. Her mother worked full time as a rheumatologist, and her father worked as a general practitioner (GP), having reduced his hours in order to provide Tina with the help she needed. Tina was undertaking an architecture degree on a 0.25 normal load, such that she was currently in the second year of her degree, although she had been enrolled for 5 years.

Tina was about 160 cm tall and of slight build. The left side of her face was red and scattered with approximately 35 small vesicles.

Current Symptoms

Tina's pain covered much of the left side of her face, sparing her lips (Fig. 9.1). It was clearly delineated along the midline of her face, with the right side of her face being completely pain-free. She described the pain as 'burning', 'tender', 'sensitive' and 'stinging'. She described pain at rest that was present all the time, although it varied from tolerable to unbearable. She described no pain on the inside of her mouth, ear, jaw, teeth, temporomandibular joint or neck. On further questioning, Tina reported no headaches but occasional migraines (approximately once a year) that seemed random and without a trigger and which would 'run their course' – head pain with aura and photosensitivity for a few hours, sleep for 12–15 hours and 'groggy' the next day. She reported no neck stiffness, no episodes of dizziness and no visual disturbances, with the exception of a watery left eye. She reported no noticeable symptoms elsewhere. On further questioning, she reported occasional pins and needles in a glove distribution around her thumb and on the pad of her index finger. She did not notice a pattern in this that related to her face symptoms.

Tina reported that touching her face was unbearable, wearing glasses was unbearable and having anything go near her face was almost unbearable. She reported that nothing eased her pain except sleeping. She had devised a method to ensure she slept on her right side. She slept 7–8 hours per night and woke without an alarm. Her pain tended to get slowly worse over the course of the day. She had not noticed any other cyclical pattern in her pain (weekly, menstrual cycle, seasonal).

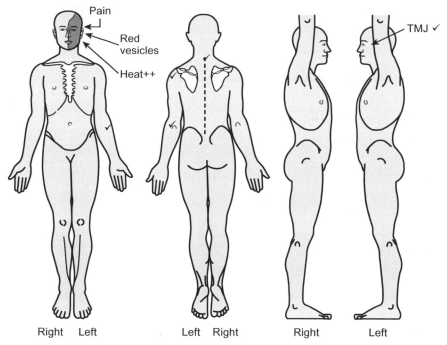

Fig. 9.1 Tina's body chart. *TMJ,* temporomandibular joint.

On further questioning, Tina reported the following:

- Mild asthma that was responsive to a steroid inhaler
- No noticeable difference in moisture between nostrils and no increase in sinus infections or a runny nose
- No increase in pain with jaw movements, chewing, eating spicy foods, arm activities such as carrying a load or bag in her hands, or neck movements and sustained postures
- A slight increase in pain after a sustained period (about 15 minutes) carrying a heavy bag using a strap over her left shoulder, which caused her to start avoiding this activity several years ago

History

All history was conveyed by Tina or her father. As a 15-year-old, Tina was waiting for her turn to bat in a softball game. She remembers that she was very anxious at the time, but she was reluctant to describe why. The injury day was a warm day in spring, and she reported suffering from some significant hay fever at the time. She was hit in the side of the face with a softball that had been hit out of the field of play. She remembered experiencing immediate stinging pain, and she sustained a small cut on the side of her face. The small scar was visible on her cheekbone about 2 cm anterior to her left ear. Over the next few days, the pain remained constant and confined to her left cheek. A bruise emerged, and Tina's father remembered it spreading across much of the side of her face.

Tina did not use any analgesics but did take a few days off school and 'took it easy'. About 4 days after the incident, she was scratched by her cat at the wound site, and the wound was reopened. She remembers immediate pain across the left side of her face at that time. The wound became infected, and Tina was placed on broad-range oral antibiotics prescribed by her father. The pain increased noticeably over the week after the cat scratch and did not resolve in line with the resolution of the infection.

The pain remained reasonably constant from that time until now. The following responses outline the consistency of her pain over the previous 9 years:

How is your pain now compared to 2 weeks after the cat scratch? 'It is the same or worse.'
How is it now compared to 5 years ago? 'It is the same or a bit worse.'
How is it now compared to 2 years ago? 'It is about the same.'

Previous Assessments

Tina had been cleared of the following: trigeminal neuralgia (neurological assessment), psoriasis, psoriatic arthritis (rheumatological assessment), Bell's palsy (neurological assessment) and temporomandibular joint injury or dysfunction (magnetic resonance imaging [MRI]; specialist physiotherapy assessment). Tina had undergone upper limb nerve conduction studies, x-ray, computed tomography (CT) scan, MRI scan and bone scan, each with no abnormalities detected.

Previous Treatments

Tina had undergone pharmacological interventions (opioids, gabapentin [nerve membrane stabilizer often called an 'antiepileptic' and often prescribed for peripheral neuropathic pain], non-steroidal anti-inflammatory drugs [NSAIDs], steroids), psychological interventions (hypnosis, meditation, cognitive-behavioural therapy, psychotherapy), a multidisciplinary pain management program, physiotherapy (temporomandibular joint manual therapy, biofeedback training, cervical spine manual therapy, cervical spine specific muscle training), acupuncture, homeopathy and craniosacral therapy. Reports from all physiotherapists who had seen her and her treating GP (not her father) were available. She described some pain relief with opioids and gabapentin, but both were intolerable because of side effects. She described no response to NSAIDs and an initial reduction in pain in response to steroids. That pain relief lasted about 3 months. She described no response to subsequent courses of steroids.

She described some help from learning to meditate and perform self-hypnosis and that she still used those techniques about once a day. She described no help from the multidisciplinary pain management program and that she found the program 'insulting' because they thought she was 'making it up'. She felt that she was worsened by the physiotherapy, particularly the muscle training (which she also found confusing because she did not have neck pain) and jaw mobilizations (which she indicated were painful because of the physiotherapist's hands on her face), and craniosacral therapy. She had been offered surgical intervention, but her mother had excluded that approach on the grounds that there was no evidence of nerve conduction compromise. This view was based on the lack of paraesthesia. No nerve conduction studies or electromyography of the face had been undertaken.

Impact of Pain on Her Life

Tina reported that her pain had had a huge impact on her life. She reported that it prevented her from attending most of her classes at school, and she attributed a low school-leaving mark to this (although note that she gained entry to a very competitive university degree). She reported that her pain prevented her from socializing because she could not bear having people or noise on her left.

She reported that her pain prevented her from wearing glasses, which made going out in the sun unpleasant. She could not wear a hat. Her left eye was often 'scratchy', sometimes watery, and she tended to squint. She reported being very self-conscious of the appearance of her face. Her pain did not prevent her from talking or eating or performing the requirements of daily living, as long as she could do them 'at her own pace'.

She described herself as being 'a bit depressed' and 'quite anxious'. She reported that previous formal assessments of both using standardized questionnaires (results not available to me) suggested that she had 'moderate depression' and 'mild anxiety'. She reported that her depression was completely due to her face pain and that it has probably made her more anxious as well.

On further questioning, Tina reported that she found noises on her left to be bothersome and difficult to listen to. Her father reported that the family had learnt to talk to Tina from her right side because she found it difficult when they talked to her from her left.

When asked, 'What do you think is causing this?', Tina stated that she did not know but that something had ruined the blood and nerve supply to her face and that, presumably, the softball and wound problem damaged these nerves. When asked, 'How do you think this will progress from here?' she reported that she was not at all confident. I asked her father the same questions, and his responses were nearly identical.

General Health

Tina reported that her general health was good. She walked at a moderate pace for 30 minutes a day. GP reports indicated no health comorbidities and no medications over time other than those listed by Tina. All screening questions regarding 'red flags' or potential indicators of more serious or sinister pathology (e.g. night pain, weight loss, constitutional symptoms, etc.) were negative.

Reasoning Question:

1. Based on the information obtained through your interview, what were your hypotheses regarding the dominant 'pain type' (i.e. nociceptive, peripheral neuropathic, nociplastic)?

Answer to Reasoning Question:

My hypothesis was that Tina's pain was being driven largely by a combination of enhanced efficacy of cortical networks that subserved her face pain and a loss of normal intracortical inhibitory drive. Of the choices you have given, my hypothesized mechanism most closely resembled nociplastic pain. That auditory stimuli seemed to modulate her symptoms offered corroboratory evidence of sensitivity and discriminative problems upstream of the somatosensory pathways. That said, I also thought that there might be primary nociceptive contributions but that it might be endogenously driven.

Reasoning Question:

2. If a nociceptive component were present, what potential 'sources of symptoms' (nociception) did you consider may be involved?

Answer to Reasoning Question:

I thought that the appearance of her face was consistent with peptidergic inflammation – vasodilation and vesicles not unlike those one sees in association with shingles. Peptidergic inflammation refers to inflammation at the terminals of nociceptors that is driven by the release of peptides from those nociceptors. This release can occur when the nociceptor is activated distally (action potentials propagate to other branches of the nociceptor) or proximally (action potentials propagate from the dorsal horn or dorsal root ganglion). In both cases, the action potentials cause the release of peptides at the terminals, and these peptides cause inflammation. My hypothesis was that this was most likely to be driven by descending facilitation because other potential drivers had been excluded by tests or had been unresponsive to therapies that I would expect to successfully modulate a primary nociceptive driver.

Reasoning Question:

3. Please discuss any potential 'contributing factors' (intrinsic or extrinsic) you hypothesized may have either predisposed to the onset of Tina's persistent pain or contributed to its maintenance.

Answer to Reasoning Question:

It is difficult to identify clear contributing factors, but the following candidate mechanisms emerged from the history:

1. Pro-inflammatory state: Tina reported being an asthmatic and suffering from hay fever. She describes a highly inflammatory response to the initial injuries. She reports 3 months of reduced pain after the first course of steroids. The pattern of spread and presenting condition appeared highly consistent with peptidergic inflammation and loss of intracortical inhibition, itself most probably associated with intracortical inflammatory mechanisms (although this is still open to conjecture). That she reported symptoms in a non-dermatomal distribution on her ipsilateral thumb and index finger implicates primary sensory cortex involvement. All of these hypotheses are to some extent speculative.

Continued on following page

2. Mood contributors: She reported being highly anxious at the time of the injury but did not expand on the reasons for that. I would hypothesize that this would put her in a 'high-threat state', itself more likely to be associated with inflammatory load and heightened activation of other protective systems. I would hypothesize that these contributors put her at elevated risk of a 'hyper-protective response'. She also reported being depressed and anxious at presentation. Both are likely to be associated with a more pro-inflammatory and hyper-protective state.

3. Cognitive contributors: Tina reported that she believed that the nerves and blood supply to her face were 'ruined'. She reported that the initial injury damaged her facial nerves. She reported attributing the several unmet expectations (e.g. a good school-leaving mark) to 'the injury'. She reported attributing several disadvantages in life (e.g. going out in the sun) to 'the injury'.

Clinical Reasoning Commentary:

As discussed in Chapters 1 and 2, 'pain type' and the neurobiological mechanisms underpinning Tina's symptoms cannot be directly measured clinically (although they can be inferred) and therefore need to be hypothesized. Clinically, such hypotheses should be linked to features in the patient's presentation, for example, as offered here, that Tina's symptoms were modulated by auditory stimuli. The presence of primary nociceptive contributions is not dismissed but, if present, is hypothesized to be centrally driven.

Although the three broad categories of 'pain type' referred to in the Reasoning Question seem to have clinical utility (although unproven) with respect to implications to other hypothesis categories, including 'precautions and contraindications to physical examination and treatment', 'management and treatment' and 'prognosis', it must be acknowledged that this categorization is a simplistic characterization of more complex neurobiological mechanisms (see Chapter 2). However, as discussed in Chapter 1, the proposed hypothesis categories should not be taken as fixed constructs; rather, they simply reflect contemporary categories of clinical judgements to consider that can assist musculoskeletal clinicians to think about their reasoning. They have evolved considerably since their inception and must continue to evolve with the evolution of our understandings, with the overall aim of assisting recognition of relevant aspects to patients' clinical presentations that are used to guide safe and effective management.

A range of potential contributing factors should be considered, including systemic factors (e.g. asthmatic and suffering from hay fever), emotional factors (e.g. anxiety) and numerous manifestations of cognitive factors (e.g. beliefs regarding nerve injury and ruined blood supply to face, negative self-concept, negative attribution that school-leaving mark is linked to injury and negative perceptions of participation restrictions, such as going out in the sun). As discussed in Chapters 1 and 4, it can be useful when listening for and explicitly screening for potential contributing factors to conceptualize them as intrinsic (physical, psychological, behavioural and hereditary) or extrinsic (environmental, social, cultural, etc.). As highlighted in this Clinical Reasoning Answer, it is often difficult to know with certainty whether or not potential contributing factors identified in the patient's story (and later, the physical examination) are in fact relevant to the patient's development and/or maintenance of the patient's symptoms and disability. Nevertheless, it is important to hypothesize about potential contributing factors that inform other areas of reasoning, particularly 'prognosis' and 'management'. The number of factors contributing to the onset and/or maintenance of symptoms and disability, the length of time they have been present and whether they can be modified combine to influence prognosis. Management almost always needs to target contributing factors for the broader aim of minimizing recurrence and future disability.

Examination

As we spoke, Tina held her head in left rotation. If I moved to Tina's left, she too would move further, as though always 'shielding' the left side of her face from me or attempting to listen with her right ear. Her left eye would squint a little when she described the initial injury and subsequent infection or when she described aggravating activities and the nature of her pain. She did not seem to have a ptosis or any demonstrable palsy.

Tina would not allow me to touch her face. On closing her eyes, she reported an increase in warmth and pain when she placed her hand near her face, and the same thing happened whether it was her own hand or mine.

Movements of the mouth (opening, clenching, lateral deviations) or head and neck (flexion, extension, rotation, lateral flexion) did not modulate her pain, with the exception of a slight aggravation when she raised her eyebrows as high as she could and a clear aggravation in full right-side flexion that caused a puckering of the skin around some sores.

She had noticeably poor fine motor control of the left hand when her hand was situated near her face. On questioning at this time, she reported that she was a 'touch-typer' but had not noticed any problems with accuracy typing with either hand.

On sitting at a computer mimicking university work, she would hold her head in approximately 35 degrees left rotation. She did not think this was the case (i.e. she felt like she was facing the midline) until her true posture was revealed via a webcam. She was able to immediately correct her posture but returned to the default 35-degree posture as soon as I asked her another question or distracted her from the task in any way.

Further Assessments
Questionnaires

Patient-specific functional scale (PSFS) (Chatman et al., 1997). The patient selects four tasks or activities she can't do now because of pain but would like to (i.e. is closely tied to short- and long-term goals). The patient then rates her ability to perform those tasks on a scale of 0–10. Final score = average of four measures. Tina selected the following tasks: computer-based university work; going out with friends; lying on her left side; wearing sunglasses. She scored 0.7 on the PSFS, indicating that she was not able to perform her desired activities.

Pain Catastrophising Scale (PCS) (Sullivan et al., 1995). This is a 13-item questionnaire. The scoring range is 0–42, with 42 indicating very catastrophic thoughts and beliefs related to pain. Tina scored 7, which is reasonably consistent with the wider pain-free population.

Pain Knowledge Questionnaire (PKQ) (Moseley, 2003b). This is a 19-item questionnaire that aims to quantify someone's understanding of the biological mechanisms that underpin pain. The scoring range is 0–19, with 19 indicating high knowledge. A revised version with fewer items is recommended for test–retest applications (Catley et al., 2013a). Tina scored 6, which is consistent with an untrained chronic pain population.

Other Tests

Auditory detection thresholds. Tina was referred to an audiology clinic for hearing tests. Perceptual detection thresholds were normal bilaterally.

Left/right neck judgement task. This task used commercially available software (Recognise, noigroup.com, Adelaide, Australia) to undertake a reaction-time task in which she was shown pictures of a female model with her head turned to either the left or right. To perform the task, one judges whether the pictured model is turned to the left or right. Tina's left/right judgement accuracy was 85% L, 96% R; Tina's reaction time in making judgements was on average 2.4 sec L, 2.2 sec R. These results reflect an accuracy that was reliably lower than a pain-free population and comparable to a chronic-neck-pain population (Stanton et al., unpublished data). Reaction time was within normal range.

Tactile acuity. Two-point discrimination threshold (TPD) was assessed with blunted calipers using three alternated ascending and descending runs, at the back of the hand, the forehead bilaterally and on the face. Results are shown in Table 9.1. Note that TPD testing evoked pain on the left side of the face.

TABLE 9.1

TWO-POINT DISCRIMINATION THRESHOLD RESULTS

Site	Two-Point Discrimination Threshold	
	Left	Right
Hand	21, 24, 20	18, 22, 20
Forehead	23, 25, 23	16, 16, 19
Cheek	41, 37, 44	16, 15, 16

Reasoning Question:

4. Tina's clinical presentation is fascinating and may initially seem unusual to some clinicians. Please discuss whether it genuinely is unusual, both in your experience and in the chronic pain literature. Also, please discuss whether your hypothesis of a dominant 'nociplastic pain type' following the interview is supported by your examination.

Answer to Reasoning Question:

I think Tina's presentation was unusual, particularly in its severity, to me and within the literature. However, I have now seen eight almost identical cases, all triggered by a similar reasonably benign facial injury. All these patients have initially not tolerated touch, and all have responded to a similar treatment approach presented later. So, my impression with Tina was that she had a centrally driven pain disorder associated with peptidergic inflammation across the left side of the face. Tina interpreted her pain as being indicative of a tissue-based pathology on her face that was triggered by the wound and subsequent infection and maintained by ongoing tissue pathology, as evidenced by the vesicles and red skin.

Notably, I think aspects of Tina's presentation are often present in people with chronic pain. For example, in my experience, it is common in people with chronic pain to have a distribution of pain that does not follow a peripheral nerve, segmental or recognized referral distribution. It is common to see peptidergic inflammation. It is less common but not rare to have such sensitivity that the area cannot be touched, except of course in frank peripheral nerve injury. After physical examination, my initial hypotheses were further supported.

Reasoning Question:

5. Based on your combined reasoning following the interview and examination, please discuss your plans for Tina's management.

Answer to Reasoning Question:

I identified the following therapeutic targets and discussed the path forward with Tina:

1. Clarify Tina's own goals for treatment and the resources available to her for taking on a long-term therapeutic journey.
2. Establish whether Tina and I both felt we had enough alignment to plan that journey.
3. Presuming alignment is established, explain the potential for her symptoms to be explained by mechanisms other than a primary pathology or ongoing injury in her face and my desire to help her explore other potential contributors to her situation.
4. Outline possible initial treatment directions and facilitate Tina's selection of her preferred direction. Presentation of each of the following options involved some preliminary discussion about the rationale and possible effects:
   a. Develop a treatment that would reinstate tactile acuity on the affected area, in an attempt to normalize what appeared to be an aberrant representation of the left side of her face.
   b. Explore other systemic factors that may be interacting with altered nervous system function manifest in the current signs and symptoms.
   c. Explore cognitive and psychosocial factors that may be interacting with altered nervous system function to manifest in the current signs and symptoms.

Clinical Reasoning Commentary:

The recognition of clinical variations or new clinical patterns occurs when clinicians are not restricted by dominant and popular paradigms of practice and rigid categorizations of clinical presentations. As stated in Chapter 1 (p. 26), 'If we only encourage logical thinking and practice within the realm of what is 'known' or substantiated by research evidence, we limit the variability and creativity of thinking that is important to the generation of new ideas'. In this case, extensive knowledge of the pain system enables recognition of altered cortical networks (e.g. loss of normal intracortical inhibitory drive as alluded to in Answer to Reasoning Question 1) as likely contributing to Tina's abnormal facial sensitivity to touch and sound and to the physical impairment in facial appearance (i.e. left side of her face was red and scattered with approximately 35 small vesicles). This ability to apply biological (and psychosocial) knowledge to a different, 'unusual' presentation, with subsequent recognition of further identical cases, exemplifies the creative, yet critical reasoning that underpins the discovery of new knowledge, or applications of knowledge, informed by research while at the same time informing future research (e.g. validation).

Hypotheses formulated from the subjective examination are 'tested' within the physical examination, providing an evolving understanding of Tina's presentation.

The focus on establishing 'Tina's goals for treatment and the resources available', determining whether there was sufficient 'alignment' between the clinician and Tina and explicit plans to provide Tina with different options for initial treatment illustrate the 'Collaborative Reasoning' strategy discussed in Chapter 1. Collaborative reasoning is underpinned by an effective therapeutic alliance encompassing rapport, empathetic sensitivity to emotions and ethical deliberations.

Treatment (Sessions 1 and 2)

Steps 1–3 of the therapeutic targets and path forward for Tina went smoothly and were covered in sessions 1 (including assessment; 60 min) and 2 (45 min, 1 week later). Tina identified goals that were very associated with relief of pain and resolution of the red and blistered appearance of one side of her face. On further discussion, she identified that the underlying goal was to increase her life satisfaction and that she perceived her pain and appearance were the major barriers.

We both felt aligned on this latter goal and proceeded to identify a target that would establish whether or not we were making ground. That target, articulated by Tina, was a 'noticeable improvement in life satisfaction in 1 month'.

At the completion of session 1, Tina was loaned a copy of a book of metaphors and stories that aimed to improve understanding of pain biology (Moseley, 2007). I outlined that my objective was to provide her with some interesting information about pain. I explained that we now know much more about pain than we did even 10 years ago and that she might be surprised to know how relevant it all was to her situation, although none of it was specifically about her or her condition.

Tina had read the whole book by her second session. The second session began with fielding any questions or interesting reflections on that material. Tina indicated that she would like to learn more and that she would like to start with the second option of the three presented to her, to 'Explore other systemic factors that may be interacting with altered nervous system function manifest in the current signs and symptoms'.

To find a method of accessing the touch system was a challenge. I provided the rationale for one option: Based on animal findings of bimodal tactile-auditory brain cells responsive to both tactile stimuli delivered to the skin on the face and auditory stimuli delivered in the space immediately adjacent to that skin, I evaluated auditory discrimination performance for stimuli delivered around the face.

Session 3 (1 Week Later)

In session 3, we began by Tina completing the Pain Knowledge Questionnaire and the Pain Catastrophizing Scale. Those data are shown in Table 9.2.

We then evaluated auditory discrimination performance. The results of that investigation are shown in Fig. 9.2.

Auditory discrimination performance. Tina was unable to localize auditory stimuli delivered in the peripersonal space around the left side of her face but was accurate when the stimuli were delivered around the right side of her face and when the stimuli were presented either side at a distance of 65 cm (i.e. beyond the space that would be associated with bimodal cell activation). This presentation raised the clear possibility that we might be able to access the tactile system using auditory stimuli.

Sessions 4–8 (Held on Consecutive Days)

Intervention consisted of two components: (i) gradual completion of a workbook that was aligned with *Explain Pain* (Butler and Moseley, 2003) (and subsequently developed into

TABLE 9.2				
PRE-ASSESSMENT AND SESSION 3 RE-ASSESSMENT OF PSFS, PCS, PKQ AND DAILY PAIN RATING				
Session	**PSFS**	**PCS**	**PKQ**	**Pain Today**
Pre-assessment	0.7	7	6	8
Session 3	0.5	8	11	6

PSFS, Patient-Specific Functional Scale; *PCS*, Pain Catastrophizing Scale; *PKQ*, Pain Knowledge Questionnaire; Pain today = pain on 0-to-10 scale, average daily score over last week.

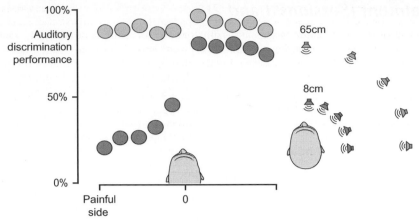

Fig. 9.2 Auditory discrimination performance with speakers situated close to the face (dark circles) or distant from the face (light circles) on the painful side of the face (on left) and the unaffected side of the face (on right).

TABLE 9.3

RE-ASSESSMENT OF PSFS, PCS, PKQ AND DAILY PAIN RATING THROUGH SESSION 6

Session	PSFS	PCS	PKQ	Pain Today
Pre-assessment	0.7	7	6	8
Session 3	0.5	8	11	6
Session 6	1	5	14	5

PSFS, Patient-Specific Functional Scale; *PCS*, Pain Catastrophizing Scale; *PKQ*, Pain Knowledge Questionnaire; Pain today = pain on 0-to-10 scale, average daily score over last week.

the *Explain Pain Handbook: Protectometer* [Moseley and Butler, 2015a]), an education approach that aimed to capture the concept of pain as a protector and the idea of an internal 'danger meter' (now operationalized as a protectometer [Moseley and Butler, 2015a]); and (ii) auditory discrimination training. Auditory discrimination training involved the presentation of tones at one of five locations around the left side of Tina's face. She was required to identify the location of each sound and was given feedback in response to each stimulus. Sessions involved the presentation of 72 stimuli and lasted approximately 30 minutes. A home training program was devised such that Tina was required to point to where a sound was delivered by her training buddy.

Results from re-assessment of the key outcome measures through session 6 are presented in Table 9.3.

Tina maintained a training diary in which she also marked the date and time of any 'flare-up'. We defined a flare-up as 'a distressing and noticeable increase in pain'. Tina's situation was monitored regularly on the basis of weekly completion of the PSFS and the daily answer, recorded in her training diary, to this question: On a scale of 0 to 10, with 0 being no pain, and 10 being the worst possible pain, on average, how was your pain today?

Reasoning Question:

6. You had indicated to Tina that your book of metaphors was not specifically about her or her condition. Would you please discuss how these sorts of resources for helping patients understand pain biology are used to facilitate their understanding with respect to their individual problems?

Answer to Reasoning Question:

In my experience, and according to our research (Moseley, 2003b; Gallagher et al., 2013), the vast majority of people with chronic pain subscribe to a structural-pathology-based understanding of pain. That view, broadly consistent with the revolutionary ideas of Rene Descartes (1644), presents pain as an event that occurs in the tissues of the body and is transmitted to the brain, where it is ultimately detected. Modern versions of that model share its dependence on a pathology in the tissues of the body. My view is that pain is best understood as a protective mechanism rather than an informant about tissue condition (Moseley and Butler, 2015b), and I would contend that there is a vast literature substantiating this perspective and refuting the structural-pathology paradigm: pain does not relate well to tissue damage even in tightly controlled experimental situations.

Explaining pain targets a shift in understanding of pain from that of an informant of tissue pathology to that of a protective mechanism. As such, pain can be modulated up by any credible evidence that protection is required and modulated down by any credible evidence that it is not. In the sense that this model of pain is not ubiquitous, the generic *Explain Pain* resources (e.g. Moseley, 2003a, 2007, 2011; Butler and Moseley, 2013; Moseley and Butler, 2015a, 2015b; Moseley and Lotze, 2015; Moseley and Butler, 2017) are suitable. In addition to the broad approach, I see that tailoring specific conceptual targets to the patient involved is very helpful, and the *Explain Pain* approach tested in randomized controlled trials (RCTs) involves this tailored approach.

There are several principles of the *Explain Pain* approach, and full review is beyond the scope of this case study, but resources are available (Moseley et al., 2012a; Moseley and Lotze, 2015) for the interested reader. Key principles include careful observation of the patient; identification of potential threats from across the mechanical (e.g. touch and movement), systemic (e.g. respiratory load), cognitive (e.g. thoughts, beliefs), environmental (e.g. places) and social (e.g. people and social situations) domains; removal of those threats wherever possible; and then graded re-exposure to threats over time.

With regard to Tina's process of reconceptualization, she was encouraged to look for situations where her symptoms were aggravated or relieved without a clear link to her proposed pathology. She, like many patients, found it easier to grasp the idea that stress might cause muscle contraction, which aggravates injury, than to grasp the idea that the threats that cause stress might also turn up pain directly. In my view, both mechanisms are likely. She was encouraged to search for relationships between her pain, redness and vesicles and events or situations in each of several domains, broadly:

1. The things she does
2. The things she says or hears other people say
3. The people she is with or engaging with
4. The places she goes
5. Patterns that coincide with social events
6. Patterns that coincide with biological rhythms or seasons

The principles of threat identification are now outlined in a patient-friendly manner in *The Explain Pain Handbook: Protectometer* (Moseley and Butler, 2015a).

Clinical Reasoning Commentary:

Musculoskeletal clinicians are arguably teachers first and foremost because the majority of clinical practice is concerned with promoting patient learning or change, in understanding/beliefs, coping, self-efficacy, health behaviours and activity/participation capability. Although this requires knowledge of broad theory (e.g. pain, healthy living/fitness, workplace/home/sport ergonomics, etc.), effectiveness in facilitating change requires advanced teaching skills. 'Reasoning about teaching' is a reasoning strategy discussed in Chapter 1 designed to facilitate awareness that teaching, like physical procedural skills, requires reasoning to plan, execute and evaluate individualized, context-sensitive teaching, including education for conceptual understanding (e.g. pain), education for physical performance (e.g. rehabilitative exercise, postural correction, sport technique enhancement) and education for behavioural change.

A key educational principle to facilitate deep learning and change is to engage the learner in a way that promotes active processing (as opposed to passive reception) of key concepts. Giving Tina the explicit 'homework' task of searching for links between her facial pain, redness and vesicles in each of the explicit domains outlined required her to reflect on and analyze (i.e. process) those relationships. As briefly discussed in Chapter 4, individuals develop their own awareness and beliefs regarding health problems ('illness perceptions') that influence their expectations, emotions (e.g. fears), behaviours and self-efficacy. Because these beliefs develop in part through learned associations, they may or may not be conscious and as such may not be immediately recognized or volunteered at the initial interview. A reflective, analytical task such as this designed to assist Tina in recognizing these relationships, and hence potential sources of threat, and giving her the necessary time to complete the task illustrate the reasoning involved in teaching and how it may even commence as part of assessment.

Reasoning Question:

7. Formal monitoring of outcomes (e.g. PSFS and training diary) is a recognized requirement of evidence-based practice. However, this does not reveal the full scope of 'monitoring' evident in expert practice. Please comment on any informal monitoring you may utilize in addition to these formal outcome measures.

Continued on following page

Answer to Reasoning Question:

I would always be asking, 'What do you reckon that means?' or 'Why do you think that happens?' or 'How might you get around that problem?'

Clinical Reasoning Commentary:

Although the importance of objective outcome measurement is emphasized in musculoskeletal therapist evidence-based practice, experienced therapists also use continual informal monitoring, as reflected in the previous examples. These or similar questions may be used in the initial assessment to understand and clarify the patient's perspectives, but returning to these sorts of questions throughout ongoing management provides an informal gauge of the patient's evolving understanding of the education provided and, for example, whether prior beliefs have shifted.

Reasoning Question:

8. What is the current evidence base for auditory discrimination training generally and specifically for patients with persistent pain? Also, what was your rationale for daily auditory discrimination training sessions?

Answer to Reasoning Question:

There is almost no evidence – the only evidence of which I am aware is the replicated case series currently under way in our research/clinical group. There are now eight patients enrolled. The idea of trialing auditory discrimination, however, was based on the growing evidence of (i) sensory discrimination deficits in people with chronic pain, and (ii) Level 2b evidence for tactile discrimination training in people with chronic pain in other anatomical regions – pain that shares common features with that described by Tina.

1. Our group has undertaken a large amount of research into tactile discrimination in people with chronic pain (Moseley, 2008; Luomajoki and Moseley, 2011; Catley et al., 2013b; Stanton et al, 2013; Wand et al., 2014) (see Catley et al., [2014] for a review). That work clearly shows anatomically specific deficits that are not explainable by deficits in tactile detection, transformation into neural signals or transmission to the brain. As mentioned earlier, the decision to trial auditory discrimination was based on (i) the fundamental science demonstrating bimodal visuo-tactile cells in both non-human primates and humans, (ii) Tina's reports concerning sound processing and (iii) the assessment of Tina's auditory discrimination performance according to the side on which the stimuli were presented (see previous discussion).

2. RCTs of tactile discrimination training have shown positive effects on phantom limb pain (Flor et al., 2001) and back pain (Wand et al., 2013); a replicated time-controlled case series (Moseley, 2005) and a randomized controlled experiment (Moseley et al., 2008b) demonstrated positive effect on pain in complex regional pain syndrome patients; other case and observational studies exist (see (Moseley and Flor, 2012; Wand et al., 2011; Moseley et al., 2012b) for relevant reviews), although the reader is cautioned to consider alternative designs to the RCT with caution (see O'Connell et al., [2015] for a review of contemporary issues relating to evidence appraisal in chronic pain).

My rationale for daily auditory discrimination training sessions was pretty simple – we are trying to shift response profiles of neurones, so the more the better, and I guess it becomes a balance between volume and burden. That recommendation reflects my best guess at where that line was.

Sessions 9–13 (Held Once Per Week)

We continued auditory discrimination training, but the emphasis was on home training. In session 12 we commenced tactile discrimination training on the face, which was now tolerable and led to only a small increase in pain, which resolved within 5 minutes of cessation of training.

Reasoning Question:

9. Please discuss your reasoning underpinning when to commence Tina's tactile discrimination training and how that training should be carried out.

Answer to Reasoning Question:

Touch-evoked pain was continually re-assessed over the course of treatment. Auditory discrimination training was replaced with tactile discrimination training once repeated touch did not evoke pain. It was presumed (although not demonstrated) that the underlying sensitivity and disinhibition hypothesized to be contributing to Tina's pain had reduced by this time.

I think it is more helpful to understand the principle behind discrimination training rather than try to remember a specific protocol because the former is defendable, but the latter really is not. The guiding principle is that the key component of training is discrimination, not stimulation. That is, the patient needs to differentiate between similar stimuli on the basis of the stimulus characteristics. This might be differentiating the location of different stimuli or the frequency, direction or modulation. The task should be pitched so as to be successful about 80% of the time. As performance increases, make the difference between stimuli smaller. For example, in a location discrimination task such as this, make the locations closer to each other. As is always the case with training, the clinician needs to find a balance between maximizing training load and avoiding cognitive overload.

Sessions 14–16 (Held Once Every 2 Weeks)

Treatment consisted of tactile discrimination training with decreasing inter-stimulus distance. By session 16, two-point discrimination threshold was comparable on both sides of her face. Session 15 focussed on giving Tina an understanding of the process of graded exposure to primary activity goals. On session 16, a plan for progressing two such activities was devised in collaboration with Tina. These activities were (i) wearing sunglasses and (ii) computer-based university work.

Reasoning Question:

10. Please discuss the neuroscience underpinning graded exposure and the practical application with Tina.

Answer to Reasoning Question:

In my view, graded exposure and response prevention are the hallmarks of successful recovery or rehabilitation in the vast majority of pain complaints. Graded exposure can be conceptualized as 'adaptation training' and exploits the fundamental biological property of adaptation to demand. The more 'hyper-protective' the biological system, the more challenging it is to present a demand that is sufficient to induce adaptation but insufficient to trigger the protective response. Others take an alternative approach to this, focusing on violating expectations of damage, and initial data are also promising (den Hollander et al., 2016) (although see Moseley, [2016]). Nonetheless, the principle has remained at the heart of my own clinical practice and research, with considerable attention being given to discovering innovative methods of finding that elusive zone. Much of my early work was in patients with complex regional pain syndrome (CRPS), in whom even imagined movements can be painful (Moseley, 2004b; Moseley et al., 2008a). There is a reasonably compelling body of work that suggests that such profound sensitivity and 'hyper-protection' reflect both increased influence of protective neural representations (for full review of neural representation theory and its application to physical therapies and graded exposure, see Moseley et al. [2012a] and Wallwork et al. [2016]) and disinhibition in sensory and motor cortices (see Di Pietro et al. [2013a, 2013b] for example reviews). One treatment, which was devised specifically for CRPS, is graded motor imagery (GMI) (Moseley, 2004a, 2006; Moseley et al., 2012a; Stanton et al., 2012; Bowering et al., 2013; O'Connell et al., 2013). GMI directly targets disinhibition and graded exposure in the motor system.

Tina's program targeted the sensory system but conformed to the same principles. Sensory discrimination training requires the brain to exploit intracortical inhibitory mechanisms. Once intracortical inhibitory control was reinstated, as reflected in Tina's performance on the task and failure of touch to evoke pain, then tactile discrimination training was commenced. Tactile discrimination training requires intracortical inhibition in the tactile processing areas, most obviously the primary sensory cortex. Although there the left/right judgement task showed reliable evidence that accuracy was decreased, this was not integrated into her treatment approach because she indicated that she did not want to do it.

Graded exposure to function involved a pre-planned time-contingent or repetition-contingent program whereby Tina spent progressively more time in previously threatening situations. For example, discrimination training was progressed by time (first incremented at 30 seconds per day); touching her face was progressed according to repetitions (from a baseline of 10 self-touches, increasing by 2 repetitions per session each day, 5 sessions a day) and according to threat (at 1 week, touch from another [father] introduced, and the same time or repetition-based progression was employed). Once the principle and justification of graded exposure was understood by Tina and her family, she planned and implemented this progression for other tasks herself.

Continued on following page

Clinical Reasoning Commentary:

The strong neuroscience rationale evident in the analysis of Tina's clinical presentation is also apparent in this answer. Application of this rationale to Tina's overall management (e.g. pain education, discrimination training, graded exposure) then requires reasoning judgements regarding 'dosage' and progression of specific treatment interventions, both of which are insufficiently researched to provide clear protocols. Tina's treatment dosage is based on baseline assessments. Although symptom provocation, tolerance and cognition (e.g. threat) are attended to in baseline assessments, a time- and repetition-contingent cautious progression (as opposed to symptom-/pain-contingent) is then followed.

TABLE 9.4

RE-ASSESSMENT OF PSFS, PCS, PKQ AND DAILY PAIN RATING OUTCOME MEASURES THROUGH SESSION 18

Session	PSFS	PCS	PKQ	Pain Today
Pre-assessment	0.7	7	6	8
Session 3	0.5	8	11	6
Session 6	1	5	14	5
Session 18	3.0	6	14	2

PSFS, Patient-Specific Functional Scale; *PCS*, Pain Catastrophizing Scale; *PKQ*, Pain Knowledge Questionnaire; Pain today = pain on 0-to-10 scale, average daily score over last week.

Sessions 17 and 18 (Held Over Consecutive Months)

Treatment focussed entirely on graded exposure and incorporated three more tasks: lying on left side, going out with friends and exercising vigorously. Tina was then given the responsibility and advice to apply the same graded-exposure approach to anything else she wanted to do.

Results of re-assessment of the key outcome measures through session 18 are presented in Table 9.4. Left/right judgements of facial postures were also re-assessed at session 18: accuracy >95% bilaterally; RT = 2.3 seconds bilaterally.

Session 19 (7 Months After Initial Presentation)

Tina reported almost complete resolution of pain. Visible signs had faded over the previous 2 months and were now not present. PSFS was 4.6/5, and average pain over the previous 7 days was 1/10. We discussed a self-management plan should she get into trouble and arranged a follow-up 3 months later. Tina presented completely recovered at 3-month follow-up (10 months after initial presentation).

REFERENCES

Bowering, K.J., O'Connell, N.E., Tabor, A., Catley, M.J., Leake, H.B., Moseley, G.L., et al., 2013. The effects of graded motor imagery and its components on chronic pain: a systematic review and meta-analysis. J. Pain 14 (1), 3–13.

Butler, D., Moseley, G.L., 2003. Explain Pain. NOI Group, Adelaide.

Butler, D., Moseley, G.L., 2013. Explain Pain, 2nd ed. NOI Group, Adelaide, Australia.

Catley, M.J., O'Connell, N.E., Berryman, C., Ayhan, F.F., Moseley, G.L., 2014. Is tactile acuity altered in people with chronic pain? A systematic review and meta-analysis. J. Pain 15 (10), 985–1000.

Catley, M.J., O'Connell, N.E., Moseley, G.L., 2013a. How good is the neurophysiology of pain questionnaire? a Rasch analysis of psychometric properties. J. Pain 14 (8), 818–827.

Catley, M.J., Tabor, A., Wand, B.M., Moseley, G.L., 2013b. Assessing tactile acuity in rheumatology and musculoskeletal medicine – how reliable are two-point discrimination tests at the neck, hand, back and foot? Rheumatology (Oxf) 52 (8), 1454–1461.

Chatman, A.B., Hyams, S.P., Neel, J.M., Binkley, J.M., Stratford, P.W., Schomberg, A., et al., 1997. The Patient-Specific Functional Scale: measurement properties in patients with knee dysfunction. Phys. Ther. 77 (8), 820–829.

den Hollander, M., Goossens, M., de Jong, J., Ruijgrok, J., Oosterhof, J., Onghena, P., et al., 2016. Expose or protect? A randomized controlled trial of exposure in vivo versus pain-contingent treatment as usual in patients with complex regional pain syndrome Type 1. Pain 157 (10), 2318–2329.

Descartes, R., 1972. L'Homme1633. In: Treatise of Man, tr. by T.S. Hall. Harvard University Press, Cambridge, MA.

Di Pietro, F., McAuley, J.H., Parkitny, L., Lotze, M., Wand, B.M., Moseley, G.L., et al., 2013a. Primary motor cortex function in complex regional pain syndrome: a systematic review and meta-analysis. J. Pain 14 (11), 1270–1288.

Di Pietro, F., McAuley, J.H., Parkitny, L., Lotze, M., Wand, B.M., Moseley, G.L., et al., 2013b. Primary somatosensory cortex function in complex regional pain syndrome: a systematic review and meta-analysis. J. Pain 14 (10), 1001–1018.

Flor, H., Denke, C., Schaefer, M., Grusser, S., 2001. Effect of sensory discrimination training on cortical reorganisation and phantom limb pain. Lancet 357 (9270), 1763–1764.

Gallagher, L., McAuley, J., Moseley, G.L., 2013. A randomized-controlled trial of using a book of metaphors to reconceptualize pain and decrease catastrophizing in people with chronic pain. Clin. J. Pain 29 (1), 20–25.

Luomajoki, H., Moseley, G.L., 2011. Tactile acuity and lumbopelvic motor control in patients with back pain and healthy controls. Br. J. Sports Med. 45 (5), 437–440.

Moseley, G.L., 2003a. A pain neuromatrix approach to patients with chronic pain. Man. Ther. 8 (3), 130–140.

Moseley, L., 2003b. Unraveling the barriers to reconceptualization of the problem in chronic pain: the actual and perceived ability of patients and health professionals to understand the neurophysiology. J. Pain 4 (4), 184–189.

Moseley, G.L., 2004a. Graded motor imagery is effective for long-standing complex regional pain syndrome: a randomised controlled trial. Pain 108 (1–2), 192–198.

Moseley, G.L., 2004b. Imagined movements cause pain and swelling in a patient with complex regional pain syndrome. Neurology 62 (1), 1644.

Moseley, G.L., 2005. Is successful rehabilitation of complex regional pain syndrome due to sustained attention to the affected limb? A randomised clinical trial. Pain 114 (1–2), 54–61.

Moseley, G.L., 2006. Graded motor imagery for pathologic pain - a randomized controlled trial. Neurology 67 (12), 2129–2134.

Moseley, G.L., 2007. Painful Yarns. Metaphors and Stories to Help Understand the Biology of Pain. Dancing Giraffe Press, Canberra, Australia.

Moseley, G.L., 2008. I can't find it! Distorted body image and tactile dysfunction in patients with chronic back pain. Pain 140 (1), 239–243.

Moseley, G.L., 2011. Teaching people about pain: why do we keep beating around the bush? Pain Manag. 2 (1), 1–3.

Moseley, G.L., 2016. More than 'just do it' – fear-based exposure for Complex Regional Pain Syndrome. Pain 157 (10), 2145–2147.

Moseley, G., Butler, D., 2015a. The Explain Pain Handbook: Protectometer. NOI Group, Adelaide, Australia.

Moseley, G.L., Butler, D.S., 2015b. Fifteen Years of explaining pain - the past, present and future. J. Pain 16 (9), 807–813.

Moseley, G.L., Butler, D.S., 2017. Explain pain supercharged. The clinician's handbook. Noigroup Publishing, Adelaide, Australia, 165pp.

Moseley, G., Butler, D., Beames, T., Giles, T., 2012a. The Graded Motor Imagery Handbook. NOI Group Publishing, Adelaide, Australia.

Moseley, G.L., Flor, H., 2012. Targeting cortical representations in the treatment of chronic pain: a review. Neurorehabil. Neural Repair 26 (6), 646–652.

Moseley, G.L., Gallace, A., Spence, C., 2012b. Bodily illusions in health and disease: physiological and clinical perspectives and the concept of a cortical 'body matrix'. Neurosci. Biobehav. Rev. 36 (1), 34–46.

Moseley, G., Lotze, M., 2015. Theoretical considerations for chronic pain rehabilitation. Phys. Ther. 95 (9), 1316–1320.

Moseley, G.L., Zalucki, N., Birklein, F., Marinus, J., Hilten, J.J., Luomajoki, H., 2008a. Thinking about movement hurts: the effect of motor imagery on pain and swelling in people with chronic arm pain. Arthritis Care Res. 59 (5), 623–631.

Moseley, G.L., Zalucki, N.M., Wiech, K., 2008b. Tactile discrimination, but not tactile stimulation alone, reduces chronic limb pain. Pain 137 (3), 600–608.

O'Connell, N.E., Moseley, G.L., McAuley, J.H., Wand, B.M., Herbert, R.D., 2015. Interpreting effectiveness evidence in pain: short tour of contemporary issues. Phys. Ther. 95 (8), 1087–1094.

O'Connell, N.E., Wand, B.M., McAuley, J., Marston, L., Moseley, G.L., 2013. Interventions for treating pain and disability in adults with complex regional pain syndrome. Cochrane Database Syst. Rev. (4), CD009416.

Stanton, T.R., Lin, C.W., Bray, H., Smeets, R.J., Taylor, D., Law, R.Y., et al., 2013. Tactile acuity is disrupted in osteoarthritis but is unrelated to disruptions in motor imagery performance. Rheumatology 52 (8), 1509–1519.

Stanton, T., Lin, C., Smeets, R., Taylor, D., Law, R., Moseley, G., 2012. Spatially-defined disruption of motor imagery performance in people with osteoarthritis. Rheumatology 51 (8), 1455–1464.

Sullivan, M.J.L., Bishop, S.R., Pivik, J., 1995. The Pain Catastrophizing Scale: development and validation. Psycholog. Ass. 7 (4), 524–532.

Wallwork, S.B., Bellan, V., Catley, M.J., Moseley, G.L., 2016. Neural representations and the cortical body matrix: implications for sports medicine and future directions. Br. J. Sports Med. 50 (16), 990–996. doi:10.1136/bjsports-2015-095356. [Epub 2015 Dec 18].

Wand, B.M., Abbaszadeh, S., Smith, A.J., Catley, M.J., Moseley, G.L., 2013. Acupuncture applied as a sensory discrimination training tool decreases movement-related pain in patients with chronic low back pain more than acupuncture alone: a randomised cross-over experiment. Br. J. Sports Med. 47 (17), 1085–1089.

Wand, B.M., Parkitny, L., O'Connell, N.E., Luomajoki, H., McAuley, J.H., Thacker, M., et al., 2011. Cortical changes in chronic low back pain: current state of the art and implications for clinical practice. Man. Ther. 16 (1), 15–20.

Wand, B.M., Stephens, S.E., Mangharam, E.I., George, P.J., Bulsara, M.K., O'Connell, N.E., et al., 2014. Illusory touch temporarily improves sensation in areas of chronic numbness: a brief communication. Neurorehabil. Neural Repair 28 (8), 797–799.

10

Targeting Treatment Distally at the Foot for Bilateral Persistent Patellofemoral Pain in a 23-Year-Old: A New Answer to an Old Problem?

Mark Matthews • Bill Vicenzino • Darren A. Rivett

Patient Interview

Ellie was a 23-year-old female who recently commenced working in a hospitality job that involved prolonged hours of standing and walking. She presented to the University of Queensland clinical Sports Injury Rehabilitation and Prevention for Health (SIRPH) research unit with a 10-year history of non-traumatic bilateral anterior knee pain symptoms, with the symptoms in the left knee more severe than the right (Fig. 10.1). Ellie had previously been a gymnast from the age of 6 years, training up to 25–35 hours per week, until the age of 12 years. She then commenced trampolining activities, training up to 6–12 hours per week, until the age of 16 years. Now Ellie worked as a bartender doing shift work for 15–20 hours per week. Outside of work, she led a sedentary lifestyle, with her hobbies including photography and laptop computer work.

Symptom Behaviour

Since commencing the new job 3 months earlier, her knee symptoms had deteriorated to the extent that she now reported a dull ache at the beginning of the shift which progressed to a tense, cramping, buzzing-like feeling by the end of the shift. Her worst symptoms occurred when ascending stairs, especially after work, with pain increasing after one to two steps, up to an intensity of 5/10 on a pain numerical rating scale (NRS; 0 = no pain; 10 = worst pain imaginable) after one flight. In the previous 7 days, Ellie rated her worst pain as being 8/10 after working more than 8 hours. Her symptoms were also aggravated when sitting for longer than 90 minutes (4/10) or driving a manual car for longer than 30 minutes, which resulted in an uncomfortable ache. Colder weather caused an increase in the knee symptoms, as did a rapid change in room temperature (e.g. when walking in/out of a large refrigerator at work). Throughout the day, Ellie's symptoms were only aggravated by activity or being in positions of knee flexion for a prolonged period of time.

Symptoms were relieved by avoiding aggravating activities, applying ice for 20 minutes after working and modifying resting knee positions. Ellie wore an elastic knee support to assist in symptom management during work. She reported audible crepitus in the left knee and to a lesser extent in the right knee, with a relieving 'crack' felt in the left knee at times after moving out of flexion from prolonged sitting.

Fig. 10.1   Body chart depicting Ellie's anterior knee pain.

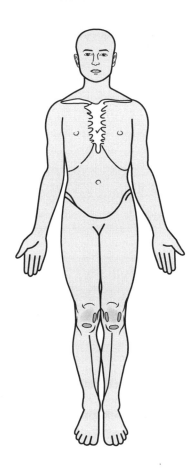

Self-Report Forms

During the assessment, Ellie completed the Kujala Anterior Knee Pain Scale (Kujala et al., 1993) scoring 68/100, which indicated a severe restriction in functional abilities due to knee pain. She also completed a Patient-Specific Functional Scale (PSFS) to evaluate her ability to perform individually selected activities (scored from 0 = 'able to do for as long as I wish', to 10 = 'unable to do') (Stratford, 1995), for which she nominated the activities of walking up/down stairs (3/10), working for greater than 8 hours (5/10) and sitting for more than 1 hour (3/10).

Ellie reported she had seen her local general practitioner for her knee pain and had not undergone any investigations. This medical practitioner essentially advised that the pain would 'go away'. She had not consulted any other healthcare professionals.

Reasoning Question:

1. Following the patient interview, and considering the chronicity of symptoms, what is your hypothesis regarding the most likely 'pain type' (nociceptive, peripheral neuropathic, nociplastic)? What is your reasoning process behind your decision?

Answer to Reasoning Question:

It was hypothesized that Ellie's pain was most likely to be predominantly of nociceptive origin. Her pain only came on with loading activities of the knee, such as negotiating stairs, and with sustained knee flexion in sitting and driving, suggesting a mechanical load-related cause for her pain. These physical activities are known to particularly increase stress at the patellofemoral joint. Ellie's report of a long history of persistent symptoms, recent deterioration with increased workloads and moderate level of symptom irritability could also suggest the presence of secondary peripheral sensitivity.

Continued on following page

Reasoning Question:

2. Can you please discuss which features of Ellie's reported history led you to your primary and secondary diagnostic hypotheses?

Answer to Reasoning Question:

The impression following the patient interview was a primary hypothesis of persistent patellofemoral pain, with a secondary hypothesis of fat-pad irritation. The primary hypothesis of persistent patellofemoral pain was supported by the exclusion of findings in Ellie's history which may be indicative of other pathologies. That is, there was no history of trauma, no mention of symptoms suggestive of ligamentous instability and little likelihood of referral of symptoms from the lumbar spine or hip. Patellofemoral pain is typically aggravated by activities that load the patellofemoral joint (e.g. squatting/crouching, stair ambulation and running) or which involve sustained knee flexion (e.g. prolonged sitting), consistent with the activities that Ellie reported to be painful.

Further supporting the primary hypothesis was Ellie's reported audible joint sounds, which is sometimes described in those with patellofemoral pain (Crossley et al., 2016a). It is thought that this noise is the result of aberrant patella motion through the trochlear groove of the femur during flexion and extension of the knee, and it may reflect the integrity of the articular cartilage (Jiang et al., 1993). It has also been suggested that audible grinding noises and/or palpable vibrations may indicate the presence of early osteoarthritic features of the patellofemoral joint on magnetic resonance imaging (MRI) in women without tibiofemoral joint changes (Schiphof et al., 2014).

The secondary hypothesis of fat-pad irritation was supported by the location and description of symptoms (anterior knee, inferior to the patella) and by the provocation of pain during dynamic activities, such as knee extension during stair ascent.

Reasoning Question:

3. It is interesting that cold environments aggravated Ellie's symptoms, yet she indicated that she used ice for pain relief, which could appear a little contradictory. Are you able to make any comment on this? Was this a consideration in determining your hypothesis regarding the dominant 'pain type'?

Answer to Reasoning Question:

The pain aggravation induced by cold ambient temperatures is not consistent with our hypothesis of a nociceptive 'pain type', but the relief of pain with ice could possibly be consistent with nociceptive pain. A study of patients with patellofemoral pain has reported that those with cold sensitivity indicate higher pain severity, tolerate less physical activity and demonstrate less improvement to lower limb stretching, vastus medialis training and patellar taping treatment (Selfe et al., 2010). Ellie's presentation did not align well with those reported findings. Perhaps in cold environments, she might have adopted more flexed lower limb postures, which she had reported were provocative of her knee pain. However, this was not explored with her at the time, and so this is purely conjecture. Regarding her use of ice to modulate patellofemoral pain, this could be subserved by a peripheral inhibitory mechanism through cooling effects on nociceptors and small-afferent-fibre function.

Pain is seldom the result of solely peripheral or solely central pathophysiology but is more likely a combination thereof. So it is conceivable that although Ellie's predominant pain presentation was nociceptive in nature, she could concurrently have had some central nervous system changes (sensitization) due to the long-term nature of her condition.

Clinical Reasoning Commentary:

It is a common clinical reasoning error for the practitioner to only consider the 'positive' or supportive clinical findings in the patient examination and to fail to give similar consideration to absent or non-supportive findings in determining likely hypotheses. This was not the case in the clinician's response to the question of which clinical features supported the primary diagnostic hypothesis of persistent patellofemoral pain where the absence of clinical features indicative of some alternative or competing hypotheses (such as knee ligamentous pathology) was given due weighting in the reasoning process. This suggests that the clinician is actively and simultaneously considering multiple diagnostic hypotheses (tissue/structural; and/or physical impairments) and ordering these based on the presence and absence of features typically to be expected in the associated clinical patterns. Pain type cannot be measured clinically and, as discussed in Chapter 1, needs to be a hypothesis based on pain science and current understanding of expected clinical patterns (see Chapter 2). Although clinical patterns are helpful, they are often not fully validated, features can overlap with other patterns and patients will not necessarily present with every feature. This is nicely illustrated in the reasoning here, where features of a nociceptive-dominant pattern are recognized along with features of central nervous system sensitization.

Physical Examination
Observation

On observation of the lower limb in bipedal stance, the hips were internally rotated, and the feet were pronated, left greater than right. The knees were in hyperextension and appeared normal, with no apparent swelling. Based on the pronated foot posture and knee hyperextension, the Beighton Hypermobility Scale was applied (Boyle et al., 2003), with Ellie scoring 6/9 with bilateral hyperextension of the 5th metacarpophalangeal joints, elbows and knees. This score indicates the presence of generalized joint laxity (Boyle et al., 2003; van der Giessen et al., 2001). Single leg stance resulted in 3/10 retropatellar pain in the left knee only. Performing a small single knee bend on the left leg resulted in 4/10 peripatellar pain, described as an 'ache', at approximately 30 degrees of flexion.

Functional Tests

Each functional test was performed either until the onset of pain or performance of 25 pain-free repetitions. These tests included squats (i.e. full deep squat/full knee flexion, onto the balls of the feet, touching the floor with hands either side of the ankles), where Ellie achieved 6/25 repetitions; step-ups onto a 25-cm step at the speed of a metronome set to 96 beats/minute (7/25 repetitions on the left, 18/25 on the right); and step-downs from a 25-cm step (2/25 repetitions on the left, 3/25 on the right).

On active range-of-motion testing with overpressure at the end range, there was full pain-free active range of motion of both knees.

Knee Tests

The patella borders were tender to palpation both medially and laterally on the left, with no swelling or joint effusion present. The Hoffa test was conducted to test for fat-pad irritation (Dragoo et al., 2012). The test is designed to irritate the fat pad by applying firm pressure via the thumb inferior to the patella outside the margin of the patellar tendon with the knee in 30 degrees of knee flexion and then in full knee extension (hyperextension). The test is regarded as positive for impingement if pain is produced during the last 10 degrees of extension indicating involvement of the fat pad in the presenting symptoms (Kumar et al., 2007), although little is known about the Hoffa test's diagnostic properties (Mace et al., 2016). The test was repeated on both the medial and lateral sides of both knees but did not reproduce Ellie's symptoms. Further testing designed to irritate the fat pad was undertaken, which involved isometric quadriceps contraction in full extension and passive extension overpressure, again with no symptoms reproduced (Dragoo et al., 2012). There was also no pain elicited on firm palpation of the proximal, mid- or distal portions of the patella tendon.

Valgus and varus ligamentous tests of the medial and lateral collateral ligaments, respectively; anterior drawer test and Lachman's test; posterior drawer test and sag sign; and McMurray's and Apley's tests were all negative for both knees, indicating that the ligamentous structures and menisci were not likely to be the source of symptoms. The patellar apprehension sign for instability was also negative. Manual compression of the patella into the trochlear groove at both 0 degrees and 20 degrees of knee flexion was positive for symptom reproduction for the left knee only. Clarke's test was performed with Ellie lying in supine, with both knees supported in slight flexion (Nijs et al., 2006). The patella was pressed distally (with the therapist's hand on the superior border of the patella), and she was instructed to gradually perform an isometric contraction of the quadriceps muscle (Malanga et al., 2003). This test is thought to actively compress and stress the articular surfaces of both the patella and the femoral trochlear groove. Reproduction of symptoms is regarded as a positive test and suggestive of a patellofemoral joint disorder, and whilst Ellie tested positive for both knees, this test's diagnostic utility is questionable (Doberstein et al., 2008). Similarly, the ability of patella mobility testing to assist in diagnosis is marginal, so no assessment of patella translation mobility was conducted (Sweitzer et al., 2010).

Foot Tests

Foot posture index (Redmond et al., 2008), navicular drop (Brody, 1990) and midfoot mobility measurements (McPoil et al., 2009) were recorded. For the foot posture index, the left foot scored +7 and the right +8, indicating a pronated foot posture bilaterally (Redmond et al., 2006). Navicular drop is measured by the change in height of the navicular tuberosity relative to the floor between a subtalar neutral posture and a relaxed stance foot posture. Ellie's navicular drop was 7 mm on the left and 9 mm on the right. Midfoot mobility is measured by recording the difference between the midfoot width in weight bearing (WB) and non-weight bearing (NWB), and is expressed as midfoot width (MFW) difference (DiffMFW = WB − NWB). Ellie's midfoot width measurements in weight bearing were 87.7 mm on the left and 87.6 mm on the right, and in non-weight bearing were 75.6 mm on the left and 76.4 mm on the right. Thus, the DiffMFW was 12.1 mm and 11.2 mm on the left and right, respectively. Ellie's change in midfoot width was more than the 11 mm previously reported to be associated with a greater benefit from foot orthoses intervention (Vicenzino et al., 2010; Mills et al., 2012).

Treatment Direction Test (TDT)

Given the findings on observation, foot posture and mobility testing, a Treatment Direction Test (TDT) was next applied. The TDT has been previously reported (Vicenzino, 2004), however, in brief, it involves applying a physical manipulation (e.g. anti-pronation taping in this case) during the client-specific impairment measure (e.g. pain-free step-ups on a 25-cm step with Ellie). According to Vicenzino (2004), if a significant improvement in the client-specific impairment measure is observed (i.e. ≥75% number of pain-free step-ups), then treatment of the foot with orthoses and exercises would have a high likelihood of success. Ellie achieved nine pain-free step-ups on the left (i.e. her most problematic knee) before the onset of her knee pain. After applying the anti-pronation tape (Fig. 10.2), Ellie was able to achieve 14 pain-free step-ups on the left, suggesting a high probability of a successful outcome with foot orthoses for Ellie.

Ankle Range of Motion

Reduced ankle dorsiflexion range has been previously associated with lower limb pathologies, including an association with aberrant hip patho-mechanics in a single leg squat task in those with patellofemoral pain (Backman et al., 2011; Collins et al., 2014; Rabin et al., 2014; Ota et al., 2014). Ellie's bent-knee ankle dorsiflexion range was measured using a modified knee-to-wall test (Larsen et al., 2016) (146 mm left and 128 mm right) and also during straight-knee ankle dorsiflexion using an inclinometer placed mid-tibia (48 degrees left and 45 degrees right).

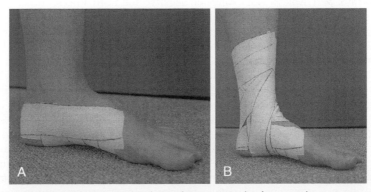

Fig. 10.2 Anti-pronation taping. A, Low dye technique (just the foot taped). B, Augmented low dye technique (with the lower leg taped).

TABLE 10.1		
MAXIMAL VOLUNTARY ISOMETRIC HIP MUSCLE STRENGTH SCORES AT BASELINE		
	0 Weeks	
	Left	**Right**
Abduction (N)	71.1	70.2
Adduction (N)	70.7	61.13
External rotation (N)	67.2	64.7

Hip Muscle Strength Tests

Deficits in hip muscle function have been associated with altered movement patterns of the lower limb (Souza and Powers, 2009a, 2009b; Powers, 2010). Recent studies have identified reduced hip muscle strength, particularly of the hip abductors and external rotators, in people with patellofemoral pain compared with an asymptomatic group (Ireland et al., 2003; Robinson and Nee, 2007; Nakagawa et al., 2012). On the basis of this evidence, maximal voluntary isometric hip strength measurements of hip abduction, adduction and external rotation were recorded (in supine lying) using a hand-held dynamometer that was fixated by a belt (Table 10.1).

Reasoning Question:

4. Can you explain how the physical examination findings supported/refuted your primary diagnostic hypothesis of persistent patellofemoral pain and your secondary hypothesis of fat-pad irritation? How did your treatment hypothesis of foot orthoses fit with these findings?

Answer to Reasoning Question:

On physical examination, Ellie presented with hyperextended knees and internally rotated femurs in standing. On observation of the knees, there was no evident swelling or enlargement of the fat pad. Ellie tested negative for fat-pad irritation on palpation and on pain reproduction techniques (Hoffa test, isometric quadriceps contraction in full extension and extension overpressure), suggesting the fat pad was not the primary source of pain. Tests were also negative for other local knee pathologies (i.e. ligamentous, tendon, etc.). Most importantly, Ellie's symptoms were reproduced with techniques that loaded and stressed the patellofemoral joint (squats, step up/down and single leg squats). Ellie also had marked tenderness on the medial and lateral borders of the patellae and symptom reproduction on Clarke's test.

When physical examination findings were taken into consideration with her patient interview and, importantly, the exclusion of other differential diagnoses, the overall findings were indicative of Ellie having bilateral persistent patellofemoral pain. Based on the findings of pronated foot posture on the foot posture index, DiffMFW ≥11 mm, and a positive response to the TDT, it was decided that foot orthoses would be the initial treatment in managing Ellie's patellofemoral pain.

Reasoning Question:

5. You performed a comprehensive assessment of foot biomechanics in this patient. Is this an assessment approach you take with all of the patients in your clinic with patellofemoral/knee pain, or were there features in the history and physical examination that led you to pursue that direction, rather than perhaps another approach?

Answer to Reasoning Question:

The focus on the foot assessment was based on Ellie's report that her most provocative activity was stair climbing, a weight-bearing-under-load task, combined with the initial observation of her marked pronated foot posture. Physical examination of stair walking confirmed it provoked her pain, and correcting her foot posture with anti-pronation taping allowed the patient to perform substantially more steps. These findings led to further examination of foot posture with the foot posture index and measures of midfoot height and weight, which confirmed her feet to be more pronated than normal. If it had not been possible to reproduce Ellie's pain on stair walking and if there had been no observable pronation of her feet, then the assessment would likely have focussed more on the knee and the hip.

Continued on following page

Clinical Reasoning Commentary:

These responses demonstrate how the clinician has come to diagnostic and treatment decisions based on a combination of knowledge/evidence derived from prior experience with similar clinical presentations and also scientific evidence obtained from the published research. Hypotheses tentatively formulated during the patient interview have now been tested in the physical examination to determine whether expected clinical findings are indeed present, based on this previously acquired experiential and empirical data. Impairments were specifically tested to determine their relevance to key presenting symptoms (such as the correction of foot pronation on the knee pain experienced during stair walking) and were not simply assumed to be supportive of the primary structural hypothesis (persistent patellofemoral pain). Similarly, it was not assumed that competing hypotheses (e.g. fat-pad irritation, ligament pathology) were not to be accepted in conjunction with or instead of the primary hypothesis but were each specifically physically tested to ensure their exclusion at this time was appropriate. In the 'hypothesis category' framework presented in Chapter 1, assessment and trial correction of foot posture represents reasoning about potential 'contributing factors', as might the assessment of femoral posture and hip strength where trial intervention may similarly have had a positive effect. Treatment decisions were therefore based on supportive derived clinical findings and applied scientific evidence built during both the patient interview and the physical examination, as well as the absence of any convincing supportive evidence for competing hypotheses.

Treatment

Ellie was provided with comprehensive information and education about patellofemoral pain. In particular, she was given an in-depth explanation of the proposed mechanisms by which excessive foot pronation might impact upon patellofemoral mechanics (Tiberio, 1987). In brief, Ellie was made aware of the effect of excessive foot pronation in inducing greater lower limb internal rotation and the flow-on effect on patellofemoral joint stress. She was further informed of the emerging evidence which suggests that a change of ≥11 mm in midfoot width (from non-weight bearing to weight bearing) is associated with a successful outcome with the use of foot orthoses and that her positive response to the anti-pronation taping technique indicated a higher probability of a successful outcome with this approach to treatment.

The foot orthoses were subsequently fitted as previously described (Vicenzino et al, 2008). In short, the fundamental aim of the fitting was to ensure the foot orthoses were comfortable in order to maximize compliance, with an overall aim of improving pain-free function. The foot orthoses fitted were commercially available, prefabricated orthotics (Vasyli International) made from ethylene-vinyl acetate with a manufacturer-specified six-degree varus wedge and arch support. Ellie was fitted with a full-length foot orthosis of the lowest density (Shore A 52 degrees) to her work footwear (sports running shoes) that were subsequently heat moulded to optimize comfort (Fig. 10.3). She was instructed to wear her work shoes during the day and at work and to remove the orthoses if they began to feel uncomfortable.

Appointment 2 (3 Days After Initial Appointment)

Ellie returned 3 days later for a review of her foot orthoses and to be taught a home exercise program. She reported that she had noticed a reduction in the severity of pain in both knees and that symptoms took longer to commence while she was working. There were no adverse effects at her foot-to-orthoses interface beyond a mild general ache. Ellie's work and casual footwear were reviewed, and all were found to have minimal heel counter-stiffness, midfoot sole sagittal stiffness (bending the midfoot in the sagittal plane) and midfoot sole frontal stability (torsional movement or twisting of the midfoot section by counter-rotating the rearfoot and forefoot components). She was asked to seek more stable footwear that would meet the requirements for her work but also complement the application of the foot orthoses.

Ellie was supplied with a second set of full-length foot orthoses of medium density (Shore A 60 degrees) that were heat moulded to optimize comfort. She was instructed to swap the foot orthoses into whatever footwear she would be wearing. This change was

Fig. 10.3 Full-length foot orthoses. *(©2017 Vionic Group LLC. Vasyli is a registered trademark used with the permission of the rights owner. All rights reserved.)*

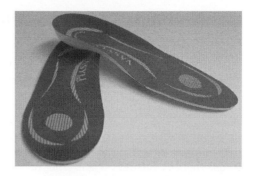

Fig. 10.4 Anti-pronation foot exercise.

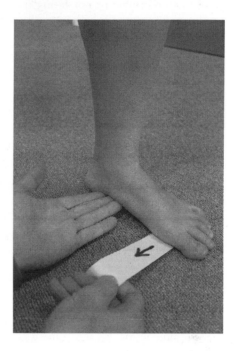

done on the basis of tolerability to the initial lower-density orthosis and a desire to provide an orthosis that would likely have a longer life.

Ellie was then taught a home exercise program consisting of anti-pronation foot exercises and calf stretches with the knee extended. The arch-forming exercises commenced in partial weight bearing (seated) with the knees flexed and bare feet flat on the floor. To help facilitate the exercise, a piece of paper or non-adhesive tape was placed under the distal end of the first metatarsal, and Ellie was instructed to maintain firm pressure on the paper/tape (in order to prevent the paper from being slid out from under the foot by the clinician) whilst keeping her toes relaxed. She was also instructed on the technique of supinating the rearfoot, which was initially assisted with manual facilitation (using finger pressure under the arch) (Fig. 10.4). This was sustained for 10 seconds and then repeated on the opposite foot. Ellie was asked to repeat the foot supination task five times for each foot, twice daily. As she became more proficient at performing this exercise, Ellie was to progress to practicing this in bipedal stance.

Finally, Ellie was asked to perform straight-knee calf stretches for 30 seconds, three times, twice daily, either by a lunge stretch against a wall or over the edge of a step whilst keeping the rearfoot in neutral supination/pronation as per the arch forming exercise. The lunge stretch against the wall involved facing the wall in step-stance with both hands on the wall and both feet flat on the floor aligned perpendicular to the wall. The lunge calf stretch was performed to a comfortable but firm stretch felt in the back of the calf. Alternatively, Ellie could lower the heel down over the edge of a step whilst maintaining a straight knee.

Appointment 3 (11 Days After Initial Appointment)

Ellie reported a notable bilateral improvement in her knee pain since the last visit. She found the foot orthoses did not fit all of her footwear, but when she was unable to fit the orthoses, she instead focused on the anti-pronation foot exercises and holding this position momentarily at various times during standing, especially at work. The anti-pronation foot exercises were reviewed and progressed from sitting to bipedal stance to bilateral isometric heel raise holds (i.e. holding heels just off the floor) whilst maintaining the rearfoot in a neutral position. Ellie was still yet to seek more supportive footwear. She was to continue to use the foot orthoses where able, particularly at work, but was to remove them if they were uncomfortable or not fitting the footwear properly and instead focus on the anti-pronation foot exercises with increasing periods of incorporating this posture during standing throughout the day.

Appointment 4 (27 Days After Initial Appointment)

Ellie returned to report significantly less knee pain, especially at work and while ascending stairs after work, which was previously the most aggravating activity and time of day. She reported that she had decided to stop wearing the foot orthoses during the previous week because she had difficulty fitting them to her footwear selection and preferred to do the anti-pronation foot exercises. She had been focusing on the exercises consistently throughout the day and particularly at work. The anti-pronation foot exercises were progressed from bipedal standing with increasing duration of isometric holds to bipedal dynamic heel raises whilst maintaining a more subtalar neutral position.

Appointment 5 (48 Days After Initial Appointment)

Ellie returned to report she was only experiencing slight twinges in her left knee at work (0.5/10). She now reported feeling no symptoms when walking up stairs and only an 'awareness' of symptoms in her left knee at other times. Importantly, her knee was not painful after work. Because Ellie was making substantial improvements, no physical re-examination or assessment was conducted.

The anti-pronation foot exercises were progressed from bipedal dynamic heel raises to single calf raises whilst maintaining a subtalar neutral position. Ellie was to perform these throughout the day as she remembered, especially at work. Ellie felt comfortable to now self-manage with anti-pronation exercises and return for review and re-assessment in 7 weeks' time.

Appointment 6 (16 Weeks After Initial Appointment)

Ellie was reviewed at 16 weeks and reported she was 'much better' on a 7-point global rating-of-change scale (much better, better, a little better, no change, a little worse, worse, much worse). On a scale of 0% (not recovered) to 100% (totally recovered), Ellie rated her knees as 100% totally recovered from her presenting knee pain. She no longer felt any pain in cold environments. On the Kujala Anterior Knee Pain Scale, she scored 100/100, and the only activity rated on the PSFS (0 = able to do for as long as I wish, 10 = unable to do) was climbing stairs (0.5/10), as Ellie had experienced a one-off slight twinge ascending stairs after work the week prior. She had now returned to doing moderate physical activity for 30 minutes, five times a week.

On retesting of the pain-free functional task of squatting, Ellie was able to complete 25/25; on step-ups onto a 25-cm step, Ellie was able to complete 25/25 on the left and 22/25 on the right with slight pain (1/10), at the speed of a metronome set at 96 beats/minute; and on step-downs, Ellie completed 25/25 on both the left and the right knee.

Ellie's maximal voluntary isometric hip strength measurements of hip abduction, adduction and external rotation were re-measured (Table 10.2), showing a bilateral increase in external rotation maximum isometric force (11% and 22% on left and right, respectively) and an increase in adduction force on the right (21%).

Interestingly, Ellie reported she felt that she subconsciously held the foot in a more neutral position that was now her new 'normal' foot posture, and a pronated foot posture now felt very awkward. On measurement of her navicular drop, it was 2 mm on the left and 1 mm on the right (compared with initial measurements of 7 mm and 9 mm, respectively). Ellie had continued to perform the single heel calf raises when she remembered to do so at work and during the day, as well as maintaining a neutral foot posture during activities of daily living, noting that this did not require much mental focus to achieve. Ellie was encouraged to keep up with the exercises she was currently doing and keep incorporating them into her activities of daily living.

TABLE 10.2

MAXIMAL VOLUNTARY ISOMETRIC HIP MUSCLE STRENGTH SCORES AT 0 AND 16 WEEKS

	0 Weeks		16 Weeks	
	Left	**Right**	**Left**	**Right**
Abduction (N)	71.1	70.2	*	*
Adduction (N)	70.7	61.13	71.2	74.1
External rotation (N)	67.2	64.7	74.8	78.7

*Unable to test maximally because back pain was present during abduction. Back pain had commenced in preceding week as a result of a fall.

Appointment 7 (32 Weeks After Initial Appointment)

When Ellie was reviewed approximately 8 months after treatment had commenced, she reported that she was still much better on a 7-point global rating-of-change scale and 100% recovered from her knee pain. Her knee pain did not limit any activity of her choice on the PSFS, and she still scored 100/100 on the Kujala Anterior Knee Pain Scale. On the pain-free functional task tests, Ellie scored 25/25 repetitions for squats, step-ups and step-downs.

On measurement of her navicular drop, it was 0 mm on both the left and right. On measurement of change in midfoot width moving from non-weight bearing to weight bearing, Ellie's midfoot difference was now 6.6 mm on the left (previously 12.1 mm at initial presentation) and 7.3 mm on the right (previously 11.2 mm). These measures were considered consistent with a less pronated foot posture type. Interestingly, the hip muscle strength had also increased (ranging from 8%–33%) from the first session (Table 10.3).

TABLE 10.3

MAXIMAL VOLUNTARY ISOMETRIC HIP MUSCLE STRENGTH SCORES AT 0, 16 AND 32 WEEKS

	0 Weeks		16 Weeks		32 Weeks	
	Left	**Right**	**Left**	**Right**	**Left**	**Right**
Abduction (N)	71.1	70.2	*	*	79.4	75.7
Adduction (N)	70.7	61.13	71.2	74.1	79.9	79.2
External rotation (N)	67.2	64.7	74.8	78.7	89.2	78.6

*Unable to test maximally because back pain was present during abduction. Back pain had commenced in preceding week as a result of a fall.

Reasoning Question:

6. Re-assessment revealed hip muscle strength had increased despite specific exercises for those muscles not being part of the treatment programme. Can you please propose the mechanism behind this increase in strength and how it may have contributed to the decrease in knee pain?

Answer to Reasoning Question:

Improved hip muscle strength was not expected because the treatment was entirely focused at the foot. The mechanism by which this happened is likely multifaceted. One such mechanism might have involved the foot exercises and orthoses inducing changes at the foot, which countered the excessive foot pronation and internal rotation of the lower limb during weight-bearing activities. The foot exercises were designed to control the amount of pronation the foot underwent in weight bearing. This was confirmed with a marked reduction in midfoot width mobility after commencing the exercises (e.g. 12.1–6.6 mm on the left foot; 11.2–7.3 mm on the right foot). This reduction in foot pronation would plausibly reduce the amount of internal rotation occurring in the lower limb, notably causing a reduction in the internal rotation and adduction of the hip during the stance phase of gait. It can be hypothesized that the hip abductor and external rotator muscles would be working at a disadvantage during the stance phase of gait with the foot pronated excessively, with concomitant increased internal hip rotation and hip adduction. The changes in foot posture observed in this case might have improved the mechanical efficiency of force production of the hip abductor and external rotator muscles by reducing the amount of lower limb internal rotation during loading in single limb stance (e.g. during gait or negotiating stairs). With improved lower limb function and reduced pain, Ellie could feasibly have moved more freely and often, leading to strength adaptations of the hip muscles. Studies have shown that isolated exercises targeting the hip abductors and external rotators have had a positive effect on patellofemoral pain (Khayambashi et al., 2012, 2014; Nakagawa et al., 2008; Fukuda et al., 2012), which might have been a means by which the foot treatment led to the observed hip muscle strength improvements.

Another mechanism might have been through unintended exercise of the hip muscles when Ellie performed the anti-pronation exercises of the foot. These exercises focussed on the coupling between the leg and foot, not just the sagittal plane of the foot in isolation. That is, the exercises involved a coupling of external rotation of the tibia with supination of the rearfoot and plantarflexion of the forefoot, rather than focussing primarily only on the foot in the sagittal plane (e.g. as with foot shortening exercises that primarily target sagittal plane posture locally at the foot). In performing these exercises, Ellie could have used her hip external rotators, which could have led to some conditioning of the hip muscles and possibly strength adaptations.

It is also feasible that the alteration in foot posture and flow-on effects to the lower limb served to de-stress the patellofemoral joint, which was posited as the nociceptive source of the patellofemoral pain. The resultant reduction in patellofemoral pain would likely lead to more efficient use of the thigh and hip muscles, which in turn might facilitate restitution of hip muscle strength.

It must be stated that it is difficult to explain how the foot treatment changed both the hip muscle strength and the patellofemoral pain, or indeed the causal direction of such effects, and that a combination of these proposed mechanisms along with others not considered may have been responsible for the observed effects.

Reasoning Question:

7. Can you please discuss Ellie's preference to exercise rather than comply with the change in footwear and how this may have influenced your management and the ultimate outcome?

Answer to Reasoning Question:

Ellie had certain requirements for work footwear; she used a variety of casual footwear and spent time in bare feet at home. During Ellie's initial session, she received a detailed explanation of active retraining of foot posture and the biomechanical effect on patellar tracking, thus addressing a potential contributor to her knee pain. After discussion of these factors and the possible long-term benefit of active versus passive intervention, she felt that an active approach with exercises was the most likely to be beneficial. Ellie felt the immediate change in her knee-pain symptoms with the anti-pronation taping at the initial appointment and the effect of the foot orthoses over the following sessions, both of which assisted with her engagement with the treatment approach and her view of progressing to active exercises. It is highly likely that an understanding of the potential mechanisms contributing to her symptoms in combination with an immediate positive response to treatment contributed greatly to Ellie's compliance and adherence to regularly performing the exercises.

Reasoning Question:

8. A midfoot width change ≥11 mm was described as being associated with a successful response to treatment aimed at the foot for those with patellofemoral pain. Are there any other factors (such as severity of symptoms, chronicity, 'pain type', age of patient, psychosocial considerations, etc.) that may need consideration in selecting your treatment approach in similar cases?

Answer to Reasoning Question:

Symptoms of patellofemoral pain are typically consistent between patients; however, biomechanical, physiological and external factors contributing to the onset of a patient's symptoms vary between individuals because of the multifactorial nature of the condition. Patients may present with one or more combinations of contributing/associated factors proximally at the hip, locally at the knee or distally at the foot and ankle.

Current evidence suggests that a multimodal treatment approach has the best outcome for reducing patellofemoral pain, but it is not a 'one-size-fits-all' approach. Of importance is a comprehensive and appropriate clinical examination to tailor the multimodal program to the patient. Identifying key characteristics that are associated with the patient's symptoms improves the optimal selection of management approach. In Ellie's case, her foot mobility indicated targeting treatment to her foot. If Ellie did not present with such a mobile foot, then evidence suggests exercises targeted more proximally at the hip to improve neuromuscular activity (Crossley et al., 2016) might be more successful. It is not unusual for these exercises to take some time to bring about an improvement, so in the meantime, it could be advantageous to consider complementary treatments to reduce pain and improve the patient's ability to be more active and adhere to the exercises (e.g. patellar taping, acupuncture, stretching).

In cases where there are severe and persistent symptoms with associated psychosocial issues, such as such as negative fear-avoidance beliefs, anxiety, depression and pain catastrophizing (Grotle et al., 2010; Crombez et al., 1999; Carroll et al., 2004), which likely mitigate against a good response to mechanically based treatments, it would be advisable to take a pain sciences approach to management. This approach would require consideration of referral to other clinicians (e.g. psychologist, pain specialist). Fundamentally, however, the key is to tailor the treatment to the individual and the presenting case and to educate the individual about his or her knee condition with the most up-to-date and relevant evidence available. It is important to involve the patient in some informed decision-making in designing the treatment plan, which can then be tailored to patient preferences and lifestyle. Crucial to a good outcome is patient confidence in the rationale behind the treatment plan to facilitate adherence, which is vital to recovery.

The key consideration in the treatment approach applied in Ellie's case was the aim of reducing pain and educating her as early as possible to help to gain her confidence in the treatment approach and to facilitate greater adherence to treatment (e.g. active exercises).

Reasoning Question:

9. Given this condition has been described as self-limiting by some authors, do you think Ellie may have recovered without any intervention? What led you to hypothesize a favourable prognosis?

Answer to Reasoning Question:

Patellofemoral pain is a common and persistent knee condition that affects teenagers and young adults (Rathleff et al., 2013a, 2013b, 2016; Collins et al., 2013; Mølgaard et al., 2011; Boling et al., 2010; Roush and Curtis Bay, 2012). Conservative treatments for patellofemoral pain, such as strengthening, stretching and functional movement retraining of quadriceps and gluteal muscles, foot orthoses, patellar taping and manual therapy, have been reported to produce modest effects of short- to moderate-term duration (Collins et al., 2008). Despite these interventions, a substantial proportion of patients still report persistent long-term symptoms (Collins et al., 2013), with approximately 1 in 4 reporting symptoms up to 20 years later (Nimon et al., 1998).

It is erroneous to consider this condition as being self-limiting, especially in adolescents, in whom patellofemoral pain could be dismissed as 'growing pains'. A substantial body of evidence points to the contrary, with 50% of 12- to 15-year-olds reporting persistent knee pain 12 months later (Rathleff et al., 2013), 55% of 15- to 19-year-olds reporting persistent pain 2 years later (Kujala et al., 1993) and, more notably, 78% of females diagnosed with patellofemoral pain during adolescence still experiencing pain after 14–20 years (Rathleff et al., 2016; Collins et al., 2013; Nimon et al., 1998). Ellie appears to be in this long-term, non-self-limiting category because she was diagnosed with patellofemoral pain at 13 years of age and has had persistent symptoms that have continued to significantly impact her life into her early 20s.

Taking in consideration the evidence highlighting that longer knee-pain duration is predictive of a poor outcome (Nimon et al., 1998; Blønd and Hansen, 1998; Collins et al., 2010), it is highly unlikely that Ellie would have recovered without any intervention. Whilst reducing the amount of knee-loading activities may change a patient's symptoms, a reintroduction of knee-loading activities will likely result in a recurrence of the symptoms. This is demonstrated in Ellie's case whereby she reported a cyclical history of improvement when activity was reduced (i.e. the knee was deloaded) but an exacerbation on attempting more activity, such as returning to hospitality work and spending more time on her feet. On commencing physiotherapy treatment, Ellie reported a significant improvement in her symptoms by appointment 3 (11 days). Given she had persistent symptoms for 10 years, it is highly unlikely this

Continued on following page

rapid improvement was a spontaneous recovery, especially because she remained improved 32 weeks later.

A favourable prognosis was indicated because Ellie responded favourably during the step-up test when an anti-pronation taping technique was applied, demonstrating an immediate effect of foot intervention on her patellofemoral pain. Over the following few weeks with foot orthoses and exercises, Ellie reported a marked improvement in her pain, which continued to be the case afterward. This is consistent with a series of studies by Barton et al. (2011a, 2011b) in which patients who demonstrated immediate improvement in a physical pain provocative test with an anti-pronation device applied were more likely to be improved weeks later (Barton et al., 2011a). In another study, Barton et al. (2011c) showed an immediate increase in the number of pain-free single leg raises and single leg squats able to be performed when those patients with a pronated foot type wore prefabricated foot orthoses. These improvements were present at follow-up (Barton et al., 2011d), indicating it was not a short-lived response. In summary, the temporal response profile seen with Ellie was commensurate with expectations and those reported in the literature. Had she not improved sufficiently, however, then management directed at the femoral posture and weakness may have been added.

Clinical Reasoning Commentary:

The importance of patient education and empowerment is well demonstrated in this case. Without a clear explanation regarding the likely cause of her knee pain and the reasons why it has persisted, Ellie may not have complied with the management program over several months and almost certainly would have been much less likely to have adhered to the tailored exercise program. Apart from the clarity and logic of the explanation provided by the clinician, the other key element in motivating Ellie to continue with the exercise program was the powerful demonstration of the effect on her knee symptoms during her most provocative activity (ascending stairs) of an anti-pronation intervention. This appears to have been the 'cognitive clincher' in Ellie understanding and believing that her persistent, decade-old problem could actually be changed for the better and that her chosen clinician could assist her to that end. Moreover, the relatively rapid improvement in her pain and function following the commencement of the exercise program provided Ellie with the knowledge that she had the 'power' to manage her symptoms herself, under the guidance of her clinician, in whom she had confidence. Ellie embraced the responsibility of taking control of her own management; however, importantly, the clinician facilitated this by allowing her to be a truly collaborative partner in the therapeutic alliance.

REFERENCES

Backman, J.L., Danielson, P., 2011. Low range of ankle dorsiflexion predisposes for patellar tendinopathy in junior elite basketball players: a 1-year prospective study. Am. J. Sports Med. 2626–2633.

Barton, C.J., Menz, H.B., Crossley, K.M., 2011a. Clinical predictors of foot orthoses efficacy in individuals with patellofemoral pain. Med. Sci. Sports Exerc. 43 (9), 1603–1610.

Barton, C.J., Menz, H.B., Crossley, K.M., 2011b. Effects of prefabricated foot orthoses on pain and function in individuals with patellofemoral pain syndrome: a cohort study. Phys. Ther. Sport 12 (2), 70–75.

Barton, C.J., Menz, H.B., Crossley, K.M., 2011c. The immediate effects of foot orthoses on functional performance in individuals with patellofemoral pain syndrome. Br. J. Sports Med. 45 (3), 193–197.

Barton, C.J., Menz, H.B., Levinger, P., Webster, K.E., Crossley, K.M., 2011d. Greater peak rearfoot eversion predicts foot orthoses efficacy in individuals with patellofemoral pain syndrome. Br. J. Sports Med. 45 (9), 697–701.

Blønd, L., Hansen, L., 1998. Patellofemoral pain syndrome in athletes: a 5.7-year retrospective follow-up study of 250 athletes. Acta Orthop. Belg. 64 (4), 393–400.

Boling, M., Padua, D., Marshall, S., Guskiewicz, K., Pyne, S., Beutler, A., 2010. Gender differences in the incidence and prevalence of patellofemoral pain syndrome. Scand. J. Med. Sci. Sports 20 (5), 725–730.

Boyle, K.L., Witt, P., Riegger-Krugh, C., 2003. Intrarater and interrater reliability of the Beighton and Horan Joint Mobility Index. J. Athl. Train 281.

Brody, D.M., 1990. Evaluation of the injured runner. Techniques in Orthopaedics 5 (3), 15.

Carroll, L.J., Cassidy, D.J., Côté, P., 2004. Depression as a risk factor for onset of an episode of troublesome neck and low back pain. Pain 107 (1), 134–139.

Collins, N., Hart, H., Garrick, L., Schache, A., 2014. Single leg squat hip pathomechanics are associated with ankle dorsiflexion restriction in people with patellofemoral pain. J. Sci. Med. Sport 18 (1), e18.

Collins, N.J., Bierma-Zeinstra, S.M., Crossley, K.M., van Linschoten, R.L., Vicenzino, B., van Middelkoop, M., 2013. Prognostic factors for patellofemoral pain: a multicentre observational analysis. Br. J. Sports Med. 47 (4), 227–233.

Collins, N.J., Crossley, K.M., Beller, E., Darnell, R., McPoil, T., Vicenzino, B., 2008. Foot orthoses and physiotherapy in the treatment of patellofemoral pain syndrome: randomised clinical trial. Br. Med. J. 337 (3), 163–168.

Collins, N.J., Crossley, K.M., Darnell, R., Vicenzino, B., 2010. Predictors of short and long term outcome in patellofemoral pain syndrome: a prospective longitudinal study. BMC Musculoskelet Disord 11, 11.

Crombez, G., Vlaeyen, J., Heuts, P., Lysensd, R., 1999. Pain-related fear is more disabling than pain itself: evidence on the role of pain-related fear in chronic back pain disability. Pain 80, 329–339.

Crossley, K.M., Callaghan, M.J., van Linschoten, R., 2016a. Patellofemoral pain. Br. J. Sports Med. 50 (4), 247–250.

Crossley, K.M., van Middelkoop, M., Callaghan, M.J., Collins, N.J., Rathleff, M.S., Barton, C.J., 2016b. 2016 Patellofemoral pain consensus statement from the 4th International Patellofemoral Pain Research Retreat, Manchester. Part 2: recommended physical interventions (exercise, taping, bracing, foot orthoses and combined interventions). Br. J. Sports Med. 50 (14), 844–852.

Doberstein, S.T., Romeyn, R.L., Reineke, D.M., 2008. The diagnostic value of the Clarke sign in assessing chondromalacia patella. J. Athl. Train. 43 (2), 190–196.

Dragoo, L.J., Johnson, C., McConnell, J., 2012. Evaluation and treatment of disorders of the infrapatellar fat pad. Sports Med. 42 (1), 51–67.

Fukuda, T.Y., Melo, W.P., Zaffalon, B.M., Rossetto, F.M., Magalhães, E., Bryk, F.F., et al., 2012. Hip posterolateral musculature strengthening in sedentary women with patellofemoral pain syndrome: a randomized controlled clinical trial with 1-year follow-up. J. Orthop. Sports Phys. Ther. 42 (10), 823–830.

Grotle, M., Foster, N.E., Dunn, K.M., Croft, P., 2010. Are prognostic indicators for poor outcome different for acute and chronic low back pain consulters in primary care? Pain 151 (3), 790–797.

Ireland, M.L., Willson, J.D., Ballantyne, B.T., Davis, I.S., 2003. Hip strength in females with and without patellofemoral pain. J. Orthop. Sports Phys. Ther. 33 (11), 671–676.

Jiang, C.C., Liu, Y.J., Yip, K.M., Wu, E., 1993. Physiological patellofemoral crepitus in knee joint disorders. Bull. Hosp. Jt Dis. 53 (4), 22–26.

Khayambashi, K., Fallah, A., Movahedi, A., 2014. Posterolateral hip muscle strengthening verses quadriceps strengthening for patellofemoral pain: a comparative control trial. Arch. Phys. Med. Rehabil. 95 (5), 900–907.

Khayambashi, K., Mohammadkhani, Z., Ghaznavi, K., Lyle, M.A., Powers, C.M., 2012. The effects of isolated hip abductor and external rotator muscle strengthening on pain, health status, and hip strength in females with patellofemoral pain: a randomized controlled trial. J. Orthop. Sports Phys. Ther. 42 (1), 22–29.

Kujala, U.M., Jaakkola, L.H., Koskinen, S.K., Taimela, S., Hurme, M., Nelimarkka, O., 1993. Scoring of patellofemoral disorders. Arthroscopy 9 (2), 159–163.

Kumar, D., Alvand, A., Beacon, J.P., 2007. Impingement of infrapatellar fat pad (Hoffa's disease): results of high-portal arthroscopic resection. Arthroscopy 23 (11), 1180–1186 e1.

Larsen, P., Nielsen, H.B., Lund, C., Sørensen, D.S., Larsen, B.T., Matthews, M., et al., 2016. A novel tool for measuring ankle dorsiflexion: a study of its reliability in patients following ankle fractures. Foot Ankle Surg. 22 (4), 274–277.

Mace, J., Bhatti, W., Anand, S., 2016. Infrapatellar fat pad syndrome: a review of anatomy, function, treatment and dynamics. Acta Orthop. Belg. 82 (1), 94–101.

Malanga, G.A., Andrus, S., Nadler, S.F., McLean, J., 2003. Physical examination of the knee: a review of the original test description and scientific validity of common orthopedic tests. Arch. Phys. Med. Rehabil. 84 (4), 592–603.

McPoil, T.G., Vicenzino, B., Cornwall, M.W., Collins, N.J., Warren, M., 2009. Reliability and normative values for the foot mobility magnitude: a composite measure of vertical and medial-lateral mobility of the midfoot. J. Foot Ankle Res. 2, 6.

Mills, K., Blanch, P., Dev, P., Martin, M., Vicenzino, B., 2012. A randomised control trial of short term efficacy of in-shoe foot orthoses compared with a wait and see policy for anterior knee pain and the role of foot mobility. Br. Med. J. 46 (4), 247–252.

Mølgaard, C., Rathleff, M.S., Simonsen, O., 2011. Patellofemoral pain syndrome and its association with hip, ankle, and foot function in 16- to 18-year-old high school students: a single-blind case-control study. J. Am. Podiatr. Med. Assoc. 101 (3), 215–222.

Nakagawa, T.H., Moriya, E.T.U., Maciel, C.D., Serrão, F.V., 2012. Trunk, pelvis, hip, and knee kinematics, hip strength, and gluteal muscle activation during a single-leg squat in males and females with and without patellofemoral pain syndrome. J. Orthop. Sports Phys. Ther. 42 (6), 491–501.

Nakagawa, T.H., Muniz, T.B., Baldon, R.D.M., Dias Maciel, C., de Menezes Reiff, R.B., Serrão, F.V., 2008. The effect of additional strengthening of hip abductor and lateral rotator muscles in patellofemoral pain syndrome: a randomized controlled pilot study. Clin. Rehabil. 22 (12), 1051–1060.

Nijs, J., Van Geel, C., Van der Auwera, C., Van de Velde, B., 2006. Diagnostic value of five clinical tests in patellofemoral pain syndrome. Man. Ther. 11 (1), 69–77.

Nimon, G., Murray, D., Sandow, M., Goodfellow, J., 1998. Natural history of anterior knee pain: a 14- to 20-year follow-up of nonoperative management. J. Pediatr. Orthop. 18 (1), 118–122.

Ota, S., Ueda, M., Aimoto, K., Suzuki, Y., Sigward, S.M., 2014. Acute influence of restricted ankle dorsiflexion angle on knee joint mechanics during gait. Knee 21 (3), 669–675.

Powers, C.M., 2010. The influence of abnormal hip mechanics on knee injury: a biomechanical perspective. J. Orthop. Sports Phys. Ther. 40 (2), 42–51.

Rabin, A., Kozol, Z., Finestone, A.S., 2014. Limited ankle dorsiflexion increases the risk for mid-portion Achilles tendinopathy in infantry recruits: a prospective cohort study. J. Foot Ankle Res. 7 (1), 48.

Rathleff, C.R., Baird, W.N., Olesen, J.L., Roos, E.M., Rasmussen, S., Rathleff, M.S., 2013a. Hip and knee strength is not affected in 12-16 year old adolescents with patellofemoral pain - a cross-sectional population-based study. PLoS ONE 8 (11), e79153.

Rathleff, M.S., Rathleff, C.R., Olesen, J.L., Rasmussen, S., Roos, E.M., 2016. Is knee pain during adolescence a self-limiting condition? Prognosis of patellofemoral pain and other types of knee pain. Am. J. Sports Med. 44 (5), 1165–1171.

Rathleff, M.S., Roos, E.M., Olesen, J.L., Rasmussen, S., 2013b. High prevalence of daily and multi-site pain—a cross-sectional population-based study among 3000 Danish adolescents. BMC Pediatr. 13 (1), 191.

Redmond, A.C., Crane, Y.Z., Menz, H.B., 2008. Normative values for the Foot Posture Index. J. Foot Ankle Res. 1, 6.

Redmond, A.C., Crosbie, J., Ouvrier, R.A., 2006. Development and validation of a novel rating system for scoring standing foot posture: the Foot Posture Index. Clin. Biomech. (Bristol, Avon) 21 (1), 89–98.

Robinson, R.L., Nee, R.J., 2007. Analysis of hip strength in females seeking physical therapy treatment for unilateral patellofemoral pain syndrome. J. Orthop. Sports Phys. Ther. 37 (5), 232–238.

Roush, J.R., Curtis Bay, R., 2012. Prevalence of anterior knee pain in 18-35 year-old females. Int. J. Sports Phys. Ther. 7 (4), 396–401.

Schiphof, D., van Middelkoop, M., de Klerk, B.M., Oei, E.H., Hofman, A., Koes, B.W., et al., 2014. Crepitus is a first indication of patellofemoral osteoarthritis (and not of tibiofemoral osteoarthritis). Osteoarthritis Cartilage 22 (5), 631–638.

Selfe, J., Sutton, C., Hardaker, N., Greenhalgh, S., Karki, A., Dey, P., 2010. Cold females, a distinct group of patellofemoral pain syndrome patients?… Patellofemoral pain syndrome: proximal, distal, and local factors, an international research retreat, April 30-May 2, 2009, Fells Point, Baltimore, MD. J. Orthop. Sports Phys. Ther. 42 (6), A42.

Souza, R.B., Powers, C.M., 2009a. Differences in hip kinematics, muscle strength, and muscle activation between subjects with and without patellofemoral pain. J. Orthop. Sports Phys. Ther. 39 (1), 12–19.

Souza, R.B., Powers, C.M., 2009b. Predictors of hip internal rotation during running: an evaluation of hip strength and femoral structure in women with and without patellofemoral pain. Am J Sports Med 37 (3), 579–587.

Stratford, P., 1995. Assessing disability and change on individual patients: a report of a patient specific measure. Physiotherapy Canada 47 (4), 258–263.

Sweitzer, B.A., Cook, C., Steadman, J.R., Hawkins, R.J., Wyland, D.J., 2010. The inter-rater reliability and diagnostic accuracy of patellar mobility tests in patients with anterior knee pain. Phys. Sportsmed. 38 (3), 90–96.

Tiberio, D., 1987. The effect of excessive subtalar joint pronation on patellofemoral mechanics: a theoretical model. J. Orthop. Sports Phys. Ther. 9 (4), 160–165.

van der Giessen, L.J., Liekens, D., Rutgers, K.J., Hartman, A., Mulder, P.G., Oranje, A.P., 2001. Validation of Beighton score and prevalence of connective tissue signs in 773 Dutch children. J. Rheumatol. 28 (12), 2726–2730.

Vicenzino, B., 2004. Foot orthotics in the treatment of lower limb conditions: a musculoskeletal physiotherapy perspective. Man. Ther. 9 (4), 185–196.

Vicenzino, B., Collins, N.J., Cleland, J., McPoil, T., 2010. A clinical prediction rule for identifying patients with patellofemoral pain who are likely to benefit from foot orthoses: a preliminary determination. Br. J. Sports Med. 44 (12), 862–866.

Vicenzino, B., Collins, N.J., Crossley, K.M., Beller, E., Darnell, R., McPoil, T., 2008. Foot orthoses and physiotherapy in the treatment of patellofemoral pain syndrome: a randomised clinical trial. BMC Musculoskelet. Disord. 9, 27.

Post-Partum Thoracolumbar Pain With Associated Diastasis Rectus Abdominis

Diane G. Lee • Mark A. Jones

Tara's Story

Tara is a physiotherapist and a mother of one child who is 13 months old. She presented with concerns about persistent, intermittent pain in her low thorax and upper lumbar regions, as well as the visual profile of her 13-month post-partum abdomen. She was looking for 'core-strengthening' guidance and thought that this would eliminate her back pain and improve the appearance of her abdomen. Tara also had questions regarding the pros and cons of a surgical repair of her abdominal wall, believing that she had a midline 'hernia' of her linea alba (LA). She had an uncomplicated pregnancy except for a series of incidents between 21 and 23 weeks when she felt a 'ripping sensation' of the LA just above the umbilicus. She felt this 'ripping' when she rolled in bed, 'moved the wrong way' or lifted heavy objects. Her baby was delivered by caesarean section after her induced labour failed to progress following 3 hours of pushing.

Tara's Current Complaints

Tara reported persistent, intermittent pain in her low thorax and upper lumbar regions, which would radiate to include her mid-thorax with increasing activity. Specifically, she felt achiness, fatigue and tenderness to touch localized to the area of the T8, T9 and T10 spinous processes. The onset of these symptoms was insidious, beginning a few months after her delivery, and localized to the thoracolumbar region initially. The symptoms progressed and spread to include the mid-thorax as she increased rotation loads through her trunk with running and kayaking. She did not report any associated, or independent, neurological symptoms such as pins/needles or numbness during any movements or loading of her trunk or extremities. On the Patient Specific Functional Scale (Horn et al., 2012; Stratford et al., 1995), she reported difficulty with lifting (6/10), running (2/10) and paddling her kayak (1/10). For this scale, 0 equals unable to perform the stated activity, and 10 equals able to perform at pre-injury levels. Essentially, she found any task that required loading, especially repetitive rotation of the trunk, aggravating. Her pain was not exacerbated by static loading tasks, such as sitting or prolonged standing.

When asked more about her experience and limitations with running, Tara said it was easier for her to rotate her thorax to the left when she ran and felt she had to 'pull her left shoulder forward' to rotate to the right. When asked about her breathing, she reported difficulty breathing during her first 2 weeks post-partum: 'I was unable to take a normal deep breath in standing. My upper abdomen would draw in and lower abdomen would pop out'. This symptom settled quickly but returned when she resumed running; she felt her breathing was 'uncoordinated'. She did not report any urinary leakage with running or any other tasks that increased her intra-abdominal pressure.

Tara's general health was good, with no precautionary medical conditions present. Historically, she reported an episode of unilateral low back and pelvic girdle pain 10 years prior that resolved when she reduced her 'volume' of dancing. She had not had her spine or thorax imaged.

Tara's Personal Profile (Social History)

Tara was currently working 4 days per week in a private orthopaedic physiotherapy practice. Outside of work and caring for her family, she cross-country skied and attended both yoga and Pilates classes. She had not been able to return to running or kayaking at her pre-pregnancy levels, two activities she missed.

Tara's Perspectives on Her Problem

Tara believed that she had an abdominal hernia due to tearing of her LA and that this was the result of the series of 'ripping sensations' she experienced in the second trimester of her pregnancy. In addition, she felt that her abdominal muscles were weak and that in compensating, she was overusing her back muscles, but she did not feel she knew how to correct this imbalance. She believed that her overused back muscles were contributing to the thoracolumbar ache and fatigue, as well as the local tenderness she experienced when the T8, T9 or T10 spinous processes were palpated. Tara also questioned whether it was possible to restore optimal strength of her abdominal wall without surgical repair of the hernia. She was coping well with both her work and home duties and did not appear overly vigilant to her pain or anxious/worried when telling her story. She was frustrated by her lack of ability to return to her pre-pregnancy levels of fitness and sport, which would seem a reasonable emotion given her circumstances.

Reasoning Question:

1. Tara's story of back pain present for approximately 15 months would be broadly classified as non-specific chronic musculoskeletal pain by many clinicians. Such presentations are frequently linked to nociplastic pain. On the basis of Tara's story, would you discuss your hypotheses regarding the dominant 'pain type' (nociceptive, neuropathic, nociplastic) in her presentation and whether you feel there were any psychosocial factors that may have contributed to the maintenance of her pain and disability?

Answer to Reasoning Question:

Although I would agree that Tara's back pain could be classified as non-specific and chronic, I didn't believe it was only due to sensitization of her CNS. When her physical, social and emotional behaviours are considered, there were no indications that she was catastrophizing, hypervigilant or demonstrating other maladaptive behaviours/beliefs associated with dominant nociplastic pain type. She continued to work 4 days per week, ski and participate in yoga and Pilates classes. Her symptoms were localized and consistent with a nociceptive pattern of aggravation; thus, it was more likely that her pain was peripherally mediated even though it was chronic. Her beliefs were realistic given the history of events during her pregnancy and worth exploring through physical examination of the abdominal wall. If she did tear the LA and does have herniation of the abdominal contents, her ability to stabilize the joints of her low back and pelvis would be compromised due to loss of the force closure mechanism (Vleeming et al., 1990a, 1990b).

Reasoning Question:

2. Given your hypothesis of a nociceptive-dominant pain type, what structures/tissues do you hypothesize as possible nociceptive sources to her pain?

Answer to Reasoning Question:

At this point in the examination, I felt the structures that were potential nociceptive sources to her pain were likely multiple and possibly enthesopathic. Nociception could be generated from one, or any combination, of attachments of several muscles directly, or indirectly through the thoracolumbar fascia, to the spinous processes of T8–T10. I did not hypothesize that the costovertebral or zygapophyseal joints of the thoracolumbar region were contributing much to her pain because 'achiness' and 'general fatigue' are not usual symptoms of an articular source of nociception.

Reasoning Question:

3. Tara indicated that she believed her lack of abdominal strength was causing her to overuse her back muscles, which then caused her symptoms. Would you please discuss your interpretation of Tara's beliefs and any associated implications for your physical examination?

Answer to Reasoning Question:

I felt that Tara's perspective of her problem was accurate in that she was likely overusing her back muscles and underusing her abdomen; however, I felt that the underlying cause of her 'abdominal weakness' and lack of improvement was less likely due to her 'core strength' and more likely due to either changes in the structure of her abdominal wall and/or her motor control strategies induced by her pregnancy.

Pregnancy and delivery present huge challenges for the abdominal wall and back. Lumbopelvic pain (Albert et al., 2001, 2002; Larsen et al., 1999; Östgaard et al., 1991, 1996), motor control changes of the abdominal wall (Beales et al., 2008; O'Sullivan et al., 2002; Smith et al., 2007; Stuge et al., 2006) and diastasis rectus abdominis (DRA) (Boissonault and Blaschak, 1988; Gilleard and Brown, 1996; Liaw et al., 2011; Mota et al., 2014) are common both during and after pregnancy. With respect to the structure of the abdominal wall, although evidence is limited, it appears that for some, recovery is not spontaneous without intervention (Coldron et al., 2008; Liaw et al., 2011; Mota et al., 2014).

From Tara's story, two aspects of abdominal wall function would need to be assessed:

1. The structural integrity of the LA and the ability of the abdominal wall to transfer load.
2. Her ability to synergistically recruit the deep (transversus abdominis [TrA]) and superficial (internal [IO] and external oblique(s) [EO] and rectus abdominis [RA]) abdominal muscles with the other muscles of her core (back and pelvic floor muscles).

Clinical Reasoning Commentary:

Consideration of pain type (e.g. nociceptive versus nociplastic) is a principal 'hypothesis category' discussed in Chapter 1, with significant implications for other clinical decision categories, such as potential sources of symptoms, precautions to examination and treatment, management and prognosis. Although chronicity is often associated with nociplastic pain/maladaptive sensitization, as highlighted in the Answer to Reasoning Question 1, this is not always the case. Maladaptive catastrophizing, hypervigilance and fears, along with social and behavioural factors, are considered here but found not to be evident, and the behaviour of symptoms is instead judged to be more consistent with a nociceptive-dominant presentation. This highlights the reality that pain and disability also can be maintained, in part or full, by continued physical stress and aggravation related to misconceptions (e.g. beliefs about the problem and what is needed, such as insufficient 'core' strength), behaviour (e.g. continued stress and aggravation from activities such as running and kayaking), environmental and social factors (not evident here) and physical factors screened later in the physical examination (e.g. alignment, mobility and control).

As discussed in Chapter 1, clinical patterns are not limited to diagnostic classifications of pathologies or syndromes; they also exist with regard to physical, environmental and psychosocial contributing factors, pain type, precautions/contraindications and prognosis. The Answer to Reasoning Question 3 reflects recognition of an evidence-informed clinical pattern of impaired motor control strategies induced by pregnancy with plans to test the hypothesis through specific physical examination assessments.

Physical Examination

Three tasks, based on Tara's goals, were chosen for evaluation; these tasks also relate to the known function of the abdominal wall:

1. Standing posture (position from which lifting and running begins)
2. Supine lying curl-up task (requires co-ordinated activation of all abdominal muscles)
3. Seated trunk rotation with and without resistance (essential for running and kayaking)

Flexion, extension and side flexion of the trunk were not tested because these cardinal plane motions, in isolation, do not specifically relate to the aggravating component (trunk rotation) of her meaningful tasks (running and paddling). In addition, no specific neuro-dynamic tests were included in this examination because there was no indication from her story that this system was contributing to her complaints or her functional limitations.

Standing Posture – Relevant Positional Findings of the Trunk

Tara was not experiencing any pain or discomfort in her thorax or upper lumbar spine at the time of this examination. In standing, her pelvis was rotated to the right in the transverse plane. Her lower thorax was rotated to the left, and her middle thorax was rotated to the right. Segmental thoracic ring shifts (L-J. Lee, 2003a) were noted in both regions of the thorax. Specifically, the 8th thoracic ring was shifted to the right, and the 9th was shifted to the left. The 4th thoracic ring was shifted to the left, and the 3rd was shifted to the right.

Reasoning Question:

4. Would you please explain the key features you assess during your analysis of standing posture and how you determine whether asymmetries identified are relevant or not to that patient's presentation?

Answer to Reasoning Question:

This is a great question and highly appropriate because many clinicians get 'bogged down' with findings that, at the end of the examination, have no clinical relevance. Meanwhile, they are overwhelmed by the information and what it all means.

Standing is the starting point for many functional tasks, including the following:

- Standing for prolonged periods of time
- Sitting
- Squatting
- Lifting
- Running
- Climbing stairs
- Reaching overhead

A quick screen of standing posture allows the clinician to interpret what happens during movement more accurately. Very few of us stand perfectly aligned, and asymmetries in multiple regions of the body are common. So, when are they relevant to the clinical picture? In short, they are relevant when the individual is held in the asymmetric position and is unable to move, or control, the asymmetric region when he or she needs to do so. For example, in standing, it is common to find the pelvis rotated in one direction in the transverse plane and the thorax rotated in the opposite direction. For a squat task, both of these transverse plane rotations should unwind, and the pelvis and thorax should align symmetrically. Loads are increased through the lumbar spine if the thorax and pelvis remain rotated in opposite directions during the squat (Al-Eisa et al., 2006).

A thoracic ring is defined as two adjacent thoracic vertebrae, the left and right ribs of the same number as the inferior vertebra, the sternum or manubrium to which the ribs attach and all the joints that connect these bones (D. Lee, 1994) (Fig. 11.1A). Each thoracic ring has the potential to rotate in the same or opposite direction to the one above/below. Thus, whereas a quick screen of the thorax is regional (lower, middle, upper), a more detailed segmental thoracic ring analysis considers the positional relationship between each thoracic ring and provides information as to which thoracic ring is 'driving' the regional rotation. Linda-Joy Lee has developed novel assessment techniques (L-J. Lee, 2003a, b, 2005, 2007, 2008, 2012) for the analysis of both position and mobility of an entire thoracic ring. These particular tests, combined with biomechanical and arthrokinematic mobility tests (D. Lee, 1993, 1994, 2003), were used to understand the clinical relevance of Tara's specific thoracic rings shifts as noted previously.

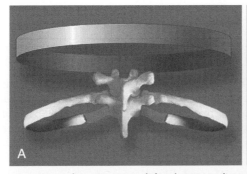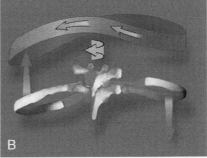

Fig. 11.1 (A) A thoracic ring is defined as two adjacent thoracic vertebrae, the left and right ribs of the same number as the inferior vertebra, the sternum or manubrium to which the ribs attach and all the joints that connect these bones (D. Lee, 1994). (B) The biomechanics of right rotation of a typical thoracic ring (D. Lee, 1993). Left lateral translation occurs in conjunction with right rotation of the thoracic ring. The right rib posteriorly rotates; the left rib anteriorly rotates; and at the end of the available range, the thoracic spinal segment rotates and side flexes to the right. Reproduced with permission from Diane G. Lee Physiotherapist Corporation©

A thoracic ring shift is another way of saying that the thoracic ring is positioned in rotation. The word 'shift' refers to the direction of translation of a thoracic ring, which is a congruent motion that occurs when the thoracic ring rotates (D. Lee, 1993) (Fig. 11.1B). This translation is easy to detect when the thoracic ring position is assessed in the mid-axillary line (L-J. Lee, 2003a, 2005, 2008, 2012).

The clinical relevance of each asymmetry is determined by correcting the rotation/shift and assessing the following:

- Whether a correction is possible or not (stiff, fibrotic or fixated joints will not allow the alignment of the thoracic or pelvic ring to correct)
- The impact of the correction on the position/alignment of the other noted asymmetries
- The impact of the correction on performance of the task being evaluated (standing posture, squat, arm elevation, one leg stand etc.)
- The impact of the correction on the patient's symptom experience (pain, tingling, burning, ability to breathe etc.)

Essentially, to understand the relationship between the thoracic rings and the pelvis, look for the 'ring' whereby the biggest resultant change in posture/position is created by a single or combined correction. Then determine if this correction also improves the alignment, biomechanics and/or control of other regions of the body during the task being evaluated.

In the Integrated Systems Model for Disability and Pain (Lee L.-J. and Lee D., 2011), this is called 'Finding the Primary Driver'. Of note, the position of the trunk (thorax and pelvis) can also be influenced by the posture/position of the lower extremity, shoulder girdle, head and neck, so the 'driver' may not be within the trunk!

Clinical Reasoning Commentary:

Postural asymmetries fall under the hypothesis category of 'contributing factors'. Like all health risk factors, they will not always result in symptoms or dysfunction because they represent only one factor within the biological and psychosocial makeup that determines health and function. Therefore, as emphasized in this answer, clinicians must have a clear rationale for each assessment performed, and because asymptomatic postural asymmetries are common, specific strategies for judging their likely relevance to an individual's presentation are essential.

Tara had five segments within her trunk that were not optimally aligned in standing: the 3rd, 4th, 8th and 9th thoracic rings, as well as the pelvis. To determine the clinical relevance of these asymmetries, a series of regional and segmental asymmetry corrections was made. When her pelvis was manually corrected (to derotate the right transverse plane rotation and center her pelvis over her feet), the alignment of both her lower and middle thorax was worse. Overall, her standing posture was worse, and she felt more twisted with this correction. This suggested that treating her pelvic alignment directly would not improve the overall posture of her trunk in standing. In addition, her ability to paddle her kayak and run would not improve if her thorax was more 'twisted'.

When the 8th thoracic ring was manually corrected (derotate/correct the segmental thoracic rotation/shift to align the adjacent rings), the position of the 9th thoracic ring improved spontaneously, as did the alignment of her pelvis. This suggested that treatment directed toward correcting the alignment of her 8th thoracic ring would improve both the 9th thoracic ring and the pelvic posture in standing. However, this correction did not change the position of the 3rd or 4th thoracic rings. Correcting the 4th thoracic ring improved the 3rd, but not the 8th or 9th rings.

Tara's standing posture improved the most when both the 4th and 8th thoracic rings were manually corrected simultaneously. None of these manual corrections provoked any symptoms in her thorax or upper lumbar spine. Conversely, Tara noticed the automatic correction in the alignment of her pelvis when her 4th and 8th thoracic rings were simultaneously aligned. She felt 'less twisted' and actually had not realized that she was twisted until the two thoracic ring corrections (4th and 8th) were released.

Correcting the alignment of two of her thoracic rings made Tara aware of the relationship between her thorax and pelvis in standing. Her existing body schema was twisted (Berlucchi, 2010), but she was unaware of this until the twist was reversed and she 'attended' to the response of her body as the correction was released. This is often a 'wow' moment for patients when they realize where they are 'living in their bodies' (i.e. acquire a new body schema). Focused attention and awareness are two key conditions necessary for change;

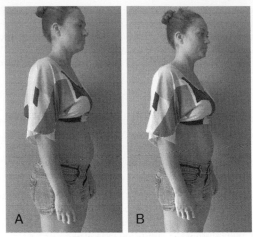

Fig. 11.2 (A) Profile of Tara's abdomen in relaxed standing. (B) Profile of Tara's abdomen using her automatic strategy for drawing in her abdomen. Note the lateral vertical line and the continued protrusion of the low belly, signs of overactivation of the superficial abdominal muscles.

these are neuroplastic principles increasingly recognized as critical for musculoskeletal rehabilitation (Boudreau et al., 2010; Snodgrass et al., 2014; van Vliet et al., 2006).

When standing, the profile of Tara's relaxed abdomen was protuberant, and when asked to 'connect to her core', excessive activation of the EO abdominals occurred. While this strategy drew her abdomen inward, it did not eliminate the protrusion completely (Fig. 11.2). Her abdomen continued to appear, and feel, highly pressurized.

When the 4th and 8th thoracic rings were manually corrected immediately prior to Tara's 'connect' cue, she noticed a decrease in the pressure sensation of her lower abdomen, and when attention was directed to the profile of her abdomen, she was pleasantly surprised at the change.

Reasoning Question:

5. Please discuss how you relate your analysis of regional and segmental postural corrections to contemporary motor control theory, and highlight what you attend to visually, kinaesthetically and via patient response in determining their relevance. Would you also comment on the current levels of evidence underpinning this assessment?

Answer to Reasoning Question:

Multiple studies suggest that the response to back pain is individual and task specific (see the review article on pain and motor control by Hodges [2011]), although there are common features to most clinical presentations. Hodges (2011, p. 222) notes that back pain patients present with a 'redistribution of activity within and between muscles (rather than inhibition or excitation of muscles in a stereotypical manner)'. All of the multisegmental muscles of the trunk contribute to movement and control, and when their activity is 'redistributed', they can produce specific vectors of force that contribute to thoracic ring shifts and pelvic rotations. Thus, Hodges states, 'If the goal of rehabilitation (e.g. using motor learning strategies) is to modify the adaptation (remove, modify or enhance) then this needs to be considered on an individual basis with respect to the unique solution adopted by the patient' (Hodges, 2011, p. 222–223).

The clinician's challenge is to determine which muscles are 'actors' (creating the primary vector of force) and which are 'reactors' (reacting to the primary vector). Increased muscle activation noted on palpation or during a certain posture (standing, sitting) or task (seated trunk rotation, single leg standing) does not mean that this muscle should be released or stretched. Releasing 'reactors' allows the primary muscle (the actor) to increase the rotation/twist (and often the symptoms). Therefore, when looking for the driver, the clinician should also pay attention to the vectors of resistance to movement encountered during specific corrections and the location, direction, length and velocity of pull of the vector upon release of the correction. This vector analysis provides further information about the underlying source of the pull (articular, myofascial, neural, visceral) (Lee D. and Lee, 2011a).

The patient is engaged (focused attention and awareness) in this entire 'correct and release' process and is asked to provide feedback on the experience. Symptoms should not increase when the driver is corrected; rather, a sense of well-being, or ease, in the body is desirable, as is an improvement in the ability to breathe or any lessening of intra-abdominal, intra-thoracic or intra-cranial pressure. Less effort should be required to perform the task when the driver is held in a corrected position and the alignment, biomechanics and control are facilitated.

I am unaware of any research that has considered changes in the 'gestalt' of the patient's experience specifically with thoracic ring corrections or any research that has investigated the impact of thoracic ring corrections on pelvic position, hip position, foot position and so forth. Currently, there are no measuring systems that are able to accurately measure segmental thoracic ring position or mobility, nor intra-pelvic mobility. These are clinical observations.

Clinical Reasoning Commentary:

Application of research evidence to practice is challenging and requires judgment regarding the applicability of findings from the population studied to your patient and their context, and whether the intervention can be replicated in the clinic. Insufficient information is often reported on precisely what was implemented in the study, including details of treatment (e.g. positions, dosage, sequence, progression), patient–therapist therapeutic alliance (e.g. rapport, collaboration) or therapeutic education (e.g. explanations, advice, instructions) to enable clinicians to replicate the assessments and management (educatively, behaviourally and humanistically) with confidence. In the absence of empirical research evidence, as acknowledged here, existing biologically plausible theory (e.g. Hodges, 2011) can be applied to clinical practice, combined with careful monitoring of individual treatment effects to guide reasoning and overall management. Although monitoring of outcomes to judge overall success will include any changes in the patient's activity (function) and participation restrictions and capabilities, monitoring (re-assessment) to determine relevance of physical findings, specific treatment interventions and progression of treatment requires attention to broader and more detailed (often qualitative) variables, as discussed here. These can include patient awareness and individual muscle activation patterns and their effects on patient symptoms, thoughts, movement control and other body sensations experienced during the functional task.

Supine Curl-Up Task

The supine curl-up task was chosen to evaluate Tara's abdominal wall and LA because this task should involve co-activation of all muscles of the abdominal wall (Andersson et al., 1997). With no cue, or instruction, Tara's automatic strategy for the supine curl-up task produced more bulging of her abdomen and asymmetric narrowing of the infrasternal angle (right side greater than left) (Fig. 11.3).

When she held the curl-up position, the left and right recti could be easily separated along the entire length of the LA (Fig. 11.4) by hand. The inter-recti distance (IRD) was two finger widths (during the curl-up), and of particular note was the lack of tension in the LA. This task did not provoke any symptoms in her thorax or upper lumbar spine.

Ultrasound imaging (UI) provided more information on Tara's abdominal wall function:

1. UI of the lateral abdominal wall during a supine curl-up using an automatic strategy: Tara had difficulty co-activating the right TrA and IO compared to the left.

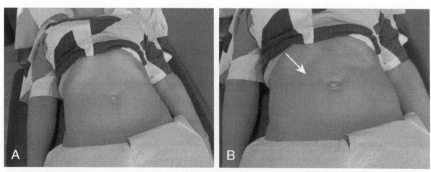

Fig. 11.3   Supine curl-up task. (A) Note the asymmetry of the infrasternal angle of Tara's rib cage at rest. (B) During the supine curl-up task using an automatic strategy, this asymmetry became more pronounced due to overactivation of part of the EO attaching to the right 8th rib (see arrow).

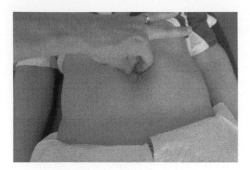

Fig. 11.4 Supine curl-up task using an automatic strategy. Minimal tension was palpable along the entire LA, and the left and right recti could be easily spread apart. The LA was easy to distort.

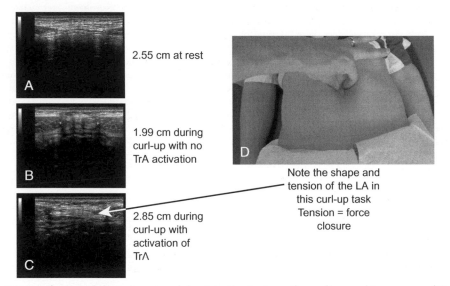

2.55 cm at rest

1.99 cm during curl-up with no TrA activation

2.85 cm during curl-up with activation of TrA

Note the shape and tension of the LA in this curl-up task

Tension = force closure

Fig. 11.5 A functional diastasis rectus abdominis: Tara's story. These ultrasound images are of Tara's LA just above the umbilicus at rest (A), during an automatic curl-up strategy (B) and during a curl-up while correcting the alignment of the 8th thoracic ring in addition to using a 'connect cue' strategy (C). Note the change in the distortion of the LA as well as the increased echogenicity as her strategy improves (D). Also note that the inter-recti distance (IRD) widens to 2.85 cm when all the abdominals co-activate; this is almost 1 cm wider than the IRD produced with her automatic strategy (1.99 cm). *LA*, Linea alba; *TrA*, transversus abdominis.

2. UI of the LA during a supine curl-up using an automatic strategy: just above the umbilicus, the IRD was 2.55 cm at rest and *narrowed* to 1.99 cm during the curl-up. The LA appeared distorted or slack, a finding consistent with the previously noted lack of palpable tension.

3. UI of the lateral abdominal wall during a supine curl-up using a 'connect to core cue' strategy: Tara was able to produce an isolated contraction of both the left and right TrA when she used imagery and cues to activate her pelvic floor (Sapsford et al., 2001); however, she was not able to sustain activation of the right TrA and perform a curl-up task *unless* she manually corrected the 8th thoracic ring (L-J. Lee, 2007) (also noted to be shifted to the right in supine lying).

4. UI of the LA during a supine curl-up while correcting the alignment of the 8th thoracic ring in addition to using a 'connect to core cue' strategy: just above the umbilicus, the IRD *widened* to 2.85 cm, and the distortion of the LA decreased (Fig. 11.5). Both of these imaging findings suggested that tension of the LA increased with this combined strategy, and this was confirmed with manual palpation.

Reasoning Question:

6. DRA assessment (manually and via ultrasound) will be less familiar to many clinicians. Please discuss this in the context of your broader motor control assessment and highlight your hypotheses regarding Tara's findings with respect to her complaints and your management.

Answer to Reasoning Question:

There is very little evidence to guide management of post-partum women with DRA (Beer et al., 2009). Which patients are appropriate for conservative treatment, and which ones will also require surgery? The distance between the left and right rectus abdominis (IRD) has been investigated in women through pregnancy and beyond, and it is thought that 100% of women have widening of the LA (increase in the IRD) during pregnancy (Gilleard and Brown, 1996; Mota et al., 2014) but that some remain abnormally widened in the post-partum period (Coldron et al., 2008; Liaw et al., 2011; Mota et al., 2014). UI is a reliable method for evaluating the IRD (Coldron et al., 2008; Mendes et al., 2007; Mota et al., 2012).

Many believe that the DRA should 'close' for restoration of optimal function of the abdominal wall (Mota et al., 2012; Tupler et al., 2011). Although this may seem intuitive, our clinical experience with over 100 women with DRA revealed that the DRA 'opened' (IRD became wider) as their abdominal wall function improved. This finding led us to question the goal of restoring strategies that merely 'close' the DRA. This was later confirmed by our research (Lee and Hodges, 2016) that suggested that the ability to generate tension of the LA is more important than the IRD and that training strategies that merely reduce the IRD may be suboptimal for function.

Pascoal et al. (2014, p. 4) noted that in post-partum women the IRD decreased during a curl-up task and suggested that

abdominal strengthening exercises contribute to the narrowing of the inter-rectus distance in postpartum women. However, research should be undertaken to evaluate which exercises are the most effective and safe for reduction of the inter-rectus distance in postpartum women.

This suggests that exercises should be chosen that reduce the IRD, in other words, close the gap. Mota et al. (2012) found that the IRD was greater during an abdominal 'drawing-in exercise' than in both the rest position and an 'abdominal crunch' in their study of post-partum women. Our results for the IRD during a curl-up task in post-partum women with DRA (Lee and Hodges, 2016) concur with the findings of both Mota et al. and Pascoal et al.; however, our conclusions from the results and recommendations for treatment differ because we also considered the distortion/laxity response of the LA during two different strategies for this task.

We investigated the LA in two conditions; an automatic curl-up strategy and a strategy with a cue to pre-contract the TrA prior to the curl-up. In our healthy, nulliparous controls, the IRD remained unchanged during the curl-up task with or without pre-activation of TrA. In other words, the LA in our healthy controls did not distort; it remained tensed. In the subjects with DRA, the IRD narrowed from the rest position during an automatic curl-up strategy and widened compared with their automatic strategy when they pre-activated TrA. These findings suggest that co-activation of the abdominals will widen the IRD and is more likely to generate tension across the LA (i.e. create less distortion).

Clinically, it appears that generating tension in the LA (create less distortion) is more important than closing the IRD. Those who can achieve co-activation strategies of the abdominal wall that are synergized with appropriate activation of the diaphragm, pelvic floor muscles and back muscles are able to transfer loads with better alignment, biomechanics and control. Clinicians often note the depth of the LA during a curl-up task and question the significance of this finding. We feel that this is merely a reflection of the distortion (laxity) of the LA during this task – the greater the distortion, the deeper you can push the LA into the abdomen (Lee and Hodges, 2016).

Tara did not have a tear of her LA (contrary to her cognitive belief). The structural integrity of the LA could be imaged throughout its entire length, and there was no herniation of abdominal contents. She did have a suboptimal motor control strategy of the abdominal muscles during the automatic curl-up task in that she had difficulty recruiting the right TrA. This asymmetric abdominal activation appeared to contribute to the distortion of the LA, resulting in insufficient tension for transferring loads. When the 8th thoracic ring shift was corrected, she was able to recruit the right TrA and co-activate it with the rest of the abdominals during the curl-up. Co-activation of all her abdominals widened the IRD resulting in less distortion of the LA.

Tara's IRD at rest (25.5 mm) classifies her as having a DRA according to Beer et al. (2009) (IRD greater than 13 mm ± 7 mm just above the umbilicus). The clinical and UI findings suggested her DRA was functional and not requiring surgery; findings from the next test would confirm or negate this hypothesis.

Continued on following page

Clinical Reasoning Commentary:

This analysis represents an example of 'inference to the best explanation' (or abduction) as discussed in Chapter 1. In the absence of research-validated criteria for deducing the effects of abdominal activation strategies (e.g. automatic curl-up versus curl-up with pre-activation of TrA) on the LA and controlled load transfer in women with DRA, extensive clinical experience led to the discovery of patterns in previously unlinked information (LA tension as opposed to IRD) through 'inference to the best explanation'. This culminated in the clinical recognition/theory that LA tension generated through abdominal wall co-activation is more important than IRD to load transfer and function. The 'clinical evidence' regarding load transfer and function was confirmed with research that investigated the effects of different activation strategies on the LA. Although research is essential to test clinical theory, clinical practice cannot be limited to research-validated knowledge (assessment and management) because it only forms one of the three elements of evidence-informed practice, the others being clinical expertise and patient values (see Chapter 5). Critical, reflective clinical reasoning, incorporating deductive and inductive inferences on the basis of what is 'known' and on consideration of the 'best explanation' when dealing with areas that are less well understood, safeguards against errors in reasoning (see Chapters 1 and 31) and enables the discovery of new knowledge. The clinical relevance and therapeutic efficacy for the individual patient, as discussed here, will always be essential to establish.

Seated Trunk Rotation With and Without Resistance

Increased effort was required for Tara to rotate her thorax to the right, and when the 8th thoracic ring shift (to the right) was manually corrected, her range of right rotation increased, and her effort to perform this task decreased (L-J. Lee, 2003a, 2012). No symptoms other than 'resistance' and 'effort' were reported during the seated trunk rotation task. A similar finding was noted with respect to the 4th thoracic ring that was shifted to the left and restricting left thoracic rotation. Left rotation of the trunk/thorax improved with manual correction of the 4th thoracic ring (range of motion improved, and the effort to perform the task was reduced). A simultaneous correction of both the 4th and 8th thoracic rings did not further improve either right or left thoracic rotation; a single ring correction was enough for each direction.

When a resisted left rotation load was applied to the trunk through her bilaterally elevated arms, marked loss of low thorax control was evident (Fig. 11.6A). In spite of the loss of regional alignment and control, no pain was provoked with this single (non-repetitive) loading task. When instructed (cued) to pre-activate TrA prior to loading, Tara's trunk control improved when resistance was applied to right trunk rotation but not to left rotation. Previous evaluation via UI revealed that the 8th thoracic ring required correction before activation of the right TrA was sustained. When the alignment of the 8th thoracic ring was corrected and its position controlled during the application of the left rotation load, Tara's low thorax/upper lumbar control, as well as her 'experience of core rotation strength', significantly improved (Fig. 11.6B). The 'gestalt' of Tara's experience in her body

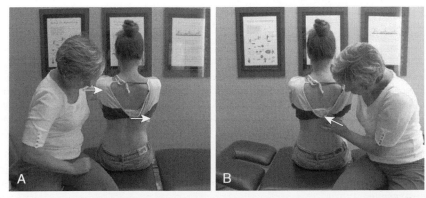

Fig. 11.6 (A) When manual resistance to left trunk rotation was applied through Tara's bilaterally elevated arms (left arrow), she was unable to control the relationship of the low thorax to the upper lumbar spine (right arrow). (B) When the 8th thoracic ring was specifically controlled (prevented from shifting to the right) Tara was able to resist left trunk rotation to a greater degree.

was related to function and performance, as opposed to the provocation/alleviation of pain during this assessment.

8th Thoracic Ring Assessment

Further testing was done to determine why the 8th thoracic ring was translated to the right/rotated to the left in standing, sitting and lying and failed to transfer loads effectively during resisted left trunk rotation. Findings from these tests resulted in the following observations/deductions:

1. The joints of the 4th and 8th thoracic rings demonstrated normal mobility and passive integrity, and testing did not provoke pain (D. Lee, 2003). This is consistent with the finding that both the 4th and 8th thoracic ring shifts were manually correctable.
2. Increased resting tone was noted in the right EO, specifically in the part of this muscle that attaches to the anterior aspect of the right 8th rib (Fig. 11.3). The attachment of the right EO to the 8th rib was tender on local palpation. The increased EO tone, and the resultant vector of force it produced on the right 8th rib, was palpable when manually correcting the alignment of the 8th thoracic ring; however, the local tenderness/discomfort was not reproduced with this manual correction, only with direct palpation. The 9th thoracic ring shift to the left corrected when the 8th ring was aligned, suggesting that its position was compensatory.
3. No apparent atrophy, or inhibition, of the deep segmental muscles pertaining to the 8th thoracic ring was palpable (i.e. multifidus/rotatores or intercostals).

Reasoning Question:

7. Please discuss your interpretation of the additional tests of the joints of the 4th and 8th thoracic rings and Tara's seated trunk rotation findings with respect to their support, or lack of support, for your previous hypotheses regarding potential 'sources of symptoms' and physical 'contributing factors'.

Answer to Reasoning Question:

I felt that Tara had developed suboptimal recruitment strategies for both mobility and control of the 4th, 8th (primary) and 9th (compensatory) thoracic rings during at least three functional tasks: standing, supine curl-up and seated trunk rotation. These suboptimal strategies were impacting her ability to transfer loads through her trunk when lifting, running and kayaking. In particular, her right thoracic rotation was limited by the 8th thoracic ring shift to the right, which may have resulted in her 'need' to pull the left shoulder forward when right rotating her thorax during running. This strategy would require more effort and could have been a contributing factor to both the fatigue and mid-thoracic pain she felt with the repetitive rotational requirement of running. The 4th and 8th thoracic ring restrictions in opposite directions of rotation would impact her mobility and strategies for kayaking, again possible factors for her muscular fatigue and aching with repetitive rotation loads.

The passive assessments of the joints of the 4th and 8th thoracic rings revealed normal mobility (consistent with the finding that the thoracic ring position and mobility could be influenced by gentle manual correction) and did not provoke her pain. In a hypothesized nociceptive-dominant presentation such as Tara's, this supports that the joints are not a pathological source of nociception; rather, they, along with the local muscles, may be overstressed and perhaps nociceptive sources secondary to her alignment and control impairments. Clinically this will require interventions targeted to her control and alignment to determine their influence.

Her sensation and belief that her 'core' was weak was likely due to dys-synergies between the abdominal muscles in that there was overactivation of the right EO and under-activation of the right TrA. This is likely a clinical example of 'redistribution of activity within and between muscles' as noted by Hodges (2011). This strategy was having an impact on her ability to generate tension in the LA throughout its length and thus control the joints of the low thorax and lumbar spine during rotation loading. This hypothesis was further supported by the findings of the resisted trunk rotation test in sitting.

The focus of this assessment was to determine why her low thorax/upper lumbar spine failed to maintain optimal alignment, biomechanics and control, as opposed to identifying the pain generators. It was hypothesized that repetitive loss of segmental control would compress/stress/irritate multiple structures (costotransverse and zygapophyseal joints, intervertebral discs, myofascial tendinous insertions etc.), pain from which is often difficult to reliably isolate.

Continued on following page

Tara had physical impairments that were relevant and proportional to her activity and participation restrictions, combined with no overt physical signs of nociplastic pain (e.g. allodynia, widespread tenderness), further supporting the previous hypothesis of a nociceptive-dominant pain type/mechanism.

Clinical Reasoning Commentary:

Hypotheses formulated during the subjective examination should be 'tested' against findings from the physical examination and again later through re-assessments to specific interventions. Here the physical findings were judged to be consistent with the previously hypothesized nociceptive-dominant pain type/mechanism. The potential for stress, and hence nociception, of multiple structures is acknowledged. However, with red flags and overt symptomatic pathology already ruled out, and both functional and spinal assessments being non-provocative, precise structural differentiation for Tara's thoracic pain was not likely possible or required. Instead, clinical 'diagnostic differentiation' of her non-specific spinal pain gives way to a focus on physical impairments that may have been contributing to her functional restrictions. Tara's pain and functional restrictions were hypothesized to be due to 'dys-synergies between the abdominal muscles'. However, it is important to recognize that judgment is not reached on the basis of neuromuscular assessment alone; rather, it is predicated on both positive and negative findings from a range of advanced clinical and manual assessments, including observation of posture, analysis of functional tasks related to her activity restrictions, thoracic ring mobility and pain provocation, observation and palpation of muscle bulk and tone and effects of thoracic ring corrections on position/alignment of other asymmetries and functional tasks being evaluated. A likely clinical pattern of muscle dys-synergy may have been recognized back in the subjective examination, but physical assessments of mobility and pain provocation were still performed, and ultimately, it is the combined picture of negative and positive findings that 'confirms' the suspected pattern.

Treatment – First Session

The EO vector (i.e. tension) that was preventing the 8th thoracic ring from moving optimally during right rotation of the thorax was released (reassessed by palpation) using a positional release technique (D. Lee and Lee, 2011b). Subsequently, the 8th thoracic ring was no longer held in left rotation/right translation (repeated standing posture assessment), and the amplitude of her active right thoracic rotation increased. Tara noticed an immediate decrease in the effort required to rotate her thorax to the right (repeated seated trunk rotation without resistance). The resting tone of the part of the EO attaching to the right 8th rib was significantly reduced on palpation. When a left rotation load was applied to the trunk through her bilaterally elevated arms, she was still unable to control her lower thorax, suggesting that her motor control strategy was still not optimal for regional control of the low thorax.

Tara was then taught a home exercise to maintain the reduced tone and optimal length specifically in this part of the EO. This required manual correction and stabilization of the right 8th rib (part of the 8th thoracic ring) as she then rotated her pelvis (and legs) to the left in supine lying. This exercise is a modified 'Wipers pose' in yoga. At the initiation of the task, inhalation is used to facilitate posterior rotation of the right 8th rib, and thus right rotation of the entire ring (Fig. 11.1B), as the legs and pelvis are taken to the left. Prior to bringing the pelvis back to neutral, exhalation is used to facilitate greater activation of the right TrA (Hodges and Gandevia, 2000).

UI is a powerful biofeedback tool (Tsao and Hodges, 2007) and was used to teach Tara more about the dys-synergies in her abdominal wall and to understand (left brain) and internalize (right brain) better ways to recruit and use these muscles for her trunk control during rotation loading (running and kayaking). Time was spent empowering her with the education and sensorial experiences she needed to continue to build a different 'brain map' for using her abdomen (Tsao et al., 2010). We talked about how this was not about 'exercise' and 'strength' but rather about motor control and muscle patterning. Better strategies needed to be 're-built' first, and then she could progress to strengthening exercises. I introduced her to the science of neuroplasticity and directed her to articles and related books on the topic for her own personal and professional learning (Boudreau et al., 2010; Doidge 2007; Siegel, 2010; Snodgrass et al., 2014; Tsao et al., 2010). She was encouraged to release her right EO and engage her right TrA frequently over the next 7–10 days, and then to integrate a pre-contraction of the deep abdominals (both TrAs) with the rest of her core muscles whenever she lifted/loaded her trunk. In addition, she was taught to correct the alignment of the 8th thoracic ring in sitting and encouraged to practice maintaining this correction (initially manually and then with imagery) as she rotated her thorax to the right. Once the 8th thoracic ring mobility and control were restored in this task, I felt she would be able to increase her loads and move toward integrating this new strategy into her running and kayaking.

This session was booked as a consultation only because Tara lived a considerable distance from my clinic and was initially interested in just one session for an opinion on appropriate exercises for her 'core' and advice on surgery. Consequently, we did not have a follow-up session for 1 month.

Reasoning Question:

8. Even simple home exercises are sometimes challenging for patients to learn. How do you facilitate this with more complex exercises such as those you taught Tara?

Answer to Reasoning Question:

Awareness, focused attention, training tasks that have meaning and massed practice of high-quality movements to normalize the sensory input and thus change the motor output are all requirements for neuroplastic changes to occur in movement behaviour. This can be achieved very quickly given the right clinical environment and sufficient time with a motivated patient. If you are able to change an individual's 'experience' of their body in a positive way, empower them to take responsibility for the next steps of their 'brain training' and use tools such as video recording their movement practice on their mobile phone, then change can occur quickly and with few appointments. The paradigm shift here is for clinicians to stop taking full responsibility for 'fixing their patients' and for patients to understand that clinicians can merely 'illuminate a path to change'. It is up to them to do the work. Tara was highly motivated and understood and accepted the work she needed to do over the next month. She left this first appointment with videos on her mobile phone of exactly what and how much she needed to do. She felt confident that she could follow through with the program and knew that she could contact me via email with any questions over the next month.

Clinical Reasoning Commentary:

This answer highlights a clear strategy underpinning the teaching for facilitating neuroplastic changes (i.e. learning) required for improved movement behaviour. 'Reasoning about teaching' is a reasoning strategy briefly described in Chapter 1 and defined as the 'reasoning associated with the planning, execution and evaluation of individualized and context-sensitive teaching, including education for conceptual understanding (e.g. medical and musculoskeletal diagnosis, pain), education for physical performance (e.g. rehabilitative exercise, postural correction, sport technique enhancement), and education for behavioural change'. Musculoskeletal clinicians are arguably teachers in the main, and our teaching to facilitate change (in cognition, behaviour, function and lifestyle) should be based on established learning theory, together with reasoning that enables adaptation to the particular requirements of each patient and in response to our re-assessment of teaching outcomes. Deep learning requires active processing of new information (e.g. patient engaged with an opportunity to ask questions, as opposed to passively being lectured), meaningful understanding (cognitively, but also in the patient's altered experiences of his or her body as highlighted in this answer), feedback and success. 'Craft knowledge' (Chapter 1) to motivate patients, facilitate understanding and promote adherence (e.g. use of mobile phone video recording to facilitate recall and practice) is often an unrecognized factor that influences our reasoning about teaching and our patient outcomes.

Follow-up – 1 Month Later
Subjective Report

Tara noticed progressive improvement in her functional abilities and significant reduction in both her low thorax and upper lumbar pain with repetitive loading tasks since learning to 're-organize the use' of her abdominal wall and regain control of her 8th thoracic ring. She reported the local tenderness at the spinous processes of T8–T10 persisted; however, the intensity and frequency of the 'achiness and fatigue' was reduced, and more activity (e.g. longer running time) was required to provoke the symptoms. She was not kayaking yet. She was pleasantly surprised at the change in her abdominal profile (Fig. 11.7).

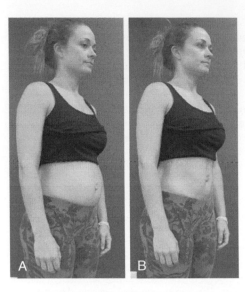

Fig. 11.7 (A) Profile of Tara's abdomen in relaxed standing 1 month after the first consultation/treatment session. (B) Profile of Tara's abdomen using her new strategy for co-activation of her 'core' muscles. Note the softening of the lateral vertical line and the absence of protrusion of her low belly, signs of a more synergistic recruitment strategy.

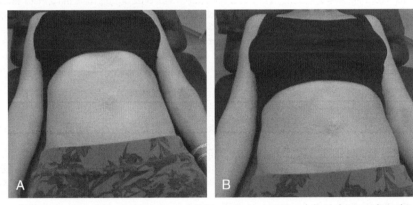

Fig. 11.8 Supine curl-up task 1 month later. (A) Note the symmetry of the infrasternal angle of Tara's rib cage at rest compared to Fig. 11.3A. (B) During the supine curl-up task, this symmetry was maintained; however, her automatic strategy still produced doming in the midline of her abdomen, suggesting the TrAs were not being recruited optimally.

Physical Examination

Standing Posture

Physical examination of her standing posture revealed better thoracopelvic alignment; her pelvis was in neutral alignment, as were her 8th and 9th thoracic rings. Because minimal attention had been directed to her 3rd and 4th thoracic rings, there was still some upper thorax asymmetry; however, it was not interfering with her lifting or running ability.

Supine Curl-Up Task

Clinically, both at rest and during her automatic supine curl-up task, the infrasternal angle was more symmetric (Fig. 11.8), suggesting that the resting tone of the left and right EO and IO was more balanced.

Without 'thinking of' pre-contracting the TrAs, doming of the abdomen was still present, and the LA still felt somewhat lax (Fig. 11.9A) (i.e. was easily distorted with finger pressure).

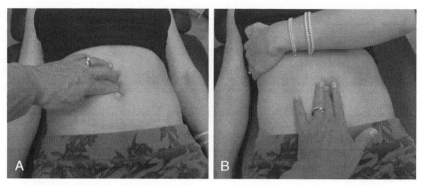

Fig. 11.9 Supine curl-up task 1 month later. (A) Minimal tension was palpable along the entire LA, and the left and right recti could still be easily spread apart. (B) Manual correction and control of the 8th thoracic ring facilitated more activation of the right TrA, evident as increased tension in the LA, reduced doming of the midline abdomen and an inability to subsequently separate the left and right recti. No more release of the right EO was required; it was time to focus on control of the 8th thoracic ring.

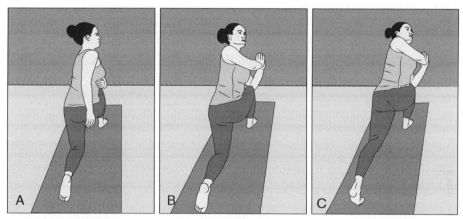

Fig. 11.10 Yoga pose *parivrtta anjaneyasana* (lunge with twist). (A) First – imagery and cues to relax the specific part of the EO attaching to the right 8th rib are facilitated by touch. Second – imagine creating space between the ribs on the right (specifically between the 8th and 9th ribs), and then gently connect, or draw, the 8th rib toward its associated vertebrae and right rotate the thorax. (B) Maintain the release, align and connect cues, and gently place the outside of the left elbow against the outside of the right knee. Press the elbow and knee toward each other. (C) Bring the awareness (focus) to the deep abdomen and connect to the deep muscles of the core, and then gently 'float' the left knee up off the ground. Maintain all this, and then lengthen up from the pelvis to the crown of the head and down to the middle of both feet.

Pre-contracting the TrAs significantly increased the palpable tension in the LA, and this was improved further by stabilizing the 8th thoracic ring (Fig. 11.9), suggesting further control was still required during this task.

No manual interventions for release of the EO were given during this treatment session. We focused on more movement training and control of the 8th thoracic ring for achieving her goal of being able to run and kayak with ease and without exacerbation of back pain. Both tasks require controlled thoracopelvic rotation, and running also requires alternate flexion and extension of the hips.

Many postures/poses in yoga are useful for rehabilitation of fundamental and functional movements. *Parivrtta anjaneyasana*, the Sanskrit name for lunge with twist (Fig. 11.10), is a useful pose, or task, for runners. To perform this pose well, thoraco-lumbo-pelvic mobility and control (both segmental and regional) are needed, as well as lower extremity mobility and control that far exceed that required for running. Tara was taught how to do this exercise or pose with optimal alignment, biomechanics and control from the 4th thoracic ring to her foot, with an emphasis on her 8th thoracic ring alignment, mobility and control when rotating to the right and the 4th thoracic ring when rotating to the left.

To do this well, she needed cues/images to relax/release the right EO, correct/align/control the 8th thoracic ring, activate the right (and left) TrA, rotate her thoracic rings congruently to the right, flex the right hip and knee and extend the left while maintaining optimal foot control and contact with the floor – no small task! Multiple myofascial slings (Vleeming et al., 1995), chains or trains (Meyers, 2001) require collaboration to do this well, and with repetition (massed practice) and focused attention (awareness), a better strategy for thoraco-lumbar-pelvic rotation mobility and control can be trained.

Considerable time was spent in this second session ensuring Tara understood the movement practice and that she continued to work on the release, alignment and control of her thoracic rings in relation to her pelvis and hips independently. She was satisfied that she would be able to progress her training on her own, and she was advised to return for follow-up advice as necessary.

Reasoning Question:

9. Recognizing you probably use a range of cues and images to facilitate a patient's understanding, awareness and efficacy for controlling the multiple components you highlight in the yoga lunge with twist exercise, would you provide your tips on cues and images you find most effective?

Answer to Reasoning Question:

This is difficult to answer because 'cues' are often based on an individual's past experiences and sometimes their culture or geography; they are highly individual. For release, words that suggest letting go or melting, lengthening, creating space between the bones of the compressed joint/region or expanding seem to work best. For connecting integrated myofascial units, words that link them together are effective, such as 'Imagine a guy wire between your left and right ASISs and find a way to connect them together', or 'Gently lift the arch of your foot and continue that gentle lift up the inside of your leg, picking up your pelvic floor; keep that, and now expand the lift up through your thorax, letting your ribs separate, and on your next exhaled breath, see if you can add a small twist between your chest and pelvis'. The nervous system appears to respond best to images and sensorial cues as opposed to 'being told what to do', and sometimes when the person does exactly what you feel is correct, you merely need to ask the person what he or she is thinking about while doing this. This way, your inventory of cues will grow; let your patients teach you how to do this. Eric Franklin's book *Dynamic Alignment Through Imagery* (1996) motivated me to try imagery with my patients with pelvic pain years ago (D. Lee, 2001). Imagery and visualization are used extensively in sport and dance for facilitating better strategies for movement.

Clinical Reasoning Commentary:

Contextualized use of metaphors as suggested here is well supported by their ability to activate sensory-motor systems, enhancing learning. The craft of teaching is again evident in this answer. Working backward from correct patterns of controlled posture and movement to the patient's particular thoughts can assist patient's recognition of unconsciously used metaphors while also building our own 'inventory of cues' for use with future patients.

Seven Months Later

I contacted Tara to ask how she was doing. Here is her emailed reply:

I am feeling really good about it all :) I am able to participate in all desired sports/ activities, though not yet to the same intensity as pre-pregnancy, but I am still steadily improving. [She also stated she was completely free from all pain in the thoracolumbar and mid-thoracic regions.]

Having said that, I have been meaning to email you and ask your clinical opinion on what you would consider a realistic expectation of what my stomach can endure with respect to another pregnancy.

We are considering trying for baby #2 very soon, and my only concern is how my stomach will tolerate the pregnancy. I know there are numerous variables and no concrete answers, but in your experience, have you seen women with a situation similar to mine come out of a second or third pregnancy with minimal progression of their diastasis, or should I be mentally prepared for things to likely be worse?

No matter what the answer, it isn't going to sway my decision to have a second baby :), but I would like to be realistic about what I am getting myself into!

There is no literature or research to provide Tara with an evidence-informed answer. No studies have yet determined what causes the LA to widen excessively in some women during pregnancy. For Tara, according to Beer et al. (2009), her IRD just above the umbilicus (her widest point) was only slightly wider (2.55 cm) than what is considered to be 'normal' (2.2 cm) (at rest). In my opinion, her minor DRA was likely caused by the dys-synergy of abdominal recruitment pre-existing her first pregnancy, and hopefully now that her abdominal musculature was more balanced and her 8th thoracic ring control was improving, her abdomen would tolerate the required expansion necessary for her second pregnancy without any long-term damage.

Reasoning Question:

10. It sounds like your prognosis for Tara was positive, both with respect to her pain as well as the ability of her LA to withstand a second pregnancy. Given Tara had 'questions regarding the pros and cons of a surgical repair of her abdominal wall' at her first appointment, please discuss your views on the indications for surgery.

Answer to Reasoning Question:

There are many subgroups of women with DRA, and treatment is highly individual (Lee and Hodges, 2016). However, in general, it can be stated that there are two kinds of patients with DRA: those we can help with physiotherapy (using a multi-modal approach to restore optimal function of the abdominal wall) and those who require surgery (recti plication [approximate the recti] and abdominoplasty [repair the skin]) and then physiotherapy (often with physiotherapy before surgery as well). When should we refer women with DRA for consideration for a surgical repair? Although research is lacking to definitively answer this question, within my clinic, we have now collectively treated over 100 women with this condition, and our combined clinical expertise suggests that surgery should be recommended in the following situations:

- If the individual shows poor control of the joints of the thorax, lumbar spine and/or pelvis during multiple functional tasks
- If the individual demonstrates optimal neuromuscular function of all muscles of the abdominal canister (assessed both clinically and via UI) but little ability for this apparent optimal strategy to control motion of the relevant joint(s)
- If the individual cannot generate tension of the LA during a contraction of the left and right TrAs or during a supine curl-up task

It appears that function can be restored *without closure, or narrowing*, of the IRD in some women with DRA, such as Tara. This finding challenges the commonly held belief that closing the DRA is a prerequisite for restoration of function. The ability to generate tension in the LA with an optimal abdominal recruitment strategy instead appears to be the factor differentiating those who require a surgical repair from those who do not.

Clinical Reasoning Commentary:

As presented in Chapter 1, the 'hypothesis category' of 'prognosis' refers to the therapist's judgment regarding his or her ability to help the patient and an estimate of how long this will take. Broadly speaking, a patient's prognosis is determined by the nature and extent of the patient's problem(s) and his or her ability and willingness to make the necessary changes (e.g. lifestyle, psychosocial contributing factors, physical contributing factors) to facilitate recovery or an improved quality of life within a permanent disability. Little research is devoted to identifying predictors for the effects of specific treatments for particular musculoskeletal conditions, although some clinical prediction rules are a relatively recent move in this direction (see Chapter 5). However, before being subjected to research, prognostic criteria for successful therapeutic management (e.g. neuromuscular retraining for DRA) must first be clinically recognized and clinically 'tested', as described in this case. To assist clinical reasoning regarding prognosis, we recommend explicitly identifying both positive and negative prognostic indicators throughout the full clinical presentation. This lessens the likelihood of an error of overfocusing on one or two key positive or negative features and facilitates a more considered decision.

REFERENCES

Al-Eisa, E., Egan, D., Deluzio, K., Wassersug, R., 2006. Effects of pelvic skeletal asymmetry on trunk movement: three-dimensional analysis in healthy individuals versus patients with mechanical low back pain. Spine 31 (3), E71–E79.

Albert, H., Godskesen, M., Westergaard, J., 2001. Prognosis in four syndromes of pregnancy-related pelvic pain. Acta Obstet. Gynecol. Scand. 80, 505–510.

Albert, H.B., Godskesen, M., Westergaard, J.G., 2002. Incidence of four syndromes of pregnancy-related pelvic joint pain. Spine 27, 2831.

Andersson, E.A., Nilsson, J., Ma, Z., Thorstensson, A., 1997. Abdominal and hip flexor muscle activation during various training exercises. Eur. J. Appl. Physiol. Occup. Physiol. 75 (2), 115.

Beales, D.J., O'Sullivan, P.B., Briffa, N.K., 2008. Motor control patterns during active straight leg raise in pain-free subjects. Spine 34 (1), E1.

Beer, G.M., Schuster, A., Seifert, B., Manestar, M., Mihic-Probst, D., Weber, S.A., 2009. The normal width of the LA in nulliparous women. Clinical Anatomy 22 (6), 706–711.

Berlucchi, G., 2010. The body in the brain revisited. Exp. Brain Res. 200, 25–35.

Boissonault, J.S., Blaschak, M.J., 1988. Incidence of diastasis recti abdominis during the childbearing year. Phys. Ther. 68 (7), 1082.

Boudreau, S.A., Farina, D., Falla, D., 2010. The role of motor learning and neuroplasticity in designing rehabilitation approaches for musculoskeletal pain disorders. Man. Ther. 15 (5), 410–414.

Coldron, Y., Stokes, M.J., Newham, D.J., Cook, K., 2008. Postpartum characteristics of rectus abdominis on ultrasound imaging. Man. Ther. 13, 112.

Doidge, N., 2007. The Brain That Changes Itself. Penguin Books, New York.

Franklin, E., 1996. Dynamic Alignment Through Imagery. Human Kinetics, Champaign, IL.

Gilleard, W., Brown, C.W., 1996. Structure and function of the abdominal muscles in primigravid subjects during pregnancy and the immediate postbirth period. Phys. Ther. 76 (7), 750–762.

Hodges, P.W., 2011. Pain and motor control: from the laboratory to rehabilitation. Journal of Electromyography and Kinesiology: Official Journal of the International Society of Electrophysiological Kinesiology 21 (2), 220–228.

Hodges, P.W., Gandevia, S.C., 2000. Changes in intra-abdominal pressure during postural and respiratory activation of the human diaphragm. J. Appl. Physiol. 89 (3), 967–976.

Horn, K.K., Jennings, S., Richardson, G., Van Vliet, D., Hefford, C., Abbott, J.H., 2012. The patient specific functional scale: psychometrics, clinimetrics, and application as a clinical outcome measure. Journal Orthopedic Sports Physical Therapy 42 (1), 30–D17.

Larsen, E.C., Wilken-Jensen, C., Hansen, A., Jensen, D.V., Johansen, S., Minck, H., et al., 1999. Symptom-giving pelvic girdle relaxation in pregnancy. I: Prevalence and risk factors. Acta Obstet. Gynecol. Scand. 78, 105–110.

Lee, D., 1993. Biomechanics of the thorax: a clinical model of in vivo function. Journal of Manual and Manipulative Therapy 1 (1), 13–21.

Lee, D., 1994. Manual therapy for the thorax. www.dianelee.ca.

Lee, D., 2001. Imagery for core stabilization. VHS produced by Diane G. Lee Physiotherapist Corporation.

Lee, D., 2003. The thorax - an integrated approach. www.dianelee.ca.

Lee, D., Hodges, P.W., 2016. Behaviour of the linea alba during a curl-up task in diastasis rectus abdominis: an observational study. Journal of Orthopaedic & Sports Physical Therapy 46 (7), 580–589.

Lee, D., Lee, L.J., 2011a. Techniques and tools for assessing the lumbopelvic-hip complex, Chapter 8 in: Lee, D. (2011), The Pelvic Girdle, fourth ed. Elsevier, Edinburgh.

Lee, D., Lee, L.J., 2011b. Techniques and tools for addressing barriers in the lumbopelvic-hip complex, Chapter 10 in: Lee, D. (2011), The Pelvic Girdle, fourth ed. Elsevier, Edinburgh.

Lee, L.J., 2003a. Thoracic stabilization and the functional upper limb: restoring stability with mobility, Course Notes. Vancouver, BC.

Lee, L.J., 2003b. Chapter 7: Restoring force closure/motor control of the thorax: In: Lee, D., The thorax – an integrated approach. www.dianelee.ca.

Lee, L.J., 2005. A clinical test for failed load transfer in the upper quadrant: how to direct treatment decisions for the thoracic spine, cervical spine, and shoulder complex. Proceedings of the Orthopaedic Symposium of the Canadian Physiotherapy Association. London, Ontario, Canada.

Lee, L.J., 2007. The role of the thorax in pelvic girdle pain. 6th Interdisciplinary World Congress on Low Back and Pelvic Pain. Barcelona, Spain.

Lee, L.J., 2008. The essential role of the thorax in restoring optimal function. Orthopaedic Symposium of the Canadian Physiotherapy Association, Montreal, Canada.

Lee, L.J., 2012. The essential role of the thorax in whole body function and the thoracic ring approach, assessment and treatment videos. Linda-Joy Lee Physiotherapist Corporation. www.ljlee.ca.

Lee, L.J., Lee, D., 2011. Clinical practice – the reality for clinicians. Chapter 7 in: Lee, D., (2011), The Pelvic Girdle, fourth ed. Elsevier, Edinburgh.

Liaw, L.J., Hsu, M.J., Liao, C.F., Liu, M.F., Hsu, A.T., 2011. The relationships between inter-recti distance measured by ultrasound imaging and abdominal muscle function in postpartum women: a 6-month follow-up study. Journal of Orthopaedic and Sports Physical Therapy 41 (6), 435–443.

Mendes, D., Nahas, F.X., Veiga, D.F., Mendes, F.V., Figueiras, R.G., Gomes, H.C., et al., 2007. Ultrasonography for measuring rectus abdominis muscles diastasis. Acta Cirúrgica Brasileira / Sociedade Brasileira Para Desenvolvimento Pesquisa Em Cirurgia 22 (3), 182–186.

Meyers, T., 2001. Anatomy Trains. Myofascial Meridians for Manual and Movement Therapists. Churchill Livingstone, Edinburgh.

Mota, P., Pascoal, A., Carita, D., Bø, K., 2014. Prevalence and risk factors of diastasis recti abdominis from late pregnancy to 6 months postpartum, and relationship with lumbo-pelvic pain. Man. Ther. 20 (1), 200–205. doi:10.1016/j.math.2014.09.002.

Mota, P., Pascoal, A.G., Sancho, F., Bø, K., 2012. Test-retest and intrarater reliability of 2-dimensional ultrasound measurements of distance between rectus abdominis in women. Journal of Orthopaedic and Sports Physical Therapy 42 (11), 940–946.

Östgaard, H.C., Andersson, G.J., Karlsson, K., 1991. Prevalence of back pain in pregnancy. Spine 16, 549–552.

Östgaard, H.C., Zetherström, G., Roos-Hansson, E., 1996. Regression of back and posterior pelvic pain after pregnancy. Spine 21, 2777–2780.

O'Sullivan, P.B., Beales, D.J., Beetham, J.A., et al., 2002. Altered motor control strategies in subjects with sacroiliac joint pain during the active straight-leg-raise test. Spine 27, E1–E8.

Pascoal, A.G., Dionisio, S., Cordeiro, F., Mota, P., 2014. Inter-rectus distance in postpartum women can be reduced by isometric contraction of the abdominal muscles: a preliminary case-control study. Physiotherapy 100 (4), 344–348. doi:10.1016/j.physio.2013.11.006.

Sapsford, R.R., Hodges, P.W., Richardson, C.A., Cooper, D.H., Markwell, S.J., Jull, G.A., 2001. Co-activation of the abdominal and pelvic floor muscles during voluntary exercises. Neurourol. Urodyn. 20 (1), 31–42.

Siegel, D.J., 2010. Mindsight. Bantam Books, New York.

Smith, M.D., Coppieters, M.W., Hodges, P.W., 2007. Postural response of the pelvic floor and abdominal muscles in women with and without incontinence. Neurourol. Urodyn. 26 (3), 377–385.

Snodgrass, S.J., Heneghan, N.R., Tsao, H., Stanwell, P.T., Rivett, D.A., van Vliet, P.M., 2014. Recognising neuroplasticity in musculoskeletal rehabilitation: a basis for greater collaboration between musculoskeletal and neurological physiotherapists. Man. Ther. 19 (6), 614–617. doi:10.1016/j.math.2014.01.006.

Stratford, P., Gill, C., Westaway, M., Binkley, J., 1995. Assessing disability and change on individual patients: a report of a patient-specific measure. Physiotherapy Canada 47, 258–263.

Stuge, B., Mørkved, S., Dahl, H.H., Vøllestad, N., 2006. Abdominal and pelvic floor muscle function in women with and without long lasting pelvic girdle pain. Man. Ther. 11 (4), 287–296.

Tsao, H., Galea, M.P., Hodges, P.W., 2010. Driving plasticity in the motor cortex in recurrent low back pain. Eur. J. Pain 14 (8), 832–839.

Tsao, H., Hodges, P.W., 2007. Immediate changes in feedforward postural adjustments following voluntary motor training. Exp. Brain Res. 181 (4), 537–546.

Tupler, J., et al., 2011. Treatment of diastasis recti and umbilical hernia with the Tupler technique. Hernia. 15 (Suppl. 1), S61.

van Vliet, P.M., Heneghan, N.R., 2006. Motor control and the management of musculoskeletal dysfunction. Man. Ther. 11 (3), 208–213.

Vleeming, A., Snijders, C.J., Stoeckart, R., et al., 1995 A new light on low back pain. In: Proceedings from the 2nd Interdisciplinary World Congress on Low Back Pain. San Diego, California.

Vleeming, A., Stoeckart, R., Volkers, A.C., Snijders, C.J., 1990a. Relation between form and function in the sacroiliac joint. Part I: Clinical anatomical aspects. Spine 15 (2), 130–132.

Vleeming, A., Volkers, A.C., Snijders, C.J., Stoeckart, R., 1990b. Relation between form and function in the sacroiliac joint. Part II: Biomechanical aspects. Spine 15 (2), 133–136.

12

A Construction Project Manager With Insidious Onset of Lateral Hip Pain

Alison Grimaldi • Rebecca Mellor • Kim L. Bennell • Darren A. Rivett

Subjective Examination

History of Current Complaint

Trish is a 48-year-old construction project manager who has been suffering from right lateral hip pain for approximately 18 months. The onset had been insidious, with no change in activity or work practices, and although the pain was intermittent at first, over time, it became constant, the intensity worsened and the impact on her life increased. Normally, she would walk four times a week for approximately 30 minutes and garden for 20–30 minutes. Walking from Trish's house unavoidably included walking up and down inclines because she lived in a hilly area, and she had been trying to walk through the pain, deliberately striding out to try to stretch the area. A number of months prior to presentation at our clinic, the pain became so marked she had to cease all walking. She had also modified or limited physical tasks involved in her work and had been hoping that the pain would resolve spontaneously. However, even with the restrictions on her activity and work, the pain continued and was now affecting her sleep, eventually prompting her to seek assistance. She had not undergone previous physiotherapy or any other intervention for her problem. Trish and her husband have three children living at home, aged 18, 15 and 12 years.

Past Medical History

Her past medical history included left inguinal and umbilical hernia repairs 4 years previously, but no other hip pain or problems. She had not experienced any significant lower back pain in the previous 10 years but had consulted a physiotherapist for back pain for a short period around the time of one of her pregnancies. Trish described this problem as a minor issue that did not require medical investigations or treatment.

Self-Report Questionnaires

Various self-report questionnaires were administered to evaluate levels of disability and self-efficacy and to screen for depression. The Patient Specific Functional Scale measures *activity limitation* on an 10-point Likert scale from 'unable to perform' to 'able to perform at the same level as prior to the injury or problem'. Trish indicated that she was having difficulty with sitting on the ground, walking on uneven or hilly terrain, sleeping, rising from sitting to standing, climbing stairs and standing on one leg to dress (see Table 12.1 for baseline responses). The Pain Self-Efficacy Questionnaire is a 10-item questionnaire that assesses the *confidence* of those with pain to perform a wide range of functions, as well as coping without medication. Trish reported moderately reduced confidence in her ability to socialize, cope without medication and increase her activity levels and reported mildly reduced confidence in engaging in leisure activities, performing household chores, enjoying

TABLE 12.1

INFORMATION FROM SELF-REPORT QUESTIONNAIRES

Self-Reported Outcomes	Initial Assessment	After 4 Weeks	After 8 Weeks	After 12 Weeks	After 26 Weeks
Pain Intensity: PNRS Over the Past Week 0 = No Pain, 10 = Worst Pain Possible					
Average pain	5	2	1	1	0
Worst pain	7	5	3	4	2
In side-lying	5	3	3	4	1
Sit-stand	4	3	1	2	0
Single leg stance	3	1	0	0	0
Walk – normal	3	0	0	0	0
Walk – fast	6	2	1	3	1
Up stairs	7	2	3	2	1
Pain Frequency: % of Time Present Over the Last Week					
Percentage	80	30	20	10	0
Patient Specific Functional Scale 0 = Unable to Perform, 10 = Able to Perform at Same Level as Before Injury or Problem					
Sitting on the ground	2	7	6	8	7
Walking uneven terrain/hills	5	8	5	8	7
Sleeping undisturbed	3	9	9	9	10
Sit-stand	8	8	9	9	10
Climb one flight of stairs	7	7	10	9	10
Single leg stance to dress	8	8	10	10	10
Global Rating of Change Scale (GROC) 11-Point Scale From 'Very Much Better' to 'Very Much Worse'					
GROC	_____	Very much better	Much better	Much better	Very much better

Normal, Normal pace; *PNRS,* Pain Numeric Rating Scale.

life and achieving life goals (see Table 12.2 for baseline responses). Trish also completed the Patient Health Questionnaire–9, which is a quick *depression assessment.* Her score was low (3 out of a possible 27), so there was no indication of a co-existing depressive illness. The three points she did score were related to difficulty sleeping – trouble falling or staying asleep, feeling tired or having little energy and having trouble concentrating on things.

Pain Behaviour

When interviewed about her pain, Trish reported that her primary area of pain was directly over the right greater trochanter (Fig. 12.1). This pain could extend approximately 75% of the distance down the lateral thigh to the knee, and sometimes in sitting with the knees crossed, the pain would extend more posterior to the greater trochanter. The pain was usually aching in nature, although at times it would feel like a hot, burning sensation. Trish also described some tenderness over the left greater trochanter, but this side was not causing her any functional difficulty. When prompted, she also recalled that she did still experience occasional central low lumbar discomfort, less than 2/10 in intensity on a Pain Numeric Rating Scale (PNRS). She had no posterior buttock or thigh pain, no pain extending past the knees and no pins and needles or numbness anywhere in the lower limbs.

Night time was particularly problematic for Trish because side-lying on either side produced pain over the right greater trochanter at an intensity of 7/10 (as measured on the PNRS). Lying on the left side also produced some tenderness over the left greater trochanter. This problem was causing considerable sleep disturbance. The only position that eased the night-time pain was lying supine, but she found it difficult to maintain this all night and would wake when she had moved onto her side in her sleep. She would often wake with her pain in the mornings, particularly if she woke on her side. Once she started moving around, the pain would reduce somewhat to an average intensity of 5/10.

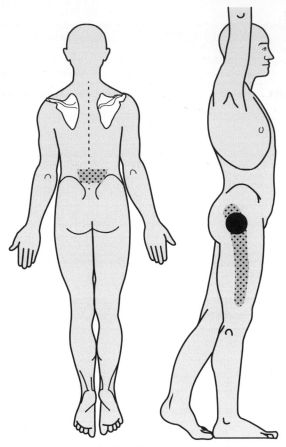

Fig. 12.1 Body chart showing the area of pain.

TABLE 12.2

INFORMATION FROM PAIN SELF-EFFICACY QUESTIONNAIRE

Pain Self-Efficacy Questionnaire

Please rate how confident you are that you can do the following things at present, despite the pain. To indicate your answer, circle one of the numbers on the scale under each item, where 0 = not at all confident, and 6 = completely confident.

	Initial Assessment	4 Weeks	8 Weeks	12 Weeks	26 Weeks
I can enjoy things, despite the pain	5	6	6	6	6
I can do most of the household chores (e.g. tidying up, washing dishes, etc.), despite the pain	5	6	6	6	6
I can socialize with my friends or family members as often as I used to do, despite the pain	3	6	6	6	6
I can cope with my pain in most situations	6	6	6	6	6
I can do some form of work, despite the pain ('work' includes housework, paid and unpaid work)	6	6	6	6	6
I can still do many of the things I enjoy doing, such as hobbies or leisure activity, despite the pain	4	4	6	5	6

TABLE 12.2					
INFORMATION FROM PAIN SELF-EFFICACY QUESTIONNAIRE (Continued)					
	Initial Assessment	4 Weeks	8 Weeks	12 Weeks	26 Weeks
I can cope with my pain without medication	3	6	6	4	6
I can still accomplish most of my goals in life, despite the pain	5	6	6	6	6
I can live a normal lifestyle, despite the pain	5	5	6	6	6
I can gradually become more active, despite the pain	3	6	5	5	6
Total	45	57	59	56	60

Trish's pain was present 80% of the time with fluctuating intensity, depending on what positions she adopted or what activities she performed. The right hip and thigh pain was aggravated by sitting, particularly with her right leg crossed over the left, or when in deeper seats where the hips were positioned below the level of the knees, such as when driving or travelling in the car. Walking at a fast pace, on uneven terrain and up hills and stairs or climbing ladders at work were also provocative for Trish's pain, causing her to deliberately avoid or minimize such tasks. Medication was the only thing that would help reduce her pain. In the week prior, she had taken non-steroidal anti-inflammatory medication three times (2 × 500 mg), and paracetamol twice (two tablets) to assist with sleeping. Her general health was otherwise unremarkable, and the only other medication she was using was for controlling pre-menstrual symptoms.

Reasoning Question:

1. What were your thoughts regarding the most likely source of Trish's pain following the subjective examination?

Answer to Reasoning Question:

Following the subjective questioning, the most likely pain source was thought to be gluteal tendinopathy, with or without associated local pathology of the bursae or iliotibial band (ITB). The key features that fit this pattern were pain and tenderness directly over the greater trochanter with pain aggravation on direct compression (lying on this side), passive compression associated with hip adduction (side-lying with the affected side uppermost, sitting with right leg crossed) and combinations of compressive and tensile load (walking at fast pace or on uneven terrain; climbing stairs, hills and ladders). It was evident that the lumbar spine would also need to be assessed due to her intermittent lower back pain and presence of lateral thigh pain. It is, however, common for patients with local soft tissue pathology at the greater trochanter to complain of pain that extends to the knee and radiates around the greater trochanter. Pain extending to the foot or the presence of pins and needles or numbness would raise suspicion of a spinal or neurogenic origin. Trish denied such symptoms.

The nature of Trish's pain was usually aching, consistent with symptomatic gluteal tendinopathy. Trish did also report that at times her pain would feel hot and burning. This type of pain description often indicates a neurogenic origin, suggesting once again that consideration should be given to other sources of nociception.

Reasoning Question:

2. Given the insidious nature of onset combined with the pain behaviour, can you please discuss your reasoning with respect to the most likely contributing factors to this episode?

Answer to Reasoning Question:

Although a sudden onset of pain is usually precipitated by a spike in tendon load such as a rapid increase in activity or a slip or fall, a gradual worsening over time suggests that the load across the tendon may have been suboptimal, leading to a gradual decline in load tolerance. Walking hills is more challenging for the lateral stability mechanism of the hip and pelvis. Trish lived in a hilly area, and all of her walking involved this higher-level challenge for which her gluteal tendons were evidently no longer optimally adapted. In response to the first signs of load failure, Trish did not reduce the load but continued to walk through the pain and with purposefully long strides, which would have amplified the loads across the lateral hip during stance phase.

Physical Examination
General Morphology

Trish was 163 cm tall and weighed 67 kg, resulting in a body mass index (BMI) of 25.2, just above the recommended healthy limit. Her hip girth measured using a tape measure at the level of the greater trochanters was 102 cm, and her waist girth was 90 cm. There was no leg-length difference when measured with a tape measure in supine lying, and in standing, there was no evidence of pelvic obliquity or scoliosis. No genu varum or valgum or significant bony torsions were evident in the lower limbs.

Posture and Function

Observation of standing posture revealed that Trish favoured a position where the pelvis was anteriorly translated relative to the ankles and shoulders, resulting in a relatively extended hip position with the centre of mass of the trunk falling posterior to the hip joint. Such a position increases load at the anterior hip, and Trish appeared to respond to that load by increasing the activity of her tensor fascia lata (TFL) muscles. Trish was asked what standing postures she tended to adopt while at work or at social functions because the posture a patient displays when under examination by a health professional may not be truly indicative of the patient's habitual standing posture, particularly during prolonged standing. Trish spends a considerable amount of time on her feet at work. She demonstrated her natural resting posture, which involved 'hanging on one hip' in adduction (Fig. 12.2). Her favoured side was the right side.

Trish's gait pattern was characterized by overstriding and heavy impact. She had a harsh, audible heel strike, leading into the right loading phase in which the pelvis dropped rapidly into a mild lateral tilt, followed by reproduction of her lateral hip pain during the late stance phase. Inadequate pelvic control in the coronal plane was also demonstrated in other single leg loading tasks such as single leg stance and single leg squat where the pelvis laterally translated and tilted, resulting in excessive hip adduction. These tasks were assessed with the non-weight-bearing foot lifted off the ground behind, allowing only 10–20 degrees of hip flexion on this side. It has been recommended that the non-weight-bearing hip should not be flexed more than 30 degrees during assessment of these tasks (Hardcastle and Nade, 1985) because the hip flexors on that side could be used to elevate the pelvis

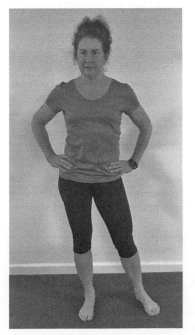

Fig. 12.2 Natural resting posture, which involved 'hanging on one hip' in adduction.

when maintained in higher ranges of hip flexion, and as a result, inadequate hip abductor function may be masked. Trunk position was also monitored because lateral trunk flexion or shift brings the centre of mass over the supporting foot, reducing the requirement for hip abductor activity, once again masking and compensating for hip abductor muscle dysfunction. Trish had an uncompensated pattern with no significant trunk translation. Her reduced lateral pelvic control in single leg stance was more evident on the right side. It also influenced both the swing and stance phases of stair climbing. As the weight-bearing hip dropped and shifted into adduction, the swing side traversed more closely to the midline of the body, resulting in a close-to-midline foot placement on the step above and therefore a position of hip adduction even before weight was transferred to this side. Further adduction occurred in her step up as weight was transferred and the body was elevated through the actions of hip and knee extension.

Reasoning Question:

3. What was your interpretation of Trish's postural tendency to overuse her TFL, and did this suggest a particular direction for treatment?

Answer to Reasoning Question:

In low load postures such as quiet, balanced bilateral standing, there should be little requirement for activation of superficial musculature. Trish, however, had high levels of palpable tension in her TFLs. Gentle manual guidance into a more neutral posture immediately resulted in relaxation of the tension in her TFLs, suggesting, firstly, that this tension was due to 'active muscle holding' rather than passive soft tissue tightness and, secondly, that postural correction may be a beneficial strategy for reducing anterior hip loading and tension within the anterior aspect of the ITB. Tensioning of the ITB, whether passive due to joint positioning, active due to recruitment of inserting or adjacent musculature, or both, may increase compressive loads on the soft tissues at the greater trochanter and, if excessive, may influence tissue health and load tolerance.

Reasoning Question:

4. Did observation of standing posture, in particular, 'hanging on one hip' in adduction, support your hypothesis regarding the source of the symptoms?

Answer to Reasoning Question:

'Hanging on one hip' in adduction is a common postural habit, and certainly everyone who stands in this manner does not develop symptomatic gluteal tendinopathy. Considered alone, this would not be considered diagnostic. However, in a clinical scenario, this postural habit is consistent with a pattern of abductor weakness or dysfunction that is typical of those with symptomatic gluteal tendinopathy. In this regard, it is supportive of the hypothesis described in the Answer to Reasoning Question 1.

Specific Tests of Gluteal Function

More formal testing of hip abductor muscle function was performed through assessment of active lag of abduction and abductor strength. Active hip abduction was assessed by positioning Trish in side-lying with the lower leg in approximately 45 degrees of hip flexion and 90 degrees of knee flexion and with a rolled towel placed under the waist angle to maintain a neutral lumbopelvic position. A plurimeter was attached to the distal lateral thigh with an elasticized strap, 5 cm above the lateral joint line. While standing behind the patient, the pelvic position was monitored with one hand over the iliac crest and the other hand free to guide the abducting leg, ensuring the femur did not flex forward. Trish was instructed to lift the leg in line with her body, maintaining neutral hip flexion/extension and rotation and avoiding hitching of the pelvis or rolling the pelvis back. End of active range was recorded at the point where she could abduct no further without compensatory movements, such as lateral pelvic tilt, hip flexion or axial rotation of the pelvis. Passive range of hip abduction was then measured while stabilizing the pelvis at the iliac crest and passively lifting the supported thigh into end-range hip abduction. The active lag of abduction is the difference between the active and passive measures.

Hip abductor isometric muscle strength testing was performed with Trish positioned in supine lying. The pelvis was strapped to the plinth with a seatbelt for stabilization, the non-test leg was flexed at the hip and knee and the test hip was abducted 10 degrees. A hand-held dynamometer was positioned above the lateral malleolus and stabilized with a seatbelt looped around the dynamometer and the end of the plinth. Trish was asked to abduct the hip against the resistance of the dynamometer, slowly ramping the contraction up to a maximal level and maintaining this isometric contraction for 3 seconds. This was repeated three times, with the highest value recorded.

Assessment of hip extensor function was performed during weight-bearing function such as squat, step up and bridge and open chain function during prone hip extension. Trish consistently demonstrated a delay or reduction in the activation of her right lower gluteus maximus muscle.

Reasoning Question:

5. Can you please explain how the information from the testing of gluteal function, in particular lag of abduction, contributed to your reasoning?

Answer to Reasoning Question:

In their role as superficial abductors, TFL and upper gluteus maximus (UGM) exert their effect via the ITB. They will be mechanically disadvantaged as the hip moves into inner range abduction and the ITB becomes relatively slack. The deeper abductors (gluteus medius and minimus) that exert their effect directly via the greater trochanter will then be primarily important for achieving movement through this inner range. Subsequently, loss of ability to move actively into inner-range abduction is likely to reflect deficiencies in these 'trochanteric abductors'. Although active range may be limited by passive joint or soft tissue restriction, the lag measurement reflects the ability of the abductors to move the hip through its available passive range.

Trish's active lag of abduction was over 20 degrees on both sides but was slightly greater on the right, reflecting poor function of the trochanteric abductors on both sides. Normative data are not available in the literature; however, clinically those with normal function can usually lift the hip into an abduction range that is within 5–10 degrees of their passive range. Trish's hip abductor strength was approximately 15% less on the right side, and both the strength test and active abduction produced a pain of 3/10 (PNRS) intensity over the greater trochanter on this side. Baseline values are reported in Table 12.3. Deficits in hip abductor muscle strength in those with symptomatic gluteal tendinopathy have been demonstrated when compared with both the asymptomatic or less symptomatic hip and a pain-free control population (Allison et al., 2016). Trish's abductor weakness and pain reproduction during strength testing was consistent with a diagnosis of gluteal tendinopathy and provided a treatment direction for the rehabilitation process.

Reasoning Question:

6. What differential diagnoses were you considering at this stage? What was the supporting and refuting evidence for each?

Answer to Reasoning Question:

The main conditions to consider with such a presentation are gluteal tendinopathy, hip joint pathology and referred lumbar pain. A battery of diagnostic tests was performed for the purpose of differential diagnosis, as described in the following sections.

Lumbar Spine Examination

All active lumbar movements were full range and pain-free. No tenderness was elicited on lumbar spine palpation, with only mild hypomobility of the thoracolumbar region detected.

Neurodynamic Examination

Straight leg raise was negative and of normal range.

TABLE 12.3

PHYSICAL OUTCOME MEASURES

Physical Measures	Initial Values			After 8 Weeks		
	Unaffected (L)	Affected (R)	PNRS	Unaffected (L)	Affected (R)	PNRS
Active hip abduction	27°	26°	3	44°	48°	0
Passive hip abduction	49°	49°		49°	51°	
Active lag	22°	23°		5°	3°	
Abductor strength	42N	36N	3	45N	46N	0

L, Left; *N*, Newtons; *PNRS*, Pain Numeric Rating Scale; *R*, right.

Hip Examination

Hip range of motion was normal and equal between sides. Both the quadrant (or scour) test and flexion adduction internal rotation (FADDIR) impingement test were negative. Other physical tests were selected for testing the hypothesis of painful gluteal tendinopathy, including sustained single leg stance; flexion, abduction, external rotation (FABER); flexion, adduction, external rotation – passive and resisted internal rotation (FADER); and hip adduction (passive and with resisted isometric abduction) (detailed results are included in the clinical reasoning discussion that follows).

In reasoning a differential diagnosis, let's first consider referred lumbar spine pain. The lumbar symptoms Trish complained of were very mild and occasional, with no temporal link between onset or variations of her lumbar symptoms and her hip and thigh pain. Furthermore, there was a lack of continuity of pain across the buttock, linking the lumbar and lateral hip and thigh regions of pain. Trish described the hip pain as emanating from the region of the greater trochanter, rather than typical radicular pain, which would tend to emanate from the spine, extend across the buttock and then down the lateral thigh. The fact that there were no symptoms past the knee and no pins and needles or numbness also reduced the likelihood of a primary lumbar issue. Trish did, however, describe a burning feeling down the right lateral thigh, which could suggest a neurogenic origin. All active lumbar movements were full and pain-free, straight leg raise was negative and of normal range and there was no tenderness on lumbar palpation, only some mild hypomobility of the thoracolumbar region. Based on these findings, the lumbar spine was considered an unlikely source of the lateral hip and thigh pain.

Second, hip joint pathology should be considered. Although lateral hip and thigh pain is commonly described by those with hip osteoarthritis (OA) (Altman et al., 1991; Lesher et al., 2008), localized pain over the greater trochanter is rarely the only or primary complaint in most clinical scenarios. Groin and posterior buttock pain are the most common types of pain associated with hip OA (Lesher et al., 2008), or the patient may describe a pain which travels between the anterior and posterior hip, indicating this by grasping the hand around the lateral hip above the greater trochanter and below the ilium – referred to as the 'C sign' (Byrd, 2007). Hip OA is also associated with loss of range of motion, particularly end-range flexion and internal rotation (Altman et al., 1991). Acetabular labral tears may also produce hip pain in the absence of OA. The most common area of pain distribution is the anterior groin region, often extending down the anterior thigh to the knee (Burnett et al., 2006). Some patients with labral tears may experience buttock pain, and just over half complain of lateral hip pain (Burnett et al., 2006). An important clinical distinction here is that the lateral pain is not generally located over the greater trochanter but rather in the anterolateral hip region between the greater trochanter and the anterior superior iliac spine. Those with labral pathology may describe pain of an aching nature; however, many patients will also experience intermittent, sharp pain in the groin or anterolateral hip, most frequently with weight-bearing pivoting (Burnett et al., 2006; Tibor and Sekiya, 2008). Mechanical descriptions such as catching, snapping or locking are also common (Burnett et al., 2006; Tibor and Sekiya, 2008). Physical tests, such as the quadrant or scour test and FADDIR, or impingement tests (flexion 90 degrees + internal rotation) are very sensitive to the presence of intra-articular hip pathologies but have poor specificity (Reiman et al., 2013). Although the lack of specificity of such tests provides low confidence in determining the precise structural source of the pain when the test is positive, sensitive tests such as these are useful for ruling out a symptomatic pathology when the result is negative.

Trish's description of her hip problem did not include groin or posterior buttock pain, sharp pains or mechanical sensations such as catching or locking. On physical examination, her hip range of motion was normal and equal between sides, and scour and impingement tests were negative. These findings indicated that an intra-articular hip pain source was an unlikely contributor to her current pain state.

Finally, gluteal tendinopathy remains. Lateral hip pain is reported to be most common in women aged over 40 years (Alvarez-Nemegyei and Canoso, 2004; Segal et al., 2007). Pain and tenderness over the greater trochanter are considered hallmark signs of local soft tissue pathology (Hoffmann and Pfirrmann, 2012; Labrosse et al., 2010; Segal et al., 2007). The literature describes pain that is provoked particularly by side-lying, but also standing on one leg, walking up hills or stairs and moving to standing after prolonged sitting (Fearon et al., 2013; Hoffmann and Pfirrmann, 2012). Traditionally referred to as trochanteric bursitis, it is now well established that gluteus medius and/or minimus tendinopathy is the most common pathology associated with lateral hip pain. However, there is often a co-existence of tendon and bursal changes, and even thickening of the iliotibial band (Bird et al., 2001; Blankenbaker et al., 2008; Cowan et al., 2003; Fearon et al., 2010; Hoffmann and Pfirrmann, 2012; Long et al., 2013). Physical tests do not accurately differentiate between these various pathologies but can be helpful in differentiating local soft tissue pathology from a more distant source, such as the spine or hip joint.

Tenderness over the greater trochanter has been shown to be the most accurate test for predicting gluteal tendon changes on magnetic resonance imaging (MRI; highest proportion of true results, either positive or negative), with the lowest negative likelihood ratio, indicating that if palpation is negative

Continued on following page

on clinical testing, the result significantly increases the likelihood that the MRI will be negative too. However, the specificity of palpation findings is low, and the positive likelihood ratio is less useful, meaning that although the test is useful for ruling out tendinopathy when the trochanter is non-tender, the trochanter may be tender in the absence of tendinopathy (Grimaldi et al., 2017). Palpation should then be used in combination with other tests that possess more useful positive likelihood ratios and positive predictive values. Physical tests, such as sustained single leg stance, FABER, FADER and hip adduction (passive and with resisted isometric abduction), can be used to increase the likelihood of a diagnosis of gluteal tendinopathy when positive, particularly the tests that include an active muscle contraction (single leg stance; FADER with resisted isometric internal rotation; adduction with resisted isometric abduction) (Grimaldi et al., 2017; Lequesne et al., 2008). These tests are described in more detail in Table 12.4. It is important to note, however, that many people without lateral hip pain have changes in their trochanteric tendons and bursae evident on MRI (Blankenbaker et al., 2008; Grimaldi et al., 2016). It is therefore important that radiological signs alone are not used for determining a pain source at the lateral hip. For a clinical diagnosis of symptomatic local soft tissue pathology at the lateral hip, the patient must be tender on palpation over the greater trochanter and be positive on at least one of the physical tests described in Table 12.4. A positive test is defined as one that reproduces the patient's pain in the region of the greater trochanter.

TABLE 12.4

DIAGNOSTIC TESTS FOR GLUTEAL TENDINOPATHY: SUSTAINED SINGLE LEG STANCE; FLEXION, ABDUCTION, EXTERNAL ROTATION (FABER), FLEXION, ADDUCTION, EXTERNAL ROTATION (FADER); HIP ADDUCTION (PASSIVE AND WITH RESISTED ISOMETRIC ABDUCTION); AND PALPATION OF THE GREATER TROCHANTER

Test	Description	Photo
A positive test is defined as reproduction of pain at the greater trochanter. Clinical diagnosis of gluteal tendinopathy = positive palpation + positive on at least 1 other test.		
Sustained single leg stance	The patient stands on one leg with fingertip support for balance. The test ceases as soon as pain is reproduced at the greater trochanter, or at 30 seconds if no pain has been reproduced before this point.	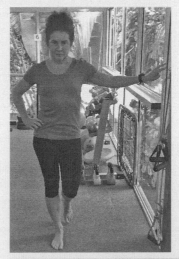
FABER	The examiner moves the hip into flexion, places the ankle above the opposite knee, stabilizes the opposite side pelvis to prevent rotation and then lowers the hip being tested into abduction and external rotation.	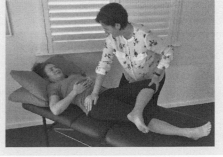

TABLE 12.4

DIAGNOSTIC TESTS FOR GLUTEAL TENDINOPATHY: SUSTAINED SINGLE LEG STANCE; FLEXION, ABDUCTION, EXTERNAL ROTATION (FABER), FLEXION, ADDUCTION, EXTERNAL ROTATION (FADER); HIP ADDUCTION (PASSIVE AND WITH RESISTED ISOMETRIC ABDUCTION); AND PALPATION OF THE GREATER TROCHANTER (Continued)

Test	Description	Photo
FADER i) Passive ii) + isometric contraction (IR)	i) The examiner moves the hip into 90° hip flexion, EOR adduction and EOR external rotation. Pain response is noted. ii) In the position from i), an isometric internal rotation contraction is added.	
Adduction i) Passive ii) + isometric contraction (ABD)	i) The patient lies on his or her side, and the examiner takes the hip to be tested into neutral hip flexion/extension, then lowers the leg over the side of the bed, taking the hip into EOR adduction. ii) In the position from i), an isometric hip abduction contraction is added.	
Palpation	The patient is positioned in side-lying with the hips flexed approximately 45°. The examiner palpates the greater trochanter for signs of tenderness.	

ABD, Abduction; *EOR*, end of range; *IR*, internal rotation.

In considering the information available for the current case study, Trish fit the population who experience lateral hip pain of local origin – female and aged over 40 years. Her description of the area, nature and aggravating factors was consistent with that outlined in the literature. Although the word 'burning' has not been used in the literature when describing the nature of tendinopathy or bursal pathology at the lateral hip, anecdotally, it is not an uncommon description in the absence of clinical or radiological signs of a neurogenic source. Such overlap in description can make differential diagnosis complicated, and each potential source must be closely considered. Trish tested positive for reproduction of her right lateral hip pain on the FADER and FADER tests with isometric internal rotation (8/10 pain reproduced on both tests), on the FABER test (6/10) and on sustained single leg stance, with lateral hip pain of 4/10 intensity reproduced within 5 seconds of single leg standing. Trish was tender on palpation of the right greater trochanter, particularly at the anterior aspect and proximal lateral aspect. There was also some milder tenderness over the left greater trochanter and a positive response to the left passive FADER test (5/10 pain).

Continued on following page

Taking all subjective and objective information into consideration, Trish's clinical diagnosis was likely right-sided gluteal tendinopathy, which may or may not have associated bursal change. Trish had some mild signs and symptoms on the left side as well, suggesting that she may have had a bilateral problem, but with the right side much more significant in terms of pain and functional limitation.

Clinical Reasoning Commentary:

Hip pain can have a number of potential sources. Clinical musculoskeletal experts are often able to recognize pain and movement patterns quickly using pattern recognition, but they will still apply hypothetico-deductive reasoning to evaluate competing hypotheses before they reach their diagnostic decision. In this case, several alternate pathologies and structural sources of pain were each tested in the light of demographic data, pain quality and location and specific physical orthopaedic test responses, among other clinical features. The knowledge supporting these reasoning processes is drawn from both the published literature – for example, studies determining the diagnostic utility of particular diagnostic orthopaedic tests – and from the clinical author's own professional craft experience gained from many years of specializing in hip problems. Of particular note is the regular recognition of the *absence of the presence* (or positivity) of key clinical findings which would be expected for a particular given diagnosis.

Although the early, preferred hypothesis of right-sided gluteal tendinopathy has been supported at the conclusion of Trish's physical examination, it has been carefully assessed against each piece of new clinical data in an open-minded and unbiased manner. Secondary hypotheses of referred lumbar spine pain and intra-articular hip joint pathology have been similarly rigorously tested and not entirely discounted at any stage. Even at the outset of treatment, these secondary hypotheses have been deemed 'unlikely contributors' rather than summarily dismissed from further reasoning, suggesting that the clinical author remains open to changing the diagnostic decision if Trish does not respond to management as hypothesized.

Reasoning Question:

7. You have performed a comprehensive physical examination. How have the results of any radiological investigations influenced your reasoning?

Answer to Reasoning Question:

Trish had been referred for MRI and radiographs of the right hip (Fig. 12.3). This information was available subsequent to her initial assessment and clinical differential diagnosis. Gluteus medius and minimus tendinosis was reported on an MRI of the right hip. The gluteus minimus tendon also demonstrated some mild calcification and partial-thickness tearing of its insertional fibres, and the underlying sub-gluteus minimus bursa was oedematous. The presence of partial-thickness tearing of the deep anterior insertional fibres of the gluteus medius and moderate oedema in the sub-gluteus maximus (trochanteric) bursa was also noted by the radiologist. With respect to articular structures, changes were rated as mildly degenerative with irregular tearing of the superior acetabular labrum but with no joint effusion. The mild degenerative joint change was confirmed on radiographs, with some subtle calcification noted adjacent to the anterior aspect of the greater trochanter, consistent with the MRI findings of gluteus minimus tendon calcification. Right hip joint changes were rated by the radiologist

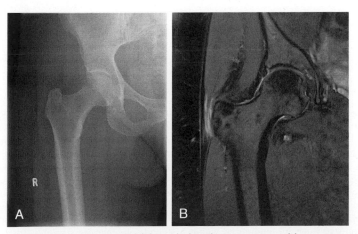

Fig. 12.3 (A) Anteroposterior radiograph of the right hip demonstrating mild joint space reduction and subtle calcific change at the anterior aspect of the great trochanter in the region of the gluteus minimus tendon attachment. (B) Coronal plane magnetic resonance image of the right hip demonstrating significant changes of the peri-trochanteric tissues as detailed in the text – note the high signal intensity (brightness/whiteness) of the soft tissues overlying the greater trochanter.

as Grade 1 (doubtful narrowing of joint space and possible osteophytes) on the Kellgren-Lawrence Scale, where 0 is no radiographic findings, and 4 is severe joint change.

When imaging information is available, it is extremely important that this information is used to augment rather than replace the clinical differential diagnosis. Fifty percent of people without lateral hip pain have gluteal tendinopathy on MRI, and 88% have some form of peri-trochanteric abnormality or increase in signal around the greater trochanter (Blankenbaker et al., 2008). Acetabular labral tears are present in 69% of an asymptomatic population of average age of 37.8 years (range 15–66), and some sign of early joint degeneration is present in 73% of this population (Register et al., 2012). Similarly, in a younger active asymptomatic population with an average age of 34 years (range 27–43), labral tears on MRI were present in 80%–85% (Schmitz et al., 2012).

Trish's imaging results helped confirm her clinical diagnosis of gluteal tendinopathy and the presence of accompanying bursal change. It also showed that she was clearly in a degenerative stage of tendinopathy, with calcification and tears evident. The mild joint change and acetabular labral tearing were in this instance considered to be irrelevant to her current pain presentation based on the differential diagnosis performed. However, a management protocol designed to improve the health of the lateral stability mechanism of the hip and pelvis and symptoms of lateral hip pain may also provide a beneficial effect for the underlying hip joint because those with hip OA also present with gluteal muscle deficits (Grimaldi et al., 2009a, 2009b).

Clinical Reasoning Commentary:

The imaging findings described here could easily be misused by the practitioner and potentially harmful to the patient. It would be very easy for a lazy 'diagnosis' to be made simply on the basis of the changes described by the radiologist. However, the clinical author has carefully avoided this reasoning error by understanding and applying the literature describing the prevalence of radiological changes in asymptomatic populations and by 'testing' the imaging findings/hypotheses in the light of the results of Trish's various physical examinations and her recounted history. Harm to the patient in such cases needs to be avoided by explaining the (in-)significance of the various changes seen on the images and by relating them back to the patient's other actual clinical findings. Taken at face value, the radiological report could have easily and unnecessarily alarmed Trish and promoted fear avoidance behaviours and a negative attitude to treatment. As seen in this case, the cultural indoctrination prevalent in Western societies that 'scientific' tests such as MRI will provide the indisputable truth often needs to be actively addressed by the musculoskeletal practitioner as part of the patient's management.

Reasoning Question:

8. What were your thoughts about the optimal approach to helping Trish manage her problems?

Answer to Reasoning Question:

There are key principles to consider in planning the management program for Trish, as described in the following sections.

Load Management

Compressive loading has been proposed to be an important aetiological mechanism for the development of insertional tendinopathy (Almekinders et al., 2003; Cook and Purdam, 2012). The tendon enthesis naturally has a higher prevalence of larger proteoglycans than the main body of the tendon, and there is a transition to cartilage-like cells at the bony interface. These features allow better adaptation to the higher incidence of compressive loads at the tendon insertion, whereas the main tendon is more adapted to high tensile loads (Cook and Purdam, 2012). However, if the tendon is exposed to excessively high levels of compression over time, adaptation may occur within the tendon to assist with controlling compressive loads – the laying down of more large proteoglycans (such as aggrecan and versican) which draw more water into the tendon, more chondrocytes and eventually osteocytes. Thickening of the bursae is likely to reflect a similar adaptation to excessive compressive loading. Compressive loading of the gluteal tendons and associated bursae occurs between the ITB and the greater trochanter in positions of hip adduction (Birnbaum et al., 2004). Daily postures that may contribute to cumulative compression include sitting with the knees crossed or together, standing 'hanging on one hip' in adduction and side-lying where the lowermost greater trochanter is compressed into the bed, and the uppermost hip rests in flexion/adduction across the body. In sitting, the depth of the seat often has an impact on lateral hip pain, with lower seats such as car seats producing more aggravation. Because the ITB merges posteriorly into the gluteal fascia, which extends up into the thoracodorsal fascia, hip flexion may also increase the tension within the ITB, particularly if there is any degree of concurrent adduction. Even 10 degrees of hip adduction can produce a nine-fold increase in compressive loading at the greater trochanter (Birnbaum et al., 2004). Load management through modification of postural and dynamic loading habits is a key component of the planned intervention.

Exercise Therapy

Exercise therapy is another key component of the planned intervention, including isometric exercise, functional strengthening in the sagittal plane and targeted abductor loading in the coronal plane.

Continued on following page

Isometric Exercise. Isometric exercises have been shown to activate segmental and extra-segmental descending pain inhibitory spinal pathways (Kosek and Ekholm, 1995; Kosek and Lundberg, 2003). Furthermore, sustained low-intensity contractions (25% of maximum voluntary isometric contraction [MVIC]) have been shown to be superior in raising pain pressure thresholds as compared with high-intensity contractions (80% MVIC) in a pain-free population (Hoeger Bement et al., 2008). Isometric contractions are now recommended for their pain-relieving qualities in the management of tendinopathy (Cook and Purdam, 2013; Rudavsky and Cook, 2014), with a regime of four 70% MVIC contractions held for 45 to 60 seconds, repeated several times a day (Rudavsky and Cook, 2014), suggested for patellar tendinopathy. However, scientific evidence based on interventional studies remains lacking, leaving the gold standard for application method yet to be determined for specific pathological conditions.

Functional Strengthening. Functional strengthening exercises are designed to provide a graduated platform for motor control retraining, abductor loading through sagittal plane tasks and generalized lower limb strengthening. Exercises move from bilateral symmetrical tasks through to asymmetrical, offset tasks, and finally on to single leg exercises providing a gradually greater challenge for the hip abductor muscles as they control femoropelvic alignment. The exercises include bridge progressions from the crook-lying positions and upright tasks progressing from double leg squats through various interim levels to step-ups.

Targeted Abductor Loading. The hip abductors are also directly targeted by providing loading in their primary plane of action – the coronal plane. These exercises, like the functional strengthening described previously, are all closed-chain exercises. Weight-bearing exercise has been demonstrated to elicit greater activation of gluteus medius than non-weight-bearing exercise (Bolgla and Uhl, 2005). Initially the loading is relatively light to establish the response to direct abductor loading. As tolerated, the loading is progressed toward a typical hypertrophy protocol employing low-velocity, high-load exercise. The high-load exercise is performed under supervision, using a spring-resisted sliding platform such as a Pilates reformer, to provide bilateral closed-chain loaded abduction. The added benefit of using the sliding platform is that hip adduction past neutral can be completely avoided, allowing provision of gradually greater tensile loads, without any compression imparted by the ITB across the greater trochanter.

Treatment
Load Management

At the initial treatment, Trish was provided with information about lateral hip pain and gluteal tendinopathy and clear advice for avoiding provocative tendon loads. As with any pain state, it was important to avoid engendering fear and hypervigilance in postural and movement patterns. Fostering an understanding of proposed mechanisms of tendon adaptation and provocation can provide the patient with a sense of power over the situation. To minimize positions of tendon compression, Trish was advised to avoid adducted sitting postures, and she also purchased a 10-degree medium-density foam wedge cushion for use in her car to reduce the amount of hip flexion during driving. She was aware that standing 'hanging in adduction' was a common posture for her at work, so she was encouraged to focus on consciously distributing her weight equally between both legs. For night time, she was advised to minimize side sleeping where possible, but if necessary, the placement of pillows between the knees and ankles to minimize adduction of the uppermost hip, and a soft mattress overlay, was suggested.

Postural retraining included standing side-on to the mirror with a plumb line for feedback. Ideally, a plumb line hanging from the greater trochanter should rest at the anterior aspect of the lateral malleolus (Peterson-Kendall et al., 2005). Trish's plumb line was hanging at least 3 cm anterior to this point, associated with her habitual anterior pelvic translation. With some instruction, Trish was trained to 'think tall' and translate the pelvis back to a more neutral posture, which had the added benefit of relieving the active holding occurring in the TFL muscles. The emphasis was on achieving a 'relaxed tall position', attaining optimal alignment with minimal muscle effort and avoiding breath-holding and 'muscle-gripping' strategies. Gait retraining followed, where optimal standing posture was first achieved and maintained before focusing on shorter strides and softer impact. Trish did well on her first attempts, but it would take time for the new posture and gait pattern to become inherent.

Exercise Therapy

Base-level exercises were also provided – low-load isometric abductor loading, two functional strengthening exercises and one dynamic abductor loading exercise.

Isometric Exercise

Low-load isometric abduction was prescribed as a first priority to assist with both pain management and early optimization of abductor muscle recruitment. Trish was prescribed low-load isometric abductor contractions performed in supine lying, consistent with a 25% MVIC application. Because Trish had demonstrated both excessive use of adduction in single leg loading tasks and increased levels of TFL activation (both of which will potentially increase compressive loading at the lateral hip), specific motor control retraining was required. The isometric exercise was performed in supine lying with a pillow beneath the knees, the hips abducted 10 degrees and a belt around the lower thighs. The abductor effort is taught as a slow 'ramp of activation' to the point of palpable active tension in the trochanteric abductor musculature but without activation of the TFL. Patients are instructed to imagine they are going to slide their legs out to the side, into abduction, just 'taking up the slack' in the belt. The activation is held for 10 seconds, or less initially if the contraction does not remain isolated to the deeper abductors. Trish was instructed to self-palpate the TFL during home exercise to ensure the recruitment remained focussed within the deep abductors. She was also taught a standing version of this exercise. Standing in slight abduction and ensuring correct pelvic position to 'turn off' the TFL, Trish again imagined she was pushing her legs out to the side, using a slow, gentle ramp of activation. Self-monitoring via TFL palpation was once again employed as a biofeedback tool. Performing the supine-lying exercise twice a day and the standing version twice during the day provided a four-times-daily isometric tendon-loading regime.

Reasoning Question:

9. Given that there seems to be no gold standard for the provision of isometric exercise, how did you determine the most appropriate format for exercise in Trish's case?

Answer to Reasoning Question:

For this intervention, a low-intensity format (approximately 25% MVIC) was chosen for the following reason. The structure and function of the multi-layered hip abductor muscle synergy are quite different from the quadriceps mechanism, where all synergists insert into the one tendon. The gluteus medius and minimus muscles insert via discrete tendons into the greater trochanter, whereas the more superficial abductors, TFL and UGM exert their abductor force via the overlying ITB. Excessive use of the superficial 'ITB tensioners' may then increase the risk of excessive compressive load of the underlying soft tissues at the greater trochanter. Although maintaining the hip in abduction should eliminate this risk, in everyday functional tasks requiring single leg loading, the hip necessarily adopts some degree of adduction to balance the body weight. In those with lateral hip pain, the TFL has been demonstrated to be hypertrophied (Viradia et al., 2011), and gluteus medius and minimus atrophied (Pfirrmann et al., 2005). A low-intensity isometric contraction allows the patient to control the level of muscle recruitment, targeting the trochanteric abductors rather than the ITB tensioners. The exercise therefore aims to both enhance motor control and provide pain relief.

Clinical Reasoning Commentary:

There is no gold standard in musculoskeletal practice for many diagnostic tests and interventions. Clinicians make informed decisions based on current available empirical and biological evidence (as shown in the Answer to Reasoning Question 9), as well as being based on their own clinical experience with similar presentations, underpinned by sound reasoning skills. In this instance, the exercise dose chosen was to a large degree determined by consideration of the specific anatomy of the hip region structures involved, rather than by simply extrapolating protocols developed for other regional clinical problems with differing anatomies and functional demands. It also demonstrates consideration of the patient's preferences and goals of self-managing the condition and self-controlling his or her pain relief.

Functional Strengthening

Two closed-chain bilateral loading tasks were also prescribed – double leg bridging and double leg squatting. In bridging, where the patient adopts the crook-lying position and uses the hip extensors to lift the pelvis from the resting surface, Trish tended to predominantly use her hamstrings rather than her lower gluteus maximus to extend the hips. Her position was therefore modified to bring the feet closer to the buttocks, using a shortened position to disadvantage the hamstrings and shift the dominant activity back to the gluteus maximus. She was taught to self-palpate her gluteal contraction in the retro-trochanteric region, aiming to activate her lower gluteus maximus to initiate a force through the heels and maintain this during subsequent raising and lowering of the pelvis. Double leg mini-squats were also taught, with a focus on appropriate patterning of the lower kinetic chain. The squat pattern is initiated with hip flexion and forward trunk inclination, as opposed to a trunk-upright, knee-forward squat that provides little stimulus for the gluteus maximus. The lumbar spine remains in a neutral position, and control of lower limb alignment is trained to avoid adduction or internal rotation of the femurs. Equal weight bearing is also an important construct for this exercise. Pain often results in protective unloading, resulting in further atrophy and reduced muscular support for the limb. After some practice in front of the mirror, Trish could comfortably perform a mid-range bilateral squat with equal weight bearing and appropriate alignment control. Again, appropriate gluteal contraction was self-palpated, and pushing through the heels was a useful cue to facilitate lower gluteus maximus activation. Endurance was assessed with respect to how many repetitions could be performed while maintaining ideal alignment control and muscle activation strategies.

Targeted Abductor Loading

Trish was also taught to perform controlled sidestepping, a gentle dynamic hip abductor exercise designed to provide a base for heavier loading in the coronal plane that would be instituted over the following weeks. The exercise involves controlled sidestepping in a step-touch pattern – a small step to one side with a controlled push from the weight-bearing side, landing on the lead leg and eccentrically controlling the pelvis to prevent excessive side-shift or pelvic drop on landing. The 'push' leg is then lifted and brought to a neutral hip position (not into adduction), touching the foot to the ground underneath the hip to re-establish balance, then repeating to the other side. Self-monitoring in a mirror is useful to ensure ideal pelvic control and also avoidance of trunk lateral flexion or drop of the femurs into internal rotation/adduction on landing and pushing off.

Trish was instructed that none of her exercises should provoke her trochanteric pain and advised to check technique; reduce speed, range and/or effort to eliminate discomfort; or call to seek further guidance if any pain provocation occurred. Details regarding exercise specifics, such as repetitions and hold times, are outlined in Table 12.5. Trish was supplied with a DVD that included lectures on her condition and reinforcement of written advice provided regarding load management, as well as videos of all her exercises. Also provided were printed exercise sheets with colour photographs and a booklet to record exercise adherence and comments regarding any difficulties encountered.

Treatment 2 (1 Week Later)

At the second visit, Trish reported that her average pain had already dropped from 5/10 to 3/10 and that she was much more comfortable at night, allowing her a better night's sleep. She was very pleased with this early response. Postural alignment control and gait were reassessed, and although Trish was able to correct adequately with conscious effort, without focussed attention, she quickly reverted to her habitual patterns. Emphasis was therefore placed on the importance of regular self-correction every day to ensure these became 'default' patterns. Exercise technique for all exercises prescribed on day 1 was checked and guidance given for fine-tuning motor control strategies. Trish was performing well, allowing for increases in repetitions and hold times (see Table 12.5) and progression to two single-leg-biased closed-chain exercises.

Functional Strengthening Progressions

Offset bridging was added, which entails performing a bridge with one foot close to the buttocks and one positioned further away. The hip extensors of the close-side foot perform the majority of the work, with the weight of the far-side leg *resting* through that foot. A level position of the pelvis must be maintained throughout the exercise, requiring activation

TABLE 12.5

HOME EXERCISE PROGRAMME

	Exercises	Week 1	Week 2	Week 3	Week 4	Week 5	Week 6	Week 7	Week 8
Isometrics	Static abduction in supine lying	1 × 5 bd, 5-s hold	1 × 7 bd, 10-s hold	1 × 10 bd, 10-s hold	1 × 10 bd, 10-s hold	1 × 10 bd, 10-s hold	1 × 10 bd, 10-s hold	1 × 10 bd, 10-s hold	1 × 10 bd, 10-s hold
	Static abduction in standing	1 × 5 bd, 5-s hold	1 × 5 bd, 10-s hold	1 × 10 bd, 10-s hold	1 × 10 bd, 10-s hold	1 × 10 bd, 10-s hold	1 × 10 bd, 10-s hold	1 × 10 bd, 10-s hold	1 × 10 bd, 10-s hold
Bridging	Double leg bridging	1 × 7	1 × 10	1 × 10	1 × 10	1 × 10	1 × 10	1 × 10	1 × 10
	Offset bridging		1 × 5	1 × 5					
	Single foot hover				1 × 5	1 × 7	1 × 10	1 × 10	1 × 10
Functional	Double leg squats	1 × 7, ~45° HF	1 × 10	1 × 10, ~60° HF	1 × 10	1 × 10, ~90° HF	1 × 5	1 × 3	1 × 10
	Offset squats		1 × 5, 50% BW, ~45° HF	1 × 5, 70% BW	1 × 5, 90% BW, ~60° HF	1 × 5, 90% BW, Decrease support	90% BW, No support	90% BW, ~90° HF	
	Single leg standing			2 ×, 15-s hold	4 ×, 15-s hold	4 ×, 15-s hold	4 ×, 15-s hold	4 ×, 15-s hold	4 ×, 15-s hold
	Single leg squats				Decrease support	No support, 1 × 3, ~60° HF	1 × 5	1 × 7, ~90° HF	1 × 10, No support
	Step-ups				1 × 5, 12 cm	1 × 5, Higher 20 cm	Decrease support, 1 × 5	1 × 5, Decrease support	1 × 5, No support
Abd	Sidestepping	1 × 7	1 × 10	1 × 10	1 × 10	1 × 10	1 × 10	1 × 10	1 × 10
	Doorway side slides			1 × 5 ea, Red band	1 × 5 ea, Red band	1 × 5 ea, Red band	1 × 7 ea, Red band	1 × 5 ea, Green band	1 × 5 ea, Green band
Walk	On flat, moderate pace, shorter strides, soft impact				1 × 10 min, 1 × 10 min	1 × 11 min, 1 × 12 min	1 × 13 min, 1 × 15 min, 1 × 16 min	1 × 20 min, 1 × 22 min	1 × 24 min, 1 × 26 min, 1 × 25 min

ea, each; *bd*, Twice daily; *BW*, body weight; *cm*, centimetre; *Decrease support*, reduce pressure through hand; *HF*, hip flexion; *min*, minute; *No support*, remove hand support; *s*, second.

of the anterior gluteus medius and minimus to act as hip internal rotators to prevent relative hip external rotation around the primary weight-bearing hip. In a similar fashion, offset squatting was added. This is similar to the double leg squat, except the ball of one foot is positioned slightly behind the line of the primary weight-bearing side. Upper limb support is also allowed initially, on the side opposite the front leg, to allow for optimization of alignment control, which is the primary objective. The 'hips-back, trunk-forward' pattern continues as per a double leg squat, but there is heavier requirement from the hip abductors of the front side to prevent pelvic shift or tilt into hip adduction. Trunk lateral deviation must also be avoided.

Treatments 3–14 (Weeks 3–8)

Trish's management plan moved from early load-management, isometric exercises and motor control retraining to a graduated loading phase to build strength and improve the capacity of the gluteal tendons to tolerate tensile loading. Over the next 6 weeks, Trish attended the clinic twice weekly for supervised exercise sessions and further progressions of her home programme. She would perform all of her exercises each morning, with the additional isometric exercises throughout the remainder of the day. Tuesdays and Thursdays were 'high-load' days where she attended the clinic, and on Saturday morning she would complete two sets of her single-leg-biased weight-bearing exercises, providing a total of 3 high-load days to stimulate strength changes. Posture and gait patterns were checked regularly to ensure these gradually became automatic patterns – for Trish, this took approximately 4 weeks.

Outcomes After 4 Weeks of Intervention

At the end of week 4, Trish was asked to complete the self-report questionnaires again. Details are presented in Table 12.1. At this point, her average pain was 2/10, with a maximum of 5/10 over the previous week. Perhaps even more importantly, her pain frequency had dropped from 80% to 30%, and her *ability* to sleep through the night had risen from 3/10 to 9/10. Substantial functional improvements were also reported for her other patient-specific issues of sitting on the ground and walking on uneven terrain. From the Pain Self-Efficacy Questionnaire, the first 4 weeks of the management programme saw a large, 12-point improvement in her confidence surrounding her ability to socialize, exercise, perform home duties and cope without medication (Table 12.2).

Functional Strengthening Progressions

Table 12.5 outlines progressions and specific details of the exercise programme. Bridging was progressed to a single foot hover, where one foot was slowly lifted from the supporting surface while the pelvis remained level. Functional weight-bearing exercises were progressed to include single leg stance, single leg squat and step-ups. For all of these exercises, strict control of hip adduction was the priority, so upper limb support was always used initially to facilitate this goal, and the range of squatting and height of the step was initially low. As control improved, range of movement was increased, and upper limb support was reduced and finally removed. Pain over the greater trochanter during any of these single-leg-biased exercises was not allowed, as it indicated that compressive load at the lateral hip was not being adequately controlled.

Targeted Abductor-Loading Progressions

Targeted abductor loading at home was progressed from sidestepping to band side-slides. This involved standing sideways in a doorway with an elastic resistance band around the ankles and one foot on a hand towel sliding on a polished floor into a position of hip abduction. The start position was a shallow double leg squat position. One leg abducts and the knee straightens, but with the emphasis on the lateral movement of the femur into hip abduction. Weight does not transfer with the moving leg, and pelvic control must be maintained on the non-moving side. During supervised sessions in the clinic, higher levels of abductor loading could be effectively imparted through the use of a spring-resisted sliding platform (Fig. 12.4). Bilateral abduction was performed by Trish in both an upright position with the knees slightly 'soft' and in a double leg squat position. Movements were

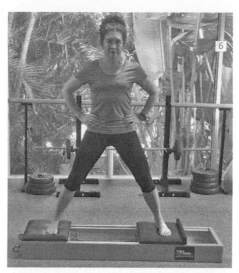

Fig. 12.4 Abductor loading exercise – bilateral spring resisted abduction in standing (sometimes referred to as 'skating'). Springs resist the movement of one plate as the patient stands on the sliding platform (TWS slider or Pilates Reformer) and pushes equally with both legs to achieve equal bilateral hip abduction. In this manner, heavy slow loading of the hip abductors can be performed. Details regarding the protocol used are given within the text and tables.

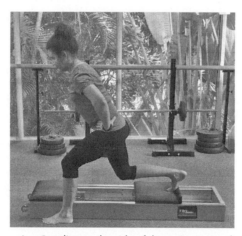

Fig. 12.5 The 'scooter' exercise. Standing to the side of the spring-resisted platform, the patient places one foot on the platform as pictured, adopts a shallow squat position and then pushes the platform back against spring resistance by extending the hip. The hip and knee of the other grounded side and the trunk remain stationary throughout the exercise. The perturbation of the moving leg requires multiaxial control around the stationary hip, resulting in loading of the gluteus medius and minimus in their important role in modulation of frontal and axial plane femoro-pelvic movement.

performed slowly with three to four for each movement phase. The muscular challenge was gradually increased over the weeks, such as by increasing range of motion and adding hold time in inner range, both increasing time under load. Spring resistance was set at a 'light' level for warm-up sets (Borg 11–12), and for the slow, high-load sets, the resistance was initially at a 'somewhat hard' to 'hard' level (Borg 13–15) until an acceptable 24-hour response to loading was established and was then increased toward the 'hard' to 'very hard' level (Borg 14–17) (Borg, 1982).

Another exercise known as the 'scooter' was also included as part of the strengthening programme. In this exercise, the patient stands to the side of the sliding platform in an offset-squat-type posture, similar to riding a scooter, with one foot on the moving plate. The weight-bearing side remains stationary, and lumbopelvic and lower limb alignment control in all three planes must be sustained under the perturbing load of the moving leg pushing back against resistance into hip and knee extension (Fig. 12.5). Initially, the sustained squat was relatively shallow, with the depth of the squat gradually increased to a maximum of 90 degrees of hip flexion. Upper limb support in the way of a single stick held in the hand opposite the main weight-bearing side was allowed in the early weeks and removed in the latter weeks of training. Spring resistance was also increased over time. Details of the supervised exercise programme are available in Table 12.6.

General Activity

With respect to general activity, Trish was advised that she could return to walking on a flat surface for 10 minutes in week 4 of the programme. She walked this distance twice in week 4 to confirm she had no negative response that night or the following morning. There were no negative effects, so she was advised to slowly build her walking distance by 1–2 minutes each session, 2–3 sessions per week, allowing at least 1 day of rest between sessions. Her walking progressions are reported in Table 12.5.

Outcomes After 8 Weeks

After 8 weeks of exercise and load management, Trish's pain was on average 1/10 and a maximum of 3/10 (PNRS) and was present for only 20% of the preceding week. Her pain self-efficacy improved another 2 points, related to an improvement in her enjoyment of hobbies and leisure-time activities. In the eighth week, Trish had been able to walk for a total of 75 minutes with no negative consequences. This successful outcome is consistent with the results of a recently published randomised clinical trial (Mellor et al., 2018).

Considerable improvements in the physical measures of active lag and isometric abductor strength were also achieved (Table 12.3). Active hip abduction range in side-lying improved 17–18 degrees on both sides, reducing the active lag to only 3–5 degrees, which was an excellent outcome for abductor function and reflected substantial gains in the ability of the trochanteric abductors to shorten into inner-range abduction. Isometric hip abductor strength increased on the affected right side by just over 20% over the eight-week intervention, bringing strength to approximately equal between sides. The optimization of hip abductor function was now also observable in functional single-leg-loading tasks. Reduced lateral shift and tilt of the pelvis was evident on both sides during single leg stance, single leg squat and stair climbing, likely due to the shift in the length–tension relationship of the abductors, which were now able to work efficiently in a more shortened range, and the specific attention paid to alignment control during the motor control retraining. Trish's lower gluteus maximus was now displaying good levels of activation and early onset during hip extension tasks, both open and closed chain. Appropriate postural positioning and gait technique were now displayed consistently.

Reasoning Question:

10. Trish appeared to have a very good medium-term outcome from the intervention you prescribed. Can you provide any insight into her long-term prognosis?

Answer to Reasoning Question:

Trish was sent the self-report questionnaires at 3 and 6 months to monitor her longer-term response (see Table 12.1 for details). Progress continued after completion of the programme, and at 6 months, she reported that she really didn't notice the pain anymore on a daily basis, and if she ever did feel anything, it was at a maximum intensity of 2/10 (PNRS). At this point there was no further sleep disturbance, and on her Patient Specific Functional Scale, only sitting on the ground and walking on uneven terrain continued to show a 3-point deficit. Trish now achieved a full score on the Pain Self-Efficacy Questionnaire, reflecting complete confidence in her ability to perform a wide range of functions, including household chores, socializing and work and recreational activities, as well as coping without medication. Trish kept up her activity levels, initially just continuing her walking, but by 6 months she had returned to vigorous physical activity, regularly attending two 1-hour boxing sessions per week without pain exacerbation. Evidence of long term success of this education and exercise approach for management of gluteal tendinopathy has been demonstrated in a high quality randomised clinical trial, where a success rate of approximately 80% at 8 weeks, was maintained at 12 months (Mellor et al., 2018).

Continued on following page

TABLE 12.6

SUPERVISED EXERCISE PROGRAMME

	Weekly Session	Week 3	Week 4	Week 5	Week 6	Week 7	Week 8
Bilateral Abduction in Upright	Session 1	1 × 5; Spr:R 1 × 10; Spr:R+Y Small range	1 × 5; Spr:R 1 × 10; Spr:R+Y Moderate range *Increase range*	1 × 5; Spr:R 1 × 10; Spr:R+Y Full range *Increase range*	1 × 5; Spr:R 1 × 10; Spr:R+Y Full range 5-s hold on reps 5 and 10	1 × 5; Spr:R 1 × 10; Spr:R+Y Full range 5-s hold on reps 5 and 10	1 × 5; Spr:R 1 × 10; Spr:R+Y Full range 5-s hold on reps 5 and 10
	Session 2	1 × 5; Spr:R 1 × 10; Spr:R+Y Small range	1 × 5; Spr:R 1 × 10; Spr:R+Y Moderate range	1 × 5; Spr:R 1 × 10; Spr:R+Y Full range 5-s hold on reps 5 and 10 *Add hold time*	1 × 5; Spr:R 1 × 10; Spr:R+YH Full range 5-s hold on reps 5 and 10 *Increase spring res*	1 × 5; Spr:R 1 × 10; Spr:R+YH Full range 5-s hold on reps 5 and 10	1 × 5; Spr:R 1 × 10; Spr:R+YH Full range 5-s hold on reps 5 and 10 *Increase spring res*
Bilateral Abduction in Mini-Squat	Session 1	1 × 5; Spr:R 1 × 10; Spr:R+Y Small range	1 × 5; Spr:R 1 × 10; Spr:R+Y Moderate range *Increase range*	1 × 5; Spr:R 1 × 10; Spr:R+Y Full range 5-s hold on reps 5 and 10 *Increase range and add hold time*	1 × 5; Spr:R 1 × 10; Spr:R+YH Full range 5-s hold on reps 5 and 10 *Increase spring res*	1 × 5; Spr:R 1 × 10; Spr:R+YH Full range 5-s hold on reps 5 and 10	1 × 5; Spr:R 1 × 10; Spr:R+YH Full range 5-s hold on reps 5 and 10
	Session 2	1 × 5; Spr:R 1 × 10; Spr:R+Y Small range	1 × 5; Spr:R 1 × 10; Spr:R+Y Moderate range	1 × 5; Spr:R 1 × 10; Spr:R+Y Full range 5-s hold on reps 5 and 10 *Add holds*	1 × 5; Spr:R 1 × 10; Spr:R+YH Full range 5-s hold on reps 5 and 10 *Increase spring res*	1 × 5; Spr:R 1 × 10; Spr:R+YH Full range 5-s hold on reps 5 and 10	1 × 5; Spr:RY 1 × 10; Spr:R+YH Full range 5-s hold on reps 5 and 10
Scooter	Session 1		1 × 5; Spr:R WB HF: ~45° Stick for support	1 × 5; Spr:R 1 × 10; Spr:R+Y WB HF: ~60° Stick for support *Deeper lunge*	1 × 5; Spr:R 2 × 7; Spr:R+Y WB HF: ~60° Stick for support *Increase reps*	1 × 5; Spr:R 1 × 10; Spr:R+YH WB HF: ~90° Stick for support *Increase spring res* *Deeper lunge* *Reduce reps*	1 × 5; Spr:R 1 × 10; Spr:R+YH WB HF: ~90° No support
	Session 2	1 × 5; Spr:R WB HF: ~45° Stick for support	1 × 5; Spr:R 1 × 10; Spr:R+Y WB HF: ~45° Stick for support *Increase reps*	1 × 5; Spr:R 1 × 10; Spr:R+Y WB HF: ~60° Stick for support	1 × 5; Spr:R 2 × 8; Spr:R+Y WB HF: ~60° Stick for support *Increase reps*	1 × 5; Spr:R 1 × 10; Spr:R+YH WB HF: ~90° No support *Remove support*	1 × 5; Spr:R 1 × 10; Spr:R+YH WB HF: ~90° No support

1 × 5, 1 set of 5 repetitions; 1 × 10, 1 set of 10 repetitions; HF, hip flexion; R, red (heavy resistance); reps, repetitions; res, resistance; s, seconds; Spr, spring; Y, yellow (light resistance); YH, yellow high (increases resistance by half a spring); WB, weight bearing.

The key to long-term control of this condition appears to be in appropriate load management, including control of postural and movement habits and maintaining an adequate amount of slow tensile loading to maintain a homeostatic situation within the tendon. Trish was warned to remain aware of good postural positioning and gait technique and to avoid slipping back into bad habits in the longer term. Trish was also advised to continue a maintenance home exercise programme three times per week and that she could gradually increase her activity levels, abiding by the principles of slow increases in load, allowing time for tendon adaptation and monitoring the 24-hour response to loading. She was also advised that if she had time out of her normal activity routine, for example, due to illness or holidays, she should slowly return to her normal activities via a graduated return to the activity plan, allowing the tendon time to adapt. Any exacerbation should be dealt with appropriately by immediate adjustments to loading and returning to the early exercise programme.

The importance of education cannot be understated. At the onset of Trish's original pain, she did not reduce her load but instead purposely pushed through the pain and even increased her stride length while walking, further exacerbating the problem. Although there is currently a strong emphasis in clinical practice on fear reduction around pain, musculoskeletal practitioners should not lose sight of the value of listening to early nociceptor-driven warnings. If Trish abides by the principles of long-term management with which she has been provided, she should be able to avoid or quickly resolve future exacerbations.

Clinical Reasoning Commentary:

Education about pain is currently very much in vogue in musculoskeletal practice, largely as a result of work undertaken in response to poor outcomes for patients with persistent spinal pain. It has become clear that for many such patients, simply applying a nociceptive-driven structural pathology or impairment pain model is not adequate as it usually is for non-chronic presentations. Changes of a psychosocial nature must be assessed and addressed, as appropriate, in persistent pain cases. However, it is unfortunate that sometimes the messages of Lorimer Moseley (see Chapter 2) and other influential authors in the brain–pain paradigm shift are inappropriately applied in practice – firstly, that it is counterproductive to touch the patient or use 'hands-on' interventions lest patients remain focussed on fear of physical structural damage and, second, that the patient's attention should not be drawn to the pain lest it reinforce pain-avoidance behaviours. Underpinning both of these misinterpretations is the misassumption that physical impairments are not relevant in the chronic stage of a patient's presentation and therefore should not be addressed.

In the case of Trish, despite having experienced pain for 18 months, she has responded very well to a mix of education addressing erroneous understandings about the causes and management of her pain and physical interventions targeting various impairments in her muscular control and strength. The practitioner has used a combination of verbal, visual and 'hands-on' or tactile cues to enable Trish to correct these impairments. In addition, as highlighted earlier by the clinical author, 'listening to early nociceptor-driven warnings' has allowed Trish to understand and minimize those behaviours which have contributed to the onset and maintenance of her symptoms. Trish was not fearful of these behaviours and associated symptoms because she had been educated to understand their significance and empowered to self-manage her pain.

REFERENCES

Allison, K., Vicenzino, B., Wrigley, T., Grimaldi, A., Hodges, P., Bennell, K., 2016. Hip abductor muscle weakness in individuals with gluteal tendinopathy. Med. Sci. Sports Exerc. 48 (3), 346–352.

Almekinders, L.C., Weinhold, P.S., Maffulli, N., 2003. Compression etiology in tendinopathy. Clin. Sports Med. 22, 703–710.

Altman, R., Alarcon, G., Appelrouth, D., Bloch, D., Borenstein, D., Brandt, K., et al., 1991. The American College of Rheumatology criteria for the classification and reporting of osteoarthritis of the hip. Arthritis Rheum. 34, 505–514.

Alvarez-Nemegyei, J., Canoso, J.J., 2004. Evidence-based soft tissue rheumatology: III: trochanteric bursitis. J. Clin. Rheumatol. 10, 123–124.

Bird, P.A., Oakley, S.P., Shnier, R., Kirkham, B.W., 2001. Prospective evaluation of magnetic resonance imaging and physical examination findings in patients with greater trochanteric pain syndrome. Arthritis Rheum. 44, 2138–2145.

Birnbaum, K., Siebert, C.H., Pandorf, T., Schopphoff, E., Prescher, A., Niethard, F.U., 2004. Anatomical and biomechanical investigations of the iliotibial tract. Surg. Radiol. Anat. 26, 433–446.

Blankenbaker, D.G., Ullrick, S.R., Davis, K.W., De Smet, A.A., Haaland, B., Fine, J.P., 2008. Correlation of MRI findings with clinical findings of trochanteric pain syndrome. Skeletal Radiol. 37, 903–909.

Bolgla, L.A., Uhl, T.L., 2005. Electromyographic analysis of hip rehabilitation exercises in a group of healthy subjects. J. Orthop. Sports Phys. Ther. 35, 487–494.

Borg, G., 1982. Ratings of perceived exertion and heart rates during short-term cycle exercise and their use in a new cycling strength test. Int. J. Sports Med. 3, 153–158.

Burnett, R.S., Della Rocca, G.J., Prather, H., Curry, M., Maloney, W.J., Clohisy, J.C., 2006. Clinical presentation of patients with tears of the acetabular labrum. J. Bone Joint Surg. Am. 88, 1448–1457.

Byrd, J.W., 2007. Evaluation of the hip: history and physical examination. N. Am. J. Sports Phys. Ther. 2, 231–240.

Cook, J.L., Purdam, C., 2012. Is compressive load a factor in the development of tendinopathy? Br. J. Sports Med. 46, 163–168.

Cook, J.L., Purdam, C.R., 2013. The challenge of managing tendinopathy in competing athletes. Br. J. Sports Med. 48 (7), 506–509.

Cowan, S.M., Bennell, K.L., Hodges, P.W., Crossley, K.M., McConnell, J., 2003. Simultaneous feedforward recruitment of the vasti in untrained postural tasks can be restored by physical therapy. J. Orthop. Res. 21, 553–558.

Fearon, A.M., Scarvell, J.M., Cook, J.L., Smith, P.N., 2010. Does ultrasound correlate with surgical or histologic findings in greater trochanteric pain syndrome? A pilot study. Clin. Orthop. Relat. Res. 468, 1838–1844.

Fearon, A.M., Scarvell, J.M., Neeman, T., Cook, J.L., Cormick, W., Smith, P.N., 2013. Greater trochanteric pain syndrome: defining the clinical syndrome. Br. J. Sports Med. 47, 649–653.

Grimaldi, A., Mellor, R., Nicolson, P., Hodges, P., Bennell, K., Vicenzino, B., 2016. Utility of clinical tests to diagnose MRI-confirmed gluteal tendinopathy in patients presenting with lateral hip pain. Br. J. Sports Med. 51, 519–524.

Grimaldi, A., Mellor, R., Nicolson, P., Hodges, P., Bennell, K., Vicenzino, B., 2017. Utility of clinical tests to diagnose MRI-confirmed gluteal tendinopathy in patients presenting with lateral hip pain. Br. J. Sports Med. 51 (6), 519–524.

Grimaldi, A., Richardson, C., Durbridge, G., Donnelly, W., Darnell, R., Hides, J., 2009a. The association between degenerative hip joint pathology and size of the gluteus maximus and tensor fascia lata muscles. Man. Ther. 14, 611–617.

Grimaldi, A., Richardson, C., Stanton, W., Durbridge, G., Donnelly, W., Hides, J., 2009b. The association between degenerative hip joint pathology and size of the gluteus medius, gluteus minimus and piriformis muscles. Man. Ther. 14, 605–610.

Hardcastle, P., Nade, S., 1985. The significance of the Trendelenburg test. J. Bone Joint Surg. Br. 67, 741–746.

Hoeger Bement, M.K., Dicapo, J., Rasiarmos, R., Hunter, S.K., 2008. Dose response of isometric contractions on pain perception in healthy adults. Med. Sci. Sports Exerc. 40, 1880–1889.

Hoffmann, A., Pfirrmann, C.W., 2012. The hip abductors at MR imaging. Eur. J. Radiol. 81, 3755–3762.

Kosek, E., Ekholm, J., 1995. Modulation of pressure pain thresholds during and following isometric contraction. Pain 61, 481–486.

Kosek, E., Lundberg, L., 2003. Segmental and plurisegmental modulation of pressure pain thresholds during static muscle contractions in healthy individuals. Eur. J. Pain 7, 251–258.

Labrosse, J.M., Cardinal, E., Leduc, B.E., Duranceau, J., Remillard, J., Bureau, N.J., et al., 2010. Effectiveness of ultrasound-guided corticosteroid injection for the treatment of gluteus medius tendinopathy. AJR Am. J. Roentgenol. 194, 202–206.

Lesher, J.M., Dreyfuss, P., Hager, N., Kaplan, M., Furman, M., 2008. Hip joint pain referral patterns: a descriptive study. Pain Med. 9, 22–25.

Long, S.S., Surrey, D.E., Nazarian, L.N., 2013. Sonography of greater trochanteric pain syndrome and the rarity of primary bursitis. AJR Am. J. Roentgenol. 201, 1083–1086.

Mellor, R., Bennell, K., Grimaldi, A., Nicolson, P., Kasza, J., Hodges, P., et al., 2018. Education plus exercise versus corticosteroid injection use versus a wait and see approach on global outcome and pain from gluteal tendinopathy: prospective, single blinded, randomised clinical trial. BMJ. 361, k1662. doi:10.1136/bmj.k1662.

Peterson-Kendall, F., Kendall-McCreary, E., Geise-Provance, P., Rodgers, M., Anthony Romani, W., 2005. Muscles Testing and Function With Posture and Pain. Lippincott Williams and Wilkins, Philadelphia.

Pfirrmann, C.W., Notzli, H.P., Dora, C., Hodler, J., Zanetti, M., 2005. Abductor tendons and muscles assessed at MR imaging after total hip arthroplasty in asymptomatic and symptomatic patients. Radiology 235, 969–976.

Register, B., Pennock, A.T., Ho, C.P., Strickland, C.D., Lawand, A., Philippon, M.J., 2012. Prevalence of abnormal hip findings in asymptomatic participants: a prospective, blinded study. Am. J. Sports Med. 40, 2720–2724.

Reiman, M.P., Goode, A.P., Hegedus, E.J., Cook, C.E., Wright, A.A., 2013. Diagnostic accuracy of clinical tests of the hip: a systematic review with meta-analysis. Br. J. Sports Med. 47, 893–902.

Rudavsky, A., Cook, J., 2014. Physiotherapy management of patellar tendinopathy (jumper's knee). J. Physiother. 60, 122–129.

Schmitz, M.R., Campbell, S.E., Fajardo, R.S., Kadrmas, W.R., 2012. Identification of acetabular labral pathological changes in asymptomatic volunteers using optimized, noncontrast 1.5-T magnetic resonance imaging. Am. J. Sports Med. 40, 1337–1341.

Segal, N.A., Felson, D.T., Torner, J.C., Zhu, Y., Curtis, J.R., Niu, J., et al., 2007. Greater trochanteric pain syndrome: epidemiology and associated factors. Arch. Phys. Med. Rehabil. 88, 988–992.

Tibor, L.M., Sekiya, J.K., 2008. Differential diagnosis of pain around the hip joint. Arthroscopy 24, 1407–1421.

Viradia, N.K., Berger, A.A., Dahners, L.E., 2011. Relationship between width of greater trochanters and width of iliac wings in tronchanteric bursitis. Am. J. Orthop. 40, E159–E162.

13

A Pain Science Approach to Postoperative Lumbar Surgery Rehabilitation

Adriaan Louw • Ina Diener • Mark A. Jones

Subjective Examination
History

Six months ago, Dean, a 59-year-old male, arrived at the physical therapy clinic for consultation. He complained of low back pain and accompanying right lateral leg and foot pain. He denied any specific injury or accident but described, rather, a progressive worsening of episodic back and leg pain for the past 5 years. He recalled developing his first episode of back pain spontaneously and experienced intermittent episodes since then. The episodes had progressed to being more frequent and longer lasting, ultimately with the development of increased pain and numbness in the right leg. As the symptoms progressed, he received various conservative treatments, including chiropractic adjustments, medication (non-steroidal anti-inflammatories and muscle relaxants), physical therapy (stretches and exercises) and a session of massage therapy. All seemed to help for a while but then failed to provide more than a few days of relief.

Personal Circumstances

Dean is married with three grown children. His work involves driving a delivery truck, requiring prolonged sitting and lifting/carrying loads varying from 2 to 20 kg. Outside his employment, Dean is a 'hobby farmer' – owning some land where he plants various small crops and raises some livestock. Given the persistence of his symptoms, he was referred to our clinic for specialized spinal care and consultation to see what options may be available for his back and leg pain.

Area and Behaviour of Symptoms

On questioning. Dean stated that when the back and leg pain first started, he could find ways to ease the pain. However, at present, he described a constant, variable, deep ache across the low back (L4–S1 area) and a burning, constant pain in the right leg with accompanying intermittent feelings of numbness. The leg pain was by far the most severe of the two pains (L5 and S1 dermatomes) (Fig. 13.1). Dean did not report any paraesthesia in his leg or foot, and the rest of his body chart was unremarkable. The leg symptoms were exacerbated with standing more than 5 minutes and walking more than 10 minutes, and they eased considerably with sitting, within a few minutes. He also reported moderate morning and afternoon stiffness in the low back and difficulty sleeping at night due to the leg pain. The low back pain intensified with transitional movements – from sitting to standing and vice versa, as well as getting in and out of the truck during a working day.

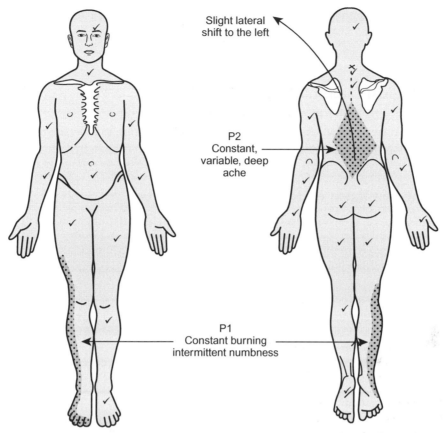

Fig. 13.1 Body chart illustrating areas of back and leg pain and leg numbness. The ticks indicate areas of no symptoms.

General Health, Medication and Oswestry Disability Index Score

Dean's general health (medical intake questionnaire) revealed no major medical issues, except being a smoker for the past 40 years. He denied any significant medical tests or treatments in his past. His current medication was a membrane-stabilizing drug (Lyrica™), which Dean believed helped his sleep somewhat. His intake forms revealed an Oswestry Disability Index (ODI) score of 54% (severe disability) and a pain rating (Numeric Rating Scale [NRS]) of 7/10. No red flags were detected.

Physical Examination

Observation

- Dean walked in slight flexion and seemed to be in moderate distress.
- Standing demonstrated mild trunk-forward flexion (he reported this eased his pain) with decreased lumbar lordosis. Dean experienced increased back pain when asked to correct the forward-flexed posture and stand more erect.
- A mild lateral mid-lumbar shift to the left was evident in standing. The low back and leg pain both increased with shift correction.

Active Movement Tests (Resting Symptoms as per Fig. 13.1 – Constant Leg and Low Back Pain)

Lumbar spine ranges of movement (estimated percentage of expected normal range of movement) and pain responses were as follows:

- Flexion 50%; reported stiffness > pain; no change in back or leg pain
- Extension 20%; increased back pain and leg pain to 8/10
- Side bend right 20%; reproduced right leg pain 8/10
- Side bend left 75%; no pain

Neurological Examination (Butler, 2000)

- Decreased right gastrocnemius reflex
- Decreased strength big toe extension (L5) and ankle eversion (S1) on the right
- Decreased sensation dorsal aspect of the big toe (L5) and lateral border of the foot (S1) on the right

Straight Leg Raise (SLR) (Butler, 2000)

- Left 60 degrees; no symptoms reproduced, 'muscular tightness' in posterior thigh stops the movement
- Right 20 degrees; reproduced 'the leg pain' – increased with ankle dorsiflexion, hip adduction and hip internal rotation

No further examination was conducted, and following discussion with (and consent from) Dean, the primary care physician was consulted. Based on the clear neurological findings, worsening presentation and failure of previous physical therapy treatments, it was decided in collaboration with his primary care physician to have Dean undergo imaging studies to rule out any red flags.

Reasoning Question:

1. Please discuss your decision to forego further physical examination and treatment and instead consult Dean's primary care physician, highlighting the key features that prompted that judgement.

Answer to Reasoning Question:

Dean presented with a worsening neurological deficit and limited effect of prior rehabilitation in altering his symptoms. The signs and symptoms indicated progressive degenerative spinal stenosis with nerve root involvement (Kovacs et al., 2011; Backstrom et al., 2011; Tran de et al., 2010):

- Insidious onset
- Progressive in nature
- Neurological signs and symptoms consistent with right-sided L5 and S1 nerve root involvement
- Progressive worsening function
- Movements/postures associated with increasing space of the intervertebral foramen (flexion, shift, sitting) eased his symptoms.
- Loading tasks and closing positions of the intervertebral foramen and postures increased his symptoms (walking, standing, extension, side-flexion toward the involved side).
- Leg symptoms were worse than those of the low back.

Due to his progressive neurological deficit, failed previous conservative care and significant, worsening pain and disability, it was reasoned additional conservative care would likely result in little added benefit. Although not extensive, these treatments had included a manual therapy and exercise approach, which typically feature as key elements of treatment for a patient with spinal stenosis, yet did not yield significant benefit in Dean's case.

Additionally, he had not reported any formal imaging to explore possible causes of the progressive worsening. There were several reasons to undertake imaging:

1. Help aid in diagnosis of the cause of his potential worsening symptoms
2. Screen for any red flags
3. Provide a baseline of any degenerative changes in his spine to be compared with potential future imaging to establish progression
4. Needed for potential invasive treatments, such as surgery and/or epidural steroid injections

Given Dean's symptoms had been present for years and were seemingly worsening specific to neurological deficit, there was an added concern that the nerves might undergo permanent changes, which might in turn result in permanent deficits. It is well established that permanent changes may occur with persistent irritation of and/or mechanical interference with neural tissue (Lundborg et al., 1983; Lundborg and Dahlin, 1996).

Clinical Reasoning Commentary:

The clinical reasoning underpinning the decision to consult Dean's primary care physician incorporates judgements across several of the 'hypothesis categories' discussed in Chapter 1. These include hypotheses regarding 'sources of symptoms' and 'pathology' (e.g. recognition of a clinical pattern of progressive degenerative spinal stenosis with nerve root involvement), 'precautions and contraindications to physical examination and treatment' (e.g. progressive neurological deficit, significant pain and disability, lack of formal imaging to explore causes of progressive worsening and rule out red flags, concern for permanent change to neural tissue and potential for permanent deficits), 'management' (e.g. surgery and/or epidural steroid injections) and 'prognosis' (e.g. failure of previous conservative care incorporating appropriate interventions). These judgements do not necessarily occur in a sequential or linear manner (i.e. one hypothesis category considered at a time or in any particular order). That is, information obtained can inform several hypotheses (e.g. same information that elicits hypothesis of nerve root involvement also has implications for 'precautions', 'management' and 'prognosis'). Similarly, it is common for the clinician to ask a question with a particular focus or hypothesis category in mind (e.g. source and associated pathology versus psychosocial), but the patient's response provides something different or more than was asked, requiring flexibility in reasoning so that potentially relevant information is not missed (see discussion of 'dialectical reasoning' in Chapter 1). Indeed, the skilled clinician commonly will need to consider multiple hypotheses across multiple categories at many stages of the evolving patient encounter.

In the subsequent weeks, Dean underwent magnetic resonance imaging (MRI) of his lumbar spine, which revealed severe degenerative spinal stenosis at the L4/5 and L5/S1 intervertebral foraminae, a disc bulge at L5/S1 and low-grade anterolisthesis at L5/S1 (Fig. 13.2).

Given these imaging findings and progressive pain and disability, Dean underwent a series of three epidural steroid injections, which failed to alter his symptoms. He ultimately underwent an L5/S1 decompressive laminectomy and discectomy, along with a transforaminal lumbar interbody fusion (TLIF) at L5/S1 to decompress the S1 nerve root and remove degenerative changes (Ostelo et al., 2003c). The lamina (right side) was removed, followed by a decompressive removal of the disc material around the L5 and S1 nerve roots. On each level (L5 and S1), two pedicle screws were inserted through the pedicles on each side, followed by connecting rods between L4 and L5. Dean remained in the hospital for 3 days to monitor his recovery, and after inpatient physical therapy (walking, transfers, non-rigid low back brace instruction), he was discharged with instructions to progressively wean himself off the brace over the next 4 weeks. Additionally, he was advised to restrict lifting to 4 kg and avoid driving more than 2 hours at a time, and he was encouraged to walk 3-4 times per day.

Four weeks after surgery, Dean attended a follow-up visit with the spinal surgeon. At the follow-up, he presented with limited active lumbar motion, low back pain, persistent pain in the L5 and S1 dermatomes (50% less than preoperative pain) and persistent difficulty

Fig. 13.2 Patient magnetic resonance imaging (MRI) scan prior to surgery.

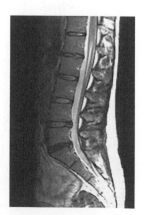

sleeping due to the leg pain. At this point the surgeon recommended physical therapy for postoperative rehabilitation. Dean was referred with a script stating: '*Evaluate and treat as necessary – TLIF/decompression L5/S1. Focus on stabilization, pain control and function*'.

Postoperative Physical Therapy Appointment 1 (5 Weeks Post-op)

Subjective Examination

Dean presented with low-grade (3/10 NRS), constant, variable low back pain, as well as leg pain corresponding to the L5 and S1 dermatomes (5/10 NRS). He had no numbness but did report intermittent pins and needles on the side of his foot (Fig. 13.3).

He reported no change in his medical history from the original preoperative consultation and that he was still using membrane-stabilizing medication to help sleep. He had discontinued any use of pain medication. His ODI score (50%) revealed severe disability (Hakkinen et al., 2007), and his Fear Avoidance Beliefs Questionnaire (FABQ) for physical activity (FABQ-PA) and work (FABQ-W) revealed high fear-avoidance scores (22 and 35, respectively) (Fritz and George, 2002). Dean had not returned to work but was motivated to resume his normal activities, including his truck driving and farming. He was walking up to 1 km 3–4 times per day. Although these walks initially eased his pain, any walk > 1 km started increasing his pain, and hence he walked more frequently for shorter distances rather than less frequently for longer distances. Upon further questioning, Dean revealed an overall anxiety and uncertainty regarding his persistent pain levels after surgery. Although he reported some relief of pain, he was under the impression he would be relatively 'pain-free' after surgery and was concerned the pain might in fact increase over time.

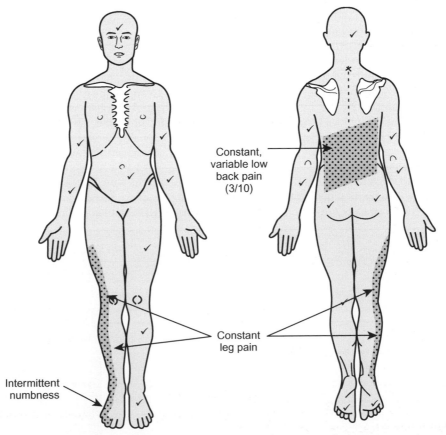

Fig. 13.3 Postoperative body chart. The ticks indicate areas of no symptoms.

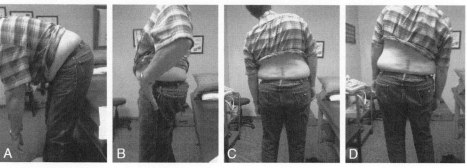

Fig. 13.4   Active lumbar range of motion after surgery. (A) Flexion. (B) Extension. (C) Left side-bending. (D) Right side-bending.

Physical Examination

Observation

- Walked in slight trunk flexion
- Loss of lumbar lordosis in standing and walking
- Surgical scar off-center over the L2–S2 area

Active Movement Tests (Resting Pain 3/10)

Lumbar spine ranges of movement (estimated percentage of expected normal) and pain responses (Fig. 13.4) (Maitland et al., 2005):

- Flexion 75%; stopped by report of stiffness, no pain reported
- Extension 10%; stopped by pain in his back (up to 7/10)
- Side bend left 25%; no pain
- Side bend right 25%; no pain

Neurological Examination

- Testing of left and right lower extremities (sensation, reflex and strength) – intact, equal bilaterally (Butler, 2000)

SLR (Butler, 2000)

- Left 60 degrees; stopped by tightness in hamstrings
- Right 45 degrees; reproduced his postero-lateral leg pain to mid-calf, increased with ankle dorsiflexion, hip adduction and hip internal rotation

Hip Joint Passive Range-of-Movement Screening

- Hip flexion within normal limits, left = right
- External rotation normal, no symptoms elicited, left = right
- Internal rotation 50% of normal bilaterally, stiffness > pain, left = right (pain around the greater trochanter)
- Combined flexion/adduction plus compression (i.e. 'quadrant' test [Maitland et al., 2005)]: no symptoms reproduced, left = right

Tinnell Test of the Tibial Nerve (Walsh and Hall, 2009a)

- Positive for pain provocation right tibial nerve (posterior knee midline and posterior tarsal tunnel)
- No sensitivity or pain provocation of tibial nerve palpation on the left leg

Motor Control (Richardson et al., 2004, Puentedura et al., 2009)

Dean was instructed and asked to perform a spinal stabilization 'draw-in' maneuver to assess his ability to activate his stabilization mechanism while lying supine with knees bent to minimize stress to the lumbar spine. Before the maneuver, he was asked to ensure his spine was in the most comfortable position close to mid-range by repeating end-range positions of anterior and posterior pelvic tilting and finding the most comfortable position midway between the two extremes. When Dean tried to perform the draw-in maneuver, visual inspection revealed various compensatory strategies, including excessive inspiration, overuse of superficial muscles and unwanted pelvic movement.

Reasoning Question:

2. Please discuss your hypotheses and supporting evidence (from Dean's presentation and research) at this stage regarding the presence of nociceptive, neuropathic and/or nociplastic pain types.

Answer to Reasoning Question:

Dean's postoperative clinical presentation was consistent with persistent neuropathic pain of the L5 and S1 nerve roots, due to mechanical sensitivity (no conduction abnormalities) (Smart et al., 2012a, 2012b, 2012c, 2009). This interpretation is supported by the persistent high level of pain, presence of night pain, easing of symptoms with walking (a natural 'slider exercise' for the sciatic nerve and aerobic exercise) and symptom reproduction with the SLR and Tinnell tests (Smart et al., 2012a, 2012b, 2012c, 2009; Walsh and Hall, 2009b). Biologically, it is well established that mechanical (e.g. stenosis, bone spurs) and inflammatory (e.g. disc herniation) mechanisms can lead to demyelinization of the proximal nerve root, resulting in an exposed and thus sensitive nerve root, along with activation of the dorsal root ganglion (Saal et al., 1990; Piperno et al., 1997). This sensitization (both mechanical and physiological) of the nervous system has been implicated as a source of persistent pain following lumbar surgery (Piperno et al., 1997; Ulrich et al., 2007). In Dean's case, the surgery decompressed the nerve root, resulting in a favorable neurological outcome with abolition of weakness, numbness and decreased reflexes.

Reasoning Question:

3. What was your interpretation of Dean's scores on the FABQ and his perspectives on his current status (e.g. understanding, cognitions, feelings/coping and interest/motivation/self-efficacy) with respect to your management and his prognosis?

Answer to Reasoning Question:

With the advent of the 'yellow-flags' research (Kendall et al., 1997; Grotle et al., 2006), much attention has been given to fear avoidance, and thresholds have been established in regard to the likelihood of returning to work. It is proposed that FABQ-W scores >34 and FABQ-PA scores >14 are associated with a higher likelihood of not returning to work (Fritz and George, 2002; Burton et al., 1999). In Dean's case, he exceeded both work and physical activity subscale thresholds, putting him at risk of not returning to work. Given the physical demands of both his truck-driving job and 'hobby farming', it seemed reasonable for him to have such high FABQ scores. In addition, Dean experienced persistent pain after surgery, which he reported as being contrary to his expectations. With unexpected pain after surgery, fear increases (Louw et al., 2009; Toyone et al., 2005). It has been shown that surgeons often provide patients with an expectation of little to no pain after surgery (Louw et al., 2009; Toyone et al., 2005), which seems contrary to current evidence and experience (Louw et al., 2014b). Dean seemingly had good attitudes regarding returning to work and function and appeared highly motivated, yet this 'unexpected' pain may have increased his FABQ scores as evident in his scores. In line with Dean's plan of care, the psychosocial issues would feature as a key issue needing to be addressed because it is well established that pain, fear and pain catastrophization may negatively impact motor control (Moseley and Hodges, 2005, 2006; Moseley et al., 2004).

Reasoning Question:

4. What was your interpretation of Dean's physical examination findings regarding possible sources of 'symptoms' and 'pathology', and likely 'contributing factors' to his activity and participation restrictions?

Answer to Reasoning Question:

Dean's postoperative physical examination revealed limited movement, increased sensitization and positive decompression of the neurovascular structures. Nociceptive contributions, supported by the presence of appropriate, consistent and pain provocative physical impairments, were likely from the following:

• The surgical site/incision
• Altered biomechanics and load on adjacent joints/tissues (spinal levels above and structures below, such as the sacroiliac joints and hips joints)

  Peripheral neuropathic mechanisms were also likely to be contributing:

• Pain from a sensitive peripheral nerve due to sustained compression, chemical irritation and demyelinization
• Reperfusion hyperalgesia likely associated with increased movement and blood flow which may increase nerve sensitization (Butler, 2000)

  In addition, fear-avoidance has been correlated to decreased movement and was likely a significant contributing factor to his limited movement and activity/participation restrictions.

Clinical Reasoning Commentary:

Preoperative neurological deficits and imaging evidence of relevant pathology would have fulfilled contemporary medical criteria for neuropathic pain (Haanpaa et al., 2011; Cruccu et al., 2010; Treede et al., 2008). However, postoperatively, a clinical pattern of 'neuropathic pain mechanical sensitivity' was recognized that is important to inform selection of specific treatment strategies.

As recommended in Chapter 4, assessment of Dean's 'perspectives' (i.e. psychosocial status) has included information obtained through both specific questioning in the patient interview and through the use of validated questionnaires. Although understanding patients' perspectives is important to management (e.g. guiding contextualized therapeutic neuroscience education), questionnaires such as the FABQ provide added quantitative measures with predictive validity for important considerations such as returning to work. Patient perspectives exist along a continuum from positive to negative and are highly individual (Pincus and Morley, 2001). Dean's high FABQ scores were judged 'reasonable', suggesting they may be on the lesser end of a stress continuum and potentially amendable. The judgement that Dean had 'good attitudes regarding returning to work and function and appeared highly motivated' illustrates this important attention to positive perspectives that strengthen the prognosis.

Clinical reasoning from the subjective examination is then continued throughout the physical examination, as evident in previous hypotheses regarding nociceptive and peripheral neuropathic pain types being supported through interpretation of physical examination findings. Possible sources of nociception (e.g. spinal joints, sacroiliac joints, hip joints) and potential contributing factors (e.g. altered biomechanics and load) are hypothesized, and patient perspectives (e.g. Dean's fear-avoidance) are further supported and correlated with decreased physical movement.

Management

After discussion of the examination findings and Dean's specific goals (returning to work and hobby farming), it was decided to approach the management in two phases. The first phase would focus on pain control, with progression to the second phase focusing on motor control and function.

Phase 1: Pain Control

The primary goal of the first phase was to address Dean's persistent pain and his high level of fear avoidance. If his pain and fear of pain could be lessened, along with improved pain-free movements and improved sleep, this should optimize his second phase rehabilitation. To obtain improvements in the neuropathic pain, strategies known to help decrease nerve sensitization were utilized, including therapeutic neuroscience education, range-of-movement exercises, neural tissue mobilization and aerobic exercise.

Phase 2: Motor Control and Function

The plan of care aimed to introduce motor control as soon as Dean's pain, fear and movement capabilities were improving at a satisfactory level. Considering his persistent history of low back pain, high levels of fear and difficulty performing low-level spinal stabilization, it was decided to focus on a more generalized co-contraction of the lumbo-pelvic muscles without undue focus on isolating specific contractions/muscle groups (Louw and Puentedura, 2013).

Treatment

Upon completion of the evaluation, treatment commenced with a brief therapeutic neuroscience education session. It was decided to use a section of a recently developed preoperative neuroscience educational program/booklet to help explain the concept of a hypersensitive nervous system (Louw et al., 2013, 2014a; Louw, 2012) as the reason why Dean still experienced pain after the surgery. To facilitate the learning experience, he was provided with various images, examples and metaphors aimed at explaining the function of acute pain and the concept of sensitization (Table 13.1).

TABLE 13.1		
EXAMPLES, METAPHORS AND IMAGES USED TO EXPLAIN THE FUNCTION OF ACUTE PAIN AND THE CONCEPT OF SENSITIZATION TO THE PATIENT		

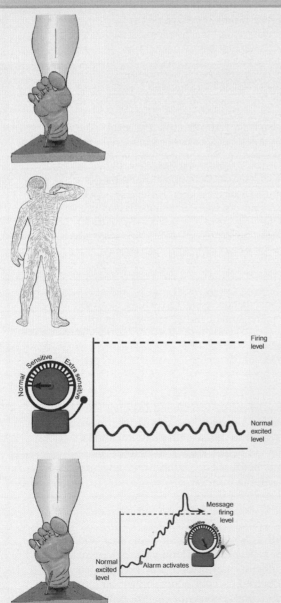

Visual example of a nail in the foot
- If you step on a rusted nail, what would you want to know about it? Why?
  - Get help
  - Tetanus shot
  - Take the nail out
  - Be careful of nails
- How do you know there's a nail in your foot?
- The message travels from the foot to the spinal cord, then on to the brain.
- The brain produces pain to grab your attention and get you to take care of the problem.

Human body nervous system
- This is the body's nervous system.
- It contains 400 individual nerves, totaling 70+ kilometers.
- All the nerves are connected like highways.

Alarm metaphor of the electrical activity of the nervous system
- All 400 nerves have a little bit of electricity flowing through them.
- This is normal and shows you're alive.
- Nerves are like our alarm systems, designed to send us danger messages when there's a threat, such as stepping on a rusted nail.

Activation of the alarm system with the nail in the foot
- So, when you step on a rusted nail, the alarm in your foot goes off.
- The alarm sends a danger message to your brain.
- The brain produces pain to grab your attention and get you to take care of the problem.

TABLE 13.1

EXAMPLES, METAPHORS AND IMAGES USED TO EXPLAIN THE FUNCTION OF ACUTE PAIN AND THE CONCEPT OF SENSITIZATION TO THE PATIENT (Continued)

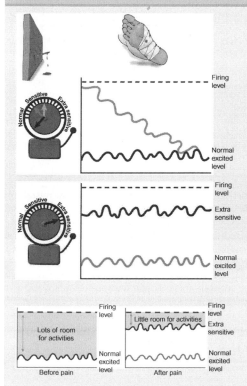

Calming of the alarm system after removal of the threat
- Once you take the nail out, the alarm should go back down.
- The alarm goes down slowly.
- You will likely feel discomfort or pain in the foot for a day or two.
- This is normal.
- Once the alarm is back to its normal level, it's ready for the next danger.

Graphic example of a sensitized nervous system
- This is key: In approximately one in four people, the alarm does not go back down.
- The alarm (nervous system) stays extra-sensitive.
- If pain lasts beyond the normal healing time, it is likely due to an extra-sensitive alarm.
- Your extra-sensitive nervous system may be a big part of your pain, limited movement and sensitivity.

Explanation of sensitization and function
- An extra-sensitive alarm system can impact your life considerably.
- In the days before pain. you had lots of room for movement and activities without causing pain.
- Since you developed pain, it takes far less activity or movement before you experience pain.
- The limited activity and movement is not necessarily due to injury or tissue damage but an extra-sensitive alarm system.

This first neuroscience education session aimed to address Dean's beliefs regarding his problem and his pain that appeared to underpin his fear-avoidance behavior. This was a brief 10-minute session that focused on one message: that a part of Dean's pain experience was likely due to an extra-sensitive nervous system and not injured tissues. The overall aim of the therapeutic neuroscience education sessions was to appropriately pace the education/exposure to information as well. It was thus decided to stop at this point and provide him with the following homework:

1. Continue walking and aim to add 1–2 minutes every other day, not contingent on pain.
2. Review the information provided to him regarding neuroscience education, and upon his return, ask any questions he may have about the information.
3. Think about what factors in his case (life, surgery, job, etc.) would be a reason as to why his 'alarm system' has remained 'extra-sensitive' as opposed to returning to a normal resting level.

Before leaving, Dean was provided with an explanation of the plan of care that had been discussed and agreed upon – continued therapeutic neuroscience education, stabilization improvement over time, range-of-movement exercises and an aerobic exercise program. In line with the surgeon's instructions, he was scheduled to attend physical therapy two times per week for 4 weeks, after which time he would have a follow-up consultation with his surgeon.

Reasoning Question:

5. We know that fear and anxiety are increasingly recognized as contributing to persistent pain and disability in chronic conditions, but what is known about post-surgical conditions?

Answer to Reasoning Question:

Following surgery, patients truly believe they will be pain-free (Louw et al., 2009; Toyone et al., 2005). Emerging evidence points to issues surrounding surgeon education and patient expectations (Louw et al., 2012). With persistent pain and disability after surgery, fear and anxiety increases (Armaghani et al., 2013; Badura-Brzoza et al., 2005). It is well established that the perioperative time is filled with high levels of fear and anxiety. This increased fear and anxiety in turn have been shown to correlate to surgical outcomes (Toyone et al., 2005; Ostelo et al., 2003a, 2003b). This is also evident in the increased activity of pharmaceutical companies investigating the use of drugs associated with calming the nervous system for patients prior to surgery, with the hope of improving outcomes associated with surgery (Yu et al., 2013; Zakkar et al., 2013; Siddiqui et al., 2014). Dean's case can be seen as such – a patient who underwent surgery and even though the mechanical decompression yielded positive results (in SLR, strength, sensation, etc.), he presented with high levels of fear, sensitization of the tissues and uncertainty about his recovery.

Clinical Reasoning Commentary:

Psychosocial factors (e.g. patient perspectives such as maladaptive fear and anxiety) are mistakenly considered by some to only be relevant to chronic pain and disability. The clinical reasoning regarding Dean's perspectives in this case, supported by the research cited in this answer, highlights the adverse impact of fear and anxiety on post-surgical pain and disability. As discussed in Chapters 1, 3 and 4, negative psychosocial factors can contribute to unhelpful patient beliefs, thoughts, emotions and behaviours associated with pain and disability in all patient presentations, from acute to chronic. As such, contemporary musculoskeletal practice necessitates that clinicians develop psychosocial assessment, management and reasoning knowledge and skills, including referral pathways for when adverse psychosocial factors are considered beyond the individual clinician's scope of practice or capabilities.

Appointment 2 (4 Days Later)

Re-assessment

Dean returned 4 days later for his second visit. Subjectively, he reported that after the first session he was somewhat overwhelmed and fatigued, but since then he has felt 'a lot better'. He reported a general feeling of less anxiety, sleeping better and even less pain. Active range-of-movement measurements remained unchanged. Upon questioning, he reported completing his home exercise program of walking, reviewing the neuroscience education booklet and reflecting on factors that may have caused his 'alarm system' to remain extra-sensitive. When asked if he had any questions regarding the pain education, he only had one: 'How do you know this happened with me?' – referring to why his nervous system had remained extra-sensitive.

This was answered as follows:

Great question – there are several ways we can determine this:

1. *You told us you were able to do quite a bit before the pain and surgery, for example, driving, sitting, etc. Now, after only a few minutes, the alarm system goes off.*
2. *Your physical examination showed us you are very sensitive to movement of your spine and leg. Furthermore, remember when I poked around the knee and ankle? Those are nerves, and they are quite sensitive. It is also important to realize that tissues heal and that the sensitivity of the tissue is likely due to a sensitive alarm system versus damaged tissue.*
3. *Pregabalin (Lyrica™) is a medicine designed to calm nerves down. It is likely that some of the improvement since your surgery has been due to this, and the treatment we have planned should further help calm the sensitivity in your nerves.*

The next step was to review the factors he identified in keeping his tissues sensitive. Dean revealed that he had thought about it but had struggled to come up with anything except being worried about his ability to return to his job. At this point the concept of alarm-system activation, briefly explained at the first visit, was reviewed again. In addition, the most common factors (yellow flags) (Kendall et al., 1997; Kendall and Watson, 2000) associated with persistent low back pain (persistent pain, fear, job issues, various explanations

TABLE 13.2

THE MOST COMMON FACTORS (YELLOW FLAGS) ASSOCIATED WITH PERSISTENT LOW BACK PAIN

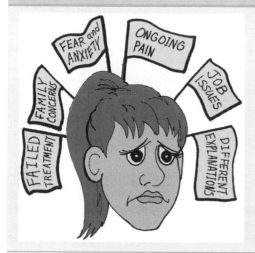

Biopsychosocial yellow flags increasing sensitization of the nervous system

- Why did your alarm system stay extra-sensitive?
- Everything you have gone through during your pain experience has kept the alarm system extra-sensitive. For example:
  - Dealing with pain every day adds stress and can cause issues at home or work.
  - Treatments are not working; otherwise, you would not be here.
  - You've been given several different explanations for your pain, which causes confusion.
- As long as you are stressed, confused, afraid, etc., your alarm is likely to remain extra-sensitive.

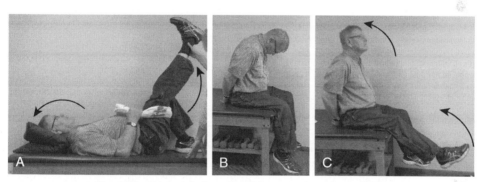

Fig. 13.5 (A) Straight leg raise slider. (B and C) Slump slider.

for pain, etc.) were discussed and applied to his situation (Table 13.2). Dean acknowledged that this made perfect sense and that he could now see why he had become so sensitive. It was decided to conclude this visit's neuroscience education at this point (after 10 minutes) to allow time to add the range-of-movement exercises and not overwhelm him with too much information.

The remainder of this second session consisted of a variety of range of movement exercises for the spine and hips as per the plan of care, as well as neurodynamic sliders (SLR and slump) (Coppieters and Butler, 2007). This included the following exercises in supine lying:

- Trunk rotations with knees bent
- Single-knee-to-chest stretches
- Double-knee-to-chest stretches
- Piriformis muscle stretches (hip flexion/adduction with external rotation)
- SLR sliders (see Fig. 13.5)

Dean was advised to perform all stretches to the point of feeling a strong stretch or even mild discomfort (which was expected). Instruction additionally utilized the neuroscience education concept of sensitization versus tissue injury, encouraging Dean to realize that some discomfort was likely due to a sensitive nervous system and that tissue injury would not occur.

Upon completion of the visit, Dean's home exercise program was reviewed, with his walking increased by 1–2 minutes every other day and the spine, hip and slider exercises to be performed three times per day. Again, he was also asked to think about the neuroscience education material and return with any questions.

Appointment 3 (4 Days Later)
Re-assessment and Treatment

Subjective re-assessment revealed that Dean had further reductions in both his pain and anxiety and had followed all his home exercises without any problems. He still reported intermittent issues with sleeping comfortably at night. On physical re assessment, his spinal range of movement remained unchanged, but his right SLR improved considerably from 45 degrees to 55 degrees, with a subjective report of less pain.

Dean had no specific questions and felt he had a 'good understanding' of what was going on with his problem. To test the depth of his understanding, he was asked to summarize verbally why he was experiencing pain. In doing so, he was able to integrate key elements of the neuroscience education provided to date with only minor corrections required. Prior to reviewing and progressing his range-of-movement exercises, Dean was given his next neuroscience education homework of summarizing in 2–3 sentences his new understanding of his postoperative pain and then reviewing and memorizing that explanation. The aim was for him to develop a concise, accurate understanding of, or mantra for, his pain experience.

Next, Dean's home exercises were reviewed to ensure he was performing the tasks as instructed. Because his SLR was improving, only one additional exercise was added: slump sliders in sitting (Fig. 13.5).

Appointment 4 (1 Week Later)
Re-assessment

Dean returned for his fourth visit reporting overall decreased pain and improved walking. This was also the first time he reported a definite increase in sleep duration and less waking at night to find a comfortable position. He was now walking up to 40 minutes twice a day; however, he did report some pain toward the end of the walking sessions and being very sore afterward and even later in the day. He had no questions or concerns regarding his home exercises. His physical tests revealed a right SLR of 55 degrees and active lumbar flexion improved to within normal limits. Side flexion and extension remained unchanged.

Dean was then asked to verbalize his understanding of his pain experience that he had memorized:

A few months ago I hurt my back. The nerves in the area woke up like an alarm system to protect me and guide me to seek help. Ultimately I had surgery to correct some tissue issues. The surgery was a success. The nerves in my back and leg, however, have remained extra-sensitive to protect me. This is normal and a big part of why I still feel pain in the back and leg after surgery. I am now attending therapy to get better and help calm the sensitive nerves down.

Dean was complimented on his good understanding, and the plan for progressing with the neuroscience education was then discussed.

Treatment

The aim was to build on the previous neuroscience education sessions by reviewing some concepts and expanding Dean's understanding of strategies that could be used to further calm his sensitive nerves. As with the other neuroscience education sessions, examples, metaphors and images were used to facilitate the learning process. The key points discussed and images used are outlined in Table 13.3.

TABLE 13.3

EXAMPLES, METAPHORS AND IMAGES TO FACILITATE UNDERSTANDING OF STRATEGIES THAT CAN BE USED TO CALM THE NERVOUS SYSTEM

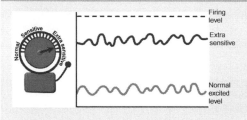

Extra-sensitive alarm system
- When you have an injury, or the brain thinks there's a threat, the body's alarm system (nervous system) wakes up.
- After the threat is removed, the system usually calms back down.
- In one in four people, the alarm system does not return to the normal resting place, but remains extra sensitive. This is usually due to:
  -Fear
  -Ongoing pain
  -Failed treatments
  -Different explanations for pain
  -Various stressors

This is not uncommon and is intended to protect you.

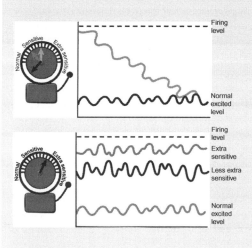

Calming of the nervous system
- The question now is, How do we calm the nervous system?
- How do we get it back to the normal resting level?
- The answer is that you've already started the recovery process.

Graphic depiction of desensitizing the nervous system
- Education is therapy.
- If you understand that a significant part of your pain is likely due to an extra-sensitive nervous system, your alarm system starts to calm down.
- As you learn about your pain today, your brain will see less of a threat, and your nervous system will start to calm down.
- As the system calms down, pain actually eases.
- Remember that it will not suddenly return to normal; it's a complicated alarm system and will go down little by little to keep protecting you.

Calming effect of moderate aerobic exercise on a sensitive nervous system
- Exercise will also help calm your nervous system.
- Remember in school when you were stressed while studying for a big test? What was the best thing to do? Go for a run or bike ride. After some exercise, you felt calm and more relaxed.
- Blood and oxygen calm the nerves. Easy, gentle aerobic exercise pumps blood and oxygen around the nerves, which helps calm them down.
- No need to run marathons or climb mountains:
  -A brisk walk 4–5 times per week for 20–30 minutes is more than enough.

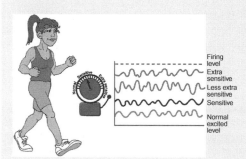

Continued on following page

TABLE 13.3

EXAMPLES, METAPHORS AND IMAGES TO FACILITATE UNDERSTANDING OF STRATEGIES THAT CAN BE USED TO CALM THE NERVOUS SYSTEM (Continued)

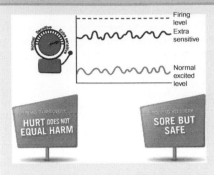

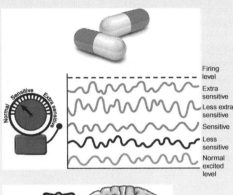

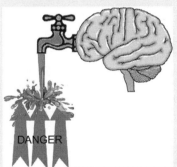

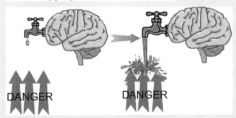

Mantras associated with a sensitized nervous system

- Many people in pain are afraid of exercise because they think exercise causes pain and pain means injury.
- Let's clear up some common misconceptions:
  - Hurt does not equal harm.
  - You may be sore, but you are safe.
  - Understand that your alarm system is extra-sensitive, and when you move or exercise, the alarm is merely telling you that your body is moving – nothing is being injured.
  - Pain that is understood and expected to some degree is not a threat and will actually decrease and eventually go away.
  - Think of the soreness you feel after a good workout.

Example of pharmaceutical effect on desensitizing the nervous system

- The third way we can help calm nerves down is using medicine.
- All questions about your medicine should be directed to your doctor.
- If your extra-sensitive alarm system limits your movement, exercise and therapy, these medications may help kick-start your progress.
- Over time, medicine should be tapered and ceased with the help of your doctor.

Endogenous mechanisms' effect on nociception depicted as a 'wet brain'

- Did you know the brain produces pain medicine as well?
- The brain has the most powerful drug cabinet in the world; we call this a wet brain.
- A wet brain is filled with lots of healthy drugs that flush down to ease incoming danger messages and the pain experience.

Picture describing the process of enhancing the endogenous mechanisms of the brain

- In people with ongoing pain, the pain medicine in their brain has dried up.
- Why is this? To protect you. The brain takes away the pain medicine to make you more sensitive so that you'll do something about it.
- How do we turn a dry brain into a wet brain?
  - Knowledge – understanding more how pain works and what pain really means
  - Aerobic exercise
  - Sleep
  - Meditation and relaxation
  - Breathing
  - Manual therapy
- There are many things we can do to help you with your pain.

Dean's current presentation of pain toward the end of his walks and the latency of increased pain afterward was considered a risk for him developing a 'boom–bust' pattern of experiencing flare-ups after doing too much, which causes many patients to react by then doing too little. To avoid this, the concept of pacing was introduced (Table 13.4). It was decided to cut all his current walking sessions down to 25–30 minutes (which he said felt really good) and instead add more walks as opposed to increasing duration. By avoiding the 'boom–bust' cycles while continuing tissue conditioning exercises, cognitive restructuring through neuroscience education and appropriate load precautions in his job, it was hoped he would be able to gradually improve his physical capacity while decreasing his central nervous system sensitivity. As he continued to recover, the duration of walking would be revisited.

Due to the lengthy neuroscience education session, it was decided not to add any additional exercises at this time. Dean was asked to think about and review the new information discussed and return with any questions he may have. He was instructed to continue with the current home exercise program and change his walking program as described.

Appointment 5 (1 Week Later)

Re-assessment

Dean reported 'no change' from the last session and once again felt he understood the neuroscience information quite well. His outcome measures were re-administered at this time:

- ODI: 28% (reduced from 50% at initial postoperative visit)
- Numeric Rating Scale
  - Low back: 2/10 (reduced from 3/10 at initial postoperative visit)
  - Leg: 1/10 (reduced from 5/10 at initial postoperative visit)
- FABQ
  - Work subscale: 18 (reduced from 35)
  - Physical Activity subscale: 14 (reduced from 22)

Physical re-assessment revealed the following:

- Right SLR 60 degrees; similar range of movement to left SLR with mild ache in the leg
- Active lumbar flexion within normal limits
- Active lumbar side-bending and extension unchanged

Treatment

Considering Dean's progress (in pain, fear, movement and function), it was decided to initiate spinal stabilization exercises. This was in line with the original plan of care. Given his active movements, aggravating and easing factors and better performance (ability to find his neutral spinal posture and correctly activate his deep stabilizing muscles) in supine lying compared to other positions, it was decided to start spinal stabilization exercises in a supine-lying position with knees bent. Dean was instructed in spinal stabilization as an exercise program aimed at retraining motor control versus strength and also allowing for movement and function. Consistent with the neuroscience education, he was not told he was 'weak' or needed 'strengthening' but rather that these were exercises to help him move and function better. While performing the co-contraction, he was monitored and taught to recognize and avoid any unwanted movements or recruitment patterns (e.g. excessive use of inspiration or loss of lumbo-pelvic control). Once Dean was able to independently perform the co-contractions correctly in supine lying, he was tested on whether he could perform these in sitting while maintaining correct breathing and lumbo-pelvic control. Dean demonstrated sufficient control in sitting to include this in his early-stage exercises. His updated home exercise program now included the following:

- Continually think about the neuroscience education, and if any questions arise, ask them at the next session.

TABLE 13.4

EXAMPLES, METAPHORS AND IMAGES USED TO EXPLAIN THE CONCEPTS OF PACING

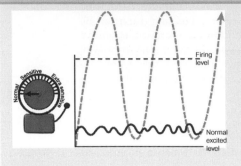

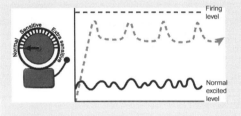

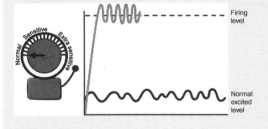

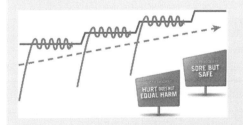

'No-pain, no gain' cycle
- One of the biggest reasons people in pain hurt with exercise or daily tasks is they do too much.
- Movement and activity are important, but you need to pace yourself.
- If you go too hard and crash through the pain, you may be sore for hours or days after the exercise.
- After you recover, you go at it again, paying the same price.
- After this cycle repeats several times, you'll likely get frustrated and give up.
- Pace yourself. A 20-minute brisk walk that feels good with no significant soreness afterward is much better than an hour-long walk that leaves you in pain for a day or two.
- Movement and activity without significant pain will help your system calm down.

'If it hurts, don't do it' cycle
- In the opposite case, many people fear and avoid pain.
- They stop any and all activities short of pain.
- They focus on 'when do I feel pain?', which actually increases their pain.
- This method hinders progress, which will leave them discouraged.
- Over time, it will take less and less activity to trigger the alarm system.

Graded exposure
- So...what should we do?
- Tease it. Nudge it. Touch it.
- Perform a task or exercise up to the point you feel some discomfort.
- Pace yourself.
- Do not be afraid of pain, but respect it.
- Don't stop short, but don't crash right through.
- With your newfound knowledge of how pain works, you won't fear pain, and it will start to ease.
- This allows for gradual increase in activity and exercise.

Graded exposure and pacing
- How do you eat an elephant? One bite at a time.
- The same goes for any exercise program or task.
- Start small.
- Every other day, add a small part.
- Day by day, your time, distance, duration, etc. will increase.
- A 3-minute walk becomes a 4-minute walk, becomes a 5-minute walk, becomes a 5K and eventually becomes the Boston Marathon.

- Continue the walking program to 30 minutes maximum, and if time allows, add short additional walks.
- Continue the home exercises for range of movement and neurodynamics.
- Add spinal stabilization exercises; every 2 hours, do 10 minutes of co-contractions varying between supine lying and sitting, always starting by first finding the neutral lumbar-pelvic position and correct breathing pattern. Dean was also asked to cue himself to practice these frequently by not answering his cell phone unless he first performed a co-contraction of the stabilizing muscles, thus incorporating it into his daily routine.

Reasoning Question:

6. Given the different philosophies and debate regarding motor control re-training, would you briefly outline your approach for patients such as Dean?

Answer to Reasoning Question:

Dean's case highlights our thoughts on pain and spinal stabilization. It is well established that motor control is influenced by pain. We believe, based on the body of evidence, biologically and through clinical experience, that for presentations such as Dean's, pain needs to be controlled and addressed before motor control. For example, it has been shown that high levels of fear and catastrophization associated with pain significantly impact motor control during spinal stabilization exercises. Furthermore, the premotor and motor cortices are both involved in pain processing in the pain neuromatrix, which impacts the execution of motor control. It was thus reasoned that a reduction of pain, and associated fear and catastrophization, prior to focusing extensively on motor control would be a wise clinical move. This does not imply the absence of pain but a progressive lessening of the pain experience. By addressing Dean's understanding of pain and his associated fear avoidance, restoration of motor control will likely be more successful.

Once pain was being addressed with Dean, we incorporated motor control attending to the following:

1. Finding a 'neutral spine' position:
   Similar to the test described in the examination, Dean was shown the task and repeated the task to ensure a comfortable mid-range of movement position was found to commence spinal stabilization exercises.
2. Initiation of the motor control mechanisms:
   Dean was taught a co-contraction of the abdominal and back muscles, ensuring limited pelvic motion while observing for any unwanted contraction of other compensatory muscles or holding his breath. Co-contractions were first performed in a comfortable position (i.e. supine lying with knees bent) and then progressed to other static positions, such as sitting, quadruped and standing. Co-contractions were initially performed for 5 seconds and progressed by increasing co-contractions for longer periods to work on endurance (Richardson et al., 2004; Puentedura et al., 2009), thereby making the exercises time contingent rather than pain contingent. The decision to focus on static positions was aimed at minimizing stress on the surgical level and not excessively increasing the pain experience.
3. Functional (closed-kinetic-chain) exercises and activities:
   Once Dean was able to perform co-contractions in various static positions without any undue increased pain or use of accessory movements/strategies, functional tasks associated with his jobs (truck driving and farming) would then be added, which would likely include the following:
   • Sitting with upper extremity use
   • Lunges
   • Squats
   • Trunk movements
   • Lifting

In line with the current controversies in regard to spinal stabilization, the co-contractions taught were general in approach rather than specifically focusing on a selected muscle/muscle group.

Clinical Reasoning Commentary:

The therapeutic neuroscience education used with Dean is consistent with current practice guidelines (Nijs et al., 2011). Facilitating more adaptive pain beliefs reduces fear avoidance and helped prepare Dean for progression to a spinal stabilization program. Although the stabilizing exercises taught follow existing motor control theory and evidence, they also follow contemporary theory on cognition-targeted motor control training (e.g. Nijs et al., 2014). Throughout the course of management, it is also clear that Dean was fully 'on board' with respect to understanding the rationale and aims of the various interventions and was an active collaborator in his recovery rather than simply a passive recipient of therapy/treatment. He is successfully being provided with the understandings and tools to cope and increasingly self-manage his problem, auguring well for his functional recovery and ongoing prognosis.

Appointments 6, 7 and 8 (Over the following 2 Weeks)

In the subsequent sessions, Dean continued to improve in regard to pain, function and range of movement. Spinal stabilization was progressed to include more closed-kinetic-chain activities to promote function. A key emphasis of his stabilization program now was increasing the duration of the co-contractions to work on endurance. Functional tasks were chosen to mimic his truck-driving job, with the dosage of each of the following functional exercises based on assessment of his baseline capacity to perform the exercise with control:

- Seated with arm use:
  - No weights; various planes
  - Weights; various planes
- Seated with leg use:
  - Moving feet in various directions
- Steps
- Lunges
- Squats
- Lifting

Upon completion of the eighth visit, Dean had reached the end of his prescribed therapy per the surgeon's initial referral. A re-examination was completed to allow the writing of a progress report:

- Low back pain (NRS): 2/10
- Leg pain (NRS): 1/10
- ODI: 18%
- FABQ:
  - Work subscale: 10
  - Physical Activity subscale: 8
- Dean reported being able to sleep through the night. He still experienced most 'soreness' and stiffness in the morning and after sitting > 60 minutes.
- No report of neurological symptoms
- Dean was anxious to return to work. He felt he could drive quite easily. He also thought he would have some issues (as expected) getting in/out of the truck but felt he would be fine.

Appointments 9, 10, 11 and 12 (Over the Following 4 Weeks)

The surgeon was pleased with Dean's progress. Repeat x-ray showed bone consolidation occurring at a satisfactory rate. The surgeon permitted Dean to resume work with a lifting restriction of 15 kg and requested he continue stabilization and functional training once per week for 4 weeks.

The subsequent therapy sessions continued, with the stabilization program focusing on increased weight, endurance and mimicking functional tasks. The home exercise program (range of movement, neural mobilization, stabilization exercises) was maintained to further ease the sensitive nervous system while increasing Dean's functional capacity. With his work schedule, walking was now limited to twice a day for 30 minutes. After 4 weeks, Dean still had 1–2/10 low back pain but described it as 'normal due to sensitivity', and all psychometric measures scored zero. Active lumbar range of movement revealed flexion within normal limits, extension 50% (stiffness > pain), side-bending left and right 75% (stiffness > pain) and SLR of 60 degrees and pain-free bilaterally.

Dean was discharged from further treatment but encouraged to continue with his home program.

Reasoning Question:

7. From your experience and any supporting research, do you think the pre-surgical patient education, particularly pain education, influences the post-surgical pain and disability experience?

Answer to Reasoning Question:

Intuitively, it seems logical. This belief is fueled by the ever-increasing activity surrounding perioperative strategies aimed at reducing pain and disability, including drugs, patient education and relaxation. In a randomized controlled trial (Louw et al., 2014b), we randomly allocated patients getting ready to undergo surgery for radiculopathy (similar to Dean) to either receive preoperative education as usual by the surgeon (usual care) or the surgeon's education and a 30-minute preoperative neuroscience educational session on the neurobiology and neurophysiology of pain. All patients underwent surgery and were tracked for 1 year after surgery in regard to back pain, leg pain, fear avoidance, pain catastrophization, function, pain knowledge, surgical experience and healthcare utilization. At the 1-year outcome, no statistical differences were found in regard to back pain, leg pain, fear avoidance, pain catastrophization, pain knowledge or function. The interesting part, however, was that despite similar pain and dysfunction, the patients who received preoperative pain science education reported significantly more successful surgical experiences on various levels. In addition, these patients spent 45% less on health care (medical tests and treatments) in the first year after surgery, despite having similar pain and disability, indicating a true behavioural change.

Patients are interested in pain and are able to understand the neuroscience of pain, and this premise extends to spinal surgery patients.

Clinical Reasoning Commentary:

Clinical reasoning regarding treatment progression in the clinic and research investigating the effectiveness of therapeutic interventions both require a broad spectrum of outcome measures to detect change and inform practice. Although patient education has historically always been a part of musculoskeletal clinical management, it perhaps has not always been used as a genuine therapeutic intervention capable of effecting change. Therapeutic education addressing patient cognitions (e.g. understanding, attributions, threat appraisal, self-efficacy), health and pain behaviours (e.g. activity avoidance or excess, medication use, lifestyle modification), exercise (e.g. postural, control of movement, mobility, pain management) and ergonomics/technique (for home, work, sport, etc.) should be underpinned by explicit reasoning informing the choice and manner of delivery of educational messages (i.e. 'reasoning about teaching' as discussed in Chapter 1). Like all clinical practice, it should be guided by research (e.g. regarding learning and pain/lifestyle education), then contextually applied to the individual patient with re-assessment of learning and other measures of change.

REFERENCES

Armaghani, S.J., Lee, D.S., Bible, J.E., Archer, K.R., Shau, D.N., Kay, H., et al., 2013. Preoperative narcotic use and its relation to depression and anxiety in patients undergoing spine surgery. Spine 38, 2196–2200.

Backstrom, K.M., Whitman, J.M., Flynn, T.W., 2011. Lumbar spinal stenosis-diagnosis and management of the aging spine. Man. Ther. 16, 308–317.

Badura-Brzoza, K., Matysiakiewicz, J., Piegza, M., Rycerski, W., Hese, R.T., 2005. [Sociodemographic data and their influence on anxiety and depression in patients after spine surgery]. Przegl. Lek. 62, 1380–1383.

Burton, A.K., Waddell, G., Tillotson, K.M., Summerton, N., 1999. Information and advice to patients with back pain can have a positive effect. A randomized controlled trial of a novel educational booklet in primary care. Spine 24, 2484–2491.

Butler, D.S., 2000. The Sensitive Nervous System, Adelaide, NOI Group.

Coppieters, M.W., Butler, D.S., 2007. Do 'sliders' slide and 'tensioners' tension? An analysis of neurodynamic techniques and considerations regarding their application. Man. Ther. 13 (3), 213–221.

Cruccu, G., Sommer, C., Anand, P., Attal, N., Baron, R., Garcia-Larrea, L., et al., 2010. EFNS guidelines on neuropathic pain assessment: revised 2009. Eur. J. Neurol. 17, 1010–1018.

Fritz, J.M., George, S.Z., 2002. Identifying psychosocial variables in patients with acute work-related low back pain: the importance of fear-avoidance beliefs. Phys. Ther. 82, 973–983.

Grotle, M., Vollestad, N.K., Brox, J.I., 2006. Screening for yellow flags in first-time acute low back pain: reliability and validity of a Norwegian version of the Acute Low Back Pain Screening Questionnaire. Clin. J. Pain 22, 458–467.

Haanpaa, M., Attal, N., Backonja, M., Baron, R., Bennett, M., Bouhassira, D., et al., 2011. NeuPSIG guidelines on neuropathic pain assessment. Pain 152, 14–27.

Hakkinen, A., Kautiainen, H., Jarvenpaa, S., Arkela-Kautiainen, M., Ylinen, J., 2007. Changes in the total Oswestry Index and its ten items in females and males pre- and post-surgery for lumbar disc herniation: a 1-year follow-up. Eur. Spine J. 16, 347–352.

Kendall, N., Watson, P., 2000. Identifying psychosocial yellow flags and modifying management. In: Gifford, L.S. (Ed.), Topical Issues in Pain 2. CNS Press, Falmouth.

Kendall, N.A.S., Linton, S.J., Main, C.J., 1997. Guide to assessing psychosocial yellow flags in acute low back pain: risk factors for long term disability and work loss, Wellington, Accident Rehabilitation & Compensation Insurance Corporation of New Zealand and the National Health Committee.

Kovacs, F.M., Urrutia, G., Alarcon, J.D., 2011. Surgery versus conservative treatment for symptomatic lumbar spinal stenosis: a systematic review of randomized controlled trials. Spine 36, E1335–E1351.

Louw, A., 2012. Your Nerves Are Having Back Surgery. OPTP, Minneapolis.

Louw, A., Butler, D.S., Diener, I., Puentedura, E.J., 2012. Preoperative education for lumbar radiculopathy: a Survey of US Spine Surgeons. Int. J. Spine Surg. 6, 130–139.

Louw, A., Butler, D.S., Diener, I., Puentedura, E.J., 2013. Development of a preoperative neuroscience educational program for patients with lumbar radiculopathy. Am J. Phys. Med. Rehabil 92, 446–452.

Louw, A., Diener, I., Landers, M.R., Puentedura, E.J., 2014a. Preoperative pain neuroscience education for lumbar radiculopathy: a multi-center randomized controlled trial with one-year follow-up. Spine 39 (18), 1449–1457.

Louw, A., Diener, I., Landers, M.R., Puentedura, E.J., 2014b. Preoperative pain neuroscience education for lumbar radiculopathy: a multicenter randomized controlled trial with 1-year follow-up. Spine 39, 1449–1457.

Louw, A., Louw, Q., Crous, L.C.C., 2009. Preoperative Education for Lumbar Surgery for Radiculopathy. S Afr. J. Physiother. 65, 3–8.

Louw, A., Puentedura, E.J., 2013. Therapeutic Neuroscience Education. OPTP, Minneapolis, MN.

Lundborg, G., Dahlin, L.B., 1996. Anatomy, function, and pathophysiology of peripheral nerves and nerve compression. Hand Clin. 12, 185–193.

Lundborg, G., Myers, R., Powell, H., 1983. Nerve compression injury and increased endoneurial fluid pressure: a 'miniature compartment syndrome'. J. Neurol. Neurosurg. Psychiatry 46, 1119–1124.

Maitland, G., Hengeveld, E., Banks, K., English, K., 2005. Maitland's Vertebral Manipulation. Elsevier, London.

Moseley, G.L., Hodges, P.W., 2005. Are the changes in postural control associated with low back pain caused by pain interference? Clin. J. Pain 21, 323–329.

Moseley, G.L., Hodges, P.W., 2006. Reduced variability of postural strategy prevents normalization of motor changes induced by back pain: a risk factor for chronic trouble? Behav. Neurosci. 120, 474–476.

Moseley, G.L., Nicholas, M.K., Hodges, P.W., 2004. Pain differs from non-painful attention-demanding or stressful tasks in its effect on postural control patterns of trunk muscles. Exp. Brain Res. 156, 64–71.

Nijs, J., Paul van Wilgen, C., Van Oosterwijck, J., et al., 2011. How to explain central sensitization to patients with 'unexplained' chronic musculoskeletal pain: practice guidelines. Man. Ther. 16, 413–418.

Nijs, J., Meeus, M., Cagnie, B., 2014. A modern neuroscience approach to chronic spinal pain: combining pain neuroscience education with cognition-targeted motor control training. Phys. Ther. 94, 730–738.

Ostelo, R.W., De Vet, H.C., Berfelo, M.W., Kerckhoffs, M.R., Vlaeyen, J.W., Wolters, P.M., et al., 2003a. Effectiveness of behavioral graded activity after first-time lumbar disc surgery: short term results of a randomized controlled trial. Eur. Spine J. 12, 637–644.

Ostelo, R.W., De Vet, H.C., Vlaeyen, J.W., Kerckhoffs, M.R., Berfelo, W.M., Wolters, P.M., et al., 2003b. Behavioral graded activity following first-time lumbar disc surgery: 1-year results of a randomized clinical trial. Spine 28, 1757–1765.

Ostelo, R.W., De Vet, H.C., Waddell, G., Kerckhoffs, M.R., Leffers, P., Van Tulder, M., 2003c. Rehabilitation following first-time lumbar disc surgery: a systematic review within the framework of the Cochrane Collaboration. Spine 28, 209–218.

Pincus, T., Morley, S., 2001. Cognitive-processing bias in chronic pain: a review and integration. Psychol. Bull. 127, 599–617.

Piperno, M., Hellio Le Graverand, M.P., Reboul, P., Mathieu, P., Tron, A.M., Perrin, G., et al., 1997. Phospholipase A2 activity in herniated lumbar discs. Clinical correlations and inhibition by piroxicam. Spine 22, 2061–2065.

Puentedura, E.J., Brooksby, C.L., Wallmann, H.W., Landers, M.R., 2009. Rehabilitation following lumbosacral percutaneous nucleoplasty: a case report. J. Orthop. Sports Phys. Ther. 40, 214–224.

Richardson, C., Hodges, P., Hides, J., 2004. Therapeutic Exercise For Lumbopelvic Stabilization. Churchill Livingstone, London.

Saal, J.S., Franson, R.C., Dobrow, R., Al, E., 1990. High levels of inflammatory phospholipase A2 activity in lumbar disc herniation. Spine 15, 674–678.

Siddiqui, N.T., Fischer, H., Guerina, L., Friedman, Z., 2014. Effect of a preoperative gabapentin on postoperative analgesia in patients with inflammatory bowel disease following major bowel surgery: a randomized, placebo-controlled trial. Pain Pract. 14, 132–139.

Smart, K.M., Blake, C., Staines, A., Doody, C., 2009. Clinical indicators of 'nociceptive', 'peripheral neuropathic' and 'central' mechanisms of musculoskeletal pain. A Delphi survey of expert clinicians. Man. Ther. 15, 80–87.

Smart, K.M., Blake, C., Staines, A., Thacker, M., Doody, C., 2012a. Mechanisms-based classifications of musculoskeletal pain: Part 1 of 3: symptoms and signs of central sensitisation in patients with low back (+/-leg) pain. Man. Ther. 17, 336–344.

Smart, K.M., Blake, C., Staines, A., Thacker, M., Doody, C., 2012b. Mechanisms-based classifications of musculoskeletal pain: Part 2 of 3: symptoms and signs of peripheral neuropathic pain in patients with low back (+/-leg) pain. Man. Ther. 17, 345–351.

Smart, K.M., Blake, C., Staines, A., Thacker, M., Doody, C., 2012c. Mechanisms-based classifications of musculoskeletal pain: Part 3 of 3: symptoms and signs of nociceptive pain in patients with low back (+/-leg) pain. Man. Ther. 17, 352–357.

Toyone, T., Tanaka, T., Kato, D., Kaneyama, R., Otsuka, M., 2005. Patients' expectations and satisfaction in lumbar spine surgery. Spine 30, 2689–2694.

Tran De, Q.H., Duong, S., Finlayson, R.J., 2010. Lumbar spinal stenosis: a brief review of the nonsurgical management. Can. J. Anaesth. 57, 694–703.

Treede, R.D., Jensen, T.S., Campbell, J.N., Cruccu, G., Dostrovsky, J.O., Griffin, J.W., et al., 2008. Neuropathic pain: redefinition and a grading system for clinical and research purposes. Neurology 70, 1630–1635.

Ulrich, J.A., Liebenberg, E.C., Thuillier, D.U., Lotz, J.C., 2007. ISSLS prize winner: repeated disc injury causes persistent inflammation. Spine 32, 2812–2819.

Walsh, J., Hall, T., 2009a. Reliability, validity and diagnostic accuracy of palpation of the sciatic, tibial and common peroneal nerves in the examination of low back related leg pain. Man. Ther. 14, 623–629.

Walsh, J., Hall, T., 2009b. Reliability, validity and diagnostic accuracy of palpation of the sciatic, tibial and common peroneal nerves in the examination of low back related leg pain. Man. Ther. 14, 623–629.

Yu, L., Ran, B., Li, M., Shi, Z., 2013. Gabapentin and pregabalin in the management of postoperative pain after lumbar spinal surgery: a systematic review and meta-analysis. Spine 38, 1947–1952.

Zakkar, M., Frazer, S., Hunt, I., 2013. Is there a role for gabapentin in preventing or treating pain following thoracic surgery? Interact. Cardiovasc. Thorac. Surg. 17, 716–719.

14

A Lawyer With Whiplash

Gwendolen Jull • Michele Sterling •
Darren A. Rivett • Mark A. Jones

Patient Interview

Emma K was a 38-year-old woman who was referred to physiotherapy by her general practitioner (GP) for management of neck pain as a result of a motor vehicle crash 10 days earlier. She had no previous history of neck pain or headache. Emma was a partner in a law practice and worked full time. She was involved in various fields of law, but her predominant work was in wills and conveyancing. She was married with two children (aged 11 and 9 years).

Ten days earlier, after dropping the children off at school on her way to work, she was stationary at red lights. She heard screeching of brakes the instant before her car was hit from the rear. She felt the jolt and immediately had a sudden twinge of pain in her neck. Her car had been hit directly in the rear, and the bumper bar and boot had crushed. The police attended the accident, her car was towed to a repair shop and the police advised her to have her neck checked as a precaution. Emma felt that her neck was not too bad, so she caught a taxi to work. However, during the day, her neck pain increased progressively, and by the day's end, a headache had developed. She went home, took two Nurofen (over-the-counter anti-inflammatory) and went to bed early.

Emma had a restless night with neck pain and woke up with her neck stiff and very sore. Her husband did the school run, and Emma made an appointment with her GP. Her GP advised her to have the day off work, ordered an x-ray and asked her to return with the x-ray later in the afternoon. The x-ray revealed no lesion, and the GP diagnosed a soft tissue injury to the neck. He advised her to take Panadol Osteo (paracetamol) routinely for a few days for the pain (two tablets, three times per day); he advised that she could continue to work but should take it easy for a few days. He advised her to see him in a week if the neck pain had not subsided.

Emma returned to the GP after the week because her neck pain was not settling and, if anything, was getting worse. He prescribed Tramadol (opioid pain medication) for her pain, (two tablets, 6 hourly) and referred her for physiotherapy.

At the time of her initial consultation, Emma felt pain generally in the neck region but mostly on the right side of her neck, which, when it built up, developed into a headache (Fig. 14.1). She rated the overall neck pain intensity as around 6/10 on a visual analogue scale (VAS), with headache intensity about the same. Emma also noticed that she felt a little light-headed and unsteady when the headaches were bad.

Emma's neck pain was constant but fluctuated. It built up if she sat at the computer at work for too long (30–60 min) without moving. The pain could be sharp (VAS 8/10) if she turned her head without thinking. The sharp pain settled in a few minutes, but once the overall pain had built up, it was difficult to get relief. Headaches usually developed in the afternoon as the neck pain built up. The light-headedness was intermittent, occurring only when the headache was bad. It only lasted a few seconds or minutes, but it was bothersome. She obtained pain relief by taking medication and lying down with a hot pack for 30 minutes when she got home. She thought the Tramadol was helping. She reported no noticeable side effects, and when asked, she did not think her symptoms of light-headedness were linked with her taking Tramadol; rather, she felt this when she had a headache. She could still function at work but was anxious about her productivity because she knew she was not functioning very efficiently. The firm's paralegal had been very supportive this last week, but she could not expect that level of support indefinitely.

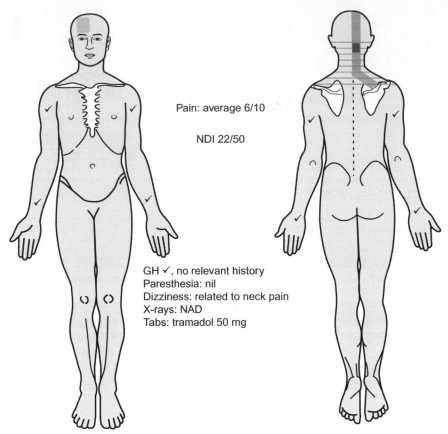

Pain: average 6/10

NDI 22/50

GH ✓, no relevant history
Paresthesia: nil
Dizziness: related to neck pain
X-rays: NAD
Tabs: tramadol 50 mg

Fig. 14.1 Body chart depicting symptoms. *GH,* Good health; *NAD,* no apparent disorder; *NDI,* Neck Disability Index; *Tabs,* tablets.

At home, Emma was still cooking, but the previous weekend, her husband and children had cleaned the house and had done the washing and shopping. Sleep was still disturbed but getting a little better. Emma slept on her side with two soft pillows. Emma said she had experienced a few dreams about the accident, and the sound of screeching brakes would wake her. Without a car, she was catching a taxi to work and requested that the driver take a specific route that avoided the intersection of the crash.

Emma was otherwise in good health, with, apart from childbirth, no other medical or surgical history. She did not participate in any formal sport but did walk with friends for exercise three times per week. Weekends were busy with the children's, household and social activities.

She had no experience with whiplash injuries, personally or professionally, but had heard they could be problematic for some people. She had not as yet lodged a claim for third-party insurance but was intending to do so to ensure that costs for the car and her treatment were covered. Emma's scores at the initial consultation are shown in Table 14.1.

Emma was screened at being of a medium risk of poor recovery, based on the Whiplash Clinical Prediction Rule (NDI score 22/50; Age: 38; Hyperarousal Symptoms 3/6 (Ritchie et al., 2015, 2013), www.recover.edu.au/recover-clinical/).

Reasoning Question:

1. After the patient interview, what was your hypothesis about the source(s) of the symptoms? What evidence supported or negated your hypothesis?

Answer to Reasoning Question:

The source of nociception was most likely in the upper cervical segments, given the area of pain as well as the referral of pain into the head. The difficulty with turning the head would suggest C1–C2

TABLE 14.1

THE PATIENT'S NECK DISABILITY INDEX AND PATIENT-SPECIFIC FUNCTIONAL SCALE SCORES AT THE INITIAL CONSULTATION

Neck Disability Index (NDI) score	22/50
Patient Specific Functional Scale (PSFS)	
Turning her head	1
Computer work (60 min)	3
Cooking (lifting pots)	5
Walking with friends	0

dysfunction. Symptoms of light-headedness and unsteadiness are more frequently (but not uniquely) associated with an upper cervical problem, and in Emma's case, they appeared to have a direct relationship to her neck pain and headache (Treleaven, 2017). They could also have a vestibular origin or could be a side effect of a concussion, although the latter was unlikely in Emma's case because she reported no knock to her head or unconsciousness at the time of the car crash.

Symptoms of dizziness and vertigo are common side effects of Tramadol use, and this could negate the hypothesis of these symptoms being a result of upper cervical spine injury. Emma was questioned about the temporal relationship of these symptoms and taking Tramadol, and there appeared to be no relationship.

Reasoning Question:

2. What were your thoughts regarding the 'pain type' (nociceptive, neuropathic or nociplastic)? How did the acute nature of the presentation in this case influence your hypothesis of the pain type involved?

Answer to Reasoning Question:

As a primary hypothesis, the neck pain was reasoned to be nociceptive, most likely with an inflammatory component (sharp pain on movement on a background of a constant aching pain). The acute nature of the pain, response to movement and posture/activity and its relationship to an injury 8 days ago guided this hypothesis. Nevertheless, the possibility that the pain could be neuropathic (high pain, irritability, constant pain, not sleeping) with involvement of the C2 nerve also had to be considered.

The headache might be reflective of CNS sensitization. Some degree of central sensitization would be expected in the acute-injury stage due to the initial excitation and sensitization of nociceptors in the cervical spine (Graven-Nielsen and Arendt-Nielsen, 2010). In Emma's case, this did not appear to be nociplastic because her pain was quite localized, and she did not demonstrate widespread hyperalgesia and pain, features proposed to be indicative of more maladaptive spreading central sensitization (Graven-Nielsen and Arendt-Nielsen, 2010). The temporal relationship of headache onset with neck injury and headache aggravation associated with pain was suggestive of a cervicogenic headache. Nevertheless, there is evidence that a whiplash injury can also trigger the onset of migraine and tension-type headaches (Drottning et al., 2002). Regardless of the headache type, all have been associated with CNS sensitization. The presence of allodynia (pain with a normally innocuous stimulus) in the physical examination would also indicate the presence of central sensitization.

Reasoning Question:

3. Was there anything in the patient interview that raised concerns about the prognosis for this patient?

Answer to Reasoning Question:

There were some features of Emma's presentation which might suggest the possibility of a poorer prognosis. These included the higher neck pain (6/10) and Neck Disability Index (NDI) scores (22/50). She was also screened at medium risk of a poorer recovery based on the Whiplash Clinical Prediction Rule. In addition, there were other signs, albeit with lesser evidence, suggestive of a poorer prognosis: immediate onset of pain and an early onset of headache and light-headedness symptoms. Emma was also experiencing some symptoms of post-traumatic stress (intrusion – dreams about the accident, wakes up with the sound of screeching brakes; avoidance – requesting the taxi driver to avoid the site of the car crash), but hyperarousal symptoms were low. The presence of these symptoms can be predictive of poor recovery (Sterling et al., 2012) and are common after a motor vehicle collision (MVC), but in most people, they resolve (Sterling et al., 2003). For Emma, these symptoms would be monitored during her physiotherapy treatment. On a positive side, there was no evidence of cold hyperalgesia, which may be associated with a poorer prognosis (Goldsmith et al., 2012).

Continued on following page

Clinical Reasoning Commentary:

As illustrated in this answer and discussed in Chapter 1, it is important to hypothesize about potential 'sources' for all symptoms, not just pain. For example, upper cervical dysfunction, vestibular, intra-cranial, secondary to a concussion and medication side effects are all recognized as potential sources for Emma's light-headedness and unsteadiness. Analysis of the relationship of symptoms temporally through the history and behaviourally through aggravating and easing factors enable preliminary hypotheses regarding potential sources. In this case, recognition of these symptoms as common with upper cervical dysfunction, combined with a direct relationship to Emma's neck pain and headache, support an upper cervical dysfunction source, whereas the specifics of the car crash don't support concussion.

Understanding pain, including types of pain, differences between acute and chronic pain, referred pain and the associated neurophysiology, is essential knowledge to musculoskeletal clinicians because clinical judgment regarding pain type has implications for other reasoning judgments, including precautions in assessment and management, management strategies and prognosis. Although both subjective and physical clinical features of pain types have been reported (see Chapters 1 and 2), as discussed here and in Chapter 2, not all sensitization is 'maladaptive', and biomarkers of nociplastic pain are still not definitive (Curatolo and Arendt-Nielsen, 2015). Nevertheless, recognition of clinical features of sensitization, as with Emma, enables appropriate caution in physical testing and physical management interventions.

Prognosis is a difficult clinical reasoning judgment, yet something every patient wants to know. The Answer to Reasoning Question 3 identifies indicators of poorer prognosis from the subjective examination, including Emma's higher neck pain intensity and neck disability scores (Walton et al., 2013), her immediate onset of pain and early onset headache and light-headedness and her symptoms suggestive of post-traumatic stress, and her Whiplash Clinical Predication Rule score placed her at medium risk of poorer recovery (Ritchie et al., 2013). As discussed in Chapter 1, in addition to research evidence regarding prognosis for different presentation categorizations, at the level of the individual patient, factors to consider throughout the subjective and physical examination and the ongoing management including the following:

- The patient's perspectives and expectations (including readiness, motivation and confidence to make changes)
- External incentives (e.g. return to work) and disincentives (e.g. litigation, lack of employer support)
- Extent of activity/participation restrictions
- Nature of problem (e.g. systemic disorder such as rheumatoid arthritis versus local ligamentous problem such as ankle sprain)
- Extent of 'pathology' and physical impairments
- Social, occupational and economic status
- Dominant pain type present
- Stage of tissue healing
- Irritability of the disorder
- Length of history and progression of disorder
- The patient's general health, age and pre-existing disorders

It is helpful to consider a patient's prognosis by reflecting on the positives and negatives as highlighted in this answer, where the immediate onset of pain and early onset of headache and light-headedness, plus symptoms of post-traumatic stress, are judged to support a poorer prognosis, whereas low hyperarousal symptoms and no evidence of cold hyperalgesia support a better prognosis.

Physical Examination

To respect Emma's pain, it was planned to limit the physical examination to that necessary to gain sufficient information to understand the nature of the disorder and to institute initial treatment.

Posture

Emma sat in a reasonable, upright posture, and postural curves from the lumbopelvic region to head position were unremarkable. Emma was holding her head quite rigidly, with some muscle guarding evident in the right neck extensors. Scapular posture revealed minor downward rotation and anterior tilt of the scapulae bilaterally.

Active Movements

Examination of cervical movements in sitting was curtailed to avoid unnecessary aggravation of pain.

- Flexion: half range with 'pulling' posterior neck
- Rotation (R): 10 degrees; acute pain (R) upper cervical region
- Rotation (L): 25 degrees; acute pain (R) upper cervical region
- Facilitating the spine to an 'ideal' upright posture and positioning the scapulae in a neutral posture had no effect on rotation range or pain.
- Extension: 5–10 degrees; painful, and Emma was reluctant to take her head any further backward.

Sensorimotor Function

Balance

- Narrow stance eyes closed – stepped out after 10 seconds

Joint Position Sense

- Testing delayed – inadequate cervical rotation range

Cervical Movement Sense

- Testing delayed

Eye Movement Control

- Eye follow – no apparent disorder
- Gaze fixation – no apparent disorder in the limited range available; contrary to a positive gaze fixation test, there was slightly improved rotation range and rhythm of movement after testing.
- Smooth pursuit neck torsion test – Testing delayed due to inadequate cervical rotation range

Sensory Testing

Sensitivity to Pressure

- Excessively tender to gentle touch on L and R sides of neck and cervicothoracic region –allodynic (R) and (L) sides
- No general tenderness to touch in arms or legs, L = R

Sensitivity to Cold

- Ice pack applied for 10 seconds over (R) side of neck – pain response 2/10

Neurological Examination

- Not indicated

Examination of Nerve Tissue Movement

- Testing delayed as not a priority

Manual Examination

Passive Physiological Intervertebral Movements (PPIVMs) in Supported Supine Lying

- Marked restriction (spasm and pain) to rotation bilaterally at C1–C2. Restriction, pain and spasm reaction to rotation at C2–C3, although lesser than C1–C2.

Passive Accessory Movement Examination

• Testing delayed

Tests of Neuromuscular Control

Craniocervical Flexion Test

• Formal testing delayed

The pattern of craniocervical flexion movement was taught and practiced in crook lying. Emma was taught to gently hold the craniocervical flexion position.

Re-evaluation of PPIVMs: pain and spasm restricting C1–C2 and C2–C3 rotation movement had reduced slightly.

Neck Extensor Muscle Testing

• Formal testing delayed; plan to incorporate into treatment as tolerated

Scapular Muscle Testing

• Formal testing delayed; plan to incorporate in treatment as a routine

Reasoning Question:

4. Your physical examination included a number of assessments of sensorimotor systems. Do you routinely perform these tests on patients presenting with neck pain after an MVC?

Answer to Reasoning Question:

Yes, the tests are performed routinely in patients following a whiplash injury. The evidence indicates that cervical sensorimotor disturbances are frequently present in whiplash-associated disorders (Treleaven et al., 2016). Light-headedness and unsteadiness are common symptoms of cervical vertigo, especially when directly related to neck pain/headache as Emma described. Tests of sensorimotor control were restricted to balance and some tests of eye movement. Other tests will be performed as cervical range of movement (ROM) improves.

When pain levels are high, as in Emma's case, it is desirous that pain is not provoked in early stages of rehabilitation. Balance training can be performed without risk of aggravating neck pain and thus can be an early component of an active rehabilitation strategy.

Reasoning Question:

5. How did you interpret the findings of the sensorimotor tests with respect to your hypotheses on the source of the symptoms and pain type? Were they consistent with your experience of similar patients?

Answer to Reasoning Question:

Failure in the test of narrow stance after 10 seconds for a person of Emma's age was interpreted as a symptom of altered cervical sensorimotor control. This fits well with the hypothesis of upper cervical segmental dysfunction, noting that the muscles of the upper cervical region have the highest concentration of muscle spindles per gram of muscle of any region in the body. The hypothesis on pain type did not particularly influence the interpretation of cervical sensorimotor dysfunction because sensorimotor dysfunction can occur with any pain type. Interestingly, idiopathic cervical vertigo can occasionally occur without neck pain.

Reasoning Question:

6. Other than being careful not to exacerbate the pain, did you identify any specific precautions or contraindications to treatment?

Answer to Reasoning Question:

The onset of neck pain was as a result of acute trauma; therefore, there are automatic precautions associated with an acute injury. Even though there is some assurance of no fracture from the x-ray report, in this acute phase, it is impossible to determine if there has been any injury which might be associated with, for example, potential instability. Thus, in this early phase, due care is required, and techniques such as high-velocity manipulation are contraindicated.

Reasoning Question:

7. Can you give your thoughts at this stage regarding the diagnosis and your planned management approach?

Answer to Reasoning Question:

The provisional diagnosis was a whiplash injury due to a rear-end MVC. VAS and NDI indicated moderate to severe pain and disability. From a biological perspective, there was pain and spasm at the C1–C2 and C2–C3 segments. It was possible this painfully restricted motion could explain the symptoms of cervicogenic headache. The articular dysfunction and associated reactions in the sub-occipital muscles could explain the cervical vertigo. From a psychosocial perspective, there were some symptoms of post-traumatic stress and some concerns/anxiety about her function at work.

Of concern, there were some indicators of a poor prognosis in Emma's history, for example, high initial pain intensity, high neck disability score, early onset of headache and post-traumatic stress symptoms. The focus of treatment at this early stage was toward educating and assuring Emma, gaining symptomatic relief (neck pain, headaches and light-headed, unsteady feelings) and a graduated return to normal activity. Lifestyle activities and treatment should be non-provocative to respect pain levels and to allow the injury to heal and settle.

Clinical Reasoning Commentary:

Features of cervical vertigo and cervical headache are highlighted in Answers to Reasoning Questions 4 and 6 and linked to physical examination planning. Clinical patterns of musculoskeletal disorders typically include the characteristic symptoms, typical behaviour of symptoms (e.g. aggravating and easing factors) and history (e.g. common mechanism of onset and progression over time). Reasoning regarding the hypothesis category 'precautions and contraindications to physical examination and management' is evident in the judgement to restrict sensorimotor testing to balance assessment and avoid/minimize pain provocation in both the physical examination and early management.

Hypotheses formulated in the subjective examination are 'tested' through the physical examination. This is evident in the Answer to Reasoning Question 4 where the findings of upper cervical dysfunction and impaired balance are judged to support the hypothesis that sensorimotor disturbance secondary to upper cervical dysfunction is the primary source of Emma's vertigo symptoms and balance impairment.

Reasoning Question 5 is aimed to further explore the hypothesis category 'precautions and con-traindications to physical examination and treatment'. Acute trauma and the potential for structural instability are highlighted as key features requiring precaution in the physical examination and con-traindications for high-velocity manipulation. As discussed in Chapter 1, clinical judgment in this hypothesis category is based on a number of factors including the following:

- Presence of symptoms that have known association with more serious pathologies (e.g. cervical arterial dysfunction, spinal cord dysfunction, cancer, etc.)
- Mechanism of onset (e.g. acute trauma)
- Dominant pain type (neuropathic and CNS sensitization typically require more caution in not flaring up symptoms)
- The patient's perspectives (anxious, fearful, angry patients, particularly with negative past medical/ physiotherapy experiences require more caution)
- Severity and irritability of symptoms
- Nature of known pathologies (e.g. rheumatoid arthritis or osteoporosis require caution due to weakened tissues)
- Progression of the presentation (e.g. rapidly worsening problems require more caution)
- Presence of other medical conditions that may masquerade as a musculoskeletal problem or co-exist and require consideration and monitoring so that musculoskeletal interventions do not compromise the patient's other health problems (e.g. cardiac and respiratory conditions)

In Answer to Reasoning Question 6, both physical and psychosocial 'diagnoses' are discussed with reference to findings in Emma's presentation supporting those judgments (hypotheses). Whereas physical diagnostic reasoning is typically prominent in most clinicians' clinical judgments, reasoning regarding patients' psychological status, factors that may have precipitated or contributed to any apparent distress and explicit physiotherapy or other health management strategies to address those factors are often less explicit. In Chapter 3, the influence of stress, coping and social factors on pain and disability is discussed, and Chapter 4 addresses assessment, reasoning and management of psychological factors in musculoskeletal practice. Both the theory in Chapter 3 and the assessment strategies in Chapter 4 are helpful resources for our enhancing psychosocial reasoning in musculoskeletal practice.

Treatment 1
Education and Assurance

A patient-centred care approach was adopted that consisted of three important components: clear communication, the provision of relevant information and patient inclusion in decision-making.

Emma was encouraged to ask any questions about any aspect of the condition that she did not understand. She indicated little knowledge of whiplash; thus, the nature of the injury was explained, and the GP's diagnosis of a soft tissue injury was reinforced and analogies made with a sprain of the ankle. Her questions regarding why x-rays had shown that nothing abnormal had been detected were carefully explained. Emma was assured that normal x-rays indicated that there was no fracture, which was good to know. The potential relationship between headaches, the sensations of light-headedness and unsteadiness and the sprain of the upper cervical region was explained. Deliberate mention was made of her waking hearing the screech of brakes, and Emma was assured that this was an understandable reaction and that it should subside with a little time. Assurance was given that there was usually reasonable recovery from the injury, but given her pain levels, it was important that pain was managed in her work and general lifestyle as well during rehabilitation. At this time, the aim was that activities were not to aggravate pain unduly. 'No pain, no gain' was not applicable in her case at this time, but the need for her to undertake some specific exercises and to continue with the daily activities that she could manage was reinforced.

The approach to physiotherapy management was discussed – to manage pain, to work to restore the neck movement and also to ensure that her muscles resumed their normal function –and to avoid mystifying the whiplash injury, the analogy with the sprained ankle was continued. The light-headed, unsteady feelings and her unsteady balance could be managed with the local treatment to her neck as well as some specific balance exercises. She was advised to take the medication that the GP had given her as prescribed (as long as she was tolerating it) because it was important that pain levels were controlled to encourage healing and gentle activity. Care was taken to include Emma in the decision-making process associated with her physiotherapy management.

Multimodal Management

Treatment initially was 'exploratory in nature' to avoid aggravating the pain. Aims were to reduce pain, encourage neck motion and facilitate muscle function. Due to the allodynia about the neck, it was decided to delay use of any manual therapy.

Movement and Muscle Facilitation

In the first instance, craniocervical flexion was taught and practiced in supine lying with the head supported in a neutral position using the feedback of the slide of the back of the head on the towel to encourage the correct sagittal plane rotation. The exercise was used to facilitate pain-free movement, facilitate the deep neck flexor muscles, maximize the reciprocal relaxation of the extensors to reduce hyperalgesia over the facet joints and mobilize the upper cervical joints in craniocervical flexion and extension. As large an amplitude of movement as possible into extension and flexion was encouraged within the limits of pain to regain movement of the joints and for the exercise to provide maximal painless afferent input into the central nervous system. Emma was also taught to use eye movement to facilitate both flexion and extension. She performed two sets of approximately five repetitions of the movement and achieved an estimated ¾ ROM of craniocervical flexion and extension without pain in the supine position.

Because movement in sitting was limited and guarded, movement was encouraged in a four-point kneeling position. The exercises aimed to facilitate the extensors generally, targeting the sub-occipital rotators and extensors and gently mobilizing the C1–C2 segment. Repetitions were limited, and all movements were to be quite comfortable. Emma was first encouraged to perform a gentle head-nodding action as if saying yes (craniocervical extension and flexion), then, secondly, to gently rotate her head to the left and right as if saying 'no'. She was encouraged to fix her gaze on a spot on the bed between her hands while doing a relaxed head rotation. Emma coped well with both sets of exercises, and they were added to a home program (see *Whiplash Injury Recovery – A Self-Help Guide* for exercise illustrations [Jull and Sterling, 2016]).

Balance

Balance exercise: narrow stance with eyes open for 30 seconds. After a rest, practice in narrow stance with eyes closed.

Posture

Emma was taught to roll her pelvis forward a little to assume a neutral lumbo-pelvic position and to gently place her scapulae in a neutral position by lifting the tips of her shoulder a few millimetres and gently spreading open her anterior chest. The posture was to be held for 10 seconds only. It was presented as an important strategy for frequent use during the day to change neck position, facilitate the deep neck flexors and gain reciprocal relaxation of the upper trapezius/levator scapulae through contraction of lower trapezius. The primary aim of the exercise at this point was not just to 'improve the patient's posture' per se, but more to facilitate movement, to reduce load on joints by change of position and to prevent/relieve tension and pain in the neck/shoulder muscles.

Home and Work Program and Advice

Emma was keen to undertake the exercise program. The home program comprised the craniocervical flexion, upper cervical extension and rotation exercises as well as the balance exercise. The initial dosage was two sets of five repetitions only to be performed twice per day. The importance of the posture exercise was reinforced, and Emma was to aim to correct her posture ideally every 15 minutes, especially while she worked on the computer. She was also advised to stand at least every 30 minutes, to move and change position.

Ways to perform work and household activities to lessen unnecessary strain were discussed and any questions answered. She asked about the use of hot packs at home, as a friend had given her one. She was advised that she could certainly use the hot pack, and safety in use was discussed. The strategy at this point was for Emma to undertake activities as tolerated but to gain a balance between rest and activity for the next several days to assist the pain to settle. She was also given an information booklet about recovery from whiplash (Jull and Sterling, 2016).

Reasoning Question:

8. You spent some time explaining Emma's problem to her using analogies and educating her about self-management. This is clearly an important component in your overall approach. Could you discuss this and strategies you use if the patient presents barriers to self-management?

Answer to Reasoning Question:

A stigma is often attached to a whiplash injury, with suggestions of malingering for financial gain. Malingering is relatively rare and can be easily detected in a physical examination by a skilled clinician. From the patients' perspective, they wish to be listened to, be understood and be assured that their neck pain is acknowledged and validated. When this does not happen, patients can become distressed and worried about their condition, which can have a harmful influence on their recovery. The physical examination and the time spent educating and assuring Emma were to ensure that she felt her neck pain was understood and that she acquired enough information to understand the injury and the way forward in her rehabilitation. Her waking at night dreaming of the accident was also discussed to assure her that this was a very understandable behaviour at this time.

Barriers to self-management could include factors such as low pain self-efficacy or passive coping skills, low mood or other personal reasons. The patient would be encouraged to nominate the barriers he or she perceived to be preventing the undertaking of a home management program. These would be discussed and the patient facilitated to develop strategies to overcome these barriers to enhance compliance. Judicious goal setting led by the patient and facilitated by the clinician, where very specific, achievable and measurable goals are set, can help overcome barriers, as can effective facilitation of the patient's problem-solving abilities. Patients are more likely to engage in any treatment if they feel included and involved in decisions around that treatment.

Reasoning Question:

9. You note a couple of psychosocial issues that had the potential to impact on the prognosis, yet unlike the physical symptoms, you didn't formally assess these. Is that your usual practice?

Continued on following page

Answer to Reasoning Question:

Yes, this is usual practice; that is, patients are not given psychological questionnaires to complete on the first appointment. This is a patient who sustained a physical injury to the neck only 8 days ago and who has been referred to a physiotherapist for management of this musculoskeletal condition. Being requested to complete psychological questionnaires on this first appointment can suggest to the patient that the clinician is thinking that the condition is psychological, and this can destroy trust and the ability to establish a therapeutic patient–clinician relationship.

Furthermore, symptoms as anxiety about getting better and coping with work and home life, fear of movement and post-traumatic stress are very normal emotional responses to the pain and the car crash at this early stage, and these can be discerned by the clinician during the patient interview without having to use questionnaires. An empathetic clinician can assist in helping the patient deal with these emotions, and the evidence indicates that they usually subside as the neck disorder subsides (Jull et al., 2013).

Questionnaires could be considered at a later stage of management if it was thought that particular psychological factors, for example, depression or symptoms of a post-traumatic stress disorder, were affecting recovery. Only after discussion with the patient would the patient be requested to complete the relevant questionnaire(s). The outcome of the questionnaire(s) would be discussed with the patient as a basis for further treatment strategies.

Clinical Reasoning Commentary:

In the Answer to Reasoning Question 7 and in the context of the stigma that can be attached to whiplash injury and implications of malingering, the authors highlight the importance of listening to and understanding patients so that their pain and disability are acknowledged and validated. Within reasoning theory, this relates to the hypothesis category 'patients' perspectives on their experience', incorporating, for example, the following factors:

- Understanding of their problem (including attributions about the cause, beliefs about pain and associated cognitions)
- Response to stressors in their lives and any relationship these have with their clinical presentation
- Effects the problem and any stressors appear to have on their thoughts, feelings, coping, motivation and self-efficacy to participate in management
- Goals and expectations for management

Listening to and acknowledging patients' pain experiences not only validates patients' perspectives, it also contributes to the clinician's evolving understanding of their psychosocial status while facilitating the patient–clinician therapeutic alliance so important to the eventual outcome. The 'empathetic' clinician, as discussed in the Answer to Reasoning Question 8, also strengthens rapport while assisting patients to deal with adverse emotions.

Initial assessment of psychosocial factors is described as occurring within the patient interview, with the recommendation that psychological questionnaires are strategically delayed until later in management. In Chapter 4, 'Assessment, Reasoning and Management of Psychological Factors in Musculoskeletal Practice', the use of psychological questionnaires is discussed, with suggestions on categories of information to screen through the patient interview that assist in understanding 'patient perspectives' and identifying when further assessment via questionnaire might be helpful. Although clinicians need to establish when and how psychosocial screening occurs in their assessment, what is critical to informing psychosocially focussed clinical reasoning is that the assessment is explicit and that assumptions that information not volunteered is not relevant are avoided.

Treatment 2 (4 Days Later)

Re-assessment

Emma reported that neck pain persisted but that, overall, it was possibly a little less (VAS ~5/10), and she felt that she could move a little better. Headaches persisted and still mainly came on in the afternoon at work. They could still make her feel light-headed. She was taking the medication, it was helping and she was not having any side effects. She found that doing the posture exercise at work was helpful, and she estimated that she did it at least twice per hour. Computer work still aggravated her neck pain. In consequence, she had reduced her hours at work a little and finished around 3 p.m., which she thought was helping.

Emma said that if she rested for 30 minutes to an hour with the hot pack when she got home from work, then she could make dinner without too many problems. The family members were supportive, for which she was appreciative. Emma was doing the exercises, and they were not aggravating her neck. She did the one on the bed and the ones on hands and knees after the shower in the morning and after her rest in the afternoon.

Physical Examination

- Rotation (R) 10–15 degrees; painful (R) upper cervical region
- Rotation (L) 45 degrees; painful (R) upper cervical region
- Balance (narrow stance eyes closed): 30 seconds
- Posture correction: performed well

Treatment

Plan: continue to progress slowly to respect pain levels. Manual therapy was added to help relieve pain and address the rotation deficit. A trial of mobilization with movement (C1–C2) alleviated some of the pain in rotation (R). Care was taken with manual handling to ensure that there was as painless manual contact as possible over the painful joints and allodynic posterior neck area. Treatment was limited to two sets of five repetitions of mobilization (to assess any adverse effect in the long term). Rotation (R) reached approximately 30 degrees.

Motion gain was reinforced by practising craniocervical rotation and flexion-extension in four-point kneeling. Cervical extension was tested in an exploratory way in this position. Emma was encouraged to flex her neck by lowering her head to look at her knees and then to curl her head and neck backward while keeping her eyes fixed on a point between her hands. She was able to lift her head back just beyond the neutral position without pain.

The craniocervical flexion exercise was checked. Emma could do the movement reasonably easily without pain. She was taught to hold to craniocervical flexion position, facilitating the hold by keeping her gaze down. She practiced 5-second holds in the first instance. Formal testing with the pressure biofeedback was further delayed because of the allodynia.

Emma practiced balance intermittently at work because it was easy to do when she stood up for relief from computer work. The balance exercise was getting easier; she could now stand for 30 seconds with feet together, eyes closed during most attempts. Thus, the balance was progressed to tandem stance with the eyes open and, as possible, with the eyes closed.

The posture exercise was checked for performance, its importance was reinforced and the home program was reviewed and updated following the day's performance.

Treatment 3 (4 Days Later)

Re-assessment

Emma noted some improvement in neck pain and movement and that afternoon headaches persisted, although the light-headed feeling had possibly decreased (Table 14.2). She was still working reduced hours, which she thought was still necessary. Her general activity was still pretty limited, but things were becoming a little easier to do. She said that she

TABLE 14.2	
THE PATIENT'S SCORES AT THE TREATMENT 3 RE-ASSESSMENT	
Visual analog scale (VAS)	Overall 4–5/10
Neck Disability Index (NDI)	18/50
Patient Specific Functional Scale (PSFS)	
Turning her head	4
Computer work (60 min)	5
Cooking (lifting pots)	7
Walking with friends	0

felt she was coping better now and getting to know the boundaries around doing things but not overdoing them. Her car had been fixed, and she was now driving again to work, although using the mirrors quite extensively. She had not yet started walking with friends as yet but thought she would try in the near future.

Emma was asked about her sleeping and her dreams. She said that sleep was still disturbed and that she still had the dreams about the car crash, but it was not every night now. She admitted that she had not attempted to drive as yet on the route where the crash occurred and was still a bit hesitant to do so.

Physical Examination

- Rotation (R) 25 degrees; pain (R) upper cervical region
- Rotation (L) 60 degrees; pain (R) upper cervical region
- Balance: tandem stance eyes open 30 seconds; eyes closed 15 seconds
- Posture correction √

Treatment

Manual therapy (mobilization with movement [C1–C2]) was repeated. Dosage increased to four sets of five repetitions – respecting the allodynia, which was subsiding. Rotation (R) reached 45 degrees.

Motion gain was again reinforced by practising and checking craniocervical rotation and flexion extension and cervical flexion and extension in four-point kneeling. Cervical extension had improved to approximately 5–10 degrees beyond the neutral position without pain.

Because the allodynia was reducing, the Craniocervical Flexion Test (CCFT) (Jull et al., 2008) was performed with feedback from the pressure biofeedback unit. Emma could perform craniocervical flexion to the fourth level (i.e. 28 mmHg) but found it difficult to hold the contraction on the second level (i.e. 24 mmHg). In consequence, Emma trained endurance at 22 mmHg and used the feedback to feel and learn the sensation of holding the muscle contraction, in preparation for practicing at home without the feedback unit.

Balance: tandem stance was continued with eyes closed – aim to consistently achieve 30 seconds.

Posture exercise: progressed by adding a manoeuvre to gently lengthen the back of the neck as the final component of posture correction. It was explained to Emma that this movement was effective in making the deep neck muscles work.

The home program was reviewed and updated following the day's performance.

Treatment 4 (1 Week Later)

Re-assessment

Emma reported that her neck pain was definitely settling, although persisting (VAS 4/10). Her headaches, although persistent, were lessening, as was the feeling of light-headedness. She had returned to her GP because she had finished the medication. In view of her improvement, he had advised her to change to taking Panadol Osteo and to continue routinely taking two tablets 8 hourly for another week or two. She had started dropping the children off at school again and had started to drive the normal route which took her through the intersection where she had had the crash. She had also resumed her walks with friends but was often a bit sore after the walk, although this was getting better. Emma also reported that she had submitted a claim to the insurance company.

Physical Examination

- Rotation (R) 35 degrees; pain (R) upper cervical region
- Rotation (L) 75 degrees; pain (R) upper cervical region
- Extension 10–15 degrees; pain (R) upper cervical region
- Balance: tandem stance, eyes closed 30 seconds

- Posture correction √
- CCFT: held 24 mmHg for five reps

Because there was now sufficient cervical ROM, testing of sensorimotor function was undertaken.

Joint Position Sense

- Testing in rotation – no apparent disorder (NAD)

Cervical Movement Sense

- Tracing an infinity sign – laser light on head, slow and with inaccuracies

Eye Movement Control

- Smooth pursuit neck torsion test – NAD

Treatment

Manual therapy (mobilization with movement [C1–C2]) repeated, dosage increased to four sets of five repetitions – still respecting the diminishing allodynia. Rotation (R) reached 45 degrees.

Motion gain was again reinforced by practising and checking craniocervical rotation and flexion extension and cervical flexion and extension in four-point kneeling. Cervical extension had improved to approximately 15 degrees beyond the neutral position without pain.

Craniocervical flexion: progressed to hold the CCFT position at 24 mmHg – with feedback and then without feedback in preparation for home practice.

Balance exercises: progressed to tandem stance on a soft surface. Emma was given a laser on loan to practice tracing the infinity sign at home. She was to practice the task while sitting.

The home program was reviewed and updated following the day's performance.

Treatment 5 (1 Week Later)

Re-assessment

Emma reported that her neck pain was continuing to improve, although it was still aggravated by computer work (Table 14.3). Her general activity was increasing, although she was careful not to overdo things. She still had headaches at work, although the feeling of light-headedness was now only very occasional. She was continuing to take Panadol Osteo routinely for work but only took them on weekends if needed. Her family was still helping with the washing and house cleaning, although she was doing more now. Her walks with her friends were becoming easier and enjoyable again. She reported that she was now driving with confidence and had no anxiety. She was no longer having dreams about the accident.

Physical examination:

- Rotation (R) 50 degrees; pain (R) upper cervical region
- Rotation (L) 80 degrees; very slight pain (R) upper cervical region

TABLE 14.3	
THE PATIENT'S SCORES AT THE TREATMENT 5 RE-ASSESSMENT	
Visual analog scale (VAS)	Overall 3/10
Neck Disability Index (NDI)	14/50
Patient Specific Functional Scale (PSFS)	
Turning her head	7
Computer work (60 min)	6
Cooking (lifting pots)	8
Walking with friends	8

- Extension 15–20 degrees; pain (R) upper cervical region
- Allodynia in neck region resolved
- Balance: tandem stance, soft surface, eyes closed 10 seconds – still challenging
- CCFT: held 26 mmHg without fatigue over multiple repetitions

Treatment

Manual therapy: a manual examination was performed, and pain and spasm were noted on postero-anterior glides over (R) C1–C2 to a greater extent than C2–C3. Manual therapy management was progressed to include (R) C1–C2 and C2–C3 postero-anterior glides without pain provocation interspersed with mobilization with movement (C1–C2 and C2–C3). Rotation (R) reached 65 degrees.

All exercises were checked for performance, and the home program was progressed to comprise the following:

- Self-application of mobilization with movement (C1–C2 and C2–C3) to enhance rotation (R)
- Craniocervical flexion to train endurance at 28 mmHg
- Extension exercises (four-point kneeling) to progress to three sets of 10 repetitions of each exercise – extension had improved to 20 degrees beyond the horizontal.
- Active extension in the sitting position was added to the program, ensuring that the extension movement was initiated with craniocervical extension and return to the upright was initiated by craniocervical flexion. Emma was to extend to the point where any pain was about to be felt and then return to the neutral position.
- Tracing the infinity sign with the laser pointer was progressed to performance in the standing position.
- Tandem stance was practiced on a soft surface, three attempts to remain for 30 seconds.

Treatment 6 (1 Week Later)

Re-assessment

Emma felt that she was on the right track; the most noticeable difference was that she hadn't experienced light-headedness, and the headaches were not so bad. She was taking Panadol Osteo routinely at lunchtime to ensure she got through the afternoon's work. For the previous week, she had been back at work full time and was managing. Practicing the posture correction regularly was becoming more of a routine, and she had started getting others in the office to practice it because she thought they all had poor sitting postures.

Physical Examination

- Rotation (R) 60 degrees; some pain (R) upper cervical region
- Rotation (L) √√
- Extension: good control through 20 degrees without pain
- Balance: tandem stance, soft surface, eyes closed 30 seconds
- CCFT: could hold 30 mmHg without fatigue over multiple repetitions

Treatment

Manual therapy management: (R) C1–C-2 and C2–C3 postero-anterior glides without pain provocation interspersed with mobilization with movement (C1–C2 and C2–C3). Rotation (R) reached 70 degrees. The technique of self-mobilization with movement (C1–C2 and C2–C3) was checked, and Emma found this a good exercise to help her move her neck.

All exercises were checked for performance, and the home program was progressed as follows:

- Continue to train craniocervical flexor endurance at 30 mmHg.
- Extension exercises (four-point kneeling) to progress to three sets of 10 repetitions of each exercise. Light bicycle helmet worn to add slight resistance.

TABLE 14.4

THE PATIENT'S SCORES AT THE TREATMENT 6 RE-ASSESSMENT

Visual analog scale (VAS)	1–2/10
Neck Disability Index (NDI)	8/50
Patient Specific Functional Scale (PSFS)	
Turning her head	9
Computer work (60 min)	8
Cooking (lifting pots)	10
Walking with friends	10

- Active extension in the sitting position to be continued to achieve control through increasing range.
- Training movement sense with laser was progressed to perform in tandem stance.
- Balance progressed to one foot standing on a soft surface.

Treatment 7 (2 Weeks Later)

Re-assessment

Emma reported that she felt more confident with her neck and that she was certainly having periods with no neck pain, but it was still sore at the end of a working day or with unguarded movements (Table 14.4). She had stopped taking the Panadol. Headaches were occasional only, and she had not experienced light-headedness.

Physical examination:

- Rotation (R) 75 degrees; slight pain (R) upper cervical region
- Rotation (L) √√
- Extension: good control through 30 degrees without pain
- Balance: tandem stance, soft surface, eyes closed 30 seconds
- CCFT: could hold 30 mmHg without fatigue over multiple repetitions

Treatment

Manual therapy management was continued as previously. Rotation (R) reached 85 degrees.

All exercises were checked for performance, and the home program was progressed as follows:

- Continue to train craniocervical flexor endurance three times per week only.
- Extension exercises (four-point kneeling) to progress to three sets of 10 repetitions of each exercise. A light weight of 200 grams was taped to the bicycle helmet.
- Active extension in the sitting position continued, with holds added in early parts of extension range.
- Add neck and trunk rotation in sitting – archery exercise: focus eyes on a point straight ahead and pretend to shoot an arrow from a bow (from both left and right sides); begin with five reps each side.
- Add alternating arm lifts in the scapular plane while maintaining good posture (three sets of 10 reps).
- Training movement sense with laser was ceased because performance was excellent.
- Balance to be practiced once or twice a week to retain performance.

Treatment 8 (2 Weeks Later)

Re-assessment

Emma reported that pain-free periods were increasing, and her main problem was if she sat at her computer too long; then her neck felt tired and achy. Headaches had resolved, and she was doing most things normally now.

Physical examination:

- Rotation (R) 85 degrees; slight pain at end of range
- Rotation (L) √√
- Extension: √ some discomfort at end of range, control fair to good
- Balance: √√

Treatment

Manual therapy management was repeated. Rotation (R) became full range and pain-free.

All exercises were checked for performance, and the home program was progressed as follows:

- Check craniocervical flexor endurance capacity once per week.
- Commence head lifts off a wall in sitting (maintain craniocervical flexion position); perform 5-second holds (two sets of five reps).
- Extension exercises (four-point kneeling) to progress to three sets of 10 repetitions of each exercise. A light weight of 250 grams was taped to the bicycle helmet.
- Archery exercise: five repetitions each direction, performed two or three times a day at work.
- Active extension in the sitting position continued, focussing on holds through extension range.
- Alternating arm lifts in the scapular plane while maintaining good posture (three sets of 10 reps, holding 250-gram weight).
- Check balance once a week.

Because Emma was coping well and rehabilitation was progressing well, it was agreed that she would self-manage and attend for a follow-up check in a month.

Treatment 9 (4 Weeks Later)

Re-assessment

Emma reported that neck pain was mild and occasional. She felt confident in performing activities but still was conscious of not sitting too long at a computer in particular. She had negotiated a settlement with the insurance company 2 weeks ago, so things were getting back to normal (Table 14.5).

Physical examination:

- Rotation (R) √√ could feel a stretch with overpressure
- Rotation (L) √√
- Extension: √ control was good; no overpressure applied because Emma still felt some vulnerability at end-range extension
- Head lift, good control
- Balance: √√
- CCFT: √√

TABLE 14.5	
THE PATIENT'S SCORES AT THE TREATMENT 9 RE-ASSESSMENT	
Visual analog scale (VAS)	0–1/10
Neck Disability Index (NDI)	3/50
Patient Specific Functional Scale (PSFS)	
Turning her head	10
Computer work (60 min)	9
Cooking (lifting pots)	10
Walking with friends	10

Treatment

Emphasis was placed on devising a maintenance program which was effective, which Emma considered was 'doable' in the long term and, to encourage compliance, was non-intrusive in her lifestyle. The importance of a maintenance program for good health of her neck was explained, and analogies were made with maintaining good general health.

Key elements were as follows:

- Continue regular performance of posture correction at work and home, to change spine and neck position and facilitate deep cervical flexor muscle activity.
- Think of neck posture in performing daily activities.
- Continue archery exercise to maintain rotation ROM of neck and trunk.

For the next month, perform the following exercises once per week to ensure that performance was maintained:

- Head nod exercise: craniocervical flexor endurance capacity
- Extension exercises (four-point kneeling)
- Head lifts off a wall in sitting (maintain craniocervical flexion position); perform five-second holds (two sets of five reps)

If into the future, Emma felt that her neck was becoming stiff or painful, she was to resume her exercise program, particularly for the neck flexors and extensors, as a prevention strategy.

Emma felt confident to self-manage and was discharged at this point.

Reasoning Question:

10. Did your treatment progress as you expected given your initial hypothesis regarding the source of symptoms and pain type?

Answer to Reasoning Question:

The treatment progressed as expected for a peripheral nociceptive source of pain in the upper cervical segments. Emma had initially higher levels of pain and disability and was screened at medium risk of poor recovery. But as her case exemplifies, they are indicators only, and certainly not all patients with initially high pain will fail to recover. Applying the analogy used with Emma, the rehabilitation program progressed in a manner similar to that for an acute grade II ankle sprain.

Reasoning Question:

11. Emma's recovery appeared to progress smoothly. How do you think the presence of more adverse psychosocial issues may have affected the recovery?

Answer to Reasoning Question:

The evidence suggests that increased symptoms of post-traumatic stress and pain catastrophizing can be linked with a poorer prognosis, although the role of other psychological features remains equivocal. The presence of more marked emotional reactions, negative thoughts or poor coping skills would have modified the approach to rehabilitation in order to lessen any adverse effect on recovery. In addition to the rehabilitation regime described, the patient would be assisted with discussion and practice of techniques to manage stress or to increase pain-coping skills as examples.

Reasoning Question:

12. How likely do you think it is that Emma will have episodes of recurrent neck pain in the future? Do you think your early recognition and management of the pain type involved had an influence on the long-term prognosis?

Answer to Reasoning Question:

Unfortunately, neck pain is characterized by its recurrent nature, whether trauma induced or idiopathic in origin. Thus, it is difficult to predict if Emma will have recurrent episodes in the future.

Knowledge of the recurrent nature of neck pain underpinned the emphasis on a maintenance exercise program and the advice that if her neck was becoming stiff or painful, she was to resume her exercise program, particularly for the neck flexors and extensors, as a strategy to abort or lessen the nature of a recurrent episode.

The early recognition and management of the pain type may not be the critical influence on the long-term prognosis. The fact that it was a peripheral nociceptive source of pain, rather than a peripheral neuropathic pain or a peripheral nociceptive source accompanied by significant and prolonged central sensitization, more likely had a favourable influence on the prognosis.

Continued on following page

Clinical Reasoning Commentary:

Although Emma's treatment progressed as the authors expected for a peripheral nociceptive source of pain in the upper cervical segments, this was guided by the thorough and systematic re-assessment of a range of outcome measures, including disability and activity and participation measures via the NDI and Patient Specific Function Scale (PSFS), symptom severity and regular monitoring of specific physical impairments. This extent of outcome re-assessment is essential to inform clinical reasoning regarding the progression of management (e.g. what to continue, what to progress and what to add) and whether prior hypotheses, for example, regarding pain type, source of symptoms and contributing factors, needed to be revised.

The Answer to Reasoning Question 12 illustrates how clinical reasoning regarding management is not limited to the immediate pain and disability but also must address strategies to minimize recurrence and manage future episodes.

REFERENCES

Curatolo, M., Arendt-Nielsen, L., 2015. Central hypersensitivity in chronic musculoskeletal pain. Phys. Med. Rehabil. Clin. N. Am. 26, 175–184.

Drottning, M., Staff, P., Sjaastad, O., 2002. Cervicogenic headache (CEH) after whiplash injury. Cephalalgia 22, 165–171.

Goldsmith, R., Wright, C., Bell, S., et al., 2012. Cold hyperalgesia as a prognostic factor in whiplash associated disorders: a systematic review. Man. Ther. 17, 402–410.

Graven-Nielsen, T., Arendt-Nielsen, L., 2010. Assessment of mechanisms in localized and widespread musculoskeletal pain. Nat. Rev. Rheumatol. 6, 599–606.

Jull, G., Kenardy, J., Hendrikz, J., et al., 2013. Management of acute whiplash: a randomized controlled trial of multidisciplinary stratified treatments. Pain 154, 1798–1806.

Jull, G., O'Leary, S., Falla, D., 2008. Clinical assessment of the deep cervical flexor muscles: the Craniocervical Flexion Test. J Manip Physiol Ther 31, 525–533.

Jull, G., Sterling, M., 2016. Whiplash Injury Recovery – A Self Help Guide. Motor Accident Insurance Commission. Available at: https://maic.qld.gov.au/rehabilitation-advice/whiplash-injury-recovery/ (Accessed 14 September 2017).

Ritchie, C., Hendrikz, J., Jull, G., et al., 2015. External validation of a clinical prediction rule to predict full recovery and continued moderate/severe disability following acute whiplash injury. J Orthop Sports Physical Ther 45, 242–250.

Ritchie, C., Hendrikz, J., Kenardy, J., et al., 2013. Development and validation of a screening tool to identify both chronicity and recovery following whiplash injury. Pain 154, 2198–2206.

Sterling, M., Hendrik, J., Kenardy, J., et al., 2012. Assessment and validation of a prognostic model for poor functional recovery 12 months following whiplash injury: a multicentre inception cohort study. Pain 153, 1727–1734.

Sterling, M., Kenardy, J., Jull, G., et al., 2003. The development of psychological changes following whiplash injury. Pain 106, 481–489.

Treleaven, J., 2017. Dizziness, unsteadiness, visual disturbances, and sensorimotor control in traumatic neck pain. J. Orthop. Sports Phys. Ther. 47 (7), 492–502.

Treleaven, J., Peterson, G., Ludvigsson, M.L., et al., 2016. Balance, dizziness and proprioception in patients with chronic whiplash associated disorders complaining of dizziness: A prospective randomized study comparing three exercise programs. Man. Ther. 22, 122–130.

Walton, D., Carroll, L., Kasch, H., et al., 2013. An overview of systematic reviews on prognostic factors in neck pain: results from the International Collaboration on Neck Pain (ICON) project. Open Orthop J 7 (Suppl. 4: M9), 494–505.

Management of Profound Pain and Functional Deficits From Achilles Insertional Tendinopathy

Ebonie Rio • Sean Docking • Jill Cook • Mark A. Jones

Subjective Assessment

Demographics and Social History

Judy, a 55-year-old post-menopausal woman, presented with a 13-month history of right-sided insertional Achilles tendon pain. She lived at home with her husband in a single-storey house with three steps at the entrance. Judy enjoyed her employment as a full-time medical receptionist, and her usual workday primarily involved sitting, but she also got up and down frequently to photocopy and file. She was previously a teacher and enjoyed the change of occupation. Prior to her Achilles pain, Judy liked to walk every day for 3.5 km and 5–6 km each day on weekends. She described a very active social life and also enjoyed Pilates twice a week. She had been unable to exercise since having her Achilles pain and had gained about 15 kg; she was unhappy about both her inability to exercise and the weight gain.

Pain Presentation

Judy presented wearing a removable rigid walking boot on her right foot that caused her to walk with a limp due to the leg-length discrepancy. Her pain was confined to the Achilles insertion at the superolateral calcaneus; there was no spreading of the pain, and she was able to localize it with one finger (Fig. 15.1). She reported no sensation changes (no pins and needles or numbness). Judy also experienced occasional pain in the lumbar region that was eased with Pilates and did not radiate to her legs. However, she had to cease Pilates because she felt her Achilles pain walking from the car to the fitness centre. She considered the lumbar pain to be unrelated to her Achilles pain. Judy also reported right knee pain that had no impact on her walking and was not painful now. She further reported also having bilateral lateral hip pain that was mildly symptomatic and aggravated at night by lying on her side. She was unsure if this preceded the Achilles pain.

Onset of Pain

Judy reported no change to her activity level preceding the onset of symptoms and no overload (e.g. increase in tendon load associated with a change in activity) or relative overload after a period of time off. However, when questioned specifically about change in load before her symptoms started, she acknowledged that she had increased her walking around that time but thought the most significant change was the purchase of new shoes. She felt that the shoes rubbed on her heel in the area of her pain, but she persisted with wearing them because the podiatrist had prescribed them. When her symptoms were not improving, the podiatrist changed her orthotics four times without any effect. Judy reported

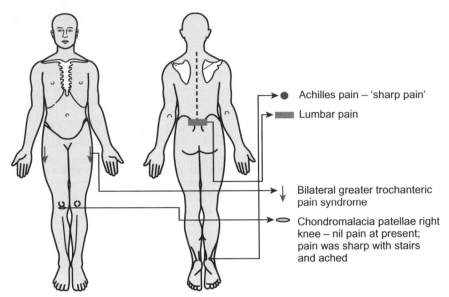

● Achilles pain – 'sharp pain'

▬ Lumbar pain

↓ Bilateral greater trochanteric pain syndrome

⬭ Chondromalacia patellae right knee – nil pain at present; pain was sharp with stairs and ached

Fig. 15.1 Body chart detailing site of symptoms.

no previous history of Achilles symptoms in either tendon or any other tendon pain or rupture.

Behaviour of Symptoms

Judy described her pain as 'agony' after walking only a few minutes without the walking boot. Her pain was worse if she had to walk up an incline, longer distances or at a faster pace. The Achilles pain was described as a grabbing pain that was highly irritable, with the pain rated as 9/10 on a numerical rating scale. Her pain was worse when walking barefoot, and flat shoes were more aggravating than shoes with a heel. She was unable to wear the shoes that she felt were linked to the onset of symptoms because of the pain. Pressure over the area was painful, especially with shoes that rubbed on her heel. The pain was worse during activity but ached afterward depending upon how far or long she had walked, and it had started to bother her at work. There was a clear relationship between greater amounts of loading and increased pain. Judy reported that her symptoms were eased by the controlled ankle movement (CAM) walker boot, and she now felt reliant on it.

Judy's morning pain and stiffness were severe; she reported crying with 10/10 pain in the morning and the pain taking hours to settle. She was now barely walking anywhere due to fear of pain and reported rarely leaving the house because her activity was so restricted, and this had helped ease her morning symptoms. When her symptoms were at their worst, she experienced night pain but had none currently.

Rest eased the Achilles pain temporarily, but it recurred once she returned to activity. During the past 13 months she had tried extended periods of rest and reduced activities (longest period was 7 weeks) but also took a non-steroidal anti-inflammatory drug (NSAID), so she was unsure if it was the rest or medication that was helpful. She reported 8 weeks of complete pain relief from a glucocorticoid injection into the painful area; however, the pain then returned to the same level.

Patient Perspectives: Expectations/Goals/ Understanding of the Problem

Judy reported fear of pain that was now limiting her activity. She did not feel that she was ever going to get better and was concerned that her only option was surgery. Judy described her tendon as being weak and likely to snap. Her husband was a radiologist, and she had

had multiple ultrasounds of her tendon, with the tendon reported as degenerative, abnormally thickened and having neovascularization. She admitted to not knowing what all this meant but thought that 'it sounded bad', and these terms concerned her. She was also fearful of not being able to walk without the walker boot.

General Health

Judy had several comorbidities and was on medication for many of them (Table 15.1), but these had been unchanged since the onset of the Achilles symptoms. She was really very keen to become active again, lose weight and try to reduce her medications. Judy had no red flags, for example, no recent loss of weight or cauda equina symptoms, nor did she have constant pain.

TABLE 15.1

MEDICATIONS THAT JUDY IS CURRENTLY TAKING AND POSSIBLE IMPLICATIONS FOR TENDON PRESENTATION

Medication	Health Issue	How It Manifests for Judy	Relevance to Tendinopathy
Plaquenil (200 mg/day)	Palindromic arthritis	Judy was referred to a rheumatologist for a persistent swelling in her right ankle. This condition is described as palindromic because the time taken to flare up is equal to the time to resolve. It is completely controlled with the medication, and she has had no further flare-ups. Her blood results were negative for rheumatoid conditions. The medication has not changed her Achilles pain.	Rheumatoid conditions are associated with insertional tendinopathy.
Xarelto (20 mg)	Atrial fibrillation – a blood thinner to reduce risk of an ischemic event	Preventative medication	Unknown
Sotalol (60 mg/day)	Atrial fibrillation, hypertrophic cardiac myopathy, high blood pressure	Preventative medication – beta blocker. Judy's blood pressure on medication is within normal limits, and she has had no history of stroke or transient ischemic events.	Unknown – there is an effect of beta blockers on the sympathetic nervous system. However, the relationship of the sympathetic nervous system to tendon pain is unknown. Any potential structural effect is also unknown.
Topamax (250 mg)	Migraines	With this medication, Judy does not suffer from migraines anymore. She has tried coming off it, and they recur.	Unknown
Crestor (5 mg)	High cholesterol	Low-density lipoproteins and overall cholesterol level was too high and not lowered after a trial of diet and exercise. The Achilles pain predates the cholesterol medication.	Cholesterol deposits in tendons – statins lower serum cholesterol as well as cholesterol in tendons; thus, there can be a change in tendon structure with the commencement of medication.

Previous Interventions

Judy had tried multiple interventions delivered by several different practitioners. After the orthotic changes by the podiatrist had not helped, she presented to the rheumatologist who managed her arthritis. The rheumatologist indicated a glucocorticoid injection would resolve the problem, and Judy had almost exactly 8 weeks of pain relief after injection before her pain returned. She then returned to the rheumatologist, who tried a second glucocorticoid injection. This time Judy felt she had missed the spot and reported it felt like she couldn't get the injection in, and she had no symptom relief. She reported losing faith in this management and then saw a sports physician who told her not to have another cortisone injection under any circumstances because the tendon might rupture. The sports physician recommended a platelet-rich plasma (PRP) injection and stated that 80% of patients get better with this treatment. Judy reported that the PRP injection was the most painful experience of her life, and her pain was worse despite resting completely for 2 weeks after the injection.

Judy then sought treatment from a physiotherapist who gave her through-range eccentric exercises off a step. The exercises were very painful to perform, and the tendon was not improving, but she was told to persist and ignore the pain because this was necessary for the tendon to recover. When the tendon pain did not settle, she was told it must be because she had poor core stability and was prescribed Pilates exercises. She was also told to try hydrotherapy, but all these made no difference. The pain failed to improve after several months of physiotherapy.

Judy visited her rheumatologist 3 months before presenting. The rheumatologist expressed annoyance that she had seen anyone else because, as the rheumatologist stated, 'I manage you'. She was advised to have another cortisone injection. She declined because she was fearful of tendon rupture. Her rheumatologist decided that the tendon must be overloaded and put her in a rigid walker boot for 6 weeks. She was not given any advice on when or how to remove the walker boot or resume activity, and 13 weeks had now passed. She was also referred to a surgeon for removal of her Haglund's morphology (the superolateral protuberance of the calcaneus). Judy saw the surgeon, who advised recovery would take more than 1 year and thus she should have the operation soon.

Three weeks ago, Judy thought she would try another physiotherapist. The assessment included hopping, jumping and lunging. These exercises were all painful, and after attempting them three times, she couldn't get out of bed for 3 days, so she didn't go back to the therapist. Judy acknowledged being nervous about what today's assessment would entail.

Reasoning Question:
1. Based on your subjective examination, please discuss your 'diagnostic reasoning' regarding the most likely 'source of nociception and associated pathology' and your hypothesis about the dominant 'pain type' (i.e. nociceptive, peripheral neuropathic, nociplastic), highlighting the clinical features supporting your hypotheses.

Answer to Reasoning Question:
The Achilles tendon insertion is the most likely source of nociception, and tendinopathy is the most probable diagnosis/pathology (Rio et al., 2015a). Morning pain and stiffness is a hallmark of Achilles tendinopathy. It is common for this to last up to 30 minutes; anything over 60 minutes may indicate a systemic contributor or cause of the tendon pain (notably, inflammatory diseases). There are two key clinical questions that support a diagnosis of Achilles tendinopathy:

- *Where is the pain?* Achilles tendon pain is localized and does not spread regardless of the length of time of the symptoms. In this case, Judy had pain at the lateral part of the insertion. Pain in the Achilles can also occur at the mid-substance, where patients commonly use two fingers to 'pinch' the area of pain.
- *What aggravates the pain?* Achilles tendon pain is aggravated by activities involving high tendon loads for the Achilles, especially energy-storage loads. Lower-energy-storage-load activities include brisk walking, whereas high-energy-storage-load activities involve running or change of direction. Activities such as cycling and swimming are low tendon load, and if these are the aggravating activities, a clinician should have a high index of suspicion that the Achilles is not the source of nociception. Tendinopathy appears to be nociceptively driven, as with Judy's presentation, and it is always intimately linked with loading. When a low-tendon-load activity is the aggravating factor, there may be another pain

source, such as neural irritation or the Achilles peritendon structures. These presentations will usually have a more diffuse pain pattern than Achilles tendon pain.

In insertional Achilles tendinopathy, movement into dorsiflexion causes compressive loading, where the tendon is compressed against the calcaneus; this can aggravate both pain and pathology (Cook and Purdam, 2012a). Activities such as stretching can cause pain because of compressive load. Walking with low-heeled shoes or bare feet is typically more aggravating than with shoes with a higher heel. The Haglund prominence is an anatomical morphology, not a deformity; it reduces load on the tendon insertion into the distal calcaneus by allowing compression of the Achilles tendon against the superior calcaneus (Benjamin et al., 2004). Removing this surgically exposes the insertion to greater load, increasing load on the tendon that has not adapted to full load on the insertion. Patients who display this morphology can have successful outcomes using rehabilitation without surgery (Fahlstrom et al., 2003; Jonsson et al., 2008).

Judy does not report any symptoms associated with a nociplastic pain type; however, it is well known that the experience of pain is modulated by conceptual and contextual factors. As such, education is critical so that language does not contribute to Judy's fear and pain experience. Therefore, increasing her understanding of tendinopathy and the rehabilitation process is likely to have a positive effect.

Posterior ankle pain has a number of differential diagnoses (Rio et al., 2015a). The key differential diagnosis is posterior ankle impingement. Patients with impingement report pain in full passive and active plantar-flexion activities, including kicking in swimming (that would not typically aggravate the Achilles tendon). The retrocalcaneal bursa is part of the Achilles enthesis and should be managed as part of an insertional Achilles tendinopathy, and is therefore not considered in any separate diagnosis. Where there is local neural entrapment or pain referral, the pain location is generally more diffuse than with Achilles tendon pathology.

Reasoning Question:

2. What is your interpretation of Judy's 'perspectives on her experience' (e.g. her understanding of her condition, fears, stress, coping, etc.)? Do you anticipate needing to address this in your management?

Answer to Reasoning Question:

Judy reported being concerned that her pain would not improve, and she was fearful of the suggested surgery. She was extremely concerned about the loading aspect of the clinical assessment because removing the boot and being examined had previously made her pain worse. Overall, she had a very poor understanding of her condition and what was the best way to improve her symptoms. It was essential, as described previously, to ensure that appropriate education and language did not contribute to her fear. It was also appropriate to consider the impact of her husband's profession (radiologist) on her views of tendon injury, as pathology and tendon pain are frequently disconnected.

Reasoning Question:

3. Please discuss the potential 'contributing factors' (intrinsic and extrinsic) to the development of Judy's problem and to her ongoing pain and disability.

Answer to Reasoning Question:

Reduction in oestrogen during menopause can contribute to tendon pathology and pain in older women. The obtained information about her menopausal status and other, sometimes associated, general health issues (see Table 15.1) was thus important to consider.

The increase in Judy's weight has implications for both load on the Achilles and for circulating cytokines associated with visceral fat deposits that in turn are associated with tendinopathy (Gaida et al., 2008). The onset of Achilles tendon pain usually coincides with a change in load, in this case a mild change in activity and footwear that may have aggravated her tendon by direct compression on the site (rubbing) or through being too low in heel height. The presence of these other comorbidities can increase the risk of developing Achilles tendon pain, with an amplified response to changes in load.

Reasoning Question:

4. Can you please highlight any aspects of Judy's presentation (e.g. pathology, clinical presentation, comorbidities, medications, previous interventions) you feel signal the need for 'precaution in the physical examination and treatment'?

Answer to Reasoning Question:

This tendon has been underloaded because Judy has been wearing a CAM walker boot for 13 weeks following several months of reduced activity. Physical tests that include high-tendon-load activities (such as hopping) are inappropriate for this tendon, and indeed she had previously had a poor response to assessment that included high-tendon-load activities. Assessment should only continue as guided by individual patient responses. Tendon pain typically increases with tendon loading; however, it is

Continued on following page

not necessary or recommended to complete all possible tests for each patient. Judy had no recent loss of weight or cauda equina symptoms, nor did she have constant pain. Her pain seemed to be of a mechanical origin because it was intimately linked with loading.

Clinical Reasoning Commentary:

Diagnostic reasoning regarding pain type, potential sources of nociception and associated pathologies commences in the subjective examination and is continued throughout the physical examination and ongoing management, where diagnostic hypotheses are tested further. As discussed in Chapter 1, these diagnoses are formulated on the basis of established (research and experience-based) clinical patterns. The specificity of musculoskeletal diagnoses varies with different problems and diagnostic tests. When the ability to identify specific sources of nociception and associated pathology is limited (e.g. non-specific low back pain), such as where overt pathology may not exist or clinical diagnostic tests lack validity to isolate sources of nociception, impairment-based diagnoses (e.g. motion segment symptom provocation, mobility and control) become the focus. In contrast, problems such as insertional tendinopathy have clearer clinical patterns, as discussed here, that can be differentiated from other sources of nociception and pathology. Although management will be largely guided by impairment based reasoning (i.e. patient's specific clinical presentation within the common clinical pattern), more accurate diagnostic classification enables more targeted research to identify effective management strategies that can then be tailored to the individual patient.

Judy's clinical presentation is judged as 'nociceptive dominant' and typical for tendinopathy that is intimately linked with loading. However, despite this, conceptual and contextual influences on the modulation of patients' pain experiences (e.g. Judy's understanding of tendinopathy and associated fear) are highlighted and linked to management reasoning regarding education and care with language that may contribute to Judy's already-expressed fears. This underscores the important reality discussed in Chapters 1, 3 and 4 that unhelpful patient perspectives, commonly associated with nociplastic pain, can present in any patient and with any dominant pain type and are therefore important to assess and manage to optimize clinical outcomes and potentially reduce the risk of progression to chronicity.

Contributing factors to the development and maintenance of patients' problems can be intrinsic or extrinsic and modifiable or non-modifiable. As discussed in Chapter 1, identification of contributing factors is important in management, both for reducing immediate symptoms and disability and for minimizing the likelihood of recurrence. Consideration of contributing factors also informs judgements regarding the hypothesis category 'prognosis'. This emphasizes the importance of undertaking medical/general health screening for comorbidities and their management, which may represent contributing factors that vary in the extent they are modifiable. Other factors such as patient weight, activity pattern and footwear are all modifiable and important to management reasoning, as are most physical impairments assessed in the physical examination (e.g. mobility, control/strength both locally and throughout the rest of the kinetic chain).

Similarly, the hypothesis category 'precautions and contraindication to physical examination and treatment' should be based on comorbidities and red flags screened, plus patients' individual clinical features, for example, those related to constancy, severity and irritability of symptoms, as well as patient perspectives such as fear.

Physical Assessment

Observation

Judy had a profound loss of muscle bulk of the right calf in both the soleus and gastrocnemius. She had an obvious Haglund morphology on both calcanea, with increased swelling over the right insertion.

Gait

Judy walked with a waddling gait and avoided pushing off on both feet. She had a reduced stride length and cadence.

Knee-to-Wall Lunge

Right – 0 cm and very painful at the end of range at Achilles insertion; left – 5 cm.

TABLE 15.2

PROGRESSIVE LOAD TEST EXAMPLES FOR THE ACHILLES (FROM LEAST PROVOCATIVE TO MOST PROVOCATIVE)

Loading Test	Description	Judy's Assessment
Double leg calf raise	Stand holding on to wall with feet in parallel. Rise up on two feet with the middle of the ankle joint over the middle of the second toe.	Able to do but uneven weight distribution. Assessment for the right was stopped at this level due to fear of severe pain.
Single leg calf raise	Stand holding on to wall with foot facing forward. Rise up on one foot with the middle of the ankle joint over the middle of the second toe.	Assessment was completed for the left leg.
Double leg jumps		Not attempted
Single leg hops	Progressing from small hops up to big hops as appropriate	Not attempted
Single leg forward hops		Not attempted

Functional Assessment

Judy had a lack of strength and power throughout the left leg when hopping; she had poor control, poor elevation and inability to hop with a consistent tempo. She was able to complete 16 heel raises on the left leg before fatiguing (Table 15.2). The right side was only assessed with four double leg heel raises that produced pain (visual analog scale [VAS] 4/10) with an uneven weight distribution (more weight on the left leg). The pain was localized to the lateral heel, and Judy could point to it with one finger. The choice to limit her assessment was, firstly, because the tendon had been unloaded in the boot and, secondly, due to her fear of being overassessed as she had been by the previous physiotherapist. When asked, she reported that she was unable to do a single leg heel raise on the right because of fear of severe pain.

No assessment of her joints was undertaken at this point because the pain was clearly tendon mediated. If there was an equivocal response to initial treatment, then further assessment of surrounding structures (such as the joints) would be undertaken.

Imaging

Although Judy had previous imaging of her Achilles, further investigation using ultrasound tissue characterization (UTC) was suggested to quantify the structural integrity of the tendon. UTC is a novel imaging modality that utilizes conventional ultrasound by capturing 600 contiguous transverse images over a 12-cm region. From this, a three-dimensional image is rendered where the stability of pixel brightness over the length of the tendon can be quantified into four echo types (van Schie et al., 2010). Previous research has validated these echo types against equine histopathological specimens (van Schie et al., 2010). It is an ideal tool to monitor tendon structure because it quantifies tendon structure and has a high degree of repeatability.

Judy's right Achilles tendon appeared focally thickened at the calcaneal insertion (Fig. 15.2), with the overall UTC echo pattern compromised compared with the contralateral Achilles. A diffuse area of disorganization was observed within the tendon (Fig. 15.3), characterized by an increase in echo type III, indicating disorganized fibrillar structure, and echo type IV, representing amorphous matrix (Table 15.3). This area of disorganization was confined to a 1-cm region at the calcaneal insertion, with the mean cross-sectional area (CSA) of the pathological lesion comprising approximately 40% of the transverse image. Her left Achilles did not appear thickened, and the overall echo pattern was within normal parameters.

Despite an area of disorganization present within the tendon, the UTC results were explained to Judy with a focus on the volume and mean CSA on aligned fibrillar structure

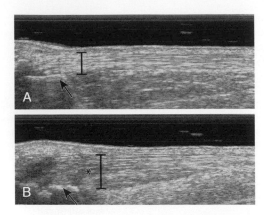

Fig. 15.2 Greyscale ultrasound views of the normal left Achilles tendon (A) and painful right Achilles tendon (B) in the sagittal plane. The right Achilles tendon is significantly thicker (at the insertion (see bar) with the presence of a hypoechoic area (asterisks). The Haglund's morphology (arrow) can be seen on both Achilles tendons.

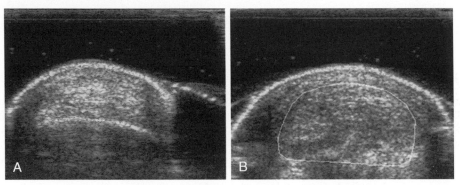

Fig. 15.3 Greyscale ultrasound and UTC images of the normal (A) and painful (B) Achilles tendons in the axial plane. (A) Left Achilles calcaneal insertion. (B) Right Achilles calcaneal insertion.

TABLE 15.3

PERCENTAGE OF DIFFERENT ECHO TYPES OF THE NORMAL (LEFT) AND PAINFUL (RIGHT) ACHILLES TENDONS

Percentage of Echo Types

Echotype	Right	Left
Type IV	2.2%	0.7%
Type III	6.6%	1.4%
Type II	30.3%	19.7%
Type I	60.9%	78.2%

(Fig. 15.4). That is, regardless of the area of pathology and increased mean CSA of disorganized echo types (echo types III and IV), Judy's right Achilles also had an increased mean CSA of aligned fibrillar structure compared with the contralateral tendon and structurally normal tendons. Previous research has shown that this is a common feature of pathological tendons (40 of the 41 pathological Achilles tendons contained similar or an increased mean CSA of aligned fibrillar structure) (Docking and Cook, 2015). It appears the pathological tendon compensates for areas of disorganization by increasing its dimensions to ensure there is sufficient aligned fibrillar structure (Docking and Cook, 2015).

Previous imaging had a negative impact on Judy's perception of her tendon. She was referred for a UTC scan to provide reassurance that her tendon could tolerate load. It was

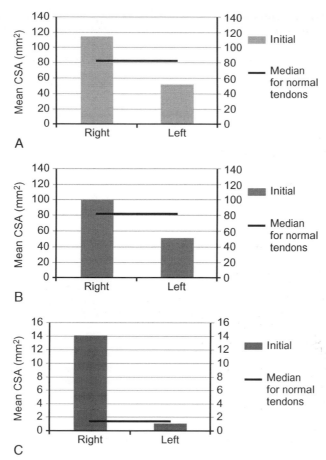

Fig. 15.4 Graphs representing the mean cross-sectional area (CSA) of total, normal and disorganized tendon tissue in the normal (left) and painful (right) Achilles tendons. The painful tendon is significantly larger, with a more disorganized structure. However, the painful tendon contains increased amounts of aligned fibrillar structure compared with the contralateral tendon and compared with a sample of structurally normal tendons (black horizontal line on graph). (A) Total mean CSA for both Achilles tendons. (B) Mean CSA of aligned fibrillar structure for both Achilles tendons. (C) Mean CSA of disorganized tendon structure for both Achilles tendons.

explained to Judy that she should not focus on the extent of disorganization because she had a sufficient amount of aligned fibrillar structure.

VISA-A Questionnaire

The Victorian Institute of Sports Assessment – Achilles (VISA-A) score documents pain and function of the Achilles tendon (Robinson et al., 2001). It was developed for mid-Achilles problems, but similarities allow its use in problems involving the insertional Achilles tendon, although it may be less sensitive to change. One hundred points is full pain-free function, 80 points suggests there is pain sufficient to affect function and 60 points indicates difficulty in function (Silbernagel et al., 2007). Judy's VISA-A score was 23 points, suggesting profound pain and functional deficits.

Reasoning Question:

5. In your Answer to Reasoning Question 1, you indicated that Judy's subjective presentation was consistent with an Achilles tendinopathy. Would you please highlight the physical examination findings that support that clinical pattern and also whether the physical examination supported your previous hypothesis regarding the dominant pain type being nociceptive?

Continued on following page

Answer to Reasoning Question:

Tendon pain frequently results in a loss of muscle bulk not only in the attached muscles (gastrocnemius and soleus) but often in other parts of the kinetic chain. In Judy's case this loss of bulk was likely to be exacerbated by the boot, which completely unloaded the musculotendinous unit. Part of the rationale for strength training in rehabilitation is to address these muscles as well as tendon capacity.

The physical examination includes tendon loading tests where increasing pain is expected with increasing tendon load. However, it is not always appropriate (as it was not in this case) to complete all of the examination, and as such, physical examination confirmation of tendinopathy was not possible, although the provocation of her localized pain with four double leg heel raises is consistent with a tendinopathy. Similarly, this specific reproduction of pain was consistent with her activity restrictions described in the subjective examination and fit with the nociceptive dominant pain type that was hypothesized.

Reasoning Question:

6. What is the relationship between UTC imaging and clinical symptoms and signs, and how do you use the UTC findings to inform your management?

Answer to Reasoning Question:

Although UTC quantifies tendon structure, it still does not correlate with clinical symptoms and pain. The disconnect between pain and structure within the tendon has been well documented in the literature (Cook et al., 2001; Khan et al., 1996).

Education is a key part of imaging and its utilization. In low back pain, the inappropriate use of imaging has been linked to 'over-medicalization', a decrease in patients' self-perceptions of health, and a contribution to fear-avoidance behaviours (Flynn et al., 2011). Judy had a classic fear response to the negative words used in imaging reports.

The UTC's ability to quantify the volume of aligned fibrillar structure can help counter any negative understandings that the patient may have about the tendon. If the tendon contains similar or an increased amount of aligned fibrillar structure compared with normal, patients easily recognize that they have enough normal tendon structure to tolerate load and that load management strategies should be embraced.

Clinical Reasoning Commentary:

Although provocation of Judy's localized pain with the double leg heel raises is considered consistent with tendinopathy, the reasoning evident in this answer highlights the value of the physical examination beyond diagnostic confirmation. In this example, the assessment is reduced to avoid aggravation of the problem and in consideration of Judy's expressed fears. A specific physical impairment is identified and measured (four double leg heel raises) that will inform exercise dosage and enable outcome monitoring of progress.

The disconnect between pain and structure within the tendon reflects the broader disconnect between musculoskeletal pain and pathology generally. Despite this limitation, confirmed pathology should not be disregarded. Pathology must be considered with respect to precautions in examination and treatment (e.g. caution with applying excessive load to tendons demonstrating significant degeneration) and with respect to evidence supporting management and prognosis. Here the UTC is used in a novel educative way whereby the aligned fibrillar structure, rather than the pathology (e.g. areas of disorganization), is highlighted to give Judy confidence in her tendon and to enhance her motivation for exercise.

Treatment

Education

Education for Judy focused on the following:

1. Debunking the myths and reducing fear around language
2. Understanding the importance of load
3. Teaching her when and how to 'listen' to her tendon

Debunking the Myths and Reducing Fear Around Language

Terminology such as *tear* or *degeneration* can have a profound impact on an individual's perception of the injury and the capacity for improvement. The UTC was vital to address Judy's fear around rupturing the tendon. Education about load helps to reduce fear of movement and empower patients. It is important to understand that tendon pain is not inflammatory. Cytokines that are present in tendinopathy may have a role in cell signaling and the pathology itself; however, their role in the clinical presentation of tendinopathy is currently unknown. Clinically, it is important that patients and clinicians understand that the approach required is different from that for an injury with classic inflammation.

Understanding the Importance of Load

It is vital to understand tendon load – both the loads that led the patient into trouble and also that load is the most important factor in the patient's rehabilitation. There are different types of load, and each has a different effect on the tendon. Tensile load maintains fibrous tissue, compressive load can form or maintain cartilage and a combination of these loads can form or maintain bone (Ingber, 2005).

High-tensile tendon load is present in any activity that requires a tendon to store and release energy. For the Achilles tendon, this may include walking, running or hopping. However, when completing these activities, there are other loads on the tendon. For example, walking uphill will increase the compressive load on the Achilles insertion by increasing the amount of dorsiflexion.

When a patient understands that tendon pain increases with excessive tendon loading, you can explain how to modify loading to reduce symptoms. For example, Judy should avoid any dorsiflexion, such as stretching, and use shoes with a substantial heel to reduce compressive loads and increase low-tensile tendon loads.

Conversely, tendon load is also the only intervention that can improve tendon pain and function and the only stimulus shown to improve tendon mechanical properties and structure (Kongsgaard et al., 2010). We often see patients who have been treated by practitioners who have an overreliance on passive therapies that fail to address tendon or kinetic chain capacity. Tendons respond slowly to load; thus, loading should be progressed in a very considered manner.

Teaching Her When and How to 'Listen' to Her Tendon

Tendons may occasionally be uncomfortable during rehabilitation. It is important that Judy listens to her tendon's response to loading. That being said, we don't advocate painful rehabilitation as has been reported with eccentric protocols (Alfredson, 2003), and in fact, early load such as isometric exercise should cause an immediate reduction in tendon pain. The tendon response in the 24 hours after activity is the most important gauge of progression. For the Achilles, it is possible to gauge progress using the length of time of morning pain or stiffness or with pain with a hop in patients who present with a higher level of function.

Response to load can vary, and it has implications for the loading program. If pain increases, the loading (or diagnosis) is wrong. If the pain response stays the same while load is increased, this is acceptable. For example, many athletes who place very high loads on their tendons in sport do not have a zero pain score the next day but are able to complete training and competition. If their pain is stable at low levels on a loading test, the tendon has not been aggravated by the load. The ideal scenario is reduction of pain with increasing load.

Instruction in Home Exercise

Judy was prescribed double leg calf raise holds with body weight in plantar-flexion. She was too fearful to start with just a single leg. This was tested in the clinic and prescribed as five isometric holds of 45 seconds each (with 2 minutes of rest between each isometric hold) (Rio et al., 2015b) because this was manageable without any muscle fasciculation. On immediate re-assessment after the isometric exercise, Judy was able to perform 25 double leg raises with a pain score of 0/10 (previously four raises at 4/10). Judy was instructed to complete these isometric holds throughout the day at work because no equipment was required. Judy was also given single leg seated calf raises twice a day, and she chose to rent a seated calf raise machine (Fig. 15.5) so that she could complete these easily at home.

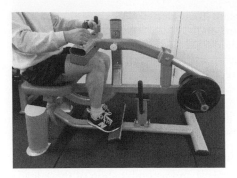

Fig. 15.5 Seated heel raise machine used for rehabilitation of Achilles tendinopathy.

Reasoning Question:

7. Judy had received a variety of treatments in the past without success. Would you provide a brief overview of the research evidence for the efficacy of the more common therapeutic interventions and discuss your reasoning for the specific exercises and dosage you selected for Judy?

Answer to Reasoning Question:

Judy had predominantly had passive treatments in the past that failed to address strength or improve capacity in the muscle–tendon unit and the kinetic chain. The standard eccentric exercise program was inappropriate because she had an insertional Achilles problem (Cook and Purdam, 2012b). Eccentric exercises over a step have been shown to not be beneficial for insertional Achilles tendinopathy due to the compression against the calcaneus in dorsiflexion (Cook and Purdam, 2012a; Jonsson et al., 2008). Judy's presentation was also too painful for the modified eccentric exercise program for insertional Achilles tendinopathy (Jonsson et al., 2008). Appropriate load exercises such as isometric load out of compression have been found to be clinically beneficial for tendon pain and has been shown to reduce pain instantly and for at least 45 minutes in a patellar tendon study (Rio et al., 2015b). Clinical experience supports that isometric load is also beneficial for other tendon pains (i.e. patellar, hamstring, gluteal tendinopathy). It is important that the load is appropriate for the individual. Seated calf raises using a machine are a good way of starting below body weight in some patients and building up. At the other extreme, some high-level athletes require the addition of external load, such as using a Smith machine whilst doing calf raises.

Glucocorticoid injections reduce tendon cell proliferation and activity (Scutt et al., 2006) and offer pain relief. However, they should never be used in isolation and without load management and tendon rehabilitation. Some studies have shown poorer outcomes when they are included in treatment, but data for the Achilles are limited (Coombes et al., 2010).

PRP is no more effective than placebo (de Vos et al., 2010) and should not be presented as a gold standard of treatment for tendinopathy.

Clinical Reasoning Commentary:

As evident here, clinical reasoning about 'management' should be evidence-informed, tailored to patients' individual presentations (e.g. with respect to mode of exercise and dosage) and monitored (re-assessed) to determine effect and guide progression.

Between Treatments

Judy was encouraged to contact the therapist with any questions or if she had any problems between appointments. Part of the education about tendon load also included information about how to use load (isometrics) to reduce pain if there was a flare-up. The morning pain score is used to indicate how the tendon responded to the loading of the day before. The decision was made by the therapist and Judy to continue in the boot for the first week and then slowly wean her off the boot by increasing walking (firstly only around the house) without it. Due to the long period of time in the boot, removing it entirely would have resulted in a large increase in tendon load to which the tendon was unaccustomed.

Second Appointment (2 Months After Initial Assessment)

Subjective Assessment

Judy reported much less fear of her tendon and was no longer wearing the boot. Judy had only taken 2 weeks to completely cease using the boot, which was faster than anticipated. However, she used the morning score to confirm that her tendon was tolerating her gradual reintroduction of walking in shoes. Her Achilles was no longer bothering her at work. She had no morning pain or stiffness. She was still bothered by walking barefoot or when wearing flat shoes or shoes that rubbed on her heel (these scenarios gave her morning pain and stiffness of 4–6/10 depending upon the length of time). She had been walking pain-free every 3 days for approximately 2–3 km, provided she wore her tennis shoes. This had been built up according to her education – that is, specific distances were not provided; instead Judy was encouraged to 'listen' to her tendon and modify or increase her load accordingly. In terms of general health, Judy had been in hospital recently for a routine colonoscopy where her heart had gone into atrial fibrillation that didn't settle, so she was admitted overnight.

Goals

Judy had planned a trip to the mountain range of the Kimberley region in northwestern Australia in 3 months' time and wanted to be able to walk every day and enjoy her holiday without pain. Her new goals also included being pain-free and being able to walk down flights of stairs normally.

Physical Assessment

On observation, Judy was in normal shoes. There was no redness of her calcaneus, and her muscle bulk had improved but still was not as large as the contralateral side. On her knee-to-wall test, she recorded 9 cm on the left side and 5 cm on the right, again an improvement from the first visit. Her gait had also improved; she was not limping and was pushing off both feet. Functionally, Judy could perform 18 calf raises on the left side, but on the right side, she was still afraid to initiate a single leg calf raise. However, she could take full body weight once in plantar-flexion (during a double leg raise with weight shifted to the right side). She was able to do more than 25 double leg raises.

Imaging

Judy was referred for a follow-up UTC scan on her right Achilles. The overall echo pattern for the right Achilles tendon had improved in comparison to the previous scan. Although the percentage of normal tendon fascicles (echo type I) was similar, a significant decrease in the percentage of echo type III and IV was observed. The diffuse pathological area at the calcaneal insertion was still apparent; however, a reduction in the mean CSA (from approximately 40% to approximately 10%) was observed, with the length remaining unchanged. A decrease in the mean CSA of disorganized tissue was observed, with the mean CSA of aligned fibrillar structure remaining similar (Fig. 15.6).

VISA-A

Her VISA-A score had increased to 63 out of 100, still indicating substantial pain and dysfunction but considerably improved from the previous time.

Treatment

Education

We continued the discussion around footwear to avoid compression at the insertion by utilizing a shoe with a substantial heel raise and to slowly increase walking load and be consistent with shoes and activity. Tendons respond poorly to change, so consistency in rehabilitation and walking load is important. Judy was reminded that the most important

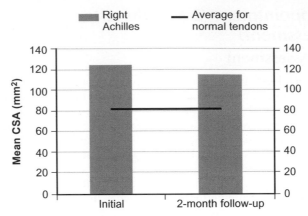

Fig. 15.6 Mean cross-sectional area (CSA) of aligned fibrillar structure for the right Achilles tendon. The graph shows the change in the amount of aligned tendon structure between the first and second visits.

time to 'listen' to the tendon was the morning after a walk. A return-to-walking plan was developed together according to tendon-loading principles.

Exercise

Judy's rehabilitation was progressed. She was to complete the isometric holds one day, followed by a double leg raise with weight shift to the right leg the next. She also completed left leg raises for a crossover strengthening effect (Kawamoto et al., 2014). If Judy had walked too much and experienced an increase in morning symptoms, she was to increase the frequency of completing the isometric holds during the day. Judy was taught how to progress these herself between the current appointment and the next appointment. She also started sit-to-stand exercises for general quadriceps and gluteal muscle function. Based on assessment of the number of repetitions Judy could perform with good control through the full kinetic chain, she was started with four sets of six repetitions and given information about progressing to encourage a strength and endurance focus.

Third Appointment (7 Months Later; 9 Months After Initial Assessment)

Subjective Assessment

Judy reported that she had had a wonderful holiday and walked at least 3 km per day and felt no pain. She avoided barefoot walking and was adherent with her exercises and walking before her holiday. Since she had returned, she had been less diligent with her exercises and reported having occasional walking pain. There was no change in her general health, and a recent checkup with her rheumatologist found everything was stable. Judy reported occasional pain at the top of the double calf raise home exercise. Footwear choice was still important, as her boots, which were very flat, aggravated her pain. She remained fearful of flat shoes and had purchased new wedge sandals for summer that had an external heel to ensure there was no compression from excessive dorsiflexion, nor did they rub on the insertion. Her current activity consisted of walking 2.5 km per day and one session of Pilates per week.

Physical Assessment

Judy had no swelling or redness over the calcaneus, and her other assessment tests were similar to the previous assessment. She was able to single leg heel raise 10 times; however, assessment of her technique revealed that she was supinating at the top of range. This decreases the load on the calf and is a 'cheat movement'. Judy was instructed on the correct

TABLE 15.4			
OVERALL ECHO PATTERN FOR RIGHT ACHILLES SHOWING IMPROVEMENT IN THE RIGHT TENDON OVER THREE VISITS			
Percentage of Echo Types			
Echotype	**Initial**	**2-Month Follow-Up**	**9-Month Follow-Up**
Type IV	2.2%	0.7%	0.7%
Type III	6.6%	2.8%	2.2%
Type II	30.3%	35.9%	33.7%
Type I	60.9%	60.6%	63.4%

way to perform calf raises and was only able to complete six repetitions with the correct technique.

Imaging

The overall echo pattern for the right Achilles was stable in comparison to the first follow-up scan (Table 15.4). Most improvement occurred between the first and second visits, with tendon structure remaining stable between the second and third visits. All four echo types were similar, with little variation observed over the length of the tendon. The diffuse area of disorganization was still apparent, and the size and length of the area of pathology had remained unchanged.

Goals and Expectations

Judy now expected to return to her pre-injury level of walking and two Pilates sessions per week. She also expressed that she now expected the tendon would get better and that she would be able to return to full activity.

Treatment

Re-education of her calf raise technique (Fig. 15.7) was undertaken to ensure appropriate alignment and calf activation to avoid posterior ankle pain. This included taking a video for Judy to watch. A trial of soft tissue work on her calf to increase knee-to-wall distance effected no change in her range of movement.

Judy's home exercises were progressed to increase her strength on both sides by (1) changing her double leg calf raise with weight shift to the right, (2) adding single right leg calf raises with isometric holds and (3) continuing to increase her walking distance.

All the education previously delivered to Judy was reiterated, and she was again told how to avoid exacerbations and what to do if one occurred. She clarified her future self-management and was happy to continue to monitor and manage her tendon.

Reasoning Question:

8. Earlier you indicated that UTC imaging does not correlate with symptoms and signs. Would you discuss the value of using imaging as an outcome measure of clinical improvement?

Answer to Reasoning Question:

If repeat imaging is utilized, it is critical that the patient's expectations are managed. A number of studies have shown that clinical improvement is not mediated by improvements in tendon structure (de Jonge et al., 2011). Importantly, the patient should be educated that the tendon is likely to remain abnormal/pathological even if the pain has improved. When repeat scanning with UTC, the ideal scenario is to hopefully see improvements in tendon structure coinciding with a decrease in pain and increase in tendon load. However, an equally suitable outcome is that the tendon's structure remains stable coinciding with a decrease in pain and increase in tendon load. Explaining to the patient that the tendon's ability to return to normal is limited and that the tendon will find a state of equilibrium is of critical importance in minimizing negative psychological outcomes with imaging.

Continued on following page

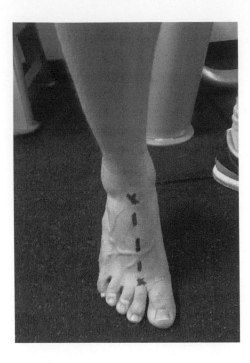

Fig. 15.7 Simple markings on the foot and instructions to keep the marks aligned throughout the heel raise movement will ensure that a quality movement occurs and strength gains are maximized.

Clinical Reasoning Commentary:

The value of imaging as an outcome measure is clarified, and its value as a resource for education is re-emphasized. 'Reasoning about teaching', a 'clinical reasoning strategy' (i.e. focus) discussed in Chapter 1, emphasizes that teaching, like all management tools, needs to be tailored to the individual patient and re-assessed to evaluate the patient's understanding (learning) and other effects (e.g. altered fear and behavior).

No further appointments were made, and Judy was advised to continue to increase her exercises as able with the ongoing goal of being able to complete 20 single leg calf raises at least three times a week.

REFERENCES

Alfredson, H., 2003. Chronic midportion Achilles tendinopathy: an update on research and treatment. Clin. Sports Med. 22, 727–741.

Benjamin, M., Moriggl, B., Brenner, E., Emery, P., McGonagle, D., Redman, S., 2004. The 'enthesis organ' concept: why enthesopathies may not present as focal insertional disorders. Arthritis Rheum. 50, 3306–3313.

Cook, J., Purdam, C., 2012a. Is compressive load a factor in the development of tendinopathy? Br. J. Sports Med. 46, 163–168.

Cook, J.L., Khan, K.M., Kiss, Z.S., Coleman, B.D., Griffiths, L., 2001. Asymptomatic hypoechoic regions on patellar tendon ultrasound: a 4-year clinical and ultrasound followup of 46 tendons. Scand. J. Med. Sci. Sports 11, 321–327.

Cook, J.L., Purdam, C., 2012b. Is compressive load a factor in the development of tendinopathy? Br. J. Sports Med. 46, 163–168.

Coombes, B.K., Bisset, L., Vicenzino, B., 2010. Efficacy and safety of corticosteroid injections and other injections for management of tendinopathy: a systematic review of randomised controlled trials. Lancet 376, 1751–1767.

De Jonge, S., De Vos, R.J., Weir, A., Van Schie, H.T.M., Bierma-Zeinstra, S.M.A., Verhaar, J.A.N., et al., 2011. One-year follow-up of platelet-rich plasma treatment in chronic Achilles tendinopathy: a double-blind randomized placebo-controlled trial. Am. J. Sports Med. 39, 1623–1629.

De Vos, R.J., Van Veldhoven, P.L., Moen, M.H., Weir, A., Tol, J.L., Maffulli, N., 2010. Autologous growth factor injections in chronic tendinopathy: a systematic review. Br. Med. Bull. 95, 63–77.

Docking, S., Cook, J., 2015. Pathological tendons maintain sufficient aligned fibrillar structure on ultrasound tissue characterization (UTC). Scand. J. Med. Sci. Sports 26 (6), 675–683. doi:10.1111/sms.12491.

Fahlstrom, M., Jonsson, P., Lorentzon, R., Alfredson, H., 2003. Chronic Achilles tendon pain treated with eccentric calf-muscle training. Knee Surg. Sports Traumatol. Arthrosc. 11, 327–333.

Flynn, T.W., Smith, B., Chou, R., 2011. Appropriate use of diagnostic imaging in low back pain: a reminder that unnecessary imaging may do as much harm as good. J. Orthop. Sports Phys. Ther. 41, 838–846.

Gaida, J., Cook, J., Bass, S., 2008. Adiposity and tendinopathy. Disabil. Rehabil. 30, 1555–1562.

Ingber, D.E., 2005. Tissue adaptation to mechanical forces in healthy, injured and aging tissues. Scand. J. Med. Sci. Sports 15, 199–201.

Jonsson, P., Alfredson, H., Sunding, K., Fahlstrom, M., Cook, J., 2008. New regimen for eccentric calf muscle training in patients with chronic insertional Achilles tendinopathy: results of a pilot-study. Br. J. Sports Med. 42, 746–749.

Kawamoto, J.E., Aboodarda, S.J., Behm, D.G., 2014. Effect of differing intensities of fatiguing dynamic contractions on contralateral homologous muscle performance. J. Sports Sci. Med. 13, 836–845.

Khan, K.M., Bonar, F., Desmond, P.M., Cook, J.L., Young, D.A., Visentini, P.J., et al., 1996. Patellar tendinosis (jumper's knee): findings at histopathologic examination, US, and MR imaging. Victorian Institute of Sport Tendon Study Group. Radiology 200, 821–827.

Kongsgaard, M., Qvortrup, K., Larsen, J., Aagaard, P., Doessing, S., Hansen, P., et al., 2010. Fibril morphology and tendon mechanical properties in patellar tendinopathy: effects of heavy slow resistance training. Am. J. Sports Med. 38, 749–756.

Rio, E., Mays, S., Cook, J., 2015a. Heel pain: a practical approach. Aust. Fam. Physician 44 (3), 96–101.

Rio, E., Kidgell, D., Purdam, C., Gaida, J., Moseley, G.L., Pearce, A.L., et al., 2015b. Isometric exercise induces analgesia and reduces inhibition in patellar tendinopathy. Br. J. Sports Med. 49 (19), 1277–1283. doi:10.1136/bjsports-2014-094386.

Robinson, J.M., Cook, J.L., Purdam, C., Visentini, P.J., Ross, J., Maffuli, N., et al., 2001. The VISA-A questionnaire: a valid and reliable index of the clinical severity of Achilles tendinopathy. Br. J. Sports Med. 35, 335–341.

Scutt, N., Rolf, C.G., Scutt, A., 2006. Glucocorticoids inhibit tenocyte proliferation and tendon progenitor cell recruitment. J. Orthop. Res. 24, 173–182.

Silbernagel, K.G., Thomee, R., Eriksson, B.I., Karlsson, J., 2007. Continued sports activity, using a pain-monitoring model, during rehabilitation in patients with Achilles tendinopathy: a randomized controlled study. Am. J. Sports Med. 35, 897–906.

Van Schie, H., De Vos, R., De Jonge, S., Bakker, E., Heijboer, M., Verhaar, J., et al., 2010. Ultrasonographic tissue characterisation of human Achilles tendons: quantification of tendon structure through a novel non-invasive approach. Br. J. Sports Med. 44, 1153–1159.

16

Cervicogenic Headache

Toby Hall • Darren A. Rivett • Mark A. Jones

Subjective Examination

Jean is a 42-year-old female working part-time from home as an information technologist managing a small website business. She does this while looking after her two young children (aged 6 and 4 years), one of whom had some early developmental delay but was now progressing well. Jean had previously been very active, with a rigorous exercise routine and regularly swimming in a swim club, but this stopped just before the birth of her first child and had not resumed due to time constraints, so she was no longer physically active. Her young children had previously caused her to wake frequently during the night, which had led to a poor pattern of sleep, which had been maintained in recent times.

History

Jean had a 5-year history of left-sided-dominant daily frontal headache together with a general non-specific headache, which made her head feel tight (Fig. 16.1). She had an episodic history of neck pain prior to the headache onset related to a whiplash injury 10 years ago, which is also shown in Fig. 16.1. Headache and neck pain now both occur together. Symptoms had plateaued in the previous few years and were rated at 58/100 on the Headache Disability Inventory, indicating a substantial burden. Headache, rather than neck pain, was the major complaint and reason for physiotherapy consultation.

Jean found that sitting for more than 30 minutes while working on her laptop with the laptop resting on her lap provoked the headaches. Lifting and carrying her children, heavy shopping bags or other loads also provoked her headache. Self-reported stress was also a factor, particularly associated with managing a small business with two young children. She had also been stressed by the developmental delay in her younger child. This was not helped by the fact that her husband was not able to help her with household duties or child care due to his long work hours. There were no associated features such as aura, nausea or photophobia, but she occasionally had light-headedness, which she could not relate to a specific aggravating activity or movement. It did not appear to be postural related, nor was it a feeling of vertigo.

Medical investigations included a computed tomography (CT) scan of the brain 5 years previously and x-rays of her neck after the whiplash injury 10 years ago. Her general practitioner (GP) had referred her to a neurologist 5 years ago, who had arranged the CT scan and who also diagnosed tension-type headache. Medication had been trialed at that time, but Jean self-medicated with over-the-counter analgesics (Panadol), often on a daily basis. Despite this, the headache had increased to the point that it occurred daily, with an average intensity of 5/10. Jean was otherwise healthy, and there were no other features indicating red or yellow flags apart from the stress that she was undergoing while managing a family and working from home. When questioned about associated features in the jaw, she denied any difficultly with jaw function or any symptoms associated with jaw movement.

Reasoning Question:
1. What were your hypotheses at this stage regarding the dominant 'pain type' (nociceptive, peripheral neuropathic, nociplastic)? What evidence supported or negated your hypothesis?

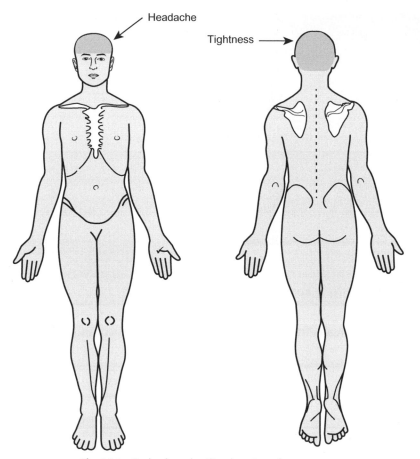

Fig. 16.1   Body chart detailing location of symptoms.

Answer to Reasoning Question:

With the information gained thus far, nociplastic appeared to be the dominant 'pain type'. There is increasing evidence that headache is a spectrum comprising different headache forms but with common underlying pathophysiology (Cady, 2007; Watson and Drummond, 2014; Watson and Drummond, 2016). The common feature among the spectrum of headache disorders is sensitization of the trigeminocervical nucleus (Bartsch and Goadsby, 2003). In fact, central sensitization of the trigeminocervical nucleus appears to be necessary for headache to arise from impairment of the cervical spine (Chua et al., 2011). This nucleus is the region where afferents converge from the cervical spine with afferents from the trigeminal system.

Sensitization of the trigeminocervical nucleus is likely to be caused by prolonged nociceptive inputs from the periphery; hence, the role of the periphery should not be ignored (Fernandez-de-Las-Penas and Courtney, 2014). Potentially, there was evidence of a peripheral driver in this case with lifting children and shopping bags and working on a laptop provoking symptoms. Perhaps peripheral input was arising from the cervical spine, associated with the whiplash injury 10 years ago. Despite this, the presence of poor sleep, de-conditioning, lack of exercise and stress are also potent contributing factors to nociplastic pain, which can lead to sensitization of the trigeminocervical nucleus and headache (Nijs et al., 2014; Noseda et al., 2014).

Clinical Reasoning Commentary:

As discussed in Chapter 2, mechanisms of central sensitization are involved to some extent in all pain types. Although understanding 'normal' mechanisms of central sensitization versus nociplastic pain mechanisms identifying environmental, psychological, social and physical factors that may be contributing to sensitization and maintenance of symptoms and disability, as reflected in this analysis, is the key to planning management interventions that target those factors. As described in this answer, these represent hypothesized 'contributing factors' in the hypothesis categories framework presented in Chapter 1.

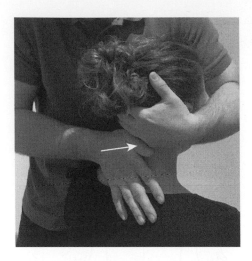

Fig. 16.2 Headache SNAG: The head is fixed while horizontal posteroanterior pressure is applied through the spinous process of C2.

Physical Examination

On physical examination, Jean sat with a kyphotic thoracic and lumbar spine and forward head posture. When standing, she adopted a swayback posture with generally low muscle tone. Her scapulae were bilaterally depressed with both clavicles horizontal, well below the normal 10-degree angle to the horizontal (Ha et al., 2013). The scapulae were also bilaterally protracted to approximately 45 degrees and tilted forward to 30 degrees, both more than optimal.

Correcting her sitting posture, by altering the pelvis, spine, scapular and head position, felt 'easier', and Jean's headache/neck pain were immediately reduced but not eliminated. Furthermore, neck movement increased in the range of lateral flexion and rotation when the scapular and spine position was corrected (Ha et al., 2011).

It was decided that a Mulligan Headache SNAG (Hing et al., 2015) would be trialed early in the physical examination. The rationale for the Mulligan approach is to determine whether manual glide force applied to the symptomatic motion segment can eliminate pain. The Headache SNAG involves the therapist contacting the C2 spinous process with the little finger of one hand while gentle horizontal pressure is applied by the opposite arm through the thenar eminence applied directly to the finger overlying the spinous process (Fig. 16.2). It is important to stabilize the patient's head during the sustained pressure on C2. Pressure is maintained for at least 10 seconds. This technique caused an immediate increase in symptoms. A Reverse Headache SNAG (reversing the Headache SNAG direction of glide) had no effect on symptoms, whereas applying a modified Headache SNAG at C3 with pressure directed at 45 degrees to the horizontal plane immediately reduced the symptoms.

Reasoning Question:

2. Please discuss your aims when using the Mulligan assessment techniques.

Answer to Reasoning Question:

The Mulligan technique is a useful tool to help quickly identify the presence of cervical involvement in headache disorders. In the presence of cervicogenic headache (CGH) features (evidenced here by the presence of neck pain associated with headache, physical activity provoking headache and limitation of cervical movement), it is useful to trial symptom alteration techniques. This is particularly helpful if the patient presents with headache pain at the time of the assessment. If the symptoms can be altered by manual force applied in different directions to the upper neck, then this suggests a cervical contribution to headache. Failure to alter symptoms is an indication that the cervical articular structures are less likely to be involved as the pain source.

Jean also had features that potentially indicated a postural abnormality contributing to headache symptoms, which was another reason to trial the Mulligan technique. A Mulligan Headache SNAG could be seen to correct a forward head posture, at least locally between the occiput and the C2 vertebra. As headache was immediately provoked by the headache SNAG this often indicates an impairment at the C2/C3 spinal segment as the pain source. This can be explained by the fact that a horizontal glide force increases C2/C3 facet joint compression loading due to the oblique nature of the articular surfaces at that level. In addition, the horizontal force also has an effect of increasing flexion at C0/C1. Hence, based on this information, in this case, at least part of the problem might have been coming from C2/C3 and possibly also C0/C1, but further tests would be required to substantiate this.

Clinical Reasoning Commentary:

In relating the aims of the Mulligan techniques discussed in this answer to the clinical reasoning theory presented in Chapter 1, these techniques can be seen to inform 'diagnostic' reasoning, both with respect to classification of headache type and for identification of specific segmental impairment in cervical motion segments. Symptom provocation to the localized physical stress of the SNAG supports reasoning regarding 'source of symptoms' and is biomechanically related to postural correction, therefore also informing reasoning regarding potential physical contributing factors and management (in this case, posture). Symptom alleviation (or reduction) to the SNAG (i.e. 'applying a modified Headache SNAG at C3 with pressure directed at 45 degrees to the horizontal plane immediately reduced the symptoms') informs reasoning regarding management.

Active and Combined Cervical Movements

Upper Cervical Spine Retraction and Protraction

Active head retraction was reduced to half the expected normal range of movement (ROM) and provoked neck pain which was increased with gentle overpressure into retraction (Fig. 16.3). Protraction range was increased and was also symptomatic. These movements predominantly occur in the upper cervical spine, with maximal movement occurring at C0/C1 and C1/C2 into flexion during retraction and extension during protraction (Ordway et al., 1999; Takasaki et al., 2010). Hence pain provocation increases suspicion of an upper cervical movement problem.

Cervical Spine Flexion and Extension

Plane axial cervical movements were also problematic. Extension of the whole cervical spine caused localized neck pain, and there was poor control of movement, with a tendency to 'collapse' the neck, associated with a focus of movement in the mid- and upper cervical spine with lack of movement in the cervicothoracic junction. Supporting Jean's head during extension and controlling the movement reduced the pain associated with extension. Similarly, correcting the spine and scapula posture also improved extension control and reduced symptoms.

Fig. 16.3 Active upper cervical spine retraction guided by the therapist to ensure pure retraction to minimize flexion occurring in subaxial segments.

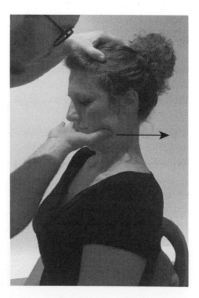

Cervical Spine Rotation and Lateral Flexion

Cervical lateral flexion and rotation bilaterally gave a feeling of tightness in the neck muscles contralaterally and appeared restricted in range. Correcting the scapular and spine posture improved the cervical rotation and lateral flexion movement markedly to near full range, which was pain-free (Fig. 16.4). This information, taken together with the evidence of poor extension control, indicated that the symptoms might be associated with issues of motor control of the spine and scapulae, although it did not discount articular impairment. It is possible that cervical segmental movement impairment may be compensated for by movement at adjacent vertebral levels (Bogduk, 2002). This might explain why a large survey of 4293 adults failed to find any difference in cervical ROM when comparing those with chronic neck pain to those without (Kauther et al., 2012).

There was little movement in the upper thoracic spine during any cervical movement.

Cervical Spine Combined Movement

Combined movement testing of the upper cervical spine revealed increased neck pain on retraction with left rotation (Fig. 16.5A). This movement is thought to bias the C0/C1 motion segment (Edwards, 1992) due to the predominance of sagittal movement at this level (Karhu et al., 1999). Hence pain provocation during this movement indicates the need for further testing at this level and the potential for symptom provocation. Further testing also identified that rotation to the left with C2 stabilized with the addition of upper cervical flexion was also provocative (Fig. 16.5B). The movement of head and upper neck rotation with C2 fixed predominantly occurs at C1/C2 (Takasaki et al., 2011; Osmotherly et al., 2013). Hence, further tests are required to evaluate symptoms arising from C1/C2. Finally, with C3 stabilized, the addition of upper cervical extension and ipsilateral lateral flexion also increased neck pain. Due to the ipsilateral nature of coupling in the cervical spine (Cook et al., 2010), the possibility of C2/C3 segmental involvement is further raised.

Segmental Mobility and Pain Provocation Tests

Segmental Movement Tests

In a seated position, examination of upper cervical left rotation with C2 stabilized was reduced in range to approximately 5 degrees (Fig. 16.6AB). The segmental range of rotation for this test is reported as approximately 10 degrees when measured using magnetic resonance imaging (MRI) in a laboratory setting (Osmotherly et al., 2013). However, typically, in a clinical test environment, the normal rotation range is 10–15 degrees to each side. Stabilizing C3 also gave a similar range of rotation.

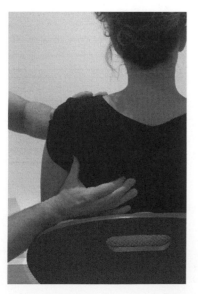

Fig. 16.4 Scapula correction with hand contact on the inferior angle and acromion: Correction is based on the individual patient presentation and response.

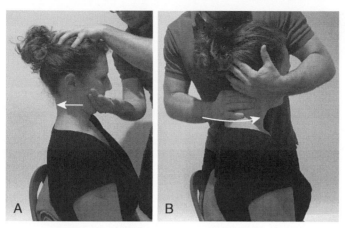

Fig. 16.5 Combined movement evaluation. (A) C0/C1 combining flexion with rotation to the left. (B) C1/C2 combining left rotation with flexion.

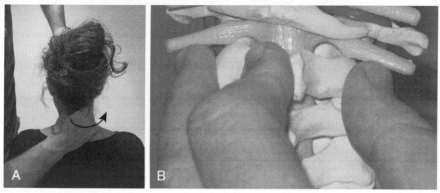

Fig. 16.6 Hand placement for fixation of C2 vertebra during axial rotation in the upper cervical spine.

Segmental examination revealed hypomobility at C0/C1, C1/C2 and C2/C3 vertebral levels. The flexion-rotation test was positive, with a subjective estimate of 20 degrees to the left side, which is much less than the expected range of 44 degrees to each side (Ogince, 2003; Hall and Robinson, 2004). A positive test is reported as range less than 33 degrees (Hall et al., 2010). Palpation of the C2 spinous process indicated that it was centrally located, not deviated. It has been suggested that a deviated C2 spinous process is indicative of dysfunction of the C2/C3 vertebral segment and is associated with headache (Macpherson and Campbell, 1991).

Segmental Pain Provocation Tests

Passive accessory movements were performed in both prone and supine positions. Headache was reproduced on palpation of the left posterior arch of C1 when the neck was positioned in upper cervical spine retraction with a few degrees of left rotation (Fig. 16.7). Local neck pain only was reproduced on palpation of the C2 and C3 articular pillars on the left side, despite the neck being placed in a provocative position for the C1/C2 and C2/C3 vertebral segments. This indicates the greater potential for C0/C1 segmental involvement over C1/C2 and C2/C3. Caution is required when interpreting headache reproduction on palpation. Recently it was shown that headache could be provoked from palpation of the neck in people with migraine and tension-type headache (Watson and Drummond, 2012).

Muscle Function

Cranio-cervical Flexion Test

The preliminary observation of posture and movement control indicated potential for impairment of motor control as a contributing factor to the patient's symptoms. The

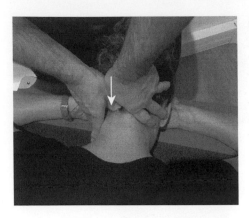

Fig. 16.7 Palpation over the C1 left posterior arch with the neck in flexion.

cranio-cervical flexion test has been shown to be a valid (O'Leary et al., 2007) and reliable (Chiu et al., 2005) measure of function of the anterior neck muscles. Research has established that patients with neck pain disorders, including CGH (Jull et al., 2007), when compared with controls, have altered motor control during cranio-cervical flexion characterized by reduced activity in the deep cervical flexors and increased activity in the superficial flexors. In Jean's case, there was a reduction in her ability to perform the cranio-cervical flexion test, with marked substitution of superficial muscles, particularly the hyoid muscles and sternocleidomastoid. Even the smallest movement of the head induced inappropriate superficial neck flexor muscle activity. This information, taken together with the apparent lack of neck movement and pain on palpation of the upper cervical spine, is highly diagnostic of CGH (Jull et al., 2007). In that study, the presence of these three factors had very high levels of sensitivity and specificity in identifying people with CGH from those with migraine, tension-type headache or asymptomatic controls.

In addition to the poor deep neck flexor muscle control, Jean was also unable to correctly position the scapulae unilaterally or bilaterally without inappropriate muscle activity of the latissimus dorsi and rhomboid muscles. Muscle length was reduced in the sub-occipital extensors and pectoralis minor bilaterally, and there were trigger points provoking headache in the levator scapulae, as well as tender points in the sternocleidomastoid and upper trapezius bilaterally. Prevalence of trigger points in neck muscles is not isolated to people with CGH; these occur in many other headache forms, including tension-type headache, migraine and cluster headache (Calandre et al., 2006, 2008; Alonso-Blanco et al., 2011).

Neurodynamic Tests

Neurodynamic tests were carried out in both sitting and supine positions. With the patient seated, upper cervical spine retraction was assessed with the patient's knees flexed to 90 degrees and then in a slumped spine position with her knees fully extended. Retraction was more painful and restricted in range in the slumped position compared to upright position. This is a useful screening tool to identify neural tissue mechanosensitivity as the limiting factor for retraction. Cervical flexion during retraction elongates the cervical neuromeningeal tract; hence, increased neural tissue mechanosensitivity is likely to be identified quickly by this test. Confirmation of a neural tissue pain disorder requires further neurodynamic tests and supporting evidence of pain on palpation of upper cervical neural tissue (Hall et al., 2008). While testing passive range of upper cervical spine flexion in supine, positioning the arms in a neural provocative position of bilateral shoulder abduction to 90 degrees increased Jean's neck pain and also reduced available range, but headache was not provoked. The greater occipital nerve at the occiput was moderately sensitized bilaterally to gentle non-noxious mechanical pressure. The prevalence of neural tissue mechanosensitivity in people with CGH is approximately 8% (Zito et al., 2006), but it also appears in people with migraine (von Piekartz et al., 2007).

Temporomandibular Joint

Temporomandibular dysfunction is common in people with CGH (von Piekartz and Ludtke, 2011). Such dysfunction is usually associated with impairment of upper cervical spine movement (Grondin and Hall, 2015). Hence, evaluation of the jaw region is important in the clinical evaluation of headache. Evaluation for temporomandibular dysfunction was carried out by evaluating range of movement, joint sounds and symptoms associated with jaw opening as well as sensitivity to palpation of the jaw muscles. No significant features of temporomandibular dysfunction were identified.

Special Tests

Due to the subjective report of light-headedness, tests for cervical arterial dysfunction were performed according to the current International Federation for Orthopaedic Manipulative Physical Therapists (FOMPT) guidelines (Rushton et al., 2014), and these tests were unremarkable. Furthermore, in light of the history of neck trauma and light-headedness, tests for cranio-cervical ligament integrity were also performed and revealed no abnormality. One study found evidence of significant ligament damage of the tectorial membranes, alar and transverse ligaments in up to one-third of cases of people who had suffered whiplash injury on average 6 years after trauma (Kaale et al., 2008). Smooth pursuit eye tests and tests for proprioception and head repositioning were not conducted at this time due to time constraints and were planned for subsequent follow-up sessions if required.

Reasoning Question:

3. Please discuss how you would classify Jean's headache, and also comment on any physical factors identified in your physical examination that you hypothesize may have been contributing to the maintenance of her headache.

Answer to Reasoning Question:

Headache is both a symptom and a disease (Dodick, 2010); hence, diagnosis can be challenging. Differential diagnosis based on symptoms alone can be problematic, and there is often misdiagnosis (Pfaffenrath and Kaube, 1990; Moeller et al., 2008). To explain this, it has been postulated that headaches form a spectrum, with shared common pathophysiological mechanisms (Cady et al., 2002). It has also been suggested that CGH forms part of this spectrum (Watson and Drummond, 2012). Despite the similarity in the mechanisms underlying different headache forms, it appears that physical treatment is not effective for all forms of headache (Biondi, 2005; Bronfort et al., 2010). Manual therapy can be effective for tension-type headache and CGH, but there is less evidence for effect in migraine (Chaibi and Russell, 2012; Sun-Edelstein and Mauskop, 2012). It appeared clear to me that Jean had a number of issues that were contributing to her chronic headache symptoms and that she should respond to physical intervention. The common difficulty in diagnosis is distinguishing between migraine without aura and CGH. Making diagnosis even more challenging is that an individual patient typically has more than one type of headache (Amiri et al., 2007).

In Jean's case, there was substantial evidence supporting a diagnosis of CGH together with medication-overuse headache and potentially tension-type headache. With respect to potential physical contributing factors identified in the physical examination, there was a clear link between her less-than-optimal spine and scapular posture and neck symptoms. Previous studies have raised questions regarding the link between posture and headache, with some studies reporting an association (Watson and Trott, 1993; Budelmann et al., 2013), which is not substantiated by others (Treleaven et al., 1994; Dumas et al., 2001; Zito et al., 2006). One explanation for this might be the wide variation in cervical posture seen in asymptomatic people (Miyazaki et al., 2008). Hence, a common postural abnormality is unlikely to be seen in headache. Despite this, a clear link was established between Jean's posture and pain by examining the effect of altering her posture on symptoms and neck movements, which were positively influenced by the correction. There was also clear evidence of movement impairment in the cervical vertebral segments capable of provoking referred head pain (Bogduk and Govind, 2009). Palpation of these impaired motion segments induced neck pain and headache. In addition, it was possible to alleviate neck pain and headache by manual therapy techniques. As well as the evidence of articular and myofascial dysfunction, there was also evidence of neural tissue mechanosensitivity. Table 16.1 defines the International Headache Society diagnostic criteria for CGH (Sjaastad et al., 1998). Based on these criteria, Jean satisfies the majority of requirements for a diagnosis of CGH (Antonaci et al., 2001) as indicative of 'probable' CGH.

Continued on following page

TABLE 16.1

INTERNATIONAL HEADACHE SOCIETY DIAGNOSTIC CRITERIA FOR CERVICOGENIC HEADACHE (SJAASTAD, ET AL., 1998)

Major criteria	I. Symptoms and signs of neck involvement
	  a. Precipitation of comparable symptoms by:
	    neck movement and/or sustained, awkward head positioning, and/or
	    external pressure over the upper cervical or occipital region
	  b. Restriction of range of motion in the neck
	  c. Ipsilateral neck, shoulder or arm pain
	II. Confirmatory evidence by diagnostic anaesthetic block
	III. Unilaterality of the head pain, without side shift

Head pain characteristics	IV. Moderate-severe, non-throbbing pain, usually starting in the neck Episodes of varying duration, or fluctuating, continuous pain
Other characteristics of some importance	V. Only marginal or lack of effect of indomethacin Only marginal or lack of effect of ergotamine and sumatriptan Female gender Not infrequent history of head or indirect neck trauma, usually of more than medium severity

Other features of lesser importance	VI. Various attack-related phenomena, only occasionally present, and/or moderately expressed when present:
	  a. Nausea
	  b. Phono- and photophobia
	  c. Dizziness
	  d. Ipsilateral 'blurred vision'
	  e. Difficulties swallowing
	  f. Ipsilateral oedema, mostly in the periocular area

TABLE 16.2

CLASSIFICATION OF MEDICATION-OVERUSE HEADACHE (HEADACHE CLASSIFICATION COMMITTEE OF THE INTERNATIONAL HEADACHE, 2013)

Medication-Overuse Headache

A.	Headache present on ≥15 days/month.
B.	Regular overuse for >3 months of one or more drugs that can be taken for acute and/or symptomatic treatment of headache. 1. Simple analgesics on >15 days/month on a regular basis for >3 months. 2. Ergotamine, triptans, opioids or combination analgesics on >10 days/month on a regular basis for >3 months. 3. Any combination of ergotamine, triptans, analgesics and/or opioids >15 days/month on a regular basis for >3 months without overuse of any single class alone.
C.	Headache has developed or markedly worsened during medication overuse.

In addition to the identified impairments, there was evidence of medication-overuse headache as defined in Table 16.2 (Headache Classification Committee of the International Headache, 2013). In this situation, the first priority is to reduce the frequency of medication as a tool for headache management.

Medication-overuse headache is one of the most common causes of chronic headache (Grande et al., 2008) that is often unrecognized. Over 50% of people with chronic headache, defined as headache on more than 15 days per month, have medication overuse headache (Grande et al., 2008; Jonsson et al., 2011). Medication-overuse headache is diagnosed if over-the-counter medication (or prescribed headache medication) is taken for headache on more than 15 days per month for 3 consecutive months.

Reasoning Question:

4. Given the number of potential contributing factors to Jean's headaches, how did this support/negate your initial hypothesis regarding the 'pain type' following the subjective examination?

Answer to Reasoning Question:

The initial thoughts were that nociplastic was the 'pain type' because this is the necessary mechanism underlying many kinds of headache. For example, sensitization of the trigeminocervical nucleus distinguishes a patient with neck pain due to a painful C2/C3 facet joint from another who has the same problem but who has headache as well as neck pain (Chua et al., 2011). Hence nociplastic pain, in the sense one would consider in fibromyalgia, for example, was not present. There was no evidence of widespread sensitivity on palpation of the cervical spine or orofacial region, and headache could only be provoked by very specific palpation on C1 in a very specific position of the neck, and not through palpation of other impaired levels. In addition, symptoms were modifiable through alteration in posture and through specific manual therapy techniques. Hence there was sufficient central sensitization affecting the trigeminocervical nucleus to induce referred pain into the head from noxious stimulation of the cervical spine but not sufficient to cause widespread pain and widespread mechanical allodynia and hyperalgesia.

Clinical Reasoning Commentary:

Diagnostic reasoning is evident in the answers to both Reasoning Questions 2 and 3. Diagnostic classification, particularly with respect to pathology and pathophysiology, is de-emphasized by some due to the recognition that pathology typically cannot be confirmed from the clinical examination; pathology can exist but be asymptomatic; symptoms can be present without overt pathology; and symptomatic pathology can have varied presentations. As discussed in Chapter 1, these are valid cautions that highlight the need for a balance in pathology and impairment focused reasoning. However, it is still important to hypothesize about pathology, or in this case, categorization of headache type and associated pathophysiology and pain mechanisms. This is evident in the answer to Reasoning Question 2, where categorization of headache, based on internationally accepted criteria, informs reasoning in other categories of judgement, such as 'management' and 'prognosis' (e.g. evidence for the effectiveness of manual therapy is stronger for tension-type and CGH than for migraine). Whereas medical diagnostic reasoning focusses primarily on pathology and disease classification, 'diagnosis' in musculoskeletal practice can be broader and include hypotheses regarding potentially relevant physical impairments that if symptomatic may represent 'sources of symptoms' (in this case, nociception) and when asymptomatic may reflect 'contributing factors' to the development and/or maintenance of the patient's symptoms and disability. The clinical reasoning challenge is to establish whether asymptomatic physical impairments, for example, in posture, flexibility, muscle control and strength, are contributing to a patient's presentation. Clearly such impairments are common in asymptomatic individuals. They can also be present but not necessarily contribute to the presentation of patients who are symptomatic. Hypotheses regarding potential physical contributing factors are strengthened when modification of a factor results in a clear and consistent change in symptoms. It then requires management intervention directed at the factor with re-assessment of both the physical impairment and the functional restrictions to warrant proceeding with that management. Although this empirical approach cannot categorically confirm the role any physical factor has in a patient's symptoms and disability, it provides a systematic method for selection and when indicated, progression of management of potential contributing factors unique to each patient.

As discussed in the previous Clinical Reasoning Commentary and in Chapter 2, the mechanism of central sensitization is normal or adaptive in many pain presentations. This highlights the need to attempt to distinguish those presentations from what has been labelled 'dysfunctional pain' (Woolf, 2011, p. s5) or more recently nociplastic pain (IASP, 2017). As discussed in the answer to Reasoning Question 3, this requires knowledge of the expected clinical pattern for nociplastic pain. The classification of the hypothesis category 'pain type' presented in Chapter 1 is most likely too simplistic and currently not possible to confirm clinically. However, like most clinical reasoning, it can still be hypothesized based on current thinking, so the hypothesized pain type can then inform other clinical judgements, such as 'precautions', 'management' and 'prognosis'.

Appointment 1

The first priority was to reduce the frequency of medication use. This requires providing information to the patient about the association between medication overuse and headache. In simple terms, in the presence of medication-overuse headache, chronic analgesic exposure leads to CNS hyper-excitability, which can perpetuate headache – so the greater frequency in daily medication use, the more the problem develops. It's a vicious cycle. The aim is to achieve a decision by the patient to cut down on the medication with a firm plan. Explicit recommendations were reduction in headache medication toward 'safe levels', and information about possible difficulties and gains including that medication-overuse headache usually gets worse before it improves 1–2 weeks after withdrawal.

It is not a physiotherapist's role to alter prescription medication. However, because Jean was inadvertently abusing over-the-counter painkillers, I was comfortable in not referring Jean to her GP for this aspect of care. This might be necessary if the patient cannot cope with the short-term increase in headache associated with reducing medication. In addition, if the patient were overusing prescription medication, then this would require medical consultation. Recently, a randomized controlled trial found that a brief intervention of advice was effective in reducing medication-overuse headache. In that study, patients were allocated to receive either usual care from their GP or a brief intervention of advice. Chronic headache was resolved in 50% of the cases receiving the brief intervention, but only 6% of those receiving usual care (Kristoffersen et al., 2016).

In addition to providing this information and to address the cervical spine impairments, correction of the maladaptive postural control was instigated first, as this was felt to be the main driver. This involved correction of the pelvis, head, scapular and spinal posture in sitting, increasing to progressively longer periods. In my experience, this alone can be sufficient to break the cycle of postural abnormality, inducing stress on the cervical spine, which causes pain and deterioration of muscle function. A recent study (Beer et al., 2012) found that a 2-week programme aimed at improving trunk posture in sitting was sufficient to improve the pattern of neck muscle activation on subsequent evaluation.

In addition to postural correction, exercises were prescribed to improve the function of the cervical muscles. A randomized controlled trial found that specific exercises for the deep neck flexor and axioscapular muscles were sufficient to improve CGH symptoms (Jull et al., 2002). This large multicenter trial compared different forms of intervention given over 12 sessions. Manual therapy and specific exercise were both substantially better than usual care from the GP. The combination of manual therapy with specific exercise was better still.

Exercises to improve craniocervical flexion and axioscapular control were given, with a plan to progress these over time. This exercise consisted of craniocervical flexion held for five seconds and repeated five times, with an emphasis on minimal movement to improve deep cervical flexor muscle activation while minimizing the activity of the hyoids and sternocleidomastoid muscles. Because of the poor level of control of these muscles, the exercises were very gentle in nature. During this first treatment session, considerable time was spent showing the patient the required movement of the cervical spine and scapula passively to achieve the correct pattern of activation. Based on personal experience, this commonly helps the patient to develop a better sense of the required movement and gentle nature of the exercise. Jean was encouraged to do these exercises at least twice per day, and on an hourly basis adopt the corrected posture of the trunk and scapula for 5-second holds repeated five times. The aim was to be more aware of the posture during the day.

Appointment 2 (1 Week Later)

The next treatment session took place 1 week later. Jean reported that she understood and accepted the problem of overusing pain medication. However, she had noticed an increase in headache symptoms with her reduction in medication but was prepared to put up with this in the short-term. Despite the exacerbation of headache, she felt that the correction of her posture had helped reduce the severity of her symptoms, and she was determined to continue to reduce her reliance on medication. Jean was advised that she could see her GP if she felt that she could not cope with a change in pain medication but that this was probably not going to be necessary because she was already well on the way to breaking the cycle.

Jean was also given extensive pain education using simple diagrams and verbal explanation, particularly regarding the association between trigeminocervical nucleus sensitization and headache. She was also given advice about computer workstation ergonomics and advised to stop using her laptop while having it resting on her lap. Further advice was given about the effects that inadequate sleep (Kovacs et al., 2014), increased stress and lack of exercise have on sensitization of the trigeminocervical nucleus. She was advised to gradually take up exercise again, choosing cycling as her preferred option.

Specific mobilization of the impaired joints was commenced at this second treatment session. Mobilization of the C0/C1 was seen as the first priority. A posteroanterior mobilization was carried out with the neck positioned in upper cervical spine flexion. Although this was painful, it did not reproduce the headache in this position. Throughout five repetitions, the pain on palpation subsided. A recent study has shown that upper cervical palpation techniques can reduce the sensitivity of the trigeminocervical nucleus (Watson and Drummond, 2014). In that study, the blink reflex was measured before and after noxious stimulation of the upper cervical spine by palpation. Repeated application of the stimulus induced a gradual reduction in severity of pain and also a reduction in sensitivity of the trigeminocervical nucleus as measured by the blink reflex.

In addition to the accessory mobilization technique, a modified Mulligan Headache SNAG was applied. This technique was applied at the C3 level using a self-SNAG cervical strap. This cushioned strap was hooked under the spinous process of C3, with Jean holding the strap with both arms. The strap was angled upward, toward her eyes, to follow the cervical facet plane, which is approximately 45 degrees at the C2/C3 level. Jean was instructed to retract her head against the pressure of the strap on C3 (Fig. 16.8). Applying the headache SNAG relieved Jean's headache symptoms, which was a positive reinforcement for her to repeat the exercise regularly during the day. She was advised to sustain a gentle pressure through the cervical self-SNAG strap onto C3 for up to 10 seconds and repeat this five times per day. Jean understood that the exercise was to relieve headache symptoms and she should stop if pain increased.

In addition to these treatments, the postural correction exercises given in the first treatment session were reviewed and fine-tuned. The cranio-cervical flexion exercise was also checked for accuracy. There was a small increase in the ability to achieve flexion of the high cervical spine without substitution of the hyoid and sternocleidomastoid muscles.

Appointment 3 (1 Week Later)

The next treatment session took place 1 week later. Jean reported an improvement in her headache severity and frequency. In fact, her headache had reduced to a level lower than prior to commencing treatment. The headache frequency was similar, but the intensity of the pain was less. She put this down to reducing her medication, taking control of her posture and relieving her headaches with the Headache self-SNAG. She also felt empowered by the combination of treatment approaches. She felt that her headaches were now more under her own control. She had also discussed the situation of lack of exercise with her

Fig. 16.8 Modified self-SNAG with a cervical self-SNAG strap.

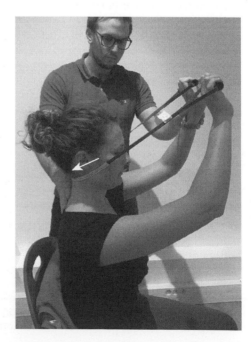

husband. They agreed to find more time so that Jean could exercise on her bike three times per week.

Assessment of cervical range of motion indicated an increase in physiological range of upper cervical spine retraction, which was no longer painful. Combined movement evaluation was less provocative and there was greater movement when compared with the initial evaluation. Palpation of C1 in neutral position indicated reduced sensitivity. Palpation of C1 in upper cervical spine flexion with left rotation was no longer provocative for headache. Despite these changes, the range of cervical rotation to the left with the spinous process of C2 fixed was still only 5 degrees. The flexion-rotation test was still symptomatic and reduced in range with an estimated range of 20 degrees to the left side.

Due to the improvement of sensitivity on palpation of C1, specific mobilization of the C0/C1 segment was progressed toward flexion with left rotation. Additional mobilization at the C1/C2 vertebral segment was commenced by the use of a cervical self-SNAG strap. This exercise is shown in Fig. 16.8 and has been shown to be effective in reducing headache in people with a positive flexion-rotation test and features of CGH (Hall et al., 2007). Jean was shown how to place the strap around the posterior arch of C1, applying tension to the strap horizontally forward toward the corner of her mouth, following the horizontally orientated articular surface at C1/C2. The other end of the strap is angled downward, passing around the back of the neck and is held lightly onto the abdomen. It is important not to apply too much tension to the strap. As the patient actively rotates the head toward the left, the strap is pulled forward with the left hand, with tension maintained gently, keeping the strap aligned with the corner of the mouth to ensure the correct direction of glide through C1. The head movement is carried out to the end range, pausing to apply overpressure for 1–2 seconds and then returning to the start position. The movement was repeated two times on the first occasion due to the large range of motion at the C1/C2 level and the propensity for exacerbation if the technique is performed too frequently or too vigorously. Applying the C1/C2 self-SNAG, the flexion-rotation test was repeated and found to be approximately 35 degrees in range to the left. Jean was advised to do this exercise at home in the evening and morning with two repetitions only. She was advised to stop if there was any exacerbation of her symptoms or if she felt any dizziness or other features.

In addition to these treatments, the postural correction exercises were reviewed with renewed emphasis and encouragement to maintain and build on the improvements gained. Jean was able to control her neck movement much better during the cranio-cervical flexion exercise and was able to achieve a larger range of upper cervical flexion without substituting with her superficial muscles. She was advised to increase the duration of the holds to 10 seconds repeated five times.

Appointment 4 (1 Week Later)

The next treatment session again took place 1 week later. Jean reported headache only twice in the previous week, and the intensity of the pain was less. Neck pain had also diminished from the first session. With her improved sitting posture and better work environment, Jean was able to work for longer on her computer before experiencing neck pain. The Headache Disability Index score was reduced to 42/100. It has been reported that a 30-point change is required to reflect an improvement in headache disability (Jacobson et al., 1995).

Active cervical range of motion was improving in all directions, although extension was still poorly controlled. Combined movement evaluation revealed poor range of extension combined with side-flexion when C3 was stabilized. The flexion-rotation test had improved from the previous treatment sessions, indicating improved C1/C2 movement. Palpation of C1 and C2 articular pillar with the cervical spine in neutral position was much less painful compared with the first treatment session. Despite this, the C3 articular pillar was still painful, and it was more painful with the neck side-flexed and extended and more painful when the pressure was inclined cranially, indicating potential impairment of the C2/C3 segment.

Because the C2/C3 joint had not improved with mobilization and exercise to this point, a decision was made to add mobilization of the C2/C3 vertebral segment. This was accomplished by applying a C2/C3 rotation SNAG in sitting. The pad of the left thumb was placed on the articular pillar of C3 on the left side. The right thumb reinforced the pressure with inclination roughly 45 degrees to the horizontal, toward Jean's eyes. With this pressure maintained, Jean was instructed to rotate her head to the left side until full-range cervical rotation was achieved. This movement was painless and was repeated six times, with three sets.

In addition to these procedures, the postural correction exercises were reviewed. In an effort to improve Jean's cervical spine extension control, she was shown how to achieve extension with better control. She was advised to use the feedback of the position of the lower cervical spine during extension as a guide to good extension control. To do this, she palpated the C5 spinous process with the tips of her middle fingers and was instructed to keep the spinous process against the fingertips by retraction first followed by extension. With this feedback, Jean was able to improve her cervical extension control for a small ROM into extension, up to 10 degrees only. She was advised to repeat this exercise for 10 movements at a time and to do this several times per day. At no time was the exercise to be painful. This exercise requires good deep neck flexor muscle control and can be seen as a progression of the exercises Jean was currently doing with the cranio-cervical flexion exercise in supine. Because her ability to perform controlled cranio-cervical flexion had improved, she was now asked to perform the flexion movement to end range, or approximately 15 degrees of upper cervical spine flexion.

Jean had virtually ceased all medication. This was the first time in many years that she had not taken medication for headache.

Appointments 5–8 (Weekly Intervals)

The following treatment sessions continued to take place at weekly intervals. This was in part due to the difficulty that Jean had in making more frequent appointments, but this was not considered to be an issue because the treatments provided were largely self-management and required time to assess the impact on the frequency of headache.

Jean reported a reduction in headache frequency to one headache per week by the fifth treatment session, which was further reduced to once per fortnight by the sixth session. She continued with her general exercise programme, riding her bike for an hour three times per week. She was also making a conscious effort to walk more often, walking with her children to school rather than driving.

At the eighth treatment session, Jean had full pain-free ROM in her neck in all directions, including retraction and protraction of the upper cervical spine. In addition, she had improved cervical extension control without pain, with much better control over the movement, no longer collapsing into extension.

Segmental mobility tests revealed 40 degrees of rotation to the left during the flexion-rotation test. This was still approximately 5 degrees less range than to the right side. Passive physiological movement tests were hypomobile at C2/C3 but appeared normal in range at C0/C1. Palpation continued to be painful at C1 with the neck in flexion and left rotation, but this was much less symptomatic when compared with this test on the fourth treatment session. Headache was no longer reproduced on palpation of C1 in flexion-rotation left. Palpation of C2 and C3 in neutral spine position was much less painful than in previous sessions. However, when the head and neck were positioned in upper cervical spine extension and left-side flexion, the C3 vertebra was now the most symptomatic when compared with palpation at C1 and C2.

Jean was able to adopt a much better posture, although she still needed reminding about this; when distracted, she tended to go back to her old 'poor' posture (depressed/protracted scapula, flexed trunk and protracted upper cervical spine). Cervical motor control was much improved. Deep neck flexor function as evaluated by the cranio-cervical flexion test in supine was now full range, with minimal substitution from the hyoid muscles. She was able to maintain an inner-range position of upper cervical spine flexion in supine for 10 seconds and was able to repeat this up to five times without substitution.

Neurodynamic tests and nerve trunk palpation were re-evaluated at the beginning of the eighth treatment session. Upper cervical spine flexion in a slump position was no longer painful. In supine lying, upper cervical spine flexion carried out with the arms positioned in 90 degrees abduction was no longer restricted in comparison to the first treatment session. Palpation of the greater occipital nerve, however, was still more sensitive on the left compared to the right side.

Based on these findings, it was apparent that the measures taken to this point had been successful. Jean was very happy with her progress because she no longer required medication. Medication-overuse headache could now be discounted as a cause of remaining headache. In addition, she was exercising on a regular basis, and her fitness levels had increased. She was also able to alter her posture at will. As mentioned, however, she still needed reminding to correct her posture, something she recognized as a problem when she was distracted. In addition, cervical spine ROM and sensitivity on palpation of the upper cervical spine was much improved. There appeared to be a continued small impairment of the C1/C2 segmental rotation. In addition, the C2/C3 was also still mildly restricted in movement and was still painful on palpation.

During these treatment sessions, a C2/C3 self-SNAG was introduced. In this seated technique, Jean was shown how to place a cervical self-SNAG strap around the C2 vertebral level on the right side, pulling the strap up toward her eye with the left hand. The other end of the strap was angled around the back of the neck and held loosely with the right hand. Jean was instructed to pull the strap with her left hand while she rotated her head to the left. The pressure from the strap exerted left rotation force on the C2/C3 segment. This technique was pain-free during the movement. Jean was advised to perform this exercise 10 times in a session at home and to perform three sets during the day. If exacerbation of pain was experienced, she was to stop this exercise.

Further Management

Jean made good progress over a total of 10 treatment sessions. At the final consultation, her neck disability score had dropped to 10/100, much more than the 30-point change required to reflect a change in headache disability (Jacobson et al., 1995). Jean had stopped taking medication completely. Her sleep pattern was much improved. She was able to sit and work on her desktop computer for extended periods of time without neck pain, and headache was reduced to once per fortnight at a 3/10 level. Finally, she had increased her exercise programme, either walking to school with the children twice a day or riding a bike three times per week with a group of friends for an hour each time.

Reasoning Question:

5. Given your analysis of the multifactorial nature of Jean's symptoms requiring several approaches to management, can you elaborate on your timing for selecting each of the approaches?

Answer to Reasoning Question:

I initially decided that the primary drivers for Jean's headache were the overuse of analgesics and her poor posture. Medication overuse could be increasing central sensitivity, priming the input from postural stress on the cervical spine, which had been affected by the previous whiplash injury. Hence, addressing these two components was seen to be a priority and was easily modifiable and could be incorporated into her busy lifestyle. Manual techniques and other exercise to address upper cervical spine impairments may well have had beneficial effects initially, but these could not be expected to have lasting effects unless the primary drivers were addressed. The lifestyle and psychological contributing factors of lack of sleep and exercise as well as stress and anxiety were additional but smaller factors which may take time to modify and therefore are unlikely to have such a quick response. However, the treatment was seen as a 'package', rather than one aspect predominating. Each factor perhaps addressed a small component of the overall problem. Addressing these individually might not have had much effect. But when these factors were combined, the cumulative effect perhaps increased the overall efficacy in reducing symptoms. An example of this is seen in patients with neck pain. Education combined with exercise was more powerful than education alone (Brage et al., 2015).

Reasoning Question:

6. Can you comment on how psychosocial issues may have influenced the outcome of Jean's management? Did you employ any specific strategies to address this aspect of the problem?

Answer to Reasoning Question:

There is some information that Jean had some stressors with respect to her work and family situation. She identified this herself as an issue in the initial interview, so it was very easy to bring this to her attention, confirming her suspicion that stress and anxiety, sleep deprivation and lack of exercise can have a substantial impact on pain in general as well as headache (Noseda et al., 2014). It was explained to her that she had the chance to control both peripheral nociceptive input through changes to posture and ergonomics, as well as exerting volitional control over top-down mechanisms (Nijs et al., 2014). Talking about these factors with her perhaps allowed her to then have legitimacy in discussing these issues with her husband and looking for a means for change. Her husband was very supportive of jointly finding ways to reduce psychosocial stresses in the family, to enable Jean to return to exercise and to develop a more normal pattern of sleep.

Clinical Reasoning Commentary:

With the multitude of interactions possible between biological, psychological, social and environmental factors, identification of risk factors to the development of musculoskeletal symptoms, impairment and disability is less clear than, for example, cardiac disease. Clinical judgement regarding where to commence management should prioritize those factors identified in the patient's presentation that are well supported by research, such as Jean's overuse of analgesics in this case. With less research evidence support, but a clear positive symptom response with Jean, posture is also addressed in the initial management. Although cost-effectiveness of musculoskeletal therapy requires that management addresses all factors hypothesized as contributing to the patient's symptoms and disability, introducing different interventions progressively over time enables some evaluation of the contribution of each.

The answer to Reasoning Question 5 reflects the psychosocial (or 'narrative') reasoning in this case. The extent to which musculoskeletal therapists screen for psychosocial factors contributing to patients' symptoms and disability varies considerably. Specific suggestions for both assessment and management of social and psychological factors are discussed in Chapters 3 and 4, respectively. Central to the management of psychosocial factors, as discussed here, is education. Education can have multiple aims, including facilitating awareness and understanding of the problem and of pain, facilitating conceptual change in beliefs, promoting more adaptive coping strategies, promoting self-management and strengthening self-efficacy, reducing fear and other negative emotions and facilitating restoration of activity and participation.

This case illustrates the value of an evidence-based, clinically reasoned approach to examination and management of headache.

REFERENCES

Alonso-Blanco, C., Fernandez-de-las-Penas, C., Fernandez-Mayoralas, D.M., de-la-Llave-Rincon, A.I., Pareja, J.A., Svensson, P., 2011. Prevalence and anatomical localization of muscle referred pain from active trigger points in head and neck musculature in adults and children with chronic tension-type headache. Pain Med. 12 (10), 1453–1463.

Amiri, M., Jull, G., Bullock-Saxton, J., Darnell, R., Lander, C., 2007. Cervical musculoskeletal impairment in frequent intermittent headache. Part 2: subjects with concurrent headache types. Cephalalgia 27 (8), 891–898.

Antonaci, F., Ghirmai, S., Bono, G., Sandrini, G., Nappi, G., 2001. Cervicogenic headache: evaluation of the original diagnostic criteria. Cephalalgia 21 (5), 573–583.

Bartsch, T., Goadsby, P.J., 2003. Increased responses in trigeminocervical nociceptive neurons to cervical input after stimulation of the dura mater. Brain 126 (Pt 8), 1801–1813.

Beer, A., Treleaven, J., Jull, G., 2012. Can a functional postural exercise improve performance in the cranio-cervical flexion test? A preliminary study. Man. Ther. 17 (3), 219–224.

Biondi, D.M., 2005. Physical treatments for headache: a structured review. Headache 45 (6), 738–746.

Bogduk, N., 2002. Biomechanics of the cervical spine. In: Grant, R. (Ed.), Physical Therapy of the Cervical and Thoracic Spine. Churchill Livingstone, St Louis, pp. 26–44.

Bogduk, N., Govind, J., 2009. Cervicogenic headache: an assessment of the evidence on clinical diagnosis, invasive tests, and treatment. Lancet Neurol. 8 (10), 959–968.

Brage, K., Ris, I., Falla, D., Sogaard, K., Juul-Kristensen, B., 2015. Pain education combined with neck- and aerobic training is more effective at relieving chronic neck pain than pain education alone – A preliminary randomized controlled trial. Man. Ther. 20 (5), 686–693.

Bronfort, G., Haas, M., Evans, R., Leiniger, B., Triano, J., 2010. Effectiveness of manual therapies: the UK evidence report. Chiropr. Osteopat. 18 (1), 3.

Budelmann, K., von Piekartz, H., Hall, T., 2013. Is there a difference in head posture and cervical spine movement in children with and without pediatric headache? Eur. J. Pediatr. 172, 1349–1356.

Cady, R.K., 2007. The convergence hypothesis. Headache 47 (Suppl. 1), S44–S51.

Cady, R., Schreiber, C., Farmer, K., Sheftell, F., 2002. Primary headaches: a convergence hypothesis. Headache 42 (3), 204–216.

Calandre, E.P., Hidalgo, J., Garcia-Leiva, J.M., Rico-Villademoros, F., 2006. Trigger point evaluation in migraine patients: an indication of peripheral sensitization linked to migraine predisposition? Eur. J. Neurol. 13 (3), 244–249.

Calandre, E.P., Hidalgo, J., Garcia-Leiva, J.M., Rico-Villademoros, F., Delgado-Rodriguez, A., 2008. Myofascial trigger points in cluster headache patients: a case series. Head Face Med. 4, 32.

Chaibi, A., Russell, M.B., 2012. Manual therapies for cervicogenic headache: a systematic review. J. Headache Pain 13 (5), 351–359.

Chiu, T.T., Law, E.Y., Chiu, T.H., 2005. Performance of the craniocervical flexion test in subjects with and without chronic neck pain. J. Orthop. Sports Phys. Ther. 35 (9), 567–571.

Chua, N.H., van Suijlekom, H.A., Vissers, K.C., Arendt-Nielsen, L., Wilder-Smith, O.H., 2011. Differences in sensory processing between chronic cervical zygapophysial joint pain patients with and without cervicogenic headache. Cephalalgia 31 (8), 953–963.

Cook, C., Brown, C., Isaacs, R., Roman, M., Davis, S., Richardson, W., 2010. Clustered clinical findings for diagnosis of cervical spine myelopathy. J Man Manip Ther 18 (4), 175–180.

Dodick, D.W., 2010. Pearls: headache. Semin. Neurol. 30 (1), 74–81.

Dumas, J.P., Arsenault, A.B., Boudreau, G., Magnoux, E., Lepage, Y., Bellavance, A., et al., 2001. Physical impairments in cervicogenic headache: traumatic vs. nontraumatic onset. Cephalalgia 21 (9), 884–893.

Edwards, B., 1992. Manual of Combined Movements: Their Use in the Examination and Treatment of Mechanical Vertebral Column Disorders. Churchill Livingstone, Edinburgh.

Fernández-de-Las-Penas, C., Courtney, C.A., 2014. Clinical reasoning for manual therapy management of tension type and cervicogenic headache. J Man Manip Ther 22 (1), 44–50.

Grande, R.B., Aaseth, K., Gulbrandsen, P., Lundqvist, C., Russell, M.B., 2008. Prevalence of primary chronic headache in a population-based sample of 30- to 44-year-old persons. The Akershus study of chronic headache. Neuroepidemiology 30 (2), 76–83.

Grondin, F., Hall, T.M., 2015. Upper cervical range of motion is impaired in patients with temporomandibular disorders. Cranio. 33 (2), 91–99.

Ha, S.M., Kwon, O.Y., Weon, J.H., Kim, M.H., Kim, S.J., 2013. Reliability and validity of goniometric and photographic measurements of clavicular tilt angle. Man. Ther. 18 (5), 367–371.

Ha, S.M., Kwon, O.Y., Yi, C.H., Jeon, H.S., Lee, W.H., 2011. Effects of passive correction of scapular position on pain, proprioception, and range of motion in neck-pain patients with bilateral scapular downward-rotation syndrome. Man. Ther. 16 (6), 585–589.

Hall, T., Briffa, K., Hopper, D., 2008. Clinical evaluation of cervicogenic headache: a clinical perspective. J Man Manip Ther 16 (2), 73–80.

Hall, T.M., Briffa, K., Hopper, D., Robinson, K., 2010. Comparative analysis and diagnostic accuracy of the cervical flexion-rotation test. J. Headache Pain 11 (5), 391–397.

Hall, T., Chan, H.T., Christensen, L., Odenthal, B., Wells, C., Robinson, K., 2007. Efficacy of a C1-C2 self-sustained natural apophyseal glide (SNAG) in the management of cervicogenic headache. J. Orthop. Sports Phys. Ther. 37 (3), 100–107.

Hall, T., Robinson, K., 2004. The flexion-rotation test and active cervical mobility – a comparative measurement study in cervicogenic headache. Man. Ther. 9 (4), 197–202.

Headache Classification Committee of the International Headache, S, 2013. The International Classification of Headache Disorders, 3rd edition (beta version). Cephalalgia 33 (9), 629–808.

Hing, W., Hall, T., Rivett, D., Vicenzino, B., Mulligan, B., 2015. The Mulligan Concept of Manual Therapy: Textbook of Techniques. Elsevier Australia, Sydney.

IASP Taxonomy 2017, IASP Publications, Washington, D.C., viewed December 2017, https://www.iasp-pain.org/Taxonomy.

Jacobson, G.P., Ramadan, N.M., Norris, L., Newman, C.W., 1995. Headache Disability Inventory (HDI): short-term test-retest reliability and spouse perceptions. Headache 35 (9), 534–539.

Jonsson, P., Hedenrud, T., Linde, M., 2011. Epidemiology of medication overuse headache in the general Swedish population. Cephalalgia 31 (9), 1015–1022.

Jull, G., Amiri, M., Bullock-Saxton, J., Darnell, R., Lander, C., 2007. Cervical musculoskeletal impairment in frequent intermittent headache. Part 1: subjects with single headaches. Cephalalgia 27 (7), 793–802.

Jull, G., Trott, P., Potter, H., Zito, G., Neire, K., Shirley, D., et al., 2002. A randomized controlled trial of exercise and manipulative therapy for cervicogenic headache. Spine 27 (17), 1835–1843.

Kaale, B.R., Krakenes, J., Albrektsen, G., Wester, K., 2008. Clinical assessment techniques for detecting ligament and membrane injuries in the upper cervical spine region–a comparison with MRI results. Man. Ther. 13 (5), 397–403.

Karhu, J.O., Parkkola, R.K., Komu, M.E., Kormano, M.J., Koskinen, S.K., 1999. Kinematic magnetic resonance imaging of the upper cervical spine using a novel positioning device. Spine 24 (19), 2046–2056.

Kauther, M.D., Piotrowski, M., Hussmann, B., Lendemans, S., Wedemeyer, C., 2012. Cervical range of motion and strength in 4,293 young male adults with chronic neck pain. Eur. Spine J. 21 (8), 1522–1527.

Kovacs, F.M., Seco, J., Royuela, A., Melis, S., Sanchez, C., Diaz-Arribas, M.J., et al., 2014. Patients with neck pain are less likely to improve if they suffer from poor sleep quality. A prospective study in routine practice. Clin. J. Pain 31 (8), 713–721.

Kristoffersen, E.S., Straand, J., Vetvik, K.G., Benth, J.S., Russell, M.B., Lundqvist, C., 2016. Brief intervention by general practitioners for medication-overuse headache, follow-up after 6 months: a pragmatic cluster-randomised controlled trial. J. Neurol. 263 (2), 344–353.

Macpherson, B.C., Campbell, C., 1991. C2 rotation and spinous process deviation in migraine: cause or effect or coincidence? Neuroradiology 33 (6), 475–477.

Miyazaki, M., Hymanson, H.J., Morishita, Y., He, W., Zhang, H., Wu, G., et al., 2008. Kinematic analysis of the relationship between sagittal alignment and disc degeneration in the cervical spine. Spine 33 (23), E870–E876.

Moeller, J.J., Kurniawan, J., Gubitz, G.J., Ross, J.A., Bhan, V., 2008. Diagnostic accuracy of neurological problems in the emergency department. Can. J. Neurol. Sci. 35 (3), 335–341.

Nijs, J., Malfliet, A., Ickmans, K., Baert, I., Meeus, M., 2014. Treatment of central sensitization in patients with 'unexplained' chronic pain: an update. Expert Opin. Pharmacother. 15 (12), 1671–1683.

Noseda, R., Kainz, V., Borsook, D., Burstein, R., 2014. Neurochemical pathways that converge on thalamic trigeminovascular neurons: potential substrate for modulation of migraine by sleep, food intake, stress and anxiety. PLoS ONE 9 (8), e103929.

O'Leary, S., Falla, D., Jull, G., Vicenzino, B., 2007. Muscle specificity in tests of cervical flexor muscle performance. J. Electromyogr. Kinesiol. 17 (1), 35–40.

Ogince, M., 2003. Sensitivity and specificity of the flexion rotation test. In: Proceedings of the World Confederation for Physical Therapy, Barcelona, Spain.

Ordway, N.R., Seymour, R.J., Donelson, R.G., Hojnowski, L.S., Edwards, W.T., 1999. Cervical flexion, extension, protrusion, and retraction. A radiographic segmental analysis. Spine 24 (3), 240–247.

Osmotherly, P.G., Rivett, D., Rowe, L.J., 2013. Toward understanding normal craniocervical rotation occurring during the rotation stress test for the alar ligaments. Phys. Ther. 93 (7), 986–992.

Pfaffenrath, V., Kaube, H., 1990. Diagnostics of cervicogenic headache. Funct. Neurol. 5, 159–164.

Rushton, A., Rivett, D., Carlesso, L., Flynn, T., Hing, W., Kerry, R., 2014. International framework for examination of the cervical region for potential of Cervical Arterial Dysfunction prior to Orthopaedic Manual Therapy intervention. Man. Ther. 19, 222–228. https://doi.org/10.1016/j.math.2013.11.005.

Sjaastad, O., Fredriksen, T.A., Pfaffenrath, V., 1998. Cervicogenic headache: diagnostic criteria. The Cervicogenic Headache International Study Group. Headache 38 (6), 442–445.

Sun-Edelstein, C., Mauskop, A., 2012. Complementary and alternative approaches to the treatment of tension-type headache. Curr. Pain Headache Rep. 16 (6), 539–544.

Takasaki, H., Hall, T., Kaneko, S., Ikemoto, Y., Jull, G., 2010. A radiographic analysis of the influence of initial neck posture on cervical segmental movement at end-range extension in asymptomatic subjects. Man. Ther. 16 (1), 74–79.

Takasaki, H., Hall, T., Oshiro, S., Kaneko, S., Ikemoto, Y., Jull, G., 2011. Normal kinematics of the upper cervical spine during the Flexion-Rotation Test - in vivo measurements using magnetic resonance imaging. Man. Ther. 16 (2), 167–171.

Treleaven, J., Jull, G., Atkinson, L., 1994. Cervical musculoskeletal dysfunction in post-concussional headache. Cephalalgia 14 (4), 273–279, discussion 257.

von Piekartz, H., Ludtke, K., 2011. Effect of treatment of temporomandibular disorders (TMD) in patients with cervicogenic headache: a single-blind, randomized controlled study. Cranio. 29 (1), 43–56.

von Piekartz, H.J., Schouten, S., Aufdemkampe, G., 2007. Neurodynamic responses in children with migraine or cervicogenic headache versus a control group. A comparative study. Man. Ther. 12 (2), 153–160.

Watson, D.H., Drummond, P.D., 2012. Head pain referral during examination of the neck in migraine and tension-type headache. Headache 52 (8), 1226–1235.

Watson, D.H., Drummond, P.D., 2014. Cervical referral of head pain in migraineurs: effects on the nociceptive blink reflex. Headache 54 (6), 1035–1045.

Watson, D.H., Drummond, P.D., 2016. The role of the trigemino cervical complex in chronic whiplash associated headache: a cross sectional study. Headache 56 (6), 961–975.

Watson, D.H., Trott, P.H., 1993. Cervical headache: an investigation of natural head posture and upper cervical flexor muscle performance. Cephalalgia 13 (4), 272–284, discussion 232.

Woolf, C.J., 2011. Central sensitization: implication for diagnosis and treatment of pain. Pain 152, s2–s15.

Zito, G., Jull, G., Story, I., 2006. Clinical tests of musculoskeletal dysfunction in the diagnosis of cervicogenic headache. Man. Ther. 11 (2), 118–129.

17

Shoulder Pain: To Operate or Not to Operate?

Jeremy Lewis • Eric J. Hegedus • Mark A. Jones

Appointment 1
Subjective Examination

Social History

Alison was referred by a sports and exercise medicine consultant for assessment and management of a recalcitrant right shoulder problem. Alison is a 48-year-old high school teacher who is married and has three teenage children. She was educated to university level, having obtained an undergraduate degree in history. She reported that she sits for approximately 8 hours per day (in total), and until the recent episode of pain, participated in exercise an average of three to four times each week. Her exercises consisted of cardiac and strength training at the gym, walking, gardening, occasional outdoor bicycling and a passion for playing social tennis.

Area and Behaviour of Symptoms

Alison described that she experienced symptoms as per the body chart (Fig. 17.1).

No paraesthesia or numbness was experienced in either the upper or lower limbs. No headaches, scapular or cervicothoracic region symptoms were reported. Deep and occasionally sharp pain in the lateral region of the right shoulder was constant but varying between 3 and 4 out of 10 on a numerical pain rating score (NPRS), where 10 was defined as the worst pain imaginable. Pain would increase up to a maximum of 6–7/10 during activities involving shoulder elevation, dressing (including hand behind back) and driving (especially turning to the left). Alison reported that repeated movements of her right shoulder as may be required during the initial assessment could lead to a substantial increase in resting pain that may settle in minutes or hours or possibly longer. Although she preferred to be a 'side-to-side' sleeper, at present, sleeping was confined to lying on her back or left side (both with one pillow under the head) and supporting her right arm on a folded pillow when on the left side (as she had been previously recommended).

History

On the first visit, Alison reported that she had been suffering from recurring shoulder pain for more than 2 years. Prior to this episode there was no history of any cervical or shoulder symptoms. She was unable to specify any specific macro-trauma event prior to onset, but Alison associated her initial shoulder pain with a period when she and her partner spent a number of days stripping wallpaper and repairing and painting walls and ceilings in a house that they were renovating. Following this activity, she described experiencing twinges in her right (dominant side) shoulder when performing activities such as blow drying her hair (an activity that might take 10–15 minutes), where the dryer was held in her left hand and brush in her right, and occasionally when elevating her arm such as when reaching to a high shelf or writing on the whiteboards at school. She described these

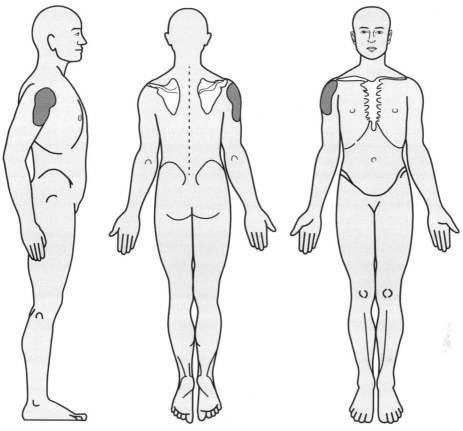

Fig. 17.1 Area of symptoms.

symptoms as very mild and as an annoyance, and she did not take any medications or seek treatment.

A few weeks after the home renovations, she reported playing tennis on an outside court. Leading up to this match, where she was competing against a more experienced player, she had not played tennis for more than 4 months. She considered this match physically demanding for her. She reported that she did not experience any symptoms on the day of the match, but upon waking the next morning, experienced substantial right shoulder pain. She did not remember if pain was present at rest but was certain it was felt during movement, such as when dressing and driving, describing that her first turn out of the driveway was to the left, and this was extremely painful. These symptoms continued for many days, and she eventually booked an appointment with her family physician, who diagnosed 'subacromial impingement syndrome' and prescribed a course of non-steroidal anti-inflammatory drugs (NSAIDs). During the initial treatment period of 3 to 4 weeks, Alison reported she was 20–30% better (she had also avoided provocative activities as much as she was able during this period), but no further improvement was made. As improvement had plateaued, her family doctor performed a landmark-guided injection of 'steroids', which hurt for a day or so but resulted in a substantial reduction in symptoms. Approximately 3 weeks later and feeling close to 100% reduction in pain, and being concerned that the protracted lack of use of her shoulder would result in a frozen shoulder (recently experienced by a friend), she went swimming. She had completed a 'few laps' (freestyle) of a 20-m pool and felt a sharp pain in her right shoulder on the commencement of the next lap just after her hand had entered the water. Concerned, she stopped swimming. and symptoms described as being 'more or less' identical to those after the tennis match started again. She was prescribed another course of NSAIDs, which had limited benefit, and was referred to physiotherapy, followed by a self-referral to osteopathy.

Treatments were as follows: recommendations to rest and ice her shoulder, soft tissue techniques, taping, acupuncture and shoulder mobilization procedures.

Over time (possibly a few months), her symptoms had settled, but she continued to feel pain in the right shoulder, especially when she elevated her arm (she again providing washing and drying her hair and school activities as examples). During this period, Alison avoided tennis and swimming but still continued to attend her gym on average two to three times a week for static bike cycling or cross training (holding the static grips on the cross trainer, as arm movement was sometimes painful), uphill walking on the treadmill and mat exercises, but no arm weight exercises or push-ups. She would work in the garden but would avoid heavy and above-shoulder activities. Over time, she felt her shoulder symptoms were improving. Approximatively 2 months prior to attending the physiotherapy our clinic, she again played tennis for about 30 minutes. She reported purposely playing a friend who understood she had a 'weak' shoulder, and they would play gently, with no serving, just gentle backhand and forehand shots. She reported that it was cold when they played and that the court was damp, and the ball possibly slightly wet. The day following the tennis match, she again experienced substantial pain, worse this episode than anything previously. She was angry with herself for playing and frustrated as she had played 'gently', although she expressed that playing when it was cold may have contributed to the increased symptoms. Pain was constantly present and would increase on movement and cause her to wake at night if she rolled onto her right side. She would typically take more than 15–30 minutes to return to sleep, and she would need to find a comfortable position to do so. She again returned to her family physician, and although she commenced another course of NSAIDs, she was not keen on another injection and discussed onward referral. She was referred to a consultant orthopaedic surgeon who referred her for an ultrasound (US) scan and radiograph. The radiograph showed an acromial spur (Type II), and the US scan showed bursal effusion and diffuse tendinosis of the right supraspinatus tendon, as well as a bursal-side partial thickness tear of the tendon. On the basis of the protracted history of symptoms; her limited response to the injection, therapy and other non-surgical management; the imaging findings; and the clinical findings of a positive Neer sign, Hawkins test and Jobe test, an arthroscopic subacromial decompression with probable rotator cuff repair was recommended by the surgeon. Unwilling to 'rush' to surgery, she again tried osteopathy. Shortly thereafter, a friend recommended she see a sports and exercise medicine consultant, who then referred Alison to our physiotherapy clinic.

Physical Characteristics and Medical History

Alison reported her height as 1.72 m and weight as 58 kilos (body mass index [BMI] 19.6). Her weight was stable, and she had never smoked cigarettes. She drank one to two glasses of wine on average once a week, reported no allergies and ate a balanced diet.

Alison reported no comorbidities or other health concerns and had recently had a negative test for thyroid disease. Alison was still having regular menses. She had never had surgery, and with the exception of about 1 month of 'quite severe' back pain after the birth of her youngest child, she reported no other significant musculoskeletal problems. There was no family history of rheumatoid arthritis. Her father (a builder) had a protracted history of shoulder pain, but she was unsure of the diagnosis, suggesting possibly a 'frozen shoulder'.

Alison reported rarely taking medications, which included occasional paracetamol for her shoulder pain, and although she had taken omega-3 supplements in the past, she was no longer taking them or any other supplements.

Patient Perspectives

Alison did not see herself as anxious or depressed, just very frustrated and concerned about her right shoulder and the ongoing impact this was having on her life. Although uncertain that physiotherapy could help (due to the previous poor response), she wanted to 'try everything possible' before considering surgery. When asked what she was hoping to achieve from the initial and possibly subsequent physiotherapy treatments and what she would consider a positive outcome, her stated aim was 'understanding what was going wrong' and 'relief of shoulder pain and return to full shoulder activity'.

Questionnaires

Alison was requested to complete the Shoulder Pain and Disability Index (SPADI) (Roach et al., 1991), and her initial score was 68%, where 100% represents maximal pain and disability.

Reasoning Question:

1. On the basis of Alison's clinical presentation thus far, please discuss your hypotheses regarding the dominant 'pain type' (nociceptive, neuropathic, nociplastic), possible 'sources of symptoms' and 'pathology' and likely 'contributing factors' to the development and continuation of her pain and disability. Also, you appear to undertake significant screening of personal/lifestyle details (e.g. BMI, cigarette and alcohol consumption, allergies, diet, education, sitting/activity pattern and general health, including menstrual status and perception of psychological health). Would you also please briefly highlight how information acquired through these inquiries assists your analysis?

Answer to Reasoning Question:

Due to the duration and presentation of symptoms, the possibility of nociplastic pain (Coronado et al., 2014; Paul et al., 2012), and cortical changes (Ngomo et al., 2015) must be considered, although definitive clinical methods of testing such hypotheses remain uncertain due to a paucity of research evidence. However, we felt the pain type was primarily nociceptive, primarily based on previous clinical experience (Lewis, 2010; McCreesh and Lewis, 2013; Lewis, 2014a; Lewis and Ginn, 2015) and because the pain was worse on movement and localized, and there were definitive aggravating and easing factors (Smart et al., 2011). Other potential sources of symptoms were assessed, such as the cervical spine and acromioclavicular joint region, and although we could not be certain, the most likely sources of nociception were the subacromial bursa and rotator cuff tendons.

Neural elements have been identified within the rotator cuff tendons, biceps tendon and sheath, transverse humeral ligament and the subacromial bursa. A significantly richer supply of free nerve fibres has been reported in the subacromial bursa compared with the aforementioned tissue (Soifer et al., 1996). Additional research has implicated subacromial bursal tissue as a potential source of shoulder pain. In this research, patients diagnosed with subacromial pain syndrome were randomized to acromioplasty and bursectomy or to bursectomy alone, with equivalent results reported in both groups (Henkus et al., 2009). Another study reports that injections targeting the subacromial bursa in isolation were associated with a significant reduction in shoulder pain (Henkus et al., 2006). It is acknowledged that confounding factors may have influenced reported findings in these studies. Additional research has identified a host of substances in the subacromial bursa in people with subacromial pain, such as substance P and pro-inflammatory cytokines (IL-Iβ, TNF-α, VEGF) in higher concentrations than in people without subacromial pain, as well as an association between higher concentrations of substance P and the subjective experience of pain (Gotoh et al., 1998, 2002, 2001; Sakai et al., 2001; Yanagisawa et al., 2001; Voloshin et al., 2005).

The main contributing factor for Alison's pain was felt to be overload of the rotator cuff at a level beyond the tissues' physiological capacity to meet the demands of the imposed load. Overload of the rotator cuff muscles can cause fatigue, and especially when coupled with pain, this can inhibit the rotator cuff, thus producing a superior migration of the humeral head leading to compression of the subacromial bursa and rotator cuff tendons (Sharkey and Marder, 1995; Keener et al., 2009; Deutsch et al., 1996; Chen et al., 1999). Possible intrabursal and intra-fascicular tendinous friction may result in a release of nociceptive substances (Backman et al., 2011a, 2011b; Blaine et al., 2005). However, currently, there is no certainty as to the cascade of events that had occurred within the tissues that resulted in Alison's symptoms.

In our opinion, questions pertaining to lifestyle factors are essential and should be considered a mandatory component of the information acquisition from the patient. Lifestyle factors in relation to musculoskeletal conditions have recently been reviewed in detail (Dean and Söderlund, 2015a, 2015b). Increased adiposity and a high-cholesterol diet may be associated with a greater risk for tendinopathy (Gaida et al., 2009; Beason et al., 2014). Cigarette smoking also has a detrimental impact on tendon tissue (Galatz et al., 2006; Baumgarten et al., 2010; Carbone et al., 2012), as may oestrogen deficiency (Frizziero et al., 2014). Extended periods of sitting and inactivity pose a significant health risk, including risk for heart disease, diabetes, cancer and death (Blair, 2009; Weiler et al., 2010; Lee et al., 2012; Biswas et al., 2015). The size of rotator cuff tears, degree of retraction and number of tendons torn have not found to correlate with pain, but the number of comorbidities and education level are correlated (Dunn et al., 2014; Unruh et al., 2014).

Continued on following page

Clinical Reasoning Commentary:

Although validation of clinical assessment criteria for pain type is still not definitive, as discussed in Chapters 1 and 2, there is increased agreement on the clinical patterns of nociceptive, neuropathic and nociplastic pain types. The criteria for pathological neuropathic pain have been revised, and new measures of CNS sensitization are becoming available. The significance of hypothesizing about pain type, as put forward in this answer, is its implications for other hypothesis categories such as management and prognosis.

Specific sources of symptoms (nociception in this case) and pathology also cannot be definitively confirmed by clinical examination alone. This highlights the importance of having a balance in reasoning between sources of symptoms and pathology on the one hand and impairments in body function or structure on the other. Known pathology must be seriously considered and unknown pathology cautiously hypothesized for their implications for safety (in physical examination and management, as with a structural instability) and for the associated research evidence supporting therapeutic management options (e.g. tendinopathy).

Hypotheses regarding potential contributing factors similarly significantly inform management and prognosis. Attention to likely contributing factors not only alleviates many patients' persistent symptoms and disability but logically also reduces the likelihood of recurrence. However, because the relevance of contributing factors also usually cannot be definitively confirmed, care is needed to avoid the confirmation-bias error of simply attending to predetermined potential contributing factors. This can be achieved by systematic 'testing' of different factors through procedures such as the shoulder symptom modification procedure (SSMP), discussed later in this case, and through targeted interventions with careful re-assessment.

The screening of lifestyle factors, highlighted here as essential, concurs with the discussion of 'screening' in Chapter 1 as a strategy to ensure that relevant information is not missed (e.g. other symptoms, other aggravating factors, comorbidities, etc.) that may have further implications for management and prognosis, as discussed in this answer.

Physical Examination

Posture

In standing, posture was examined from the front, back and sides. The only significant finding was that the right shoulder girdle was observed to be substantially lower than the left. The angle made by the clavicle, measured by placing an inclinometer on the clavicle, was 12 degrees on the left (reference lateral end of clavicle to horizontal plane) and 2 degrees on the right. Minimal muscular atrophy was observed in the right infrascapular fossa. Palpation was unremarkable with the exception of tenderness over the region of the right long head of biceps tendon in the intertubercular sulcus. However, this region was also sensitive on the left asymptomatic side.

Active and passive range-of-movement (ROM) assessments are presented in Table 17.1. Passive accessory joint movement was not tested. Internal rotation was not tested in isolation but as part of the combined functional movement of hand behind back. Scapular dyskinesis was not assessed during active movements at this stage, but the influence of scapular posture was assessed later during the assessment. The muscle strength assessment is presented in Table 17.2.

Cervical spine active movements appeared full and did not reproduce any local or referred shoulder symptoms. The same finding was recorded after passive end-range testing (overpressure) of the cervical physiological movements and during movements combining right cervical rotation with cervical flexion, and cervical extension with left and right cervical side-flexion. Active thoracic spine extension, flexion, rotation and side-flexion were equally unremarkable. A neurological examination (sensation, reflexes, vibration sense and muscle power) was not conducted because there did not appear to be any clinical evidence of a neurological deficit. Special orthopaedic tests, such as the Neer impingement sign, Hawkins test and O'Brien active compression test (Magee, 2014), were not included in the assessment, due to repeated concerns and evidence suggesting the orthopaedic tests lack the ability to differentiate the intended anatomical structure(s) of interest (Lewis and Tennent, 2007; Lewis, 2009; Hegedus et al., 2012).

Following palpation and motion and strength measurements, the SSMP (Lewis, 2009) was applied. Because Alison had indicated that repeated movements aggravated her symptoms,

TABLE 17.1

APPOINTMENT 1 RANGE-OF-MOVEMENT IMPAIRMENT MEASUREMENTS

| | Left Shoulder | | | Right Shoulder | |
	Active ROM	NPRS /10	Passive ROM	Active ROM NPRS/10 | Base Pain ~ 3/10	Passive ROM
Flexion (LLv)	178°	0		60° (P1 – 6/10) | NI* (no attempt at further AROM)	From 60° ~ + 10° (P ~7/10)
Flexion (SLv)				82° (P1 – 4/10) | NI	
Abduction (POS) (LLv)	178°	0		70° (P1 – 5/10) | Parc to 110° (P↑ 7/10) | NI	P↑ with attempted PROM
Abduction (POS) (SLv)				76° (P1 – 4/10) | Parc to 100° (P↑ 6/10) | NI	
External rotation (with arms by the side)	38 cm	0		24 cm (P1 – 3/10)	~ + 6 cm (P↑ ~4/10)
Hand behind back	Mid-thorax	0		Lat buttocks (P1 – 6/10) | NI	
Extension	45°	0		15° (P1 – 3/10) | NI	From 15° + 8° (P↑ ~4/10)
Horizontal flexion	Fingers to CL post acromion	0		Not tested because symptoms reproduced with other movements	
Horizontal extension				Not tested because symptoms reproduced with other movements	

~, Approximately; ↑, increase; *AROM*, active range of movement; *CL*, post, contralateral posterior; *Lat*, lateral; *LLv*, long lever; *NI**, not irritable; *NPRS*, numerical pain rating scale; *P*, pain; *P1*, first increase in pain; *Parc*, painful arc; *POS*, plane of scapula; *PROM*, passive range of movement; *ROM*, range of movement; *SLv*, short lever (i.e. elbow flexed to 90 degrees).

Notes: Flexion and abduction movements led with thumb facing up toward ceiling.

*In the context of these physical findings, NI (not irritable) indicates the movement did not increase resting pain after its assessment.

resulting in substantial irritability, and because resting pain had increased to approximately 4/10 on the NPRS following the limited shoulder impairment assessment, a clinical decision was made to test components of the SSMP on resting pain and not as a response to movement. Each position was held for approximately 20–30 seconds. Table 17.3 summarizes the SSMP response on right shoulder resting pain.

Reasoning Question:

2. Please discuss your analysis of Alison's physical examination findings with respect to your previous hypotheses regarding 'pain type', 'sources of symptoms', 'pathology' and 'contributing factors', highlighting those features that support your primary hypotheses.

Answer to Reasoning Question:

The physical examination was restricted primarily due to Alison's descriptions of irritability and clinical uncertainty as to how her shoulder would respond to a more comprehensive physical assessment. Following the limited physical examination, we continued to hypothesize that the pain type was primarily nociceptive and local to the shoulder. There was no evidence of referred pain from the cervical region, neuropathic pain or overt signs of nociplastic pain. Although there was constant pain, symptoms were

Continued on following page

TABLE 17.2

APPOINTMENT 1 MUSCLE STRENGTH IMPAIRMENT MEASUREMENTS USING A HAND-HELD DYNAMOMETER

	Left Shoulder			Right Shoulder		
	MVC–B	Reps to Pain	Reps to Fatigue	MVC–M	Reps to Pain	Reps to Fatigue
10° abduction	86 N			36 N	1	NT
External rotation (with arms by side)	45 N		SL (5 kg)	10	18 N	1	NT
Internal rotation (with arms by side)	72 N			66 N	NT	NT
Elbow flexion at 90°	108 N			112 N	1	NT
Full can test	NT			NT	NT	NT
Empty can test	56 N			NT	NT	NT
External rotation at 80° abduction	NT			NT	NT	NT
Other:						

MVC–B, Maximum voluntary contraction – break; *MVC–M,* maximum voluntary contraction – make; *N,* Newton); *NT,* not tested; reps, repetitions; *SL,* side-lying.
Tests (e.g. full or empty can) performed as described in Magee (2014).

provoked in the physical examination with movement in a mechanical and consistent manner, and this presentation is consistent with descriptions of nociceptive pain (Smart et al., 2011). In addition, when the load was purposely reduced during the examination of shoulder movement from long-lever shoulder flexion and abduction to short-lever movements, combinations of less pain and greater movement were recorded, reinforcing the hypothesis that nociceptive pain was the primary pain type and was associated with tissue overload (i.e. longer moment arm resulted in a greater weight imposed on the local shoulder tissues during movement).

The main aim of the examination was not to identify a structure or structures as specific sources of symptoms but to instead identify techniques that would reduce or alleviate her symptoms. Morphologically, it is unlikely that it is possible to differentiate a particular rotator cuff tendon from the others and also from other local tissues (Clark et al., 1990; Clark and Harryman, 1992), and because of this, tests such as the Jobe test (Jobe and Moynes, 1982) (colloquially known as the 'empty can' test and designed to test the structural integrity of the supraspinatus tendon) are probably incapable of specifically testing this tendon with certainty. In addition, needle electromyographic (EMG) investigations of the full and empty can tests have demonstrated, respectively, that eight and nine other muscles are as equally activated as the supraspinatus (Boettcher et al., 2009). It is also inconceivable that these tests do not stretch and compress the overlaying subacromial bursa (Lewis, 2011).

Based on Alison's history, the main factor contributing to her protracted symptoms appeared to be cumulative mechanical loading of the rotator cuff and surrounding tissues at a physiological level beyond the structures' abilities to cope and restore homeostasis. The episode that had most recently exacerbated her symptoms was playing 'gentle' tennis on a wet court. It is highly probable that 'gentle' was her perception of how she was playing, but the imposed load was beyond the physiological limit of her shoulder tissues, and a wet ball would have further increased the load due to increased weight and the force required to effectively return the ball to the opposite side of the court. If drying and brushing her hair exacerbated her shoulder pain, then it is highly probable that even 'gentle' tennis subjected her shoulder tissues to a load beyond their physiological capacity. It is not possible to implicate any one tissue or combination of tissues with certainty because imaging and clinical tests cannot identify the specific source of symptoms with confidence (Lewis, 2009; Hegedus et al., 2008, 2012; Lewis and Tennent, 2007). However, research – albeit with risk of high levels of bias and identifiable confounding factors – has implicated the subacromial bursa as a potential source of nociception (Santavirta et al., 1992) for people experiencing constant, irritable and nocturnal pain, as Alison described.

The purpose of the SSMP (Lewis, 2009) is to systematically assess the influence of potential contributing factors, including (1) central (spinal) posture, (2) scapular position and (3) humeral head position, as well as (4) pain neuro-modulation procedures and (5) combinations of these on symptoms associated with movements, postures and activities. Examples of these physiological movements or activities include routine shoulder movements such as shoulder flexion and hand behind back and higher-level functional activities such as swimming strokes, push-ups and high-speed, explosive throwing movements or activities such as hammering or throwing. However, for people whose symptoms would be exacerbated

TABLE 17.3

PATIENT RESPONSES TO SELECTED MOVEMENTS OF SHOULDER SYMPTOM MODIFICATION PROCEDURE (SSMP)

SSMP	Right Shoulder Resting Pain
Thoracic component	No change
Active	NT
• Extension	NT
• Flexion	
Taping procedure	
Scapula component	Slight ↓ P for a few seconds
(Passive repositioning prior to active movement)	then returned ISQ
• Elevation	↑ P
• Depression	No change
• Protraction	No change
• Retraction	Slight ↓ P for a few seconds
• Posterior tilt	then returned ISQ
• Anterior tilt	↑ P
Combined: Elevation and posterior tilt	As for individual tests
Humeral head component	NT
• Active depression in standing	No change
• Active and passive depression in supine lying	NT
• Active depression (abduction)	NT
• Active depression (flexion)	Slight ↓ P for a few seconds
• AP glide	then returned ISQ
• PA glide	Worse
• AP glide with superior inclination	Slight ↓ P for a few seconds
	then returned ISQ
Pain modulation component	Reduced resting pain for a
• Spinal mobilization with arm movement (Mulligan, 1999) to lower cervical spine, with pressure applied from both sides of the spine (with arm at rest and during one movement of right shoulder flexion)	few minutes post-procedures to ~1–2/10 but then returned to 4/10
• In left side-lying (right side uppermost with arm supported on pillow), combinations of the following pressure/touch techniques:	
∘ Cervical region mobilization techniques directed to right lower cervical region (equivalent to a Maitland [1986] Grade III pressure)	
∘ Upper to mid-thoracic region mobilization techniques from midline and to right of midline (equivalent to a Maitland Grade III pressure)	
∘ Supra- and infrascapular fossae regions soft tissue techniques	

~, Approximately; ↓, decrease; ↑, increase; *AP*, anteroposterior; *NT*, not tested; *PA*, posteroanterior; *ISQ*, in status quo or no change; *P*, pain.

during repeated movement testing, the effect of SSMP procedures 1–5 may be assessed on static baseline symptoms. In this instance, the SSMP failed to meaningfully reduce Alison's symptoms.

Reasoning Question:

3. On the basis of Alison's findings from both the subjective and physical examination, and supporting research evidence, please outline your plans and associated rationale for 'management'.

Answer to Reasoning Question:

The primary initial aim of management was to reduce Alison's shoulder pain, especially the irritability she was experiencing, to allow rehabilitation and restoration of function to progress effectively without detrimentally exacerbating symptoms. Patient education and tissue load management are key priorities to achieve this.

Numerous clinical methods aimed at controlling pain have been advocated. Commonly these include soft tissue massage, passive mobilization procedures, acupuncture, acupressure, trigger point therapy, taping and electrotherapy modalities. The majority of these techniques sit within Section IV of the

Continued on following page

SSMP (i.e. the pain neuro-modulation procedure component). The clinical effectiveness of these procedures has not been unequivocally proven, and it has been challenged in many cases. Although many therapists find these techniques helpful, there may be an element of survivor bias, and research investigating the efficacy of these procedures is either non-existent or frequently short term, subject to high levels of risk of bias, equivocal and fail to report important information such as Numbers Needed to Treat. As such, clinical practice is commonly fraught with difficulty as to which techniques and procedures should be selected to control pain. In this specific case, all four sections of the SSMP failed to reduce Alison's resting pain and pain associated with her shoulder movement. In this situation, anecdotal experience has suggested that isometric muscle contractions in the direction of pain provocation may help to reduce pain (Parle et al., 2016). The use of this is described later in this case.

Clinical Reasoning Commentary:

The lack of research supporting some common therapeutic interventions for musculoskeletal pain, in part related to limitations in research design, as highlighted in the previous answer, underscores the importance of skilled and critical clinical reasoning in treatment selection and progression. Lack of evidence of statistically significant and clinically meaningful effects should be heeded when backed by high-level and high-quality studies which have been replicated with similar findings. This is especially the case when the patient's clinical presentation is clearly consistent with the inclusion/exclusion criteria for participants in these studies. Similarly, the proposed intervention needs to be consistent with that investigated in these studies, with relevant factors such as the skill level of the treating practitioner, dosage and the use or lack of use of commonly associated modalities (e.g. the prescription of simple pain-free range of motion or functional home exercises following passive joint mobilization) considered in the weighting of the research evidence.

When the quality of existing research is limited, management must be guided by the best available evidence, including the individual clinical experience of the practitioner as well as the collective professional craft knowledge, and by the critical appraisal of treatment effectiveness through thorough re-assessment and monitoring of outcomes.

After a few minutes of rest, the right shoulder resting pain level was remeasured, and active flexion (long-lever) and hand-behind-back movements were retested. The responses were clinically similar to the original assessment. Following this retesting, the response to external rotation submaximal isometric contractions (3 × 20 seconds) were assessed on resting pain, as well as right shoulder flexion (long lever) and right hand-behind-back range of motion. There was no detectable change in resting pain, but there was a definite improvement in right shoulder flexion with a 50% decrease in pain (at 60 degrees) and the same pain for right hand behind back but with an increased active range to the lumbar spinal region.

Treatment

At the end of the first assessment, the findings were discussed with Alison. It was communicated with her (with the aid of a plastic shoulder model and digital shoulder diagrams) that the underlying problem possibly involved the tendons of the rotator cuff, most likely a combination of the three tendons that contribute to external rotation of the shoulder, with potential bursal involvement. An explanation was offered when Alison asked (1) why a definitive diagnosis was not possible and (2) why the US scan results did not explain her symptoms. She also wanted to further discuss the partial-thickness tear that had been identified in the US scan and her concern that if not repaired, it would become larger and irreparable, and especially the implications that this would have for long-term pain and function. Further explanation was offered with reference to current published research investigations of imaging and outcomes of surgical and non-surgical interventions (Girish et al., 2011; Lewis, 2011; Kukkonen et al., 2014).

Following discussion Alison expressed that her main concern was the pain she was experiencing. Explanation that experiencing pain was unlikely to result in tissue damage, but as she reiterated that this was her main concern, an agreement was reached with Alison that the initial primary aim of management was to reduce her pain. A plan was agreed that Alison would, as much as possible, avoid movements that provoked pain, including drying her hair and driving. In addition to avoiding pain-provoking movements, she would perform 3 × 20-second shoulder external rotation isometric contractions, avoiding any fatigue (i.e. arm tiredness/shaking), up to five times per day and would stop if the pain between sessions increased. She was requested to continue this for 3 days and then add a second exercise that required her to slowly perform right shoulder flexion to approximately 50 degrees with the elbow flexed (i.e. short lever) and leading with her thumb. To facilitate this second exercise, she was asked to securely place an ironing board on a chair or sofa at approximately a 45-degree angle and roll her hand and forearm on a small ball along the board during the movement. If Alison felt able, she could progress this exercise by removing the board and performing unsupported, slow un-resisted short-lever low-range shoulder flexion during step-standing. She was to take approximately 3 seconds to get to 50 degrees, hold for a second or two and then slowly return to the starting position. Based on fatigue and pain responses, Alison was requested to perform the exercise three times, with a 1-minute rest, and then repeat this twice more (i.e. 9 repetitions in total on each occasion, aiming for a total of 27 repetitions each day). Pain at rest and/or during movement was not to increase as a consequence of the exercises or any routine daily activities.

Alison was also asked to start a spreadsheet recording the number of exercises she was performing, as well as documenting the night pain response and the 24-hour pain response to exercise. She would document the exercises and pain responses for a week, and then her progress would be re-assessed. She was advised to contact the clinic with any concerns or questions that might arise during the week.

Reasoning Question:

4. Please discuss the biological mechanism(s) you speculate may have underpinned the improvement in active shoulder flexion and hand behind back following the 3×20-second submaximal isometric external rotation contractions. Also, would you explain your rationale for the dosage of exercise prescribed, both biologically and on the basis of Alison's clinical presentation?

Answer to Reasoning Question:

Although some research evidence exists (Lemley et al., 2014; Hoeger Bement et al., 2008), albeit limited by the study design issues discussed in the responses to Questions 2 and 3, anecdotal clinical observations of people experiencing shoulder pain suggest that isometric contractions are a promising potential method of controlling pain. The benefit of isometric exercises as a method of controlling tendon pain has been reported in the literature (Rudavsky and Cook, 2014; Rio et al., 2013). A definitive biological explanation for this observation, if correct, is not currently available, and ongoing research is now being conducted to determine if this observation is valid and to identify the mechanisms by which these procedures may help reduce pain. For many people with shoulder pain, isometric contractions are not always beneficial and may not be associated with long-term pain reduction. However, in cases where they do contribute to pain reduction, then this may facilitate more effective exercise therapy.

Reasoning Question:

5. Please highlight the evidence regarding surgical versus non-surgical treatment outcomes for rotator cuff (RC) tendinopathy.

Answer to Reasoning Question:

Physiotherapists, as well as people suffering RC tendinopathy, should derive considerable confidence that appropriately constructed exercise therapy will achieve the same outcomes as those achieved with surgical management. Surgery has not demonstrated additional benefit for RC tendinopathy at 1-, 2- or 5-year follow-up (Haahr et al., 2005; Haahr and Andersen, 2006; Ketola et al., 2009, 2013). Holmgren et al. (2012) demonstrated that a graduated exercise program substantially reduces the need for surgery for 80% of patients who have already experienced failed non-surgical treatment. Of importance in this study, it was found that exercising into pain (up to 5/10 on the NPRS), and provided the pain had settled by the subsequent exercise session, was associated with better outcomes. For people diagnosed with atraumatic partial-thickness tears of the supraspinatus tendon involving less than 75% of the tendon, and also experiencing pain, a graduated physiotherapy exercise program was as beneficial as surgery (acromioplasty, or acromioplasty and RC repair) (Kukkonen et al., 2014). This finding suggests that attempting surgical repair of an RC tear may not improve the outcome over a well-structured physiotherapy exercise program. In another study, at the 2-year follow-up, it was reported that 75% of people diagnosed with an atraumatic full-thickness tear and experiencing shoulder pain who had undergone a graduated exercise program did not require surgical intervention (Kuhn et al., 2013).

The findings of these studies suggest that a carefully planned and graduated exercise program should achieve the same outcomes as surgery for subacromial pain/impingement syndrome and RC tendinopathy (Holmgren et al., 2012), as well as for atraumatic partial (Kukkonen et al., 2014) and full-thickness (Kuhn et al., 2013) RC tears. To achieve the outcomes reported in these studies, patients received between 6 to 19 treatments. These findings suggest that even in the presence of identified structural failure, non-surgical management is likely to be as effective as surgical intervention.

Continued on following page

Although the findings of surgical and non-surgical studies demonstrate comparable results, it is essential to emphasize that not all patients will achieve complete cessation of symptoms and restoration of normal and complete function with each intervention, highlighting the importance of discussing concepts such as Numbers Needed to Treat with patients and the need for ongoing research to further improve outcomes. It may be appropriate to develop well-thought-out care pathways with all relevant stakeholders, including patients, healthcare providers (e.g. physiotherapists and surgeons) and commissioning bodies to determine what constitutes best assessment and management, in addition to when decisions should be made to consider alternative treatments, such as surgery. For those who have failed non-surgical care, surgery should be considered and may provide a reduction in pain and symptoms and assist in restoring shoulder function. However, uncertainty persists as to the mechanisms by which surgery works (Lewis, 2011).

Interestingly, research has been published suggesting that clinical outcomes may be comparable for both those with intact and failed RC repairs following surgery (Kim et al., 2012). Placebo surgery has shown to be as effective as surgery performed to rectify structural abnormalities in other musculoskeletal conditions (Moseley et al., 2002; Sihvonen et al., 2013), and this type of research is required to better understand the benefits of subacromial decompression (SAD) and RC repairs. Moreover, relative rest and often a prolonged period of slow and graduated rehabilitation are considered important when treating RC tendinopathy, especially when tissue irritability is present or the symptoms flare easily when the tissue is loaded (Lewis, 2011, 2014a). Following SAD and RC repair, there are often considerable periods of relative rest (McClelland et al., 2005; Charalambous et al., 2010) followed by graduated rehabilitation. It may be that post-surgical guidelines requiring relative rest and slow graduated rehabilitation, controlled tendon reloading and motor control exercises actually facilitate clinical improvement, and possibly not the surgery itself (Lewis, 2015). Appropriately constructed research investigations are required to address these areas of uncertainty.

Clinical Reasoning Commentary:

The use of isometric exercise in this case is linked to both the limited supporting research available and to the practitioner's clinical experience, although the biological explanation for its suggested efficacy is currently unknown. The encouraging results of studies evaluating conservative management discussed here provide relevant evidence clinicians should factor into their management reasoning, including explanations to patients regarding the potential benefits of treatment options.

Appointment 2 (1 Week Later)

Alison returned 1 week later and reported that the night after the first assessment was worse than normal. She had woken at least four to five times, and on one occasion, she could feel her shoulder throbbing. It took an hour to return to sleep on this occasion, and that was after taking a combination of paracetamol and ibuprofen (NSAID). She had continued with the anti-inflammatory for a few days and was sure it was helping. On the second day after her first appointment, she started her external rotation isometric exercises. She did not feel these isometric exercises had helped, and so on the fifth day post-appointment, she added the shoulder flexion exercises on the ironing board. On the following day, she had substantially more pain (both at rest and with movement). Alison expressed her concern and felt she was heading for surgery. She also admitted that she had been unable to reduce her shoulder activity level, and on the evening of the day that she started her shoulder flexion exercises, she had also gone to the theatre to watch a musical and had clapped and 'danced' along (in her chair) to a few songs and felt this had also aggravated her shoulder. Her active movements were all more painful, and she expressed her concern about worsening night pain. She wanted to further discuss surgery. We discussed that for many, surgery is extremely beneficial at reducing pain and improving function. We also discussed, in slightly more detail than during the first appointment, findings from current research evidence suggesting that the benefits of exercise therapy were equivalent to SAD surgical outcomes in studies that had compared the two treatments with up to 5 years' follow-up and that research comparing exercise to surgical repair of partial-thickness tears of the rotator cuff had shown no difference in outcomes between these interventions at 1-year follow-up (Holmgren et al., 2012; Ketola et al., 2013; Haahr and Andersen, 2006; Kukkonen et al., 2014; Kuhn et al., 2013).

We also discussed that following surgery, there are often prolonged periods of relative rest (McClelland et al., 2005; Charalambous et al., 2010) and that one of the potential benefits of surgery is that it enforces a protracted period of relative rest and a graduated rehabilitation that avoids any fast or prolonged activities. The nature of tissue 'irritability' was also explained, as was the fact that for many, although not a definitive treatment, an injection can help to reduce shoulder pain and allow rehabilitation to proceed more effectively (Crawshaw et al., 2010). Her SPADI at Appointment 2 was 78%.

We also discussed that Alison had reported a very positive response to her first injection, but it was possible she progressed to a level of activity faster than her shoulder could manage. She admitted to also thinking her previous return to activity might have been too aggressive and agreed to try a second injection. After reviewing the contraindications and special precautions and also discussing the benefits and risks, Alison provided written consent for an injection. She also agreed not to drive for a week and to avoid any activities requiring rapid movements, pulling and pushing or carrying heavy items. In supine lying and under ultrasound guidance, 5 ml of lidocaine (with no steroid) was injected into the right subacromial bursa, which was well visualized and seen to distend during the procedure. The pre- and post-injection impairment measurements are detailed in Table 17.4. The form is a standard form used in our clinic, and not all movements detailed on the form are always tested. This is primarily to reduce the burden on the patient.

Alison was asked to continue only with the short-lever flexion movements on the ironing board and to perform them twice per day. As a point of education, it was explained that tendons are often more difficult to treat than bone fractures and must be given at least the same respect. There is unfortunately no 'quick fix', and it would be impossible to drive, play tennis or hammer nails into walls with a fracture of one of the shoulder bones, and equally, problems that involve the muscles and tendons sometimes also require periods of relative rest. Tendons, like fractures, need graduated rehabilitation, with the main difference being that tendons don't require immobilization as required to heal a fracture. We agreed to meet again the following week.

Reasoning Question:

6. What was your interpretation of Alison's adverse response following the first appointment with respect to biological mechanisms? Also, please discuss the indications for a subacromial steroid injection (your clinical experiential and supporting research evidence).

Answer to Reasoning Question:

Clinically, it often is difficult to determine the exact reasons for an exacerbation in a patient's symptoms. It may be due to the increased load imposed on the tissues as a consequence of the components of the assessment, postures adopted by the patient after the assessment, activities the patient was involved in before and/or after the assessment, disease progression, psychological factors and combinations of all of these possibilities. Because Alison reported a substantial increase in symptoms on the night of the first assessment and did not report any other change in activity that might explain the increase in symptoms, the exacerbation was attributed to the increased load placed on her shoulder tissues as a

Continued on following page

TABLE 17.4

PRE- AND POST-INJECTION IMPAIRMENT MEASUREMENTS

Active Right Shoulder Movement	Pre-injection		Passive ROM: Shoulder as Appropriate	Post-injection	
	ROM	NPRS		ROM	NPRS
Flexion (inclinometer)	60°	7/10	NT	70°	3/10
Abduction (inclinometer)	70°	7-8/10	NT	70°	4/10
External rotation (tape measure)	25 cm	5/10	NT	27 cm	3/10
Hand behind back	Lateral buttock	6/10	NT	Buttock	3/10
Horizontal flexion	NT		NT	NT	
Horizontal extension Other	NT		NT	NT	

NPRS, Numerical pain rating scale; *NT,* not tested; *ROM,* range of movement.

direct consequence of the assessment. The increased load imposed by the external rotation and ironing board exercise and/or her 'enthusiastic' attendance at the musical may be further examples of activities leading to physiological overload.

Currently, the definitive biological mechanisms that explain the increase in Alison's shoulder symptoms are unclear. The increase may be due to an increase in local inflammation or changes in other substances associated with pain. The evidence to explain the increase in Alison's symptoms on the basis of classic tissue inflammation alone is minimal due to a paucity of research in this area across all clinical presentations and durations of symptoms (Fukuda et al., 1990; Sarkar and Uhthoff, 1983; Santavirta et al., 1992; Millar et al., 2010). Although the increase in symptoms may be due to tissue inflammation, it may also have occurred as a result of increased expression of other potential chemical mediators, such as cytokines (Sakai et al., 2001) and neuropeptides (e.g. substance P). Higher levels of shoulder pain have been positively correlated with increased concentrations of substance P in the subacromial bursal tissue (Gotoh et al., 1998). In addition, substance P has been reported to increase tendon cell (tenocyte) numbers and may contribute to pain associated with tendinopathy (Backman et al., 2011a, 2011b). Of therapeutic relevance, exercise may decrease the expression of substance P (Karlsson et al., 2014).

In the United Kingdom, physiotherapists have been performing injections since the mid-1990s to support clinical interventions, and more recently, appropriately trained physiotherapists are performing US-guided injection procedures. Injection experience, together with the ability to participate in postgraduate training to become independent medical prescribers, has increased the scope of professional practice to provide new methods of controlling pain to support rehabilitation pathways. Crawshaw et al. (2010) have demonstrated that a subacromial corticosteroid injection and exercise, in comparison to exercise in isolation, may produce faster improvement in symptoms at 1 and 6 weeks (but not by 12 weeks) for people with moderate to severe shoulder pain. This finding suggests pain reduction may be faster for those receiving injections. In addition, injections delivered by therapists may be a cost-effective use of resources compared with exercise alone and lead to lower healthcare costs and less time off work (Jowett et al., 2013). There is, however, a concern that corticosteroid injections may be associated with deleterious effects on tendon tissue (Dean et al., 2014). Findings from other research suggest that for patients experiencing symptoms suggestive of rotator cuff tendinopathy or subacromial pain syndrome, analgesic-only injections may be as beneficial as combined corticosteroid and analgesic injections (Alvarez et al., 2005; Ekeberg et al., 2009). To potentially reduce the possible detrimental effect of corticosteroids, analgesic-only injections should be considered first in an attempt to reduce pain.

Painful tendinopathy may be associated with an increase in tendon cells known as fibroblasts or tenocytes (Cook and Purdam, 2009), and reducing proliferation of these cells may help to restore tissue homeostasis. Analgesics have been reported to reduce fibroblast numbers (Scherb et al., 2009; Carofino et al., 2012) and thus may be a mechanism for possible benefits. Considerably more research is needed in this field. This synthesis of the literature is the reason Alison received an analgesic injection and not a combined corticosteroid and analgesic injection. Much is still to be learnt about injection therapy, and it may be that dry needling or saline-only or saline-combination injections have the same benefit. Of note, ibuprofen has also been reported to reduce tenocyte expression (Tsai et al., 2004), and this may have been a reason Alison reported that taking these NSAIDs was helpful.

Clinical Reasoning Commentary:

Clinical reasoning is required to judge (hypothesize) the effects of any intervention, be it an examination procedure and/or treatment. Both aggravation and improvement in symptoms and function may occur for a variety of reasons, as acknowledged in this answer. Consequently, skilled questioning is needed for clarification of meaning when, for example, the patient reports symptom aggravation or improvement. Clarification of meaning is essential to enhance the accuracy, completeness and relevance of information obtained. Common examples of the importance of clarification of meaning are discussed in Chapter 1. Here, the analysis of Alison's increase in symptoms on the night after the first assessment without any other significant change in activity, combined with background knowledge of the recent pattern of symptom behaviour obtained in the initial subjective examination, illustrates the clarification of meaning that underpinned the judgement reached.

Increased local inflammation and/or changes in substances associated with pain are suggested as biological mechanisms that may account for the increase in Alison's symptoms, with evidence incriminating substance P singled out. Although chemical analysis is not available clinically to test such biological mechanisms for individual patients, research demonstrating an association between substance P and increased tenocyte numbers in tendinopathy, and the possibility that exercise may decrease substance P expression, provides a logical rationale for the trial of therapeutic exercise tailored to Alison's presentation. The irritability of Alison's shoulder pain alluded to on several occasions is a useful construct that enables the ease of aggravation, severity of symptom provocation and time for symptoms to settle to be used as a guide as to the desirable extent of physical examination and management, regardless of the underlying cause (Hengeveld and Banks 2014). Although the biological processes underpinning clinical presentations of irritability have not been investigated, two likely processes are sensitivity from local inflammation and/or changes in substances (such as substance P) as discussed here, as well as nociplastic pain associated sensitization. Familiarity with the clinical patterns of each process should assist in clinical differentiation.

The use of US-guided injection of an analgesic into Alison's subacromial bursa is explained not simply as a therapy on its own, which it can be and often is, but as a method of 'controlling pain to support rehabilitation pathways'. This exemplifies the multifaceted reasoning and multidimensional management necessary with most patients. Instead of simplistically pitting one therapy against another (e.g. NSAID, injection, manual therapy, exercise, etc.) as is often the case in older studies, pragmatic therapy and research attempt to address different components of patients' problems through systematic trials of different mixed interventions, in this case an injection and then exercise rehabilitation.

Assessment 3 (1 Week Later)

Alison returned the following week with a smile and reported that she had experienced a positive response. Following the injection, she was asked to state her Global Impression of Change (Kamper, 2009; Kamper et al., 2009) score, which she reported as 40% (slightly improved). In addition, her SPADI score was reduced to 36%. She reported that she had heeded the advice to return slowly to activities, and she was commended for her efforts. Alison's impairment assessment is described in Table 17.5.

Alison was requested to continue only with the short-lever right shoulder flexion exercises, without support. She was asked to perform five repetitions, two to three times each day. She was to monitor her 24-hour pain and night pain. An increase in either of these was undesirable. She was also asked to continue with her exercise diary and to attempt to change either the range of her shoulder flexion movements or the number of repetitions, but not both at the same time, and to continue to monitor the 24-hour response to her exercise.

We also discussed the importance of energy transfer from the lower limbs through the abdominal region into the shoulder, and to facilitate this discussion, she was asked to describe how she served when playing tennis. The conversation was supported with reference to studies that have demonstrated that 50% of the energy when serving comes from the lower limbs, with the shoulder only contributing 20%, and that a 25% decrease in hip-trunk force requires an additional 35% in force from the shoulder (Kibler, 1995; Sciascia and Cromwell, 2012; Seroyer et al., 2010). This suggests that if the lower limbs and trunk do not fully contribute to serving, more force would be required at the shoulder, possibly leading to an earlier point of fatigue and potential tissue failure.

Although we hadn't assessed lower limb or trunk ROM, strength and endurance, the fact that Alison had substantially decreased her normal level of exercise needed to be

---

TABLE 17.5

THIRD APPOINTMENT RANGE-OF-MOVEMENT IMPAIRMENT MEASUREMENTS

	Right Shoulder	
	Active ROM **NPRS/10 | Resting Pain ~ 1/10**	**Passive ROM**
Flexion (LLv)	100° (P1– 2/10) | NI	From ~ +15° (P ~5/10)
Flexion (SLv)	NT	NT
Abduction (POS) (LLv)	95° (P1 – 3/10) | NI	NT
Abduction (POS) (SLv)	NT	NT
External rotation	26 cm (P1 – 1.5/10)	~ + 4 cm (P↑ ~2/10)
Hand behind back	Mid lumbar level (P1 – 3/10) | NI	
Extension	NT	
Horizontal flexion	NT	

~, Approximately; ↑, increase; *LLv*, long lever; *NI*, not irritable; *NPRS*, numerical pain rating scale; *NT*, not tested; *P*, pain; *P1*, first increase in pain; *POS*, plane of scapula; *ROM*, range of movement; *SLv*, short lever (i.e. elbow flexed to 90°).

Note: Flexion and abduction movements led with thumb facing up toward ceiling.

addressed, and she agreed to slowly and carefully introduce 'rest-of-body' exercises, making one change at a time to ensure there was no adverse effect on the shoulder. We planned to meet again in 2–3 weeks, and she would be in contact with any questions in the intervening period.

Appointment 4 (3 Weeks Later)

Alison returned and indicated that she didn't feel her shoulder pain levels had improved but that she was undertaking more activity, had not experienced shoulder pain at rest or at night and was delighted that she was doing more general exercise. In addition to returning to the gym (walking on treadmill, exercise bike, seated resistance exercises for the lower limbs), she was now routinely doing her shoulder flexion exercises, regularly completing five sets of three to four repetitions with a rest of 3 minutes between sets, three to four times per day. It was reiterated that a slow approach may have better long-term outcomes. Her SPADI score remained essentially unchanged (38%). She had started driving 2 weeks previously but was using public transportation and getting lifts when able.

Right shoulder ROM was comparable to that recorded for the third appointment. Alison agreed to the SSMP being repeated, and she identified right shoulder flexion and right hand behind back as the movements to test (Table 17.6).

The SSMP is designed as a system to guide treatment selection (Lewis et al., 2015; Lewis, 2009). As a result of the SSMP, Alison was provided with a Shoulder Fixation Belt (www.LondonShoulderClinic.com) and instructed to fix it to the top of a closed door in order to provide an anteroposterior (AP) and superior glide of her right shoulder (glenohumeral joint) when standing. She was provided with a yellow (lowest grade) resistance band to hold in her left hand and place around the dorsal surface of her right hand, with her thumb facing toward the ceiling. In this position she was to continue her shoulder flexion exercises (Fig. 17.2), starting with three repetitions, followed by rest, performed in three sets twice a day every other day. Alison was to continue to build repetitions and sets and eventually progress to daily exercises, making one change at a time and recording the 24-hour response. While doing these exercises, she was encouraged to visualize herself moving her arm without pain and restriction as though she was painting a wall, brushing her hair or playing tennis. She was also to continue with her gym program.

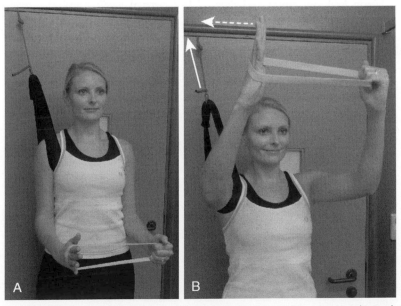

Fig. 17.2 Shoulder anterior-posterior glide with superior inclination *(solid arrow)* together with isometric external rotation *(dotted arrow)* during shoulder flexion exercises.

TABLE 17.6

SHOULDER SYMPTOM MODIFICATION PROCEDURE (SSMP) FINDINGS RECORDED DURING FOURTH APPOINTMENT (RANGE OF MOVEMENT AND NPRS SCORE)

SSMP	Right Shoulder Flexion (long lever)	Right Shoulder Hand Behind Back
Thoracic component	No change	No change
Active	No change	No change
• Extension	NT	NT
• Flexion		
Taping procedure		
Scapula component (passive repositioning prior to active movement)	Reduced pain by ~30%, P1 120°	Worse (pain more around shoulder)
• Elevation	No change	Worse
• Depression	No change	No change
• Protraction	No change	No change
• Retraction	Reduced pain by ~20%, P1 120°	Worse
• Posterior tilt		No change
• Anterior tilt	No change/? worse	Worse (pain more at front of shoulder)
• Combined: Elevation and posterior tilt	P1 120° (1/10)	
Humeral head component	No change	? slight decrease in pain ~10%
• Active depression in standing	No change	
• Active and passive depression in supine lying	? slight decrease in pain ~10%	No change/? worse
• Active depression (abduction)	No change	No change
• Active depression (flexion)	Worse	No change
• Flexion with resisted internal rotation	P1 150° (1–2/10)	P1 low thoracic region (1–2/10)
• Flexion with resisted external rotation	P1 140° (2/10)	
• AP glide	Worse	No change
• PA glide	P1 160° (2/10)	Worse
• AP glide with superior inclination	P1 165° (0.5/10)	P1 low thoracic region (1–2/10)
• AP glide with superior inclination together with resisted external rotation		P1 inferior scapula angle (1/10)
Pain modulation component	NT	NT
Summary		

AP glide with superior inclination, together with resisted external rotation, substantially increased right shoulder flexion and hand-behind-back range and was associated with a concomitant decrease in pain.

~, Approximately; *AP,* anterior to posterior; *NT,* not tested; *P,* pain; *PA,* posterior to anterior; *SSMP,* shoulder symptom modification procedure; *?,* uncertain.

Reasoning Question:

7. Please discuss your interpretation of your SSMP findings, including your choice of an additional glenohumeral-targeted exercise over a scapular-targeted exercise, and when you feel scapular exercises are indicated. Also, would you highlight the evidence (experience based and research) supporting your use of visualization in Alison's exercises?

Answer to Reasoning Question:

The SSMP is designed to help guide treatment selection. Techniques that have a beneficial effect on postures, movements and activities identified by the patient are then used as treatment. It is, of course, possible that the techniques incorporated in the SSMP will have no effect on symptoms and cannot be used to inform treatment choice. Equally, one or more techniques may have a partial effect or result in a complete cessation of symptoms. On occasion, as in this case, a beneficial effect (i.e. reduction in symptoms) was identified from a number of procedures (scapular elevation and two combined humeral head techniques). Because the combined humeral head procedures almost completely reduced the symptom of pain and restored full ROM, a clinical decision was made to use this first in treatment. It is also possible that the superior glide component of the combined AP superior glide technique using

Continued on following page

the Shoulder Fixation Belt provided an element of scapular elevation which helped to partially reduce symptoms. Other reasons why only one procedure was introduced were as follows: (1) it is difficult for most patients to find time to incorporate multiple exercises into their daily routine, and (2) the introduction of multiple exercises may lead to clinical reasoning confusion if the patient reports no response or an adverse response. As such, the most beneficial procedure identified by the SSMP was introduced first. If this had been the scapular positional change procedure, then this would have been first introduced. In reality, all exercises will involve some level of scapular muscle activity whether they are shoulder isometric exercises, shoulder movement exercises, traditional rotator cuff exercises, 'whole-body' exercises or scapular-specific exercises. It is accepted that specific exercises will recruit muscles preferentially (Boettcher et al., 2010; Wattanaprakornkul et al., 2011).

Movement visualization or imagery has been used to improve performance in dancers, musicians and athletes and may have a role to play in the management of painful shoulder conditions with pain reduction, force production and movement enhancement (Hoyek et al., 2014; Franceschini et al., 2012; Tamir et al., 2007; Ranganathan et al., 2004; Porro et al., 2007).

Clinical Reasoning Commentary:

Clinical judgement regarding where to commence treatment is challenging when, as is often the case, the examination has identified a number of potentially relevant physical impairments and in many instances psychosocial (patient perspective) issues as well. Different musculoskeletal clinicians will commence and progress therapy differently, and indeed, it may be that there are several equally effective options. Prescriptive clinical prediction rule research may provide some useful evidence to indicate likely treatment effects for some musculoskeletal problems (see Chapter 5), and this may help guide treatment selection, especially in more complex cases and for the novice practitioner. However, unless research has provided definitive guidance on the optimal therapy for a given presentation, what is essential from a clinical reasoning perspective is that management is evidence informed, tailored to patients' individual presentations and critically monitored (re-assessed) to gauge its short- and longer-term value. This is evident here as the aim of initially controlling pain is collaboratively reached with Alison and the SSMP is used to systematically evaluate the potential value of different procedures, culminating in the identification of a combined procedure that provided maximal relief of symptoms in the initial trial.

Appointment 5 (3 Weeks Later)

Alison returned reporting her Global Impression of Change as 'much improved' (citing at least 80% improvement), and her SPADI score was now 13%, meaning a low level of pain/disability (0% implies no pain and no disability). Although she felt that she was not as good as she had been after her first landmark-guided injection provided by her family physician, she was substantially better than at any time in the past few months and expressed confidence that if her progress continued, she might not need surgery. She reiterated her desire to return to 'full duties', which included playing tennis. Her impairment measurements on this occasion are detailed in Table 17.7.

Weeks 8–14

Over the next 6 weeks (weeks 8–14), Alison changed her exercise program to include graduated right shoulder external rotation eccentric, concentric and isometric exercises, commencing with her elbow 10 cm away from the side of her body and progressing in the direction of abduction toward a maximum of 80 degrees abduction. Initially her arm was supported in abduction, and gradually the support was withdrawn. Her program included combinations of strength, endurance and speed exercises. Every time she progressed (e.g. increasing speed or weight), she would initially only perform one or two sets and only repeat the program every 3 days to ensure there was no symptom aggravation. The exercises gradually incorporated lower body movements, such as shifting her body weight from the back to front legs at varying speeds. She performed these exercises in a self-directed manner, reporting in (via email or phone) every 1–2 weeks.

Alison reported at least two setbacks during this time where pain had increased during movements (but not at rest or night). She employed the strategy we had previously discussed should exacerbation occur, which was to have a 2-day rest from exercise and then restart at the immediate prior level for which she had not recorded any exacerbation in her exercise diary.

TABLE 17.7

FIFTH APPOINTMENT RANGE-OF-MOVEMENT IMPAIRMENT MEASUREMENTS

	Right Shoulder	
	Active ROM **NPRS/10 | Base Pain 0/10**	**Passive ROM**
Flexion (LLv)	165° (0.5/10) | NI	~ + 10° (1/10) | NI
Flexion (SLv)	NT	
Abduction (POS) (LLv)	170° (1/10) | NI	
Abduction (POS) (SLv)		
External rotation	34 cm (0.5/10)	~ + 2 cm (no ↑ in P)
Hand behind back	Mid-thoracic (1/10)	
Extension		
Horizontal flexion	Top of opposite shoulder (0.5/10)	+ few cm, P ↑ to 1–2/10 | NI

~, Approximately; ↑, increase; *LLv*, long lever; *NI*, not irritable; *NPRS*, numerical pain rating scale; *NT*, not tested; *P*, pain; *POS*, plane of scapula; *ROM*, range of movement; *SLv*, short lever (i.e. elbow flexed to 90°). Note: Flexion and abduction movements led with thumb facing up toward ceiling.

Appointment 6 (Week 14)

Alison's Global Impression of Change was much improved (90%), and her SPADI score was only 9% (as she still experienced 'random' occasional sharp, albeit momentary, pain). Her range of active and passive movement was essentially full and pain-free, and there was no evidence of any additional impairments such as posterior shoulder tightness. Posterior shoulder tightness was screened during this session but could have equally been screened earlier during the assessment and management process. She was washing and blow drying her hair without concern. She had also slept on the right shoulder on a number of occasions (both voluntarily and involuntarily) and reported she only would typically experience right shoulder 'stiffness' for 10 minutes in the morning if she did. Her gym program was progressing, and she had been running on the treadmill and using the cross-trainer moving her arms, as well as attempting a number of 'Zumba' classes. Alison was also able to do 10 push-ups and was able to lift 7-kg weights bilaterally (in the abduction plane of scapula to 90 degrees with a short lever, that is, with the elbow flexed to 20 degrees and leading with the thumb). In addition, she was now performing 'lawn-mower exercises' (Kibler et al., 2008) where she lifted a 5-kg weight placed in front of her left foot on a small portable step with the right shoulder in flexion and internal rotation, progressing through standing and right trunk rotation and moving the shoulder into elevation and external rotation with the elbow almost extended, then returning the weight to the step (Fig. 17.3). She had varied these movements at slower and faster paces, following the rules established previously. Alison had also been replicating both backhand and forehand tennis movements using a free-weight pulley system.

We agreed that although there had been fluctuations in her rehabilitation, she had substantially improved, and we should progress to the final, more functional stages of her program.

The final stages of rehabilitation involved combinations and progressions of the following:

1. Weight-bearing exercises on stable and unstable surfaces, and
2. Sensory-motor exercises to facilitate non-weight-bearing shoulder repositioning, pursuit and holding, using pointing tasks and a laser pointer with increasing complexity and speed (e.g. Fig. 17.4).

The final stages also involved exercises with a tennis racquet. Initially, Alison was instructed to move the racquet slowly and facilitating different tennis shots but avoiding end-range serving movements. Once she had developed confidence with this, she started

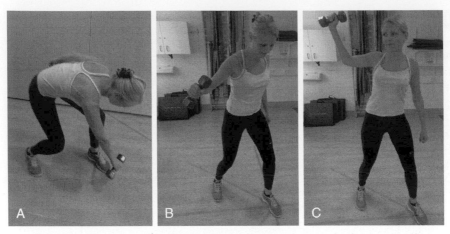

Fig. 17.3 'Lawn-mower' exercise.

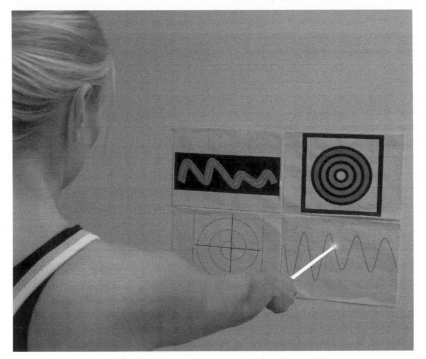

Fig. 17.4 Sensory-motor exercise with a laser pointer.

practicing on an indoor court. She employed the services of a tennis coach to train with, and three-party communications were established to set out the collaborative plan for progression. Court time was incrementally increased, starting at 5 minutes (initially twice weekly). Increased ROM and speed were gradually introduced, as were serving movements and serving speeds. Serving and end-range backhand and forehand movements were initially carefully controlled, and when incorporated into her program, only permitting a maximum of one or two movements. Over the next 6 weeks of court time, ROM, speed and repetitions were incrementally increased. There were times when Alison experienced momentary (non-irritable) sharp pain which she described as frightening, but it was not associated with any night pain or increase in 24-hour pain. Approximately 32 weeks after starting rehabilitation, Alison played her first full tennis match. It was relatively gentle, and although there were occasional twinges of pain, she finished the match and suffered no lasting ill-effects.

Toward the end of her rehabilitation, it was explained that if there was ever a gap in activity, such as serving in tennis or gardening, that it was inadvisable to restart at the same intensity and duration as she had performed on the occasion before the break in that activity. She should always restart such an activity at a lower than usual level, reducing duration, speed and intensity and build up to the desired level slowly. This rule was to be applied for other activities as well, such as painting walls.

Appointment 7 (34 Weeks After the Start of Treatment)

On her final visit, Alison reported her Global Impression of Change was much improved (95%), and her SPADI score was just 3%. The less-than-perfect score was only because she recorded the dimension of worst pain experienced in the past week at 4/10 as she had experienced momentary sharp shoulder pain when lifting a heavy suitcase off an airport carousel onto an airport trolley. At this point Alison was discharged from this program of care and invited to call or email at any time with any concerns or questions, as well as to report any deterioration in her condition. To date, more than 12 weeks after the end of treatment, she has not been in contact.

Reasoning Question:

8. Would you discuss your clinical reasoning regarding Alison's 'prognosis', commenting on both positive and negative features in her presentation?

Answer to Reasoning Question:

Alison's initial presentation, history, duration of symptoms, baseline pain scores, baseline disability scores, uncertainty over the potential benefit of non-surgical treatment, concern regarding the imaging identified structural deficit, recommendations from the orthopaedic surgeon and desire to return to a relatively high level of function collectively favoured a poor prognosis. Her motivation, level of education, good physical health and lack of identified comorbidities favoured a good prognosis.

Alison's initial favourable response to injection therapy combined with her poor response following the post-injection introduction of exercise specifically suggested it was unlikely she would respond to physiotherapy and thus supported a poor prognosis. However, later in the assessment, her positive response to the SSMP anecdotally favoured a positive prognosis, as did her eventual willingness to be patient with the process, monitor changes and respond (progress or relatively rest) to the influence of activity on her shoulder symptoms.

Clinical Reasoning Commentary:

'Prognosis' is discussed in Chapter 1 as a hypothesis category – after all, patients want and deserve to know whether the clinician thinks he or she can help them and how long it will take. Broadly speaking, a patient's prognosis is determined by the nature and extent of a patient's problem(s) and the patient's ability and willingness to make the necessary changes (e.g. lifestyle, psychosocial contributing factors, physical contributing factors) to facilitate recovery or an improved quality of life within a permanent disability. Importantly, clues about prognosis are sprinkled throughout the subjective and physical examinations, in addition to the ongoing management. As highlighted in this answer, patients commonly present with a combination of both negative and positive prognostic indicators. Conscious and balanced consideration of these indicators, and their modifiability, assists the formulation of the prognostic hypothesis. If critically followed up over time with reflection on initial and modified judgements, musculoskeletal clinicians can improve their prognostic reasoning.

REFERENCES

Alvarez, C.M., Litchfield, R., Jackowski, D., Griffin, S., Kirkley, A., 2005. A prospective, double-blind, randomized clinical trial comparing subacromial injection of betamethasone and xylocaine to xylocaine alone in chronic rotator cuff tendinosis. Am. J. Sports Med. 33, 255–262.

Backman, L.J., Andersson, G., Wennstig, G., Forsgren, S., Danielson, P., 2011a. Endogenous substance P production in the Achilles tendon increases with loading in an in vivo model of tendinopathy-peptidergic elevation preceding tendinosis-like tissue changes. J. Musculoskelet. Neuronal Interact. 11, 133–140.

Backman, L.J., Fong, G., Andersson, G., Scott, A., Danielson, P., 2011b. Substance P is a mechanoresponsive, autocrine regulator of human tenocyte proliferation. PLoS ONE 6, e27209.

Baumgarten, K.M., Gerlach, D., Galatz, L.M., Teefey, S.A., Middleton, W.D., Ditsios, K., et al., 2010. Cigarette smoking increases the risk for rotator cuff tears. Clin. Orthop. Relat. Res. 468, 1534–1541.

Beason, D.P., Tucker, J.J., Lee, C.S., Edelstein, L., Abboud, J.A., Soslowsky, L.J., 2014. Rat rotator cuff tendon-to-bone healing properties are adversely affected by hypercholesterolemia. J. Shoulder Elbow Surg. 23, 867–872.

Biswas, A., Oh, P.I., Faulkner, G.E., Bajaj, R.R., Silver, M.A., Mitchell, M.S., et al., 2015. Sedentary time and its association with risk for disease incidence, mortality, and hospitalization in adults: a systematic review and meta-analysis. Ann. Intern. Med. 162, 123–132.

Blaine, T.A., Kim, Y.S., Voloshin, I., Chen, D., Murakami, K., Chang, S.S., et al., 2005. The molecular pathophysiology of subacromial bursitis in rotator cuff disease. J. Shoulder Elbow Surg. 14, 84S–89S.

Blair, S.N., 2009. Physical inactivity: the biggest public health problem of the 21st century. Br. J. Sports Med. 43, 1–2.

Boettcher, C.E., Ginn, K.A., Cathers, I., 2009. The 'empty can' and 'full can' tests do not selectively activate supraspinatus. J. Sci. Med. Sport 12, 435–439.

Boettcher, C.E., Cathers, I., Ginn, K.A., 2010. The role of shoulder muscles is task specific. J. Sci. Med. Sport 13, 651–656.

Carbone, S., Gumina, S., Arceri, V., Campagna, V., Fagnani, C., Postacchini, F., 2012. The impact of preoperative smoking habit on rotator cuff tear: cigarette smoking influences rotator cuff tear sizes. J. Shoulder Elbow Surg. 21, 56–60.

Carofino, B., Chowaniec, D.M., Mccarthy, M.B., Bradley, J.P., Delaronde, S., Beitzel, K., et al., 2012. Corticosteroids and local anesthetics decrease positive effects of platelet-rich plasma: an in vitro study on human tendon cells. Arthroscopy 28, 711–719.

Charalambous, C.P., Sahu, A., Alvi, F., Batra, S., Gullett, T.K., Ravenscroft, M., 2010. Return to work and driving following arthroscopic subacromial decompression and acromio-clavicular joint excision. Shoulder & Elbow 2, 83–86.

Chen, S.K., Simonian, P.T., Wickiewicz, T.L., Otis, J.C., Warren, R.F., 1999. Radiographic evaluation of glenohumeral kinematics: a muscle fatigue model. J. Shoulder Elbow Surg. 8, 49–52.

Clark, J., Sidles, J.A., Matsen, F.A., 1990. The relationship of the glenohumeral joint capsule to the rotator cuff. Clin. Orthop. Relat. Res. 29–34.

Clark, J.M., Harryman, D.T., 2ND, 1992. Tendons, ligaments, and capsule of the rotator cuff. Gross and microscopic anatomy. J. Bone Joint Surg. Am. 74, 713–725.

Cook, J., Purdam, C.R., 2009. Is tendon pathology a continuum? A pathology model to explain the clinical presentation of load-induced tendinopathy. Br. J. Sports Med. 43, 409–416.

Coronado, R.A., Simon, C.B., Valencia, C., George, S.Z., 2014. Experimental pain responses support peripheral and central sensitization in patients with unilateral shoulder pain. Clin. J. Pain 30, 143–151.

Crawshaw, D.P., Helliwell, P.S., Hensor, E.M., Hay, E.M., Aldous, S.J., Conaghan, P.G., 2010. Exercise therapy after corticosteroid injection for moderate to severe shoulder pain: large pragmatic randomised trial. BMJ 340, c3037.

Dean, B.J., Lostis, E., Oakley, T., Rombach, I., Morrey, M.E., Carr, A.J., 2014. The risks and benefits of glucocorticoid treatment for tendinopathy: a systematic review of the effects of local glucocorticoid on tendon. Semin. Arthritis Rheum. 43, 570–576.

Dean, E., Söderlund, A., 2015a. Lifestyle factors and musculoskeletal pain. In: Jull, G., Moore, A., Falla, D., Lewis, J.S., McCarthy, C., Sterling, M. (Eds.), Grieve's Modern Musculoskeletal Physiotherapy, fourth ed. Elsevier, London.

Dean, E., Söderlund, A., 2015b. Role of physiotherapy in lifestyle and health promotion in musculoskeletal conditions. In: Jull, G., Moore, A., Falla, D., Lewis, J.S., McCarthy, C., Sterling, M. (Eds.), Grieve's Modern Musculoskeletal Physiotherapy, fourth ed. Elsevier, London.

Deutsch, A., Altchek, D.W., Schwartz, E., Otis, J.C., Warren, R.F., 1996. Radiologic measurement of superior displacement of the humeral head in the impingement syndrome. J. Shoulder Elbow Surg. 5, 186–193.

Dunn, W.R., Kuhn, J.E., Sanders, R., An, Q., Baumgarten, K.M., Bishop, J.Y., et al., 2014. Symptoms of pain do not correlate with rotator cuff tear severity: a cross-sectional study of 393 patients with a symptomatic atraumatic full-thickness rotator cuff tear. J. Bone Joint Surg. Am. 96, 793–800.

Ekeberg, O.M., Bautz-Holter, E., Tveita, E.K., Juel, N.G., Kvalheim, S., Brox, J.I., 2009. Subacromial ultrasound guided or systemic steroid injection for rotator cuff disease: randomised double blind study. Br. Med. J. 338, a3112.

Franceschini, M., Ceravolo, M.G., Agosti, M., Cavallini, P., Bonassi, S., Dall'armi, V., et al., 2012. Clinical relevance of action observation in upper-limb stroke rehabilitation: a possible role in recovery of functional dexterity. A randomized clinical trial. Neurorehabil. Neural Repair 26, 456–462.

Frizziero, A., Vittadini, F., Gasparre, G., Masiero, S., 2014. Impact of oestrogen deficiency and aging on tendon: concise review. Muscles Ligaments Tendons J. 4, 324–328.

Fukuda, H., Hamada, K., Yamanaka, K., 1990. Pathology and pathogenesis of bursal-side rotator cuff tears viewed from en bloc histologic sections. Clin. Orthop. Relat. Res. 75–80.

Gaida, J.E., Ashe, M.C., Bass, S.L., Cook, J.L., 2009. Is adiposity an under-recognized risk factor for tendinopathy? A systematic review. Arthritis Rheum. 61, 840–849.

Galatz, L.M., Silva, M.J., Rothermich, S.Y., Zaegel, M.A., Havlioglu, N., Thomopoulos, S., 2006. Nicotine delays tendon-to-bone healing in a rat shoulder model. J. Bone Joint Surg. Am. 88, 2027–2034.

Girish, G., Lobo, L.G., Jacobson, J.A., Morag, Y., Miller, B., Jamadar, D.A., 2011. Ultrasound of the shoulder: asymptomatic findings in men. AJR Am. J. Roentgenol. 197, W713–W719.

Gotoh, M., Hamada, K., Yamakawa, H., Inoue, A., Fukuda, H., 1998. Increased substance P in subacromial bursa and shoulder pain in rotator cuff diseases. J. Orthop. Res. 16, 618–621.

Gotoh, M., Hamada, K., Yamakawa, H., Yanagisawa, K., Nakamura, M., Yamazaki, H., et al., 2002. Interleukin-1-induced glenohumeral synovitis and shoulder pain in rotator cuff diseases. J. Orthop. Res. 20, 1365–1371.

Gotoh, M., Hamada, K., Yamakawa, H., Yanagisawa, K., Nakamura, M., Yamazaki, H., et al., 2001. Interleukin-1-induced subacromial synovitis and shoulder pain in rotator cuff diseases. Rheumatology 40, 995–1001.

Haahr, J.P., Andersen, J.H., 2006. Exercises may be as efficient as subacromial decompression in patients with subacromial stage II impingement: 4-8-years' follow-up in a prospective, randomized study. Scand. J. Rheumatol. 35, 224–228.

Haahr, J.P., Ostergaard, S., Dalsgaard, J., Norup, K., Frost, P., Lausen, S., et al., 2005. Exercises versus arthroscopic decompression in patients with subacromial impingement: a randomised, controlled study in 90 cases with a one year follow up. Ann. Rheum. Dis. 64, 760–764.

Hegedus, E.J., Goode, A., Campbell, S., Morin, A., Tamaddoni, M., Moorman, C.T., 3rd, et al., 2008. Physical examination tests of the shoulder: a systematic review with meta-analysis of individual tests. Br. J. Sports Med. 42, 80–92, discussion 92.

Hegedus, E.J., Goode, A.P., Cook, C.E., Michener, L., Myer, C.A., Myer, D.M., et al., 2012. Which physical examination tests provide clinicians with the most value when examining the shoulder? Update of a systematic review with meta-analysis of individual tests. Br. J. Sports Med. 46, 964–978.

Henkus, H.E., Cobben, L.P., Coerkamp, E.G., Nelissen, R.G., Van Arkel, E.R., 2006. The accuracy of subacromial injections: a prospective randomized magnetic resonance imaging study. Arthroscopy 22, 277–282.

Henkus, H.E., De Witte, P.B., Nelissen, R.G., Brand, R., Van Arkel, E.R., 2009. Bursectomy compared with acromioplasty in the management of subacromial impingement syndrome: a prospective randomised study. J. Bone Joint Surg. Br. 91, 504–510.

Hengeveld, E., Banks, K., 2014. Maitland's Vertebral Manipulation. Management of Neuromusculoskeletal Disorders – Volume One, eighth ed. Churchill Livingstone Elsevier, Edinburgh.

Hoeger Bement, M., Dicapo, J., Rasiarmos, R., Hunter, S., 2008. Dose response of isometric contractions on pain perception in healthy adults. Med. Sci. Sports Exerc. 40, 1880–1889.

Holmgren, T., Bjornsson Hallgren, H., Oberg, B., Adolfsson, L., Johansson, K., 2012. Effect of specific exercise strategy on need for surgery in patients with subacromial impingement syndrome: randomised controlled study. BMJ 344, e787.

Hoyek, N., Di Rienzo, F., Collet, C., Hoyek, F., Guillot, A., 2014. The therapeutic role of motor imagery on the functional rehabilitation of a stage II shoulder impingement syndrome. Disabil. Rehabil. 36, 1113–1119.

Jobe, F.W., Moynes, D.R., 1982. Delineation of diagnostic criteria and a rehabilitation program for rotator cuff injuries. Am. J. Sports Med. 10, 336–339.

Jowett, S., Crawshaw, D.P., Helliwell, P.S., Hensor, E.M., Hay, E.M., Conaghan, P.G., 2013. Cost-effectiveness of exercise therapy after corticosteroid injection for moderate to severe shoulder pain due to subacromial impingement syndrome: a trial-based analysis. Rheumatology 52, 1485–1491.

Kamper, S., 2009. Global rating of change scales. Aust. J. Physiother. 55, 289.

Kamper, S.J., Maher, C.G., Mackay, G., 2009. Global rating of change scales: a review of strengths and weaknesses and considerations for design. J. Man. Manip. Ther. 17, 163–170.

Karlsson, L., Gerdle, B., Ghafouri, B., Backryd, E., Olausson, P., Ghafouri, N., et al., 2014. Intramuscular pain modulatory substances before and after exercise in women with chronic neck pain. Eur. J. Pain 19 (8), 1075–1085.

Keener, J.D., Wei, A.S., Kim, H.M., Steger-May, K., Yamaguchi, K., 2009. Proximal humeral migration in shoulders with symptomatic and asymptomatic rotator cuff tears. J. Bone Joint Surg. Am. 91, 1405–1413.

Ketola, S., Lehtinen, J., Arnala, I., Nissinen, M., Westenius, H., Sintonen, H., et al., 2009. Does arthroscopic acromioplasty provide any additional value in the treatment of shoulder impingement syndrome?: a two-year randomised controlled trial. J. Bone Joint Surg. Br. 91, 1326–1334.

Ketola, S., Lehtinen, J., Rousi, T., Nissinen, M., Huhtala, H., Konttinen, Y.T., et al., 2013. No evidence of long-term benefits of arthroscopic acromioplasty in the treatment of shoulder impingement syndrome: five-year results of a randomised controlled trial. Bone Joint Res 2, 132–139.

Kibler, W.B., 1995. Biomechanical analysis of the shoulder during tennis activities. Clin. Sports Med. 14, 79–85.

Kibler, W.B., Sciascia, A.D., Uhl, T.L., Tambay, N., Cunningham, T., 2008. Electromyographic analysis of specific exercises for scapular control in early phases of shoulder rehabilitation. Am. J. Sports Med. 36, 1789–1798.

Kim, K.C., Shin, H.D., Lee, W.Y., 2012. Repair integrity and functional outcomes after arthroscopic suture-bridge rotator cuff repair. J. Bone Joint Surg. Am. 94, e48.

Kuhn, J.E., Dunn, W.R., Sanders, R., An, Q., Baumgarten, K.M., Bishop, J.Y., et al., 2013. Effectiveness of physical therapy in treating atraumatic full-thickness rotator cuff tears: a multicenter prospective cohort study. J. Shoulder Elbow Surg. 22, 1371–1379.

Kukkonen, J., Joukainen, A., Lehtinen, J., Mattila, K.T., Tuominen, E.K., Kauko, T., et al., 2014. Treatment of non-traumatic rotator cuff tears: a randomised controlled trial with one-year clinical results. Bone Joint J. 96-B, 75–81.

Lee, I.M., Shiroma, E.J., Lobelo, F., Puska, P., Blair, S.N., Katzmarzyk, P.T., 2012. Effect of physical inactivity on major non-communicable diseases worldwide: an analysis of burden of disease and life expectancy. Lancet 380, 219–229.

Lemley, K.J., Drewek, B., Hunter, S.K., Hoeger Bement, M.K., 2014. Pain relief after isometric exercise is not task-dependent in older men and women. Med. Sci. Sports Exerc. 46, 185–191.

Lewis, J.S., 2009. Rotator cuff tendinopathy/subacromial impingement syndrome: is it time for a new method of assessment? Br. J. Sports Med. 43, 259–264.

Lewis, J.S., 2010. Rotator cuff tendinopathy: a model for the continuum of pathology and related management. Br. J. Sports Med. 44, 918–923.

Lewis, J.S., 2011. Subacromial impingement syndrome: a musculoskeletal condition or a clinical illusion? Phy. Ther. Rev. 16, 388–398.

Lewis, J.S., 2014a. Management of rotator cuff tendinopathy. In Touch - Journal of the Organisation of Chartered Physiotherapists in Private Practice 149, 12–17.

Lewis, J.S., 2015. Bloodletting for pneumonia, prolonged bed rest for low back pain, is subacromial decompression another clinical illusion? Br. J. Sports Med. 49, 280–281.

Lewis, J.S., Ginn, K., 2015. Rotator cuff tendinopathy and subacromial pain syndrome. In: Jull, G., Moore, A., Falla, D., Lewis, J.S., McCarthy, C., Sterling, M. (Eds.), Grieve's Modern Musculoskeletal Physiotherapy, fourth ed. Elsevier, London.

Lewis, J.S., McCreesh, K., Roy, J.S., Ginn, K., 2015. Rotator cuff tendinopathy: navigating the diagnosis-management conundrum. J. Orthop. Sports Phy. Ther. in press.

Lewis, J.S., Tennent, T.D., 2007. How effective are diagnostic tests for the assessment of rotator cuff disease of the shoulder? In: Macauley, D., Best, T.M. (Eds.), Evidenced Based Sports Medicine, second ed. Blackwell Publishing, London.

Magee, D., 2014. Orthopedic Physical Assessment. Elsevier, Philadelphia.

Maitland, G.D., 1986. Vertebral Manipulation. Butterworths, London.

McClelland, D., Paxinos, A., Dodenhoff, R.M., 2005. Rate of return to work and driving following arthroscopic subacromial decompression. ANZ J. Surg. 75, 747–749.

McCreesh, K., Lewis, J., 2013. Continuum model of tendon pathology - where are we now? Int. J. Exp. Pathol. 94, 242–247.

Millar, N.L., Hueber, A.J., Reilly, J.H., Xu, Y., Fazzi, U.G., Murrell, G.A., et al., 2010. Inflammation is present in early human tendinopathy. Am. J. Sports Med. 38, 2085–2091.

Moseley, J.B., O'Malley, K., Petersen, N.J., Menke, T.J., Brody, B.A., Kuykendall, D.H., et al., 2002. A controlled trial of arthroscopic surgery for osteoarthritis of the knee. N. Engl. J. Med. 347, 81–88.

Mulligan, B.R., 1999. Manual Therapy "Nags", "Snags", "MWMs" etc. Plane View Services, New Zealand.

Ngomo, S., Mercier, C., Bouyer, L.J., Savoie, A., Roy, J.S., 2015. Alterations in central motor representation increase over time in individuals with rotator cuff tendinopathy. Clin. Neurophysiol. 126, 365–371.

Parle, P., Riddiford-Harland, D.L., Howitt, C., Lewis, J.S., 2016. Acute rotator cuff tendinopathy: does ice, low load isometric exercise, or a combination of the two produce an analgesic effect? Br. J. Sports Med. http://dx .doi.org./10.1136/bjsports-2016-096107.

Paul, T.M., Soo Hoo, J., Chae, J., Wilson, R.D., 2012. Central hypersensitivity in patients with subacromial impingement syndrome. Arch. Phys. Med. Rehabil. 93, 2206–2209.

Porro, C.A., Facchin, P., Fusi, S., Dri, G., Fadiga, L., 2007. Enhancement of force after action observation: behavioural and neurophysiological studies. Neuropsychologia 45, 3114–3121.

Ranganathan, V.K., Siemionow, V., Liu, J.Z., Sahgal, V., Yue, G.H., 2004. From mental power to muscle power–gaining strength by using the mind. Neuropsychologia 42, 944–956.

Rio, E., Kidgell, D., Moseley, L., Pearce, A., Gaida, J., Cook, J., 2013. Exercise to reduce tendon pain: a comparison of isometric and isotonic muscle contractions and effects on pain, cortical inhibition and muscle strength. J. Exerc. Med. Sport 16, e28.

Roach, K.E., Budiman-Mak, E., Songsiridej, N., Lertratanakul, Y., 1991. Development of a shoulder pain and disability index. Arthritis Care Res. 4, 143–149.

Rudavsky, A., Cook, J., 2014. Physiotherapy management of patellar tendinopathy (jumper's knee). J. Physiother. 60, 122–129.

Sakai, H., Fujita, K., Sakai, Y., Mizuno, K., 2001. Immunolocalization of cytokines and growth factors in subacromial bursa of rotator cuff tear patients. Kobe J. Med. Sci. 47, 25–34.

Santavirta, S., Konttinen, Y.T., Antti-Poika, I., Nordstrom, D., 1992. Inflammation of the subacromial bursa in chronic shoulder pain. Arch. Orthop. Trauma Surg. 111, 336–340.

Sarkar, K., Uhthoff, H.K., 1983. Ultrastructure of the subacromial bursa in painful shoulder syndromes. Virchows Arch. A. Pathol Anat Histopathol. 400, 107–117.

Scherb, M.B., Han, S.H., Courneya, J.P., Guyton, G.P., Schon, L.C., 2009. Effect of bupivacaine on cultured tenocytes. Orthopedics 32, 26.

Sciascia, A., Cromwell, R., 2012. Kinetic chain rehabilitation: a theoretical framework. Rehabil. Res. Pract. 2012, 853037.

Seroyer, S.T., Nho, S.J., Bach, B.R., Bush-Joseph, C.A., Nicholson, G.P., Romeo, A.A., 2010. The kinetic chain in overhand pitching: its potential role for performance enhancement and injury prevention. Sports Health 2, 135–146.

Sharkey, N.A., Marder, R.A., 1995. The rotator cuff opposes superior translation of the humeral head. Am. J. Sports Med. 23, 270–275.

Sihvonen, R., Paavola, M., Malmivaara, A., Itala, A., Joukainen, A., Nurmi, H., et al., 2013. Arthroscopic partial meniscectomy versus sham surgery for a degenerative meniscal tear. N. Engl. J. Med. 369, 2515–2524.

Smart, K.M., Blake, C., Staines, A., Doody, C., 2011. The discriminative validity of "nociceptive," "peripheral neuropathic," and "central sensitization" as mechanisms-based classifications of musculoskeletal pain. Clin. J. Pain 27, 655–663.

Soifer, T.B., Levy, H.J., Soifer, F.M., Kleinbart, F., Vigorita, V., Bryk, E., 1996. Neurohistology of the subacromial space. Arthroscopy 12, 182–186.

Tamir, R., Dickstein, R., Huberman, M., 2007. Integration of motor imagery and physical practice in group treatment applied to subjects with Parkinson's disease. Neurorehabil. Neural Repair 21, 68–75.

Tsai, W.C., Tang, F.T., Hsu, C.C., Hsu, Y.H., Pang, J.H., Shiue, C.C., 2004. Ibuprofen inhibition of tendon cell proliferation and upregulation of the cyclin kinase inhibitor p21CIP1. J. Orthop. Res. 22, 586–591.

Unruh, K.P., Kuhn, J.E., Sanders, R., An, Q., Baumgarten, K.M., Bishop, J.Y., et al., 2014. The duration of symptoms does not correlate with rotator cuff tear severity or other patient-related features: a cross-sectional study of patients with atraumatic, full-thickness rotator cuff tears. J. Shoulder Elbow Surg. 23, 1052–1058.

Voloshin, I., Gelinas, J., Maloney, M.D., O'Keefe, R.J., Bigliani, L.U., Blaine, T.A., 2005. Proinflammatory cytokines and metalloproteases are expressed in the subacromial bursa in patients with rotator cuff disease. Arthroscopy 21, 1076. e1–1076. e9.

Wattanaprakornkul, D., Halaki, M., Boettcher, C., Cathers, I., Ginn, K.A., 2011. A comprehensive analysis of muscle recruitment patterns during shoulder flexion: an electromyographic study. Clin. Anat. 24, 619–626.

Weiler, R., Stamatakis, E., Blair, S., 2010. Should health policy focus on physical activity rather than obesity? Yes. BMJ 340, c2603.

Yanagisawa, K., Hamada, K., Gotoh, M., Tokunaga, T., Oshika, Y., Tomisawa, M., et al., 2001. Vascular endothelial growth factor (VEGF) expression in the subacromial bursa is increased in patients with impingement syndrome. J. Orthop. Res. 19, 448–455.

18

Post-Traumatic Neck Pain, Headache and Knee Pain Following a Cycling Accident

Rafael Torres Cueco • Darren A. Rivett • Mark A. Jones

First Appointment Subjective Assessment – Part 1

Monica was a 31-year-old female who presented to the physical therapy department following a cycling fall 3 months earlier. Monica was completing her studies in tourism and had been recommended to our clinic by a fellow student. The reasons for the consultation in order of importance to Monica were as follows: pain throughout her neck that prevented her from moving it in any direction, more intense in the right occipital region; right frontotemporal headache that sometimes affected the whole head; pain in the right facial region; dull pain in the area of the right upper trapezius muscle; dizziness, nausea and a feeling of unsteadiness.

The accident had occurred when Monica was cycling through an old part of town where the streets were narrow. She took a sharp curve too fast and, on seeing a parked car, braked suddenly and fell. At the time of the fall, she recalled hitting herself hard against the ground with her left shoulder and remembered a very brief stabbing sensation in the right cervical region. She was unable to specify how she moved her neck when she fell but was sure that she did not hit her head on the ground. After the fall, only her left shoulder hurt, but she was quite shaken, realizing that at that speed, she could have killed herself if she had impacted against the car.

Three or four hours after the accident, she began to feel neck pain, especially in the right suboccipital region, as well as a slight headache in the frontotemporal region of the same side. At bedtime the pain was intense, and she took a tablet of acetaminophen (1 g). The following morning, she woke up with moderate neck stiffness, and 2 hours later her neck pain and headache reappeared. It felt like a bruised shoulder, but the pain was not severe. At that time, surprisingly, pain appeared in her right knee, which she described as a burning pain on the anterior side of her knee. When asked about the cause of knee pain or if the knee had impacted against the ground or some other element during the fall, she recalled to have discussed this with her boyfriend, and she was sure she didn't hit her knee during the accident. She did mention, however, that it was her 'bad knee', without giving further details.

The day after the accident, she went to the doctor, who ordered an x-ray of her neck, which was conducted on the same day. The x-ray revealed flattening of the cervical lordosis. The doctor said she had a 'whiplash' injury and a 'contracture' that were causing the pain. With regard to her knee pain, despite no memory of having hit her knee, she was diagnosed with 'bruising'. She was prescribed ibuprofen (400 mg), one tablet to be taken every 12 hours and was sent to a physiotherapist. The other symptoms, such as facial pain, unsteadiness and nausea, appeared gradually weeks later, after several sessions of physiotherapy.

Monica reported that after the accident, she avoided walking or cycling along the street where the accident had happened, despite it being the shortest route between her home and her boyfriend's. Indeed, 1 month later, her boyfriend, realizing that this behaviour was unusual, insisted that she resume this route. During the 3 weeks following the accident, she avoided recalling the event because she found it highly distressing.

Initially, Monica received physiotherapy treatment twice a week for about 6 weeks. For the first 2 weeks, physiotherapy sessions consisted of passive mobilization of the cervical spine and stretching exercises for her 'contracture'. Monica felt that she was not improving and that after each physiotherapy session, her neck hurt more, and her headaches were more intense. Because she felt no improvement, she insisted that she had been incorrectly diagnosed and that perhaps they were not giving her the right treatment and therefore aggravating the problem. In view of there being no improvement through the physiotherapy treatment, she was told that her problem was probably due to cervical 'instability' caused by the accident, and besides continuing with the previous passive treatment, she was prescribed isometric cervical exercises to be performed three times daily. Monica was alarmed about the 'cervical instability', and on discussing this with her mother, she said it sounded as if she might 'break her neck'. She attempted to do the exercises prescribed, but she was afraid she might make the problem worse. She also felt pain and dizziness when performing her exercises.

After a month of treatment, Monica was getting worse. Her headaches were daily, especially when sitting for over an hour, and she also felt a little dizzy throughout the whole day. She was afraid of moving her neck quickly in case she felt dizzy and fell. Her knee ached more and more, and she was afraid of going up or down stairs in case her knee failed her. Monica felt that she could hardly do anything because if she was sitting, she got dizzy, and if she moved a lot, she also felt dizzy, and her knee hurt. This prevented her from studying or carrying out everyday activities. Monica reported that this situation made her unhappy because she felt very limited in her activities.

Monica returned to her doctor, who ordered magnetic resonance imaging (MRI), which revealed a protrusion at C5–C6 with no other lesions. Her doctor diagnosed that this 'disc herniation' was the cause of her neck pain and headache. The doctor recommended that to prevent the herniation from getting worse, she should not bear weight with her arms and avoid resisted activity with her arms above her head. Although nothing should be done initially, the doctor clarified that no improvement within the following months would make surgery advisable. The doctor recommended that she abandon the physiotherapy sessions and to continue with the isometric exercises without 'overstraining' herself. Ibuprofen (600 mg) and pregabalin (Lyrica) (75 mg) twice a day for 4 weeks were prescribed for pain relief.

Following the consultation, Monica expressed her frustration: 'Now I can't even use my arms, what else? I can't strain my knee, neck or arms. I can do virtually nothing'. Monica now reported that she felt like a burden for everyone. She could not help her mother at home and was constantly angry at her boyfriend. He wanted to go out and do things, but Monica was afraid she would aggravate her injury, and the pain and dizziness made her extremely irritable about anything. She was also upset with her boyfriend because he said she was overreacting and that it could not hurt so much. Monica was frightened and kept wondering what was to become of her life if she did not recover. She needed a solution, and she felt desperate.

Monica happened to search 'disc herniation' on the Internet and read blogs posting experiences of patients who had suffered quadriplegia due to a herniated cervical disc and also that many people got worse after surgery. Monica was getting more and more scared. All the information she found suggested that her problem was serious and could become more serious. She stopped doing her exercises because she was sure they were doing her no good. She continually thought about how to avoid ending up in a wheelchair.

Following the advice of one of her mother's friends, she decided to visit another physiotherapist, who said that her neck pain was due to a joint 'injury' and that her headache was caused by trigger points in the neck muscles. The diagnosis of knee pain was also attributed to myofascial trigger points in the vastus medialis. The first session was mainly passive mobilization of the cervical spine and a gentle massage on the trapezius muscle area.

Although she felt some discomfort during the massage, she experienced a slight improvement for a few days. At the second session, she received a much more intense manual therapy treatment and dry needling in the right upper trapezius, and her neck pain and headache became much worse. The therapist proposed needling of the vastus medialis, but Monica refused. She attended a third session, but at the very start of the session, she began to feel nauseous, unsteady, dysesthetic discomfort in the sub-occipital region and right-sided facial pain. Since the 'damage' caused in the second session of physiotherapy, her neck felt colder, drafts bothered her and even at home she needed to wear a scarf. After that, she started to feel discomfort from her shirt collar in contact with her neck and inability to carry her handbag on her right shoulder because the rubbing feeling was extremely unpleasant. She eventually decided to stop physiotherapy due to the aggravation of symptoms. Headaches were now almost constant throughout the day, and she also felt discomfort on the right side of her face.

It was apparent that Monica did not really understand the different diagnoses she had been given and was least convinced about the treatment, which was very painful and, in her opinion, 'too aggressive', perhaps 'aggravating the problem'. The idea of needling didn't make sense to Monica. The manual therapy hurt, and she couldn't understand why she also required the needling. She was very unhappy with the physiotherapy. She spoke with her mother, and together they decided to stop treatment because it surely must not be doing her neck any good. The previous doctor had told her it was a herniated disc, and although she was not sure about what she had, if that was right, she couldn't see how these treatments would help. Monica subsequently gave up the physiotherapy treatment, deciding instead to rest and avoid straining her neck or knee.

For over a month Monica, was unable to attend her academic classes because the neck pain and headaches made concentration extremely difficult. At the time of the present consultation, she reported feeling very tired at the end of the day and incapable of studying. She had rejected an employment proposal as a hotel receptionist, feeling incapable of carrying out this job due to her neck and knee pain.

Monica felt terribly unhappy. She could no longer do any of the things she enjoyed. Not being able to study got her down, and she felt disappointed by having rejected an interesting job offer. She was increasingly convinced that she would not recover, and she felt depressed, not knowing what to do from now on. She woke up every day thinking about her neck pain.

She was now concerned that the physiotherapy treatment might have exacerbated her neck injuries. She had come to our clinic upon the insistence of a fellow student; however, she was fearful of undergoing further treatment.

Reasoning Question:

1. What were the salient aspects of the history that facilitated your clinical reasoning process? Did any of the history raise any concerns or suggest a likely prognosis?

Answer to Reasoning Question:

It is essential that the medical history should initially establish the date of onset of the symptoms, if the onset was acute or progressive and whether it was traumatic or not. The history of post-traumatic pain needs to be more thorough than that of non-traumatic neck pain or pain of insidious origin. The details regarding how the accident occurred and the initial symptoms reported by the patient are both relevant. The manner in which the accident occurred may help interpret the possible mechanism of injury, which is relevant for the purpose of determining the severity of injuries. The fact that her head did not hit the ground reduced the possibility of serious bone or ligament damage.

Initial symptoms experienced by the patient are also very important in order to establish a possible prognosis. Indicators of an adverse prognosis include severe cervical pain, pain which appears immediately after the accident or cervical pain accompanied by a severe headache. The occurrence of neurological signs (e.g. perioral paresthesia, Horner's syndrome, gait disorders, dizziness, etc.) may be indicative of serious neurovascular injury. Obviously, there may be many other red flags, such as loss of consciousness, dysphagia in the days following the accident and so forth.

Emotional distress at the time of the accident was also relevant. The fact that Monica was badly shaken, with a feeling of serious injury, may be associated with an adverse development of symptoms. In this case we could identify symptoms associated with post-traumatic stress syndrome and a clear fear-avoidance behavior. Signs of post-traumatic stress disorder (PTSD) are often disturbing recurrent flashbacks, avoidance of memories of the event and hyperarousal more than a month after the traumatic event (American Psychiatric Association, 2013). When patients present with PTSD-associated symptoms, they should be asked, unobtrusively, if they have previously (especially during childhood) ever experienced any kind of traumatic event.

Reasoning Question:

2. Can you comment on features from the subjective examination up to this point that you associated with 'pain type' (nociceptive, peripheral neuropathic, nociplastic)? What were the implications of this reasoning for your plans for physical examination and treatment?

Answer to Reasoning Question:

There had been a gradual evolution of Monica's symptoms 3 months following the accident, and the symptoms had worsened rather than improved. There were aspects suggestive of a pattern of a nociplastic pain type, such as tactile allodynia as evidenced by her discomfort from her shirt collar in contact with her neck and inability to carry her handbag on her right shoulder due to the extremely unpleasant rubbing feeling. Further, difficulty in concentrating is a common cognitive dysfunction in subjects with central hyperexcitability. Monica then experienced a significantly adverse therapeutic response to manual therapy and dry needling which may have also contributed to central sensitization, particularly if intense, pain-provoking interventions were performed without any prior pain education. In my experience, overly intense techniques should have never been applied. Monica was fearful of treatment, and any negative expectations can be a major barrier to successful treatment. These expectations implied that we needed to be extremely cautious during examination and treatment.

Reasoning Question:

3. What were your thoughts at this point following the first part of the assessment? How did the information fit into your clinical reasoning hypotheses?

Answer to Reasoning Question:

Monica presented with a complex clinical pattern which had many similarities with whiplash-associated disorders (WADs). Her headache might have been related to an injury to the cranio-cervical spine. It was essential to ask questions aimed to establish a differential diagnosis of headache. Frontotemporal post-traumatic headache may be of different etiologies, including cervicogenic-type headache. We also needed to identify the etiology of her right facial pain. Dizziness, nausea and a feeling of unsteadiness are common symptoms in WAD. However, it was important to rule out other etiologies. Particularly striking is the appearance of a sore right knee that Monica did not relate to an impact during the accident.

Significant distress at the time of the accident and the presence of PTSD-associated symptoms in the first month after the event are indicators of adverse prognosis. However, the facts that injuries are not secondary to a car accident and that there is no pending litigation are positive because these can confound the symptom and disability presentation. Important aspects are also the adverse outcomes from the previous physiotherapy treatment and Monica's subsequent fear of treatment. Obviously, at this time of the subjective assessment, appropriate treatment planning is crucial to a good outcome.

The first part of the subjective assessment allowed two things. Firstly, it allowed us to generate a clinical hypothesis based on inductive or heuristic reasoning. This reasoning is based on the recognition of relevant clusters of cues and contextual issues that fit a known clinical pattern. At this early stage of the subjective assessment with pieces of the information collected, the experts organize their knowledge to develop a more efficient assessment. It also illustrates an initial approach that emphasizes the patient's perspective (narrative reasoning) providing initial information about the patient's beliefs, expectations, emotions, context and the significance of the problem to the patient. Initial impressions from this information are then tested as further detail is obtained in the second part of the subjective assessment and ongoing appointments.

Clinical Reasoning Commentary:

While highlighting the importance of a structured and thorough history regarding the mechanism of onset and initial symptoms to hypotheses regarding potential severity of injury and prognosis, emphasis is also given to associated emotions at the time of onset, which, in Monica's case, were linked to potential PTSD and fear avoidance. This represents 'screening' for additional symptoms (including emotions) not spontaneously volunteered, which, as discussed in Chapter 1, is a key strategy to minimize the fast reasoning error of assuming 'what you see is all there is' (Kahneman, 2011, p. 86).

Also, as discussed in Chapter 1, there are many different areas of clinical judgement where knowledge of clinical patterns assists inductive hypothesis formation, follow-up hypothesis testing and eventual deductive clinical decisions. For example, knowledge of clinical patterns of pain type enables recognition of a likely component of nociplastic pain.

Clinical reasoning requires more than making judgements in any single 'hypothesis category' but also recognizing how judgements in one category influence judgements in others. This interconnection of hypothesis category reasoning is evident here, where a hypothesis regarding a nociplastic 'pain type' is linked to analysis of 'patient perspectives' (e.g. Monica's fear of treatment and any negative expectations

Continued on following page

associated with her past adverse treatment response), to 'prognosis' (e.g. can be a major barrier to successful treatment) and to 'precautions' (e.g. these expectations implied we needed to be extremely cautious during examination and treatment).

Pattern recognition is further evidenced in the analysis of presentation similarity to WAD; the need for differential diagnosis for the headache, the dizziness, nausea and unsteadiness symptoms; and recognition of PTSD-associated symptoms.

First Appointment Subjective Assessment – Part 2

In the second part of the case history, we asked two types of questions. Firstly, general questions such as those addressing the pain profile, trigger factors, pain rhythm, stage, previous treatment, additional tests and so forth are necessary to establish the clinical syndrome. We also asked specific targeted questions to establish a differential diagnosis to rule out alternative diagnostic hypotheses.

Current Symptoms

In order of importance, we collected each one of the patient's symptoms, assigning them a number. We asked a series of essential questions to establish the profile of pain, symptom behavior, previous history and evolution of the current clinical pattern. The profile of pain included the location, duration, rhythm and regularity, quality (descriptors), intensity, irritability, pain behavior and associated symptoms.

Map of Symptoms

In order to accurately determine the area in which the patient experiences symptoms, it is recommended to draw, on a body chart, the location of pain (Fig. 18.1). The way in which the patient points out the area where he or she feels pain may give some clues about the source of the pain. Therapists should ideally draw the areas of the symptoms themselves because the patient is often unable to express the symptoms on the drawing. However, in other cases, especially in patients with chronic pain, it may be interesting to let the patients draw their own symptoms. A color code can be useful, where red indicates pain, and yellow represents paresthesia or dysesthetic symptoms. Areas with more intense pain are solid red, whereas areas with less intense pain are shown as faded red.

Once the drawing has been completed, the patient is asked to confirm if it accurately reflects his or her symptoms.

Frequency of Symptoms

Monica reported suffering cervical pain, headache, dizziness, nausea and the feeling of unsteadiness as well as pain in her right knee every day, whereas her facial symptoms were experienced 2–3 days per week. Pain was present throughout the day, but got worse depending on the activity performed. The headache and facial symptoms always appeared with increasing neck pain.

Symptom Characteristics, Pain Descriptors and Pain Behavior

Neck Pain and Headache

Sub-occipital pain was described by Monica as a deep dull pain that, when more intense, was accompanied by ipsilateral occipital and fronto-temporal pain. The pain on the right side of the supraspinous fossa also seemed to be associated with her neck pain and was almost always triggered after sitting for a long time while studying. We asked her to rate the intensity of symptoms on a scale from 1 to 10. Firstly we obtained the average intensity of pain (NRS [A]) in the two preceding weeks and then asked her to rate the level of more severe symptoms (NRS [S]).

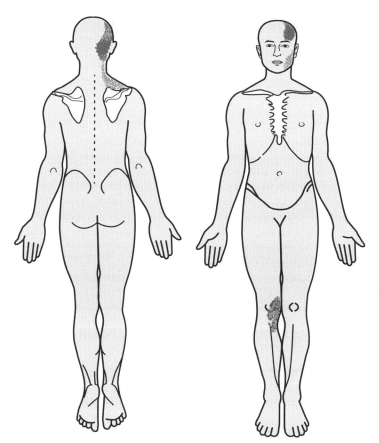

Fig. 18.1   Body chart showing areas of pain.

Monica replied that her usual suboccipital neck pain was 7/10 NRS [A], reaching 9/10 NRS [S] when it was most intense. She had pain every day but not all day. The pain was worse when she woke up in the morning and in the evenings. We asked about trigger factors and aggravating symptoms. She replied that the pain usually appeared when sitting for long periods and became worse with rotational head movements to the right and with cervical extension. She also reported that when lying on her back, she was unable to lift her head from the pillow because she no longer felt she had the strength. This was only possible by lifting her head with her hands. She also commented about problems with her pillow, sometimes struggling with her pillow position. When starting with neck pain, she folded the pillow and the pain lessened, but after a while it became uncomfortable, and she removed it. The pain seemed to be relieved in the short term and then worsened after a while. Some nights she continually placed and removed the pillow, sometimes even throwing it across the room. Neck pain was relieved a little when she lay supine with a hot pad under her neck, but she was unable to stay in that position for a long time.

She recalled that pain became worse after going to the hairdresser, where she kept her neck in extension while they washed her hair. She spent several days with severe neck and head pain and had much difficulty turning her neck to the right after this occasion.

Monica described her headache as a dull ache. The usual intensity was highly variable depending on the severity of the neck pain. Usually it was rated 6/10 and slightly worse when more intense (7/10). The headache was not pulsating or throbbing like a migraine, nor severe as in a trigeminal-autonomic headache. The nature of the pain was not consistent with occipital neuralgia because this type of pain is very short in duration and can be piercing like an electric shock. We asked Monica if sometimes she perceived a different sensation, paresthesia or a feeling of numbness in the occipital region, symptoms that often accompany occipital neuralgia, to which she answered no. Although she reported difficulties in concentrating when having a headache, the headache did not get worse or limit her normal activities of daily life, as in the case with migraine. She also replied that she only had a headache when the suboccipital pain became worse. The time pattern is also quite variable, and it might hurt for a couple of hours or, in the worst of cases, throughout the day. When asked if the headache was accompanied by nausea, phonophobia, photophobia, lacrimation or rhinorrhea (asked in simple terms), she replied that since the accident, she had become more sensitive to light and loud noises and suffered from nausea, but these symptoms remained throughout the day and did not become significantly worse when she had a headache.

When asked about facial symptoms, Monica reported that they appeared after the 'disastrous' physiotherapy session. Although she spent a week with constant facial pain, currently these facial symptoms were rare and only appeared when she had a bad headache or felt 'nervous'. In that case, even talking increased her facial pain. She explained that it was currently a difficult feeling to describe, but it felt like 'having something adhered to her face' or a numb area. We asked her if she had ever previously experienced any symptoms in that area. She told us that about 10 years ago while eating a piece of tough meat, she had experienced a stabbing feeling inside her ear, and the pain in that area had lasted for 2 weeks. Currently, she occasionally heard a click 'inside her ear' and sometimes felt as if 'her jaw is dislocated' but no pain. The pain she now felt, although somewhat similar, was not exactly the same.

Monica insisted that the dizziness and feeling of unsteadiness that she was experiencing appeared after that particular physiotherapy session when 'they hurt her so much'. We asked her to describe the dizziness and to distinguish between a feeling of rapid and spinning vertigo or a dizzy feeling of vague unsteadiness. Monica reported that it was more like a feeling of drunkenness and unsteadiness accompanied by nausea. Symptoms of dizziness, unsteadiness and nausea always appeared with neck movements, particularly by extending the neck or when quickly turning the head either right or left.

We asked Monica if she could describe what the physiotherapy session consisted of and if, during this time, they performed any cervical mobilization with a wide range of rotation or of extension or if they performed high-velocity thrust manipulation. Monica replied that there were no wide-range movements but that the physiotherapist 'pressed' very hard with his fingers, and this was extremely painful. Also, it was terrible to be needled because she had always been very afraid of needles.

Monica also reported that since the accident, she could not stand the smell of strong perfume. We then asked whether stimuli such as light, noise or temperature changes were capable of triggering her symptoms, to which she replied that since the accident, she had become less tolerant to intense noise and that cold temperature increased the pain.

Reasoning Question:

4. Can you comment on the clinical reasoning behind your second stage of the subjective assessment? Can you also outline why you are interested in a detailed description of the pain and how you used that information?

Answer to Reasoning Question:

This part of the assessment targeted diagnostic reasoning to enable the establishment of clinical hypotheses and alternative hypotheses for differential diagnosis. This diagnostic reasoning is aimed at asking 'what?', identifying how best to categorize the patient's clinical condition. This requires understanding 'how?' through analysis of clusters of signs and symptoms associated with different clinical conditions, including 'why' they are associated, that is, making sense of both the mechanism of onset and the behavior of symptoms. Importantly, the information obtained after the second stage leads to the physical examination planning.

The descriptors of the pain are one of the key issues in determining the mechanisms of pain involved. They provide key information to determine if the pain is somatic, inflammatory, neuropathic or complex. The patient was asked to use descriptors to explain her pain. The quality of pain, defined as dull, burning, stabbing, paroxysmal, pressing and so forth, provides relevant information on the type of pain and the pathophysiological mechanisms involved. It is important not to suggest words to the patient, and if the latter has difficulty finding a descriptor, I ask questions such as, What is it like? What would you compare it with?

Reasoning Question:

5. What was your process of differential diagnosis with respect to the headaches and facial symptoms Monica was experiencing?

Answer to Reasoning Question:

The differential diagnosis of headache requires asking questions about six issues: headache characteristics, time pattern (frequency and duration of the crisis), intensity, location, trigger factors and associated signs and symptoms. It is also important to understand the current diagnostic criteria for headache from the International Headache Society (ICHD-III) (Headache Classification Committee of the International Headache Society, 2013). In addition to these helpful criteria in the differential diagnosis, it is useful to know Cervicogenic Headache International Study Group (CHISG) (Sjaastad et al., 1998) criteria because they better characterize cervicogenic headache.

In this case, the headache characteristics, trigger factors and rhythm seemed to suggest cervicogenic headache; however, specific physical dysfunction detectable on physical examination should be present. Although the painful area may suggest occipital neuralgia, the pain descriptor was not consistent with neuropathic pain and did not have the characteristics of this type of headache.

It should be noted that there was no need to establish a direct relationship between neck pain and headache. The fact that a person suffers headaches and neck pain after trauma is insufficient to confirm the headache is cervicogenic. Trauma may in fact be a sensitizing mechanism which increases the frequency and intensity of the headache episodes, regardless of the type (tension-type, migraine or cervicogenic headaches).

Although facial symptoms were episodic, they required careful assessment during the physical examination. These symptoms may be associated with central sensitization. However, peripheral neuropathy needs to be ruled out, and we needed to make sure that the symptoms were not referred symptoms from the temporomandibular joint (TMJ).

Reasoning Question:

6. Were you interested in the previous physiotherapy treatment, and how did this impact your assessment and clinical reasoning about the pain mechanism involved?

Answer to Reasoning Question:

At this time of the subjective assessment, it was essential to know what happened in the physiotherapy session which significantly worsened her symptoms. Monica reported that after eight or nine sessions, the physiotherapist said that progress was very slow and that treatment should be more intense. The physiotherapist asked her to lie face down and pressed with his fingers on her neck on the painful area for a long time, causing a lot of pain. Subsequently, in the same position, he needled her 'shoulder'. Both the pressure on her neck and the needling were very painful. At the end of the session, she felt very sore and a little dizzy, but it was not until a few hours later that the neck pain and headache intensified and she started to feel nausea and a strange feeling on the left side of her face and neck. Monica's description suggested that the aggravation of symptoms was unrelated to having suffered a potentially damaging treatment but, rather, was related to the pain experienced during the session.

The disproportionate aggravation of symptoms after treatment is an indicator of a nociplastic pain type. Importantly, in patients with central sensitization, overly intense maneuvers or those which may aggravate the patient's symptoms are contraindicated (Nijs and Van Houdenhove, 2009). As discussed later in this case, osmophobia, photophobia and intolerance to cold are indicative of central sensitization. Further, the cognitive deficits she reported are extremely common among subjects with chronic pain.

Reasoning Question:

7. Monica reported dizziness as one of her symptoms. Can you comment on how you interpreted this dizziness?

Answer to Reasoning Question:

Pseudo-vertiginous sensations are symptoms commonly associated with a cervical spine pathology or dysfunction. The first difficulty the clinician has to address is the variety of names used to refer to feelings of vertigo. Terms such as *dizziness*, *loss of balance* or *unsteadiness* make it difficult to interpret the patient's symptoms. The first step is, therefore, to clarify the terminology related to vertigo.

Vertigo can be defined as a false sense of motion of the subject with respect to the surrounding environment or of the latter with respect to the subject. The most common peripheral vestibular vertigo is benign paroxysmal positional vertigo (BPPV), which is characterized by a sudden onset of rotational vertigo that typically lasts fewer than 30 seconds, triggered by changes in the position of the head. This type of vertigo may also be associated with a sudden head movement.

Dizziness is a more ambiguous term that is described as a subjective sensation of unsteadiness with no objective loss of balance. The patient refers a feeling of unsteadiness, swaying or weakness, often accompanied by nausea. Based on Monica's description of her pseudo-vertiginous symptoms, we can

Continued on following page

rule out a true vertigo of vestibular or central origin; it was therefore not necessary to conduct tests to assess vestibular function.

The symptoms were suggestive of a cervicogenic dizziness. The physical examination should differentiate whether the sense of unsteadiness is subjective (without objective loss of balance) or is accompanied by an objective loss of balance.

Clinical Reasoning Commentary:

As discussed in Chapter 1, the description of understanding and connecting the 'what', 'how' and 'why' in diagnostic reasoning is consistent with Boshuizen and Schmidt's (2008) construct of pattern recognition in experts incorporating enabling or predisposing factors, pathobiological and psychosocial processes and the resulting consequences or disability:

- Enabling conditions: conditions or constraints under which a disease or problem occurs, such as personal, social, medical, hereditary and environmental factors
- Fault: the pathobiological and psychosocial processes associated with any given disease or disability
- Consequences of the fault: signs and symptoms of the particular problem as well as its functional impact on the patient's life

This is exemplified in the discussion of information needed for differential diagnosis of headache.

Knee Pain

The next part of the assessment was directed toward her knee pain. Monica reported pain in the anteromedial region of the right knee, a burning pain, as if her knee was hot, which sometimes seemed to extend up to her thigh. The pain did not appear immediately after the accident but a few hours later. We again asked her if she hit her knee when falling, and she insisted that she did not.

We asked her when her knee hurt, and she replied that it was especially at the end of the day when she was lying on the couch watching TV. When asked what movements triggered the knee pain, she again replied that going down stairs or lying for more than half an hour. But it is 'when she is sitting on the couch' at the end of day when the pain is worst. We asked about the influence of functional activities such as walking, climbing stairs, running and so forth, and she reported that her knee hurt especially when going down stairs, and she was afraid that her knee would fail her. She was afraid that it might give way or hurt when taking weight on that leg.

When asked why it is her 'bad knee', she reported a long history of knee problems. In 2001 she suffered a complete rupture of the anterior cruciate ligament and underwent surgery. During the immediate postoperative period, she had much knee pain, and instead of improving, it got worse in the 3 weeks after surgery. She finally went back to the hospital, and an examination of the synovial fluid revealed a perioperative infection. After an arthroscopic lavage and antibiotic treatment, within weeks, she began rehabilitation. Despite physiotherapy, she developed significant knee stiffness associated with extremely severe pain every time knee mobilization was attempted. Six months later, she underwent a second arthroscopy to improve mobility. Even so, the pain and stiffness did not subside until almost a year after surgery.

In 2003, given continued pain in her right knee, she again underwent surgery. Although without significant complications, she again developed a severe painful stiffness that required intensive physiotherapy for more than 6 months. At the time of the accident, she did not present with any knee pain or knee-related functional impairment.

At this point in the conversation, Monica mentioned that, curiously, every time she saw an athlete on television injure his or her knee, her own knee hurt immediately and exactly where it usually hurt.

Imaging Tests

Imaging tests can help in the differential diagnosis. In this case, we were interested in detecting the presence of severe structural damage to the cervical spine or progression toward delayed cervical instability. Monica brought x-rays (cervical spine anteroposterior and lateral views) performed on the day of the accident that were absolutely normal and an MRI performed 1½ months after the accident. The MRI showed a diffuse bulging in the C5 disc with a decrease in signal intensity in T2. No signs of bone or ligamentous injury were evident in the cervical spine, nor delayed cervical instability.

Mood, Family History, Sleep Quality

We asked Monica how she felt, and she replied that she was angry with herself, noting, 'If I hadn't been going so fast, this wouldn't have happened to me'. She felt down; there were many things that worried her, such as missing her academic year, rejecting a job offer and the fear that neck pain and knee pain would become chronic.

She also reported that she was annoyed with her boyfriend. He said she was obsessed with her pain and had surely not hurt herself so much when falling. He belonged to an amateur cycling group and said that many people fall, and it is not that bad.

At this point we enquired if anyone in her family had developed a chronic pain syndrome, and she reported that her mother suffered migraines all her life, but Monica couldn't recall them as interfering too much with her life. We asked her about her mood before the accident, and she said it was fine. We enquired if she slept well, and she reported that she sometimes woke up at night because of the neck pain and sometimes got up in the mornings with neck pain and headache.

Current Pharmacological Treatment

Monica was currently taking pregabalin (Lyrica) 75 mg twice a day and 600 mg ibuprofen or acetaminophen 1 g only when she had a severe headache.

Reasoning Question:

8. The knee pain in this case seems a little unusual. What were your thoughts about this?

Answer to Reasoning Question:

The behavior of Monica's knee pain was not consistent with an isolated nociceptive source. Although there were mechanical features such as aggravation going down stairs and with sitting, the mechanism of 'injury' was not clear, and Monica's report that simply viewing a knee injury on TV could elicit her own knee pain supported the possibility of a 'pain memory' possibly activated due to an increase in central hyperexcitability.

Reasoning Question:

9. You gathered a lot of information in your subjective assessment. Can you summarize your conclusions about the various domains, beliefs, emotions and any personal and external factors that may be contributing to this case?

Answer to Reasoning Question:

Pursuant to this case history, it was clear that Monica had a complex clinical pattern having many similarities with a WAD. At this point it was necessary to establish Monica's clinical status, distinguishing the three domains of impairment, activity restriction and participation restriction. We also needed to identify the personal and external factors involved, and it was time to assess beliefs and behaviors (Table 18.1).

Reasoning Question:

10. You have mentioned the pain mechanisms you believed were involved in this case. Could you elaborate on this at this stage of the assessment?

Answer to Reasoning Question:

The recognition of pain mechanisms is a crucial aspect of the clinical assessment and in patient management. Classically, pain can be classified as nociceptive, inflammatory and neuropathic pain types. However, there is a type of pain that is not included in this classification, namely, complex pain, or a nociplastic pain type. Complex pain can be defined as a pain initiated by afferent input (or without any) that causes central hyper-excitability and that is self-perpetuating and persists in spite of the elimination of the nociceptive input.

Recognition of this type of pain is critical because although other types of pain exhibit a consistency between the nociceptive source and the patient's clinical expression, complex pain does not. The pattern of pain is either disproportionate to the severity of the injury or does not match any recognizable clinical pattern. Failure to identify complex pain often results in the patient receiving conflicting

Continued on following page

TABLE 18.1			
DOMAINS, BELIEFS, EMOTIONS, BEHAVIOURS AND PERSONAL AND EXTERNAL FACTORS			
Clinical Picture	**Main Problems**		
Domains	Physical dysfunction • Right suboccipital neck pain • Right-sided headache • Right-sided facial and dysesthetic symptoms • Dizziness • Dysfunctional right knee pain	Disability • Fast movements of the cervical spine • Limitation of cervical extension and left cervical rotation • Going down stairs	Handicap/participation • She cannot study due to difficulties in concentrating. • She has rejected a job offer. • She does not go out with friends.
Factors implicated	Personal factors • Post-traumatic stress disorder (PTSD) • No history of first-degree relatives with chronic pain syndrome		External factors • There is no pending litigation.
Beliefs	• She fears that maybe her knee is degenerating. • She doesn't understand her problem. • She is not sure she will recover. • She thinks it must be something really serious.		
Emotional situation	• Emotional distress • She feels terribly unhappy. • PTSD • She feels demoralized by pain. • Her boyfriend does not understand her pain.		
Behaviours	• She displays fear-avoidance behaviours: avoids moving her head for fear of vertigo and pain. • She is afraid of taking long walks and especially of going up and down stairs. • She has rejected a job offer. • She is not going out with friends.		

explanations and undergoing unnecessary explorations and ineffective treatments. For nociceptive pain, it is necessary to treat the nociceptive source or associated contributing factors, whereas for complex pain, we must focus on the central modulation mechanisms.

We have developed a tool for the identification of a pattern of nociplastic pain in the form of an algorithm based on three criteria (Nijs et al., 2014):

- Criteria 1: Pain experience disproportionate to the nature and extent of injury or pathology
- Criteria 2: Diffuse pain distribution, allodynia and hyperalgesia
- Criteria 3: Hypersensitivity of senses unrelated to the musculoskeletal system

If the first criterion plus either criterion 2 or 3 are met, this implies that the patient presents with a nociplastic pain type.

Regarding the *pain mechanisms*, suboccipital neck pain is somatic, and pain in the supraspinous fossa seemed to be somatic referred pain. The right-sided headache also appeared to be somatic referred pain from the upper cervical joints. Monica presented with central sensitization. The referred pain and tactile allodynia are a sensitization phenomenon.

The facial pain may be related to a TMJ dysfunction or peripheral neuropathic or complex pain due to nociplastic sensitisation. The pain in the right knee presented as a complex pain and an activation of the patient's previous painful memory.

Monica's symptoms were moderately severe but demonstrated high irritability. The physical examination needed to be brief and avoid reproducing symptoms.

Reasoning Question:

11. You performed a detailed subjective assessment of this patient with attention to the pain type or mechanisms involved. Can you outline how you planned the next stage of your assessment and the information you anticipated gaining at this stage? How does this information inform the prognosis?

Answer to Reasoning Question:

The subjective assessment found that Monica showed cognitive and emotional aspects that may have been contributing negatively to her prognosis, such as a misinterpretation of symptoms, expectations about treatment that were not entirely positive, catastrophic thoughts, feeling down, low self-efficacy and fear-avoidance behaviors. We needed to act on each of these issues in order to achieve a good therapeutic outcome. In particular, we needed to consider the following:

- The pattern of suboccipital neck pain may be consistent with an impairment of the facet joints and/or cranio-cervical joints (C0–C1, C1–C2).
- Although initially the facial pain does not seem to suggest temporomandibular joint dysfunction, an assessment of this joint is advisable to rule out this possibility.
- Although the anterior knee pain is likely to be associated with a pain memory, it should be physically examined to rule out relevant physical impairment and nociception.
- It was important to assess whether Monica had a motor control deficit in the cervical spine. Several tests were necessary to evaluate this.
- An assessment of vertiginous and unsteadiness symptoms should be addressed. These symptoms may be accompanied by several objective signs in the sensorimotor system, such as altered cervical kinesthetic sense, altered neck motor control patterns, standing balance dysfunction, altered oculomotor and neck vision coordination. All these impairments should be assessed.

On this first visit, the physical examination would need to be very brief and avoid causing pain, firstly due to the patient's hypothesized nociplastic pain type, and secondly because of negative expectations about treatment. In the first assessment, we aimed to primarily assess the mobility pattern and perform tests to identify somatosensory and balance-control deficits. Therefore, the examination would be very brief, and after that, the most important thing would be to take time explaining to the patient the main findings and suggested management, boosting her confidence and encouraging her involvement in treatment. Possible physical dysfunctions would not in themselves indicate an adverse prognosis as long as Monica understood her problem and decided to participate actively in her treatment.

The prognosis regarding outcome was largely determined by assessment of cognitive and emotional factors in Monica's presentation. The crucial aspect to facilitate recovery was education management to address her incorrect pain perception, catastrophic thoughts, illness perception, emotional distress, fear-avoidance behaviors, expectations for recovery and self-efficacy beliefs (Burns et al., 2003). It has also been shown that an important prognostic factor in recovery after whiplash injury is patient expectations of recovery (Carroll et al., 2009). The association between expectations for recovery and actual recovery is robust and consistent, and it can be mediated by self-efficacy beliefs (Carroll et al., 2009; Glattacker et al., 2013).

Clinical Reasoning Commentary:

A strategy to minimize errors of reasoning is to take note of clues that don't fit with a particular pattern (i.e. attend to the 'negatives'). This is evident in the author's Reasoning Question 1 answer regarding Monica's knee pain, where non-mechanical features in the behavior of the knee pain (e.g. provocation elicited by seeing another person's knee injury) are recognized as inconsistent with a clear mechanical nociceptive source of knee pain.

The answer to Reasoning Question 2 mapping Monica's clinical presentation of her impairments, activity restrictions and participation restrictions (consistent with the International Classification of Functioning, Disability and Health [ICF] biopsychosocial framework of health and disability [World Health Organization, 2001]) highlights the author's biopsychosocial perspective guiding his clinical reasoning. Clinical reasoning is significantly influenced by your paradigms of practice, and the recognition here of potential personal and environmental influences on her pain/disability experience highlights the scope of knowledge and clinical reasoning required to holistically understand her presentation.

In the Answer to Reasoning Question 3, the first author shares an algorithm to identify nociplastic pain that incorporates criteria from the history and pathology, area of symptoms, behaviour of symptoms and physical examination to assist clinicians' pattern recognition in this important hypothesis category.

Lastly, in the Answer to Reasoning Question 4, the author highlighted key features in Monica's presentation that would influence prognosis and highlight implications for the physical examination. Broadly, a patient's prognosis is determined by the nature and extent of the patient's problem(s) and his or her ability and willingness to make the necessary changes (e.g. lifestyle, psychosocial contributing factors, physical contributing factors) to facilitate recovery or improved quality of life. As discussed in Chapter 1, clues will be available throughout the subjective and physical examination and the ongoing management including the following:

- Patient's perspectives and expectations (including readiness, motivation and confidence to make changes)
- External incentives (e.g. return to work) and disincentives (e.g. litigation, lack of employer support)

Continued on following page

- Extent of activity/participation restrictions
- Nature of problem (e.g. systemic disorder such as rheumatoid arthritis versus local ligamentous such as ankle sprain)
- Extent of 'pathology' and physical impairments
- Social, occupational and economic status
- Dominant pain type present
- Stage of tissue healing
- Irritability of the disorder
- Length of history and progression of disorder
- Patient's general health, age and pre-existing disorders

Objective Assessment

Monica demonstrated a slightly swayback posture, but her neck alignment was unremarkable. In standing, no significant differences between right and left knees were observed. Notably, there was a slightly thinner right thigh.

We assessed spinal range of motion. Flexion was normal; however, during extension, her fear of extending the cervical spine became obvious.

We then performed the postural Romberg test, and although she was slightly afraid of closing her eyes, Monica kept perfect balance, without a significant increase in postural swaying. We then performed the tandem stance test, and although repeated twice, Monica was incapable of maintaining postural stability in tandem stance for more than 30 seconds (Treleaven et al., 2005; Field et al., 2008).

It was suggested that during the next visit, a dynamic posturography should be conducted to determine if unsteadiness was objective or subjective and also to quantify postural control deficits. Posturography records postural body sway on a computerized dynamometric platform. Posturography makes it possible to quantify postural oscillations and, depending on the conditions in which the test is carried out, to observe the relative contribution of each sensory system (vestibular, visual and proprioceptive) to postural control.

We completed the examination in standing by asking Monica to firstly perform bilateral arm flexion (Comerford and Mottram, 2012) followed by unilateral flexion of both arms (Sahrmann, 2011). This test was conducted because Monica avoided lifting her arms for fear of aggravating her disc herniation. It can also serve as a motor control test to assess a cervical movement control dysfunction. In the active bilateral arm flexion test, Monica was able to lift both arms without a compensatory forward head movement or extension of the cervical spine, but we observed a clear head retraction at the end of the arm elevation. This indicated Monica was subconsciously avoiding neck extension.

The unilateral arm flexion test on the right side clearly showed a compensatory motion of cervical side bending to the right of 20 degrees and a slight head retraction during arm flexion. Monica clearly demonstrated a compensatory head retraction movement.

Active Movement of the Cervical Spine

In a seated position, we asked Monica to point out the different areas of pain. She indicated with her finger the point where it hurt on the right suboccipital area; in contrast, she used all her fingers to point out the fronto-temporal area of the ipsilateral side. She gestured with her whole hand toward the area of the right upper trapezius and her face.

We asked Monica to perform neck flexion and extension in four stages (Jull et al., 2008): (1) from neutral to flexion, (2) from flexion to neutral, (3) from neutral to extension and (4) from extension to the neutral position.

In the first two stages, nothing of interest was found, but stage 3 was notably dysfunctional. Monica was practically incapable of going beyond 10 degrees of extension, limiting movement due to the pain and especially due to a striking apprehension of movement. Stage 4 could not be evaluated because there was no real movement from extension to the neutral position.

We subsequently explored right and left neck rotation. Left rotation was limited to 40 degrees and elicited moderate right suboccipital pain. Right rotation was barely 20 degrees and reproduced considerable pain in the same area. It was clear that Monica was afraid of this movement because it was done very slowly and in a guarded manner.

Cervical Spine Manual Assessment

Before performing any tests to identify the likely level of symptoms, we performed a gentle palpation of the upper trapezius and posterior neck muscles in a sitting position. Monica perceived the gentle palpation of the trapezius as painful and extremely unpleasant. She made small evasive movements and facial expressions of pain when we placed our hands on the region of the right trapezius. We felt that this was a clear patient 'overreaction' to assessment. We decided to evaluate superficial sensitivity using a cotton swab. We asked Monica to describe the sensation as we ran the swab on both sides of her face and over the region of both trapezius muscles. We insisted that she tell us if she also noticed an area with an obvious decrease in sensitivity. Monica perceived the swab rubbing the skin of both trapezius muscles as unpleasant, although more uncomfortable on the right side. When running the swab over the right side of her face, she noticed no difference from the left side.

In a seated position, we palpated the right and left neck articular pillars, and we performed a small movement of contralateral rotation (Fig. 18.2). Palpation of the right articular pillar C2–C3 and right C1–C2 was extremely painful, to such an extent that she grasped our hands to prevent us from continuing.

We decided not to conduct any manual examination of segmental or accessory movements of the cervical spine due to Monica's fear and distress and the irritability of the presentation.

Right Knee Assessment

We asked Monica to perform a bilateral squat, and although she did this fearfully, neither flexion nor returning to full extension reproduced any symptoms. We also compressed the patella while she was doing the squats to assess crepitus and pain (Waldron test), and there was no crepitus or pain. An eccentric step test (Nijs et al., 2006) with the right knee demonstrated slight valgus movement and considerable apprehension, with no report of pain.

Palpation of both knees to assess changes in temperature or any possible hidden effusion was unremarkable. Monica did, however, report that manual contact on the anterior side of her knee was unpleasant. General atrophy of the right quadriceps muscle, more marked in the oblique vastus medialis, was observed, although patella position was normal. There

Fig. 18.2 Palpation of the right neck articular pillars associating a small movement of left rotation.

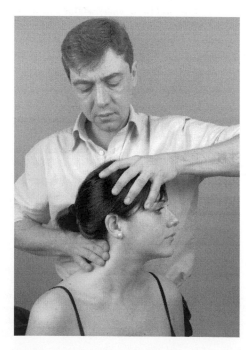

was no crepitus with mediolateral and cranio-caudal gliding of the patella. Palpation of the patellar facets, of the lower pole and Hoffa's fat pad was likewise asymptomatic. The patellar apprehension test was also negative. In supine, we performed passive flexion and extension of the right knee, and this was full and painless. We performed tibial rotation medially and laterally in full flexion without pain.

Given the high irritability of Monica's presentation, no further physical examination was pursued, and no further tests on the knee and cervical spine were conducted. We planned to assess her TMJ at the next consultation.

Reasoning Question:

12. Can you summarize your findings following your initial assessment? How did Monica's behavior in the assessment fit into your hypotheses regarding the pain mechanisms, and how would this direct treatment?

Answer to Reasoning Question:

The findings of the physical examination were the following:

1. Significant limitation of active mobility in extension and bilateral rotation of the cervical spine, most remarkably in right rotation.
2. Marked apprehension, primarily in cervical extension and right rotation. The movements were clearly guarded.
3. Superficial palpation of the right cervico-scapular region demonstrated significant tactile allodynia.
4. Palpation of the right articular pillars, together with the reproduction of pain in extension and right rotation, may suggest a symptomatic articular dysfunction in the ipsilateral cranio-cervical spine. It may also be that this is the area Monica considers vulnerable.
5. The standing in tandem test suggests a deficit in balance control.
6. The knee shows no significant signs, except for atrophy from former surgery. Tactile allodynia on the anterior side of the knee is evident.

There were some essential considerations in planning treatment. In view of her previous history, Monica was afraid of manual mobilization techniques on her neck. Adverse previous response to this type of approach ruled out the initial use of manual techniques on the cervical spine. Monica had a clear fear-avoidance behavior toward anything that involved moving her cervical spine as well as climbing stairs or sitting for over half an hour for fear of pain in her right knee.

In this clinical situation with obvious nociplastic pain, the most important aspect was to modify Monica's understanding of her pain. The first strategy would be to re-interpret the pain experience. Our aim was to help Monica understand that although there was an active nociceptive source, the central nervous system was amplifying the pain. The second strategy was to help Monica stop focusing her attention on the 'injury' and to realize how her fear-avoidance behaviors were negatively affecting the situation. Monica needed to understand that the most important part of treatment was to gain improvement in cervical spine and knee function. She needed to begin to realize that improving neck mobility could decrease her symptoms, and the best way to 'desensitize' the knee would be to start using it normally.

Given her central sensitization, the progression of the exercises, especially during the first sessions, would need to be very cautious to avoid excessive pain.

Clinical Reasoning Commentary:

The summary of physical examination findings highlights impairments in movement (e.g. limitation in cervical extension and rotation), palpation (e.g. provocation of pain with articular pillar palpation) and function (e.g. tandem balance control) as expected in 'diagnostic' reasoning of the physical examination. However, the physical examination findings also document features from the 'patient's perspectives' (e.g. marked apprehension in cervical extension and rotation; Monica's possible vulnerability during articular pillar palpation), illustrating that clinical reasoning through the physical examination is not simply a physical diagnostic process because significant cues to psychological status (patient's perspectives) are also available.

The author's clinical reasoning hypothesis of a nociplastic 'pain type' formulated in the subjective examination is then considered (i.e. 'tested') and further supported in his reasoning analysis of the physical examination (e.g. tactile allodynia).

The initial focus in the plans for management is to address Monica's perspectives or pain experience. The two strategies discussed are based on her unique pain/disability experiences (e.g. understanding of pain, overattention to the injury, fear-avoidance behaviours), illustrating a 'management' hypothesis of education based on explicit reasoning linked to specific impairments or unhelpful features from Monica's psychosocial assessment.

Treatment 1

Following the initial assessment, three exercises were prescribed to perform at home. The first two exercises were performed in the supine position, with Monica's head on a folded towel to keep the cervical spine in slight flexion to reduce her fear of performing them.

- First exercise: The first exercise involved nodding affirmatively in a supine position. In this position, Monica performed flexion and extension of the head and the neck in her pain-free range. Monica was asked to do a nodding movement from a neutral position to flexion and from flexion back to a neutral position. We insisted that she should avoid retraction of the head. It was necessary that this exercise should be in the pain-free range, at a comfortable speed that avoided both excessively fast movements and unduly slow and guarded movements.
- Second exercise: Remaining in the supine position, Monica rotated her head to the right and to the left. By keeping the cervical spine in slight flexion, these movements were expected to be performed with an increased pain-free range. As with the preceding exercise, this exercise needed to be performed in the greatest pain free-range possible, at a comfortable speed and perceived as pleasant. She was told that while performing the exercises, she could place a hot pack behind her neck if she wished.
- Third exercise: The third exercise was performed in a seated position and involved making eye movements of maximum amplitude up and down and to the right and left without moving the neck. This exercise needed to be performed several times a day. It was acceptable to feel a little dizzy when carrying this out but it was anticipated she would adapt very quickly. We insisted that these exercises were very important to gradually 'awaken' the neck muscles and to ameliorate dizziness.

Reasoning Question:

13. What did you consider were the main goals of your first treatment session? How did you explain Monica's condition to her in this session, in particular, the unusual pain behavior and severity of her symptoms?

Answer to Reasoning Question:

Having taught Monica the exercises, we explained our diagnostic findings, treatment planning and prognosis of her problem, which we believed was the most important part of the first visit. We outlined to Monica that her injury demonstrated many similarities with a WAD, which can often have a gradual onset and frequently can be associated with signs of PTSD.

It was very important that she understood that despite her pain, the injuries were not serious, as shown by the x-rays and MRI. We emphasized that she had a dysfunction in her cranio-cervical joints on the right side similar to a 'sprain'. We explained that the headache was a referred pain from the cranio-cervical joints, amplified by her central hyperexcitability. This did not imply a serious injury because it was a fairly common symptom in patients with severe neck pain. We also explained that these neck joints are involved in postural regulation. Hence, symptoms such as dizziness and the perception of unsteadiness and imbalance are very common.

We emphasized that her cervical pain was associated with fear of moving her neck and that she was using a pattern of movement that merely aggravated it. Regaining neck movement without fear would be sufficient to rid the pain. We explained that the exercises to strengthen her neck muscles would result in safer and painless movements. We insisted that her prognosis, despite the symptoms she was experiencing, would be favorable because the pathology was not serious or likely to be long term (Leaver et al., 2013).

The second relevant goal of this first session was for Monica to understand the severity of pain and symptoms and that their gradual onset related to a state of central hyper-excitability. We explained how the CNS increases our sensitivity in a situation perceived as threatening or potentially dangerous, and this is often manifested as an amplification of pain, as in her case. We explained the phenomenon of allodynia and how a tactile stimulus that should not be painful is perceived as painful and unpleasant. Other symptoms, such as pain referred to the temporal region and facial pain, were also indicative of central sensitization. For instance, a sprained ankle, often being a minor injury, can cause pain that is sometimes perceived in the whole foot and lower leg. Other indicators of nociplastic pain are intolerance to certain odors, such as strong perfume, and increased sensitivity to cold. We explained that we were confident that her 'disastrous physiotherapy' session did not really aggravate the injury. In a subject having nociplastic pain, an overly aggressive treatment can significantly amplify pain without implying

Continued on following page

an aggravation of the injury. The problem was that her therapist was not aware of her central sensitization situation.

It was also important that she rethink the pain in her right knee. She needed to understand that sometimes the pain, especially if severe and persisting for a long time, leaves a memory in the brain. Her long, painful history with her knee was a good example of such a pain memory. Simply increasing the central hyperexcitability had been sufficient to evoke her painful memory. It was important to reassure her, explaining that her pain was not associated with any change in her knee as determined by physical examination. It was an example of complex pain. The pain behavior was inconsistent because it hurt most at rest, and the pain was complex because there was no active disease in the knee itself. It was also important to understand that her pain which appeared when she saw someone hurt their knee was a fairly common phenomenon with a sensitized CNS.

At this point Monica needed to understand what factors were often associated with central sensitization. The pain was a result of an unexpected trauma, which at that time had a feeling almost of impending doom. Trauma with these characteristics favors central sensitization and PTSD. Monica was asked if she understood our explanation and if she considered it consistent with her experience.

Treatment 2

Re-assessment of Patient Pain Cognitions

At her next appointment 3 days later, Monica was worried and did not understand what we explained about central sensitization. She only did the exercises prescribed on the first day and gave up the second day because of a strong headache and had not tried again.

Monica insisted that she had a lot of pain and that her problem was related to an injury that had not been properly treated, and she failed to understand what 'sensitization' and her brain had to do with her problem. She insisted she had a *real* injury and that her problem was not psychological. Further, she had been diagnosed with cervical disc herniation, which was sufficiently important alone. She still believed that the physiotherapy session aggravated the problem because she had read on the Internet that a cervical herniation must be treated with great care. She believed the former physiotherapist was not careful. Clearly, on Monica's first consultation, she was very distressed, and perhaps we had given her too much information, which she was unable to assimilate.

It was necessary to spend almost this whole session talking to Monica in order for her to better understand her problem. If we failed to change her thinking about her pain, she would not work with us in our treatment programme. We explained that the MRI did not show a cervical hernia but a diffuse disc bulging that was usually asymptomatic and was not related to her pain pattern. We insisted that of course her pain was real, she had certainly suffered neck injury and that in no way was her pain psychological. It was very important that she understood that central sensitization is not a psychological problem but, rather, a common but exaggerated response to situations associated with considerable distress, such as the accident she experienced. Central sensitization is a neurobiological and not a psychological phenomenon. To reinforce our point, we gave the example that many women experience hormonal changes during menstruation that can result in increased sensitivity. This may be expressed as intolerance to smells, increased sensitivity to noise, increased excitability in general, and so forth, and that these changes in sensitivity cease quickly. We also explained that the problem that arises is that many patients correlate the severity of pain with a serious injury. This misinterpretation makes them reduce their activities because of fear of pain or re-injury, and thus deterioration is exaggerated.

Our management strategy involved gradually increasing her activities without fear to the level of activity prior to the accident. We insisted that both physical examination and imaging tests demonstrated that there was no serious injury. We also explained that distinguishing between organic and psychosomatic pain is a misconception. Pain and its perception have many facets, including changes in the tissues, the context in which the damage occurs and previous experiences, among others. All these aspects are able to modulate the pain experience.

At this point it was emphasized once again that sensitization can be dampened and that it would help to start movement and become active as soon as possible. At this point Monica asked whether movement would make the problem worse. Apparently, this is one of the things that worried her most. We informed her that movement helps and that the problem does not worsen with movement. We insisted that the activity would improve her situation, and in no way would it cause an injury. Monica appeared calmer following our explanation.

At the end of the second session, we reminded her about the nodding and cervical rotation exercises in supine position with the head resting on a towel, insisting that she should avoid guarded movements. The movement should be completely painless and must even be perceived as pleasant. The message repeated is that 'painless movements remove pain'.

We also reminded her about the ocular motility exercises, insisting that while reducing dizziness, they awaken the deep muscles of the neck. We planned to review Monica in 1 week.

Treatment 3

Fear-Avoidance Behaviors

Monica was calmer and reported that although she had almost the same pain, she was not so worried. The neck mobility exercises in supine position felt good, and the ocular mobility exercises, although they make her a bit dizzy, did not aggravate the pain.

We spent most of the session talking about fear-avoidance behaviors. We explained that this is the most relevant factor in the chronicity of all pain. We explained that fear of pain is more detrimental than the pain itself. It is responsible for the generation of dysfunctional movement patterns which increase rather than reduce pain. We gradually reduce our daily activity, which decreases tissue tolerance, so eventually, innocuous stimuli are able to provoke the pain. We thus develop a deconditioning syndrome that makes us more vulnerable. It also begins to interfere with our work and recreational activities, as in her case. We begin to self-marginalize ourselves socially. All this has an influence on our mood and leads to a state of increasingly low mood and an increasing feeling of being unable to control our lives. We explained that it is a vicious circle, a real 'way to perdition'. Fear of pain and catastrophic thoughts increase the perception of threat and that the body is vulnerable. It increases hypervigilance of our symptoms, increasing anxiety about our pain and increasingly reduces our activity, which ultimately leads to depression, increases our disability, determines a disuse syndrome and leads to social self-exclusion.

She needed to understand that until now, she had performed activities depending on whether the pain permitted. This type of attitude turned her into a 'slave' of her pain; in the end, this was what let her body move. Moving forward, she was instructed that she must perform activities based on the goals set rather than based on her pain.

She must go from challenging the problem from a passive coping mechanism to an active one. Success would be assured by abandoning a sick role and becoming the main promoter in her recovery process. We would help her to find strategies to accelerate this process.

We showed Monica a schematic representation of Vlaeyen's fear-avoidance model (Vlaeyen et al., 2012). This model explains how pain disability, affective distress and physical disuse develop as a result of a protective-behavior learning process. It is an easy way to describe that there are two opposing behavioral responses to an injury, avoidance and confrontation. The avoidance behavior leads to a vicious circle of pain-related fear, hypervigilance and avoidance that aggravates disability, depression and disuse. No fear and a confrontation behavior are the only way to recovery.

We gave Monica a copy of this schema and asked her to fill it with her personal pain experience and give it to us at the next session. We also gave her another sheet of paper to write down all the barriers she could identify to a full recovery, with consideration of cognitive, emotional and behavioral barriers and their personal and social consequences.

Posturography

We decided not to examine the cervical spine and performed a posturography on a computerized dynamometric platform. Posturography provides information on overall postural performance with parameters such as the surface area and length of body sway.

We performed six examinations: two in static conditions on firm surface with eyes open and eyes closed and four in dynamic conditions placing a moving plate on the platform that caused oscillations in the sagittal and coronal planes first with eyes open followed by eyes closed. On the firm surface, the sway area with eyes open was 467.6 mm^2, and the path length was 331 mm. Both values were above the normal limits (surface area 91 [39/210], path length 245 [180/310]). But the most relevant findings were that with eyes closed, the values for surface sway area and path length were completely normal, and the Romberg coefficient was below the normal value at 0.82 (normal value 2.88 [1.12/6.77]) (Fig. 18.3). A decrease in body sway is not always indicative of a good strategy for postural control. In fact, this decrease can be indicative of an excess of stiffness in patients who feel subjectively unstable (Carpenter et al., 2001). Some patients demonstrate what has been called 'postural blindness'. These patients show a smaller displacement with the eyes closed than with the eyes open, thereby showing a Romberg's coefficient below normal (2.88) (Gagey and Toupet, 1991).

This postural blindness has been interpreted as a manifestation of a failure of the integration of visual information in subjects with a postural control deficit, although it can also be the result of a hypervigilance strategy, common in patients who perceive a sense of instability and are afraid they will fall when they close the eyes.

The data obtained with the posturographic examination served to explain to Monica that her strategy of balance control was dysfunctional and associated with an excessive hypervigilance secondary to her fear of feeling dizzy or losing balance.

Treatment 4

Re-assessing Fear-Avoidance Behaviors

We talked to Monica about how things had gone since her last visit. Monica looked happier, and the explanation about 'the road to ruin' sounded convincing. She told us that she had thought a lot about the explanation about fear and avoidance behaviors and said she felt that she had been really constrained by pain and had stopped doing things she liked, and that had made her really sad. She had completed the fear-avoidance and barriers sheets (Fig. 18.4). She understood the relationship between her beliefs, fear-avoidance behaviors, negative mood and future disability.

We then discussed with her all the points of her schema of fear avoidance. Because she now understood that there was hope and that recovery was possible, she was determined to do all she could to recover because she was tired of her 'disability'. It was important to talk to her at the beginning of every session to overcome doubts and fears. The way to recovery is closely linked to a pain reconceptualization.

Assessing Neck Mobility

At this point it seemed appropriate to assess the cervical spine in more detail. In a seated position, we prompted Monica to perform right and left rotation. Left rotation was 70 degrees and referred only a slight tightness in the right suboccipital region. Right rotation had improved somewhat, and she was able to turn her neck to about 40 degrees, although

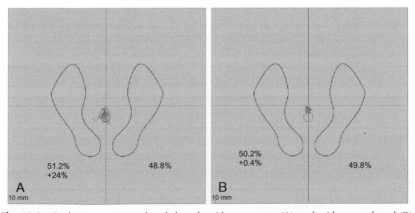

Fig. 18.3 Body sway area and path length with eyes open (A) and with eyes closed (B).

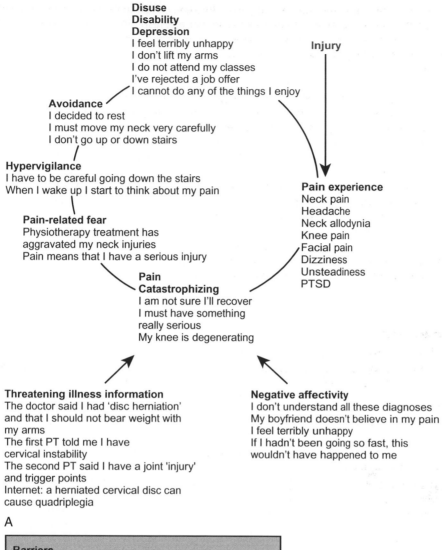

Disuse
Disability
Depression
I feel terribly unhappy
I don't lift my arms
I do not attend my classes
I've rejected a job offer
I cannot do any of the things I enjoy

Injury

Avoidance
I decided to rest
I must move my neck very carefully
I don't go up or down stairs

Hypervigilance
I have to be careful going down the stairs
When I wake up I start to think about my pain

Pain experience
Neck pain
Headache
Neck allodynia
Knee pain
Facial pain
Dizziness
Unsteadiness
PTSD

Pain-related fear
Physiotherapy treatment has
aggravated my neck injuries
Pain means that I have a serious injury

Pain
Catastrophizing
I am not sure I'll recover
I must have something
really serious
My knee is degenerating

Threatening illness information
The doctor said I had 'disc herniation'
and that I should not bear weight with
my arms
The first PT told me I have
cervical instability
The second PT said I have a joint 'injury'
and trigger points
Internet: a herniated cervical disc can
cause quadriplegia

Negative affectivity
I don't understand all these diagnoses
My boyfriend doesn't believe in my pain
I feel terribly unhappy
If I hadn't been going so fast, this
wouldn't have happened to me

A

Barriers	
Cognitive	Misconceptions about pain
Emotional	PTSD Emotional distress
Behavioural	Fear–avoidance behaviours

B

Fig. 18.4   Monica's fear-avoidance sheet (A) and barriers-to-recovery sheet (B).

that caused pain, and she was afraid to go further. Gentle palpation of the trapezius, although a little unpleasant, did not cause an evasive response. Cervical extension was still very limited, and she still showed considerable apprehension to movement. We decided not to manually assess the cervical spine in this third session.

TMJ Assessment

In this session we decided to explore the TMJ. Firstly we recorded a normal 30-mm opening and no deflection, then a 5-mm protrusion, 11 mm right laterality, 12 mm left laterality.

We asked her to open as far as possible, and we gently forced the mouth opening, reaching 54 mm. Although afraid, she felt no pain, and opening was in midline without deflections.

To record any joint noise, we placed the index fingers first in the lateral pole of both condyles and then in the mandibular angles and asked her to repeat the functional mandibular movements. We detected a very weak clicking at 20-mm opening on the right side, which was pain-free.

Load tests of the TMJs were performed in the supine position. Whilst applying cranial pressure on the mandibular angles, we asked her to perform protrusion, left and right laterality and opening movements. The right TMJ clicked only during opening. With an intraoral grip, we glided the condyle caudally, anteriorly and posteriorly. Then we directed the condyle cranially, anteriorly and posteriorly. These tests were negative. We decided not to continue TMJ assessment because there was nothing remarkable.

Examination of the TMJ was suggestive of a small asymptomatic functional displacement of the disc and not related to the facial symptoms. We therefore explained that she had a slightly hypermobile disc without clinical significance.

Sensorimotor Control Assessment

Because Monica also described dizziness, we decided to evaluate any other sensorimotor control disturbances. We choose to conduct the *smooth-pursuit neck torsion test* because it did not require extensive cervical rotation (Fig. 18.5). With the trunk turned left (implying a relative right cervical rotation) during visual tracking, we observed a small saccade movement every time she looked to the right, but most significantly, Monica began to feel dizzy and a little nauseous.

It was important that Monica began to realize that her neck was not vulnerable. We decided to do some motor control exercises in four-point kneeling to take advantage of the fact that she thought her neck was weak and needed strengthening exercises.

We started teaching her the active cervical extension in four-point kneeling (Jull et al., 2008). She was asked to move from full cervical flexion to extension of about 20 degrees while keeping the cranio-cervical region in neutral. On the first attempt, Monica demonstrated a clear head retraction. With our hands, we helped her to understand the correct position, and after two attempts, she was able to do it easily. This exercise also served to develop a subjective perception of strengthening the muscles of her neck.

The second exercise related to gaze stability with cervical rotation in a seated position. We asked her to look at a point and keep her eyes fixed on that point while rotating the

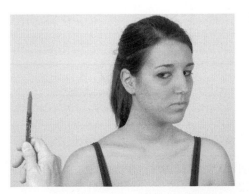

Fig. 18.5   Smooth-pursuit neck torsion.

head right and left in a range that was comfortable. To start reducing her apprehension with regard to cervical extension, we also taught her to put a rolled towel under her neck to perform the nodding and cervical rotation exercises in supine.

Because she was worried about her strange knee pain, we explained that we planned to strengthen her knee and recommended that she walk 30 minutes each day. Further, every time she sat at a table, she was to perform the exercise of going from sitting to standing several times. This exercise would assist her to realize that her knee was able to take the load.

Treatment 5

Increasing Desensitization With Active Exercises

Monica reported that her symptoms had improved. Her neck had less pain, and she was less afraid to move. She reported that the exercises felt good, although her neck felt slightly tender afterward, and she still got a bit dizzy. In the afternoons, there were times when she noticed no pain in her right knee, and she thought it was getting stronger.

We then decided to explore active cervical extension. To give her greater confidence, we placed a hand under her chin and the other holding the back of her head. We asked her to slowly extend her neck, and at approximately 20 degrees of extension, we noticed that she could control the weight of her head. We helped her return to the neutral position. As we aimed to reduce her fear of movement, we again asked her to perform cervical extension, assuring her that when she found it hard to take the weight of her head, we would help her with our hands (Fig. 18.6). During extension, this time to 30 degrees, we noticed that she could no longer support her head, and we asked her to relax her neck as much as she could, and passively, we took her to full extension until her face was almost horizontal. We took her head passively back to the neutral position. Monica was very surprised to note that when assisted in the movement, she felt no pain. We repeated this exercise. This exercise served two purposes. Firstly, it decreased her fear of moving her neck in extension, and secondly, it demonstrated to her that an important strategy to reduce neck pain was strengthening the muscles.

We then decided to prescribe an exercise to perform every 2 hours. It consisted of five flexion and extension movements, clutching her head from behind with her hands entwined, in a seated position. We asked her to try to reach maximum numbers while remaining relaxed and confident.

As she still struggled to lift her head from the pillow, we decided to evaluate the cranio-cervical flexion test (CCFT) with pressure biofeedback (Jull et al., 2008). The CCFT test was performed in supine crook-lying position. We first evaluated movement in five progressive stages of the cranio-vertebral flexion. Monica could perform this properly in the first two stages (from 20 to 22 and from 20 to 24). We then analyzed the isometric capacity in two stages, and it was evident that in the first stage, when she was attempting

Fig. 18.6 Assisted neck extension.

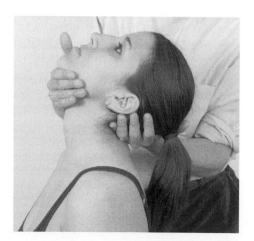

to hold the contraction, she started to retract the neck. We decided not to start the exercise with the pressure feedback and told her to incorporate an exercise that would activate her deep flexor muscles during her head flexion-extension exercises whereby she would start by keeping her head still while looking at her feet for about 10 seconds and then proceed to the flexion-extension controlled-movement exercise.

In this fifth session, we decided to introduce some manual therapy techniques. This allowed a manual approach to the tissues, but in particular, if we performed it carefully and painlessly, we would be able to reduce the patient's fear. This would allow us to further assess her articular condition at subsequent sessions.

We decided to do a global mobilization of the entire cervical spine in right and left side bending, adding a passive neck rotation of small amplitude. Then we made a very smooth side-glide segmental mobilization. After these maneuvers, we placed the fingers of both hands on the suboccipital region and conducted very light rhythmic and oscillatory pressure. The aim was to gently stimulate the tissue of the suboccipital region to induce a peripheral neuromodulation. Each treatment was immediately re-assessed, with improvement in the impairment targeted.

We spent very little time on manual exploration because if we did too much, Monica might have become afraid, recalling previous sessions with the former physiotherapist. She needed to feel calm during the session because stress may lead to fear and a subsequent increase in pain.

After the session, we reminded her about the exercises she had to do, and we agreed that she replace walking with 30 minutes of cycling along the promenade along the river near her home. We planned to review Monica in a week's time.

Treatment 6

Joint Passive Mobility Assessment Is Performed

Monica appeared to be happy. The previous session did not cause her discomfort, and she felt more confident with her neck. The first thing we re-assessed was the right cervical rotation, which was now almost 80%, with local pain at the end of the movement. Cervical extension was still limited because she was still afraid to extend the neck.

We repeated the maneuver of assisted extension with our hands three times, which was well tolerated. We decided that in sitting, she should begin performing flexion and extension of the head over the neck in a broader range of movement but without evoking pain.

We decided to evaluate joint dysfunction. First we evaluated cranio-cervical extension with the head in protraction, and Monica reported that this movement reproduced pain on the right side.

We decided to carefully perform a combined test of cranio-cervical extension, side bending and right rotation. This movement immediately evoked her right suboccipital pain. Monica demonstrated a clear closing pattern in the right craniocervical spine.

The first segmental mobility test we performed was flexion-rotation for C1. Although right rotation was painful, we did not detect any significant restriction of movement. We then evaluated the occipital glide, and although glide in extension on the right side caused discomfort, there was no evidence of restriction. The segmental mobility of C2–C3 was then evaluated. In extension, we perceived a restriction in the right articular pillar, and Monica told us that this movement caused her pain. We evaluated right side bending and obtained the same response. Initially, we evaluated left rotation, and Monica immediately reported that the mere contact of our fingers with the right articular pillar was very painful. However, left passive rotation was limited only by a few degrees. When evaluating the right rotation, we perceived a painful resistance that limited full rotation.

We decide to evaluate the accessory mobility in prone with a unilateral postero-anterior (PA), which revealed stiffness in right C2–C3 with the same painful response. Joint dysfunction of right C2–C3 appeared to be the major source of symptoms and behaved mechanically as a restriction of facet joint (limited facet joint convergence).

Given the irritability and tenderness of the right articular pillar, we decided to perform a global mobilization in rotation to the right and left, avoiding contact with her area of pain and not reaching the end range. We mobilized the cranio-cervical spine in right side bending and finally performed a gentle oscillatory mobilization of right C2–C3, doing a

PA glide with the cervical spine in mild left rotation. After a short period, we re-evaluated with a right cervical rotation and noted an increase in the range of rotation. The treatment had been very short, but it helped us identify Monica's facet dysfunction with a restriction in closing (limited facet joint coupled downslope movement) of C2–C3, which we could attribute to small post-traumatic changes in the facet joint.

We repeated the graded cranio-cervical flexion test. Monica was able to obtain correct activation of the deep cranio-cervical flexor muscles reaching the third level (26), and she could maintain a first-level (20–22) isometric contraction for 10 seconds, 10 times, without substitutions. We then used the pressure biofeedback to facilitate her performance of the exercises at home. Initially, she needed to perform the sequenced activation of level 1, 2 and 3 (three times for each one) and then 10 isometric contractions for 10 seconds in the first level.

To improve her function and reduce the fear of cervical extension, we taught her two exercises. The first was gaze stability in flexion/extension. Keeping her gaze fixed on a point would facilitate greater control of the extension movement. The second exercise was cervical extension on three levels assisted with a towel. With Monica seated, we asked her to take the edge of a towel and to let it slip across the occiput until falling approximately near the spinous process of C2. Pressing the towel in a forward and cranial direction, she had to extend her neck three times. We repeated the same exercise by changing the pressure to the mid-cervical spine and the lower cervical spine.

We mentioned that although she may note some discomfort after the exercise, it was important to continue because her neck would recover quickly. We decide to discontinue the eye motility movements.

Treatment 7

Monica reported that she had some neck pain, especially after performing the neck extension exercises. However, as she had been advised, she had not given this much consideration. Her neck felt 'freer', and she was less afraid to move, although sometimes a quick head movement made her a little dizzy. It still bothered her to carry her bag on her right shoulder after a while because it irritated her neck.

She reported her knee 'feels much stronger'. She had not experienced pain riding her bike but commented that she forgot to do the sitting and standing exercises. We reminded her that it was important to feel that her knee was strong, and after a few days, the exercise would progress to going up and down stairs. We suggested that when studying, she should slowly do the sitting and standing exercise several times every hour.

We evaluated the right rotation, which was now full range, with slight pain at the end range. Assessment of cervical extension demonstrated that she was capable of performing this with good head control to almost the middle portion of its full range.

We decided to continue with the manual treatment. We started with non-specific techniques of global mobilization in rotation first left, then right to almost the entire range. We initially performed an oscillatory treatment in opening (facet joint coupled upslope) of the right C2–C3 facet, and then with the cervical spine in slight right rotation, we mobilized the right facet joint into a downslope movement. Monica reported that the latter maneuver caused slight discomfort. We re-evaluated in right rotation, and end of range rotation was slightly uncomfortable but not painful.

We re-evaluated the CCFT and observed proper activation of the deep cranio-cervical flexors to the fourth level (28) and ability to maintain an isometric contraction at the second level (24) for 10 seconds 10 times without head retraction. In this session, we asked her to continue with the sequenced activation from level 1 to 4 (three times for each) and then 10 isometric contractions for 10 seconds on the second level. She was given an appointment for the following week.

Treatment 8

Reassuring the Patient and Improving Sensorimotor Deficits

At this appointment Monica reported that she felt somewhat worse. Her neck had bothered her, and she had experienced a headache for 2 days. Earlier in the week, she felt fine and energetic and decided to visit a couple of hotels to resume work practice. She had to travel by train, and a couple of 2-hour journeys and the rattle of the train aggravated her symptoms. Seeing objects whizzing past through the window also made her very dizzy. These symptoms indicated that we should pay more attention to her cervical sensorimotor deficits. But what was also important was to reassure Monica that these symptoms are a normal response and avoiding the provocative movements would delay her recovery. We reminded her of the vicious cycle of fear-avoidance and disuse and that the best way to desensitize her nervous system was to return as soon as possible to her normal life.

Improving Sensorimotor Deficits

We decided to assess the cervical kinesthetic sense with Roren's joint position error test (Fig. 18.7). Seated 90 cm from the target and with a laser pointer on the head, we asked her to turn left as far as she could and then return until the laser pointed to the center of the target. We asked her to repeat this twice and then do it with her eyes closed. We then asked her to perform right rotation and observed that on each attempt with her eyes closed, the laser point always went beyond the target. When we did the same test in extension, she was also unable to return to the center of the target with her eyes closed. We recommended that she do this same exercise at home once a day. This exercise has the advantage that the patient becomes less aware of the neck symptoms and concentrates on hitting the target.

In addition to these exercises, we taught Monica dissociated oculo-cervical movements in rotation and in flexion and extension. These exercises can significantly improve dizziness symptoms.

We re-evaluated the CCFT and observed proper activation of the deep cranio-cervical flexors to the fourth level (28), and she could maintain an isometric contraction at the third level (26) for 10 seconds 10 times without head retraction. In this session, we told her to only do 10 isometric contractions for 10 seconds on the third level.

To improve cervical rotation, we taught her an assisted exercise for rotation using the towel. This involved leaning to the edge of the towel on the symptomatic segment C2–C3 and performing three rotations to the left and then three to the right (Fig. 18.8). She assisted the end of each rotation by pressing with the towel.

We re-evaluated the active cervical extension exercise in four-point kneeling, and because she was able to do it without difficulty, we told Monica that it was no longer necessary to do it every day.

We also performed manual treatment of the cervical spine in this session. We started with non-specific global mobilization techniques in rotation, first left and then right. We continued with the oscillatory techniques, first into downslope movement and then upslope for the right C2–C3 facet. We finished treatment with physiological movements of C2–C3, adding a gentle hold-relax at the end range of right rotation.

Fig. 18.7 Roren's joint position error test.

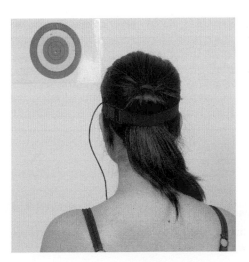

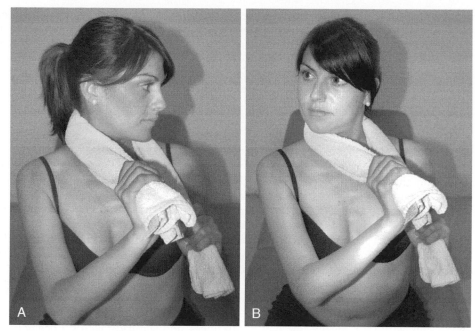

Fig. 18.8 Assisted mobilization in rotation for C2–C3.

Desensitizing the 'Bad Knee'

This week we commenced going up and down stairs. During the first week, we wanted Monica to climb to her floor using the stairs (she lived on the fourth floor) but go down in the lift. We wanted her to do this at least three times a day. The following week, we wanted her to go up and down only using the stairs.

We planned to see Monica in 2 weeks' time.

Treatment 9

Functional Exercises

Seven weeks after the first visit, Monica was beginning to feel like her former self. In the previous 2 weeks she had felt better, although she told us how she saw a woman stumbling down the subway steps and immediately felt a stabbing pain in her right knee. She was a little frightened but told herself not to allow further fear of going down stairs, and after a while, the pain disappeared. She also felt a bit stressed by her studies and no longer had much time to do the exercises. She was no longer able to cycle 30 minutes each day.

Given Monica's favorable progress and the lack of time to do the exercises, we decided to prescribe more functional exercises that she could do throughout the day that would not require extra time. We therefore discontinued the joint position error training with the target. We recommended that in prone and without a pillow, in a relaxed manner, she should attempt to maintain her head for 5 seconds at maximum rotation first left and then right. This would eliminate the fear of more eccentric positions in rotation.

During the day, we recommended that when sitting while studying, Monica should perform hourly or every 2 hours several cervico-ocular dissociation exercises in rotation and extension, and with her elbow on the table and her hand on chin, she should do several low-intensity isometric contraction exercises in flexion. She was also instructed that, a couple of times a day, when standing, she should place her feet in tandem and do cervico-ocular dissociation exercises in rotation, flexion and extension.

As manual treatment, we attempted to evaluate the accessory mobility in the prone position. Unilateral PA accessory movements over the C2–C3 right pillar demonstrated a different resistance with respect to the left and caused a little pain. It was decided to first perform unilateral PA C2–C3 starting from a left side-bending, focusing on the same segment to gain greater accessory movement. We then we conducted right side-bending with a slightly oblique thrust medially. The latter technique caused discomfort but was tolerated. Finally, we performed a thrust technique to get a joint gapping of right C2–C3 facet. We used very small-range motion which was not uncomfortable (Fig. 18.9).

We gave Monica an appointment for 3 weeks later and recommended that she try her preferred sporting activity (paddle) during the weekend. We also recommended that she spend her free time having fun with her friends and to avoid staying at home.

Treatment 10

Developing Active Coping Strategies

As soon as we saw Monica, she reported that in the previous 2 weeks, she had been playing paddle, and she could hardly believe it – she had no pain in her neck either during or after the match! When asked about her knee, she reported that she did not even think about it. One of the things that this demonstrated was that Monica had understood her problem and she was already capable of developing her own coping strategies.

She had not had suboccipital pain or headache in the previous 2 weeks, and she only felt her right trapezius a little tense after a long time studying. She only felt slight discomfort when lying face down in bed with her neck in maximum rotation to the right.

She commented that she only did the exercises when she remembered when sitting and standing, and they now made her feel confident.

At this time Monica had stopped being afraid to move her neck, and her discomfort was felt only very sporadically. She had no dizziness, and she had taken up her normal activities. She was now doing an internship at a hotel 30 minutes from her home by train. Although she sometimes got a little dizzy when looking out of the train window, these symptoms were mild and did not worry her.

We decided to re-evaluate the active movements, and we observed a symmetrical rotation on both sides. The overpressure in right rotation was only slightly uncomfortable for her. The movement from neutral to extension was performed with a correct pattern. In movement from full extension to neutral, she slightly poked her chin at the beginning of the movement.

We tested the combined movement of cranio-cervical extension, rotation and right side-bending and she only experienced discomfort when we applied overpressure.

We evaluated segmental mobility in rotation C2–C3, and at the end of the movement, a slight resistance was still perceived. When we tested the C2–C3 PA accessory movements, Monica reported that the contact with our thumbs still caused discomfort. We conducted C2–C3 PA with right side-bending, which, although uncomfortable, was well tolerated. In supine position, we performed several oscillatory movements C2–C3 in the plane of the facets with her head in right rotation.

We told her that it was likely that at some times, she might have some tenderness in her right suboccipital region, but this would eventually disappear.

We encouraged Monica to continue for some time with the exercises but mostly to be physically active.

We agreed with Monica that we could discontinue our treatment, confident that her symptoms would fully resolve over time. We did, however, recommend that she visit us in a couple of months to confirm she was not having further problems.

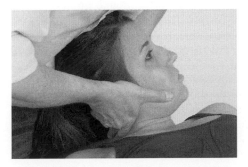

Fig. 18.9 Thrust technique to get a joint gapping of the right C2–C3 facet joint.

Reasoning Question:

14. Can you summarize your thoughts about this case and what it highlights about your clinical reasoning?

Answer to Reasoning Question:

Monica's story is not uncommon. The two most important aspects of her case are her post-traumatic neck pain and pain in the right knee.

Although the accident was a fall from a bicycle, it demonstrated the characteristics of WAD, with multiple impairments, neck pain, headache, dizziness, sensorimotor deficits and deficits in balance control. All these symptoms were amplified by a clear central hyper-excitability.

Monica's knee pain was a clear example of pain memory. The pain behavior was not consistent because it hurt going down stairs, yet the worst time of day was when she was lying on the couch. She experienced allodynia with palpation, but knee tests failed to reveal an active nociceptive source.

Key management factors for Monica were restructuring her beliefs about her injuries. Although many symptoms were clearly indicative of complex pain, a thorough and comprehensive examination, checking her imaging tests and so forth, served to increase Monica's confidence in us. In this type of presentation, we should take time to remove false misinterpretations, often transmitted by health professionals who have attended the patient. Considerable time had to be spent explaining that her pain stemmed largely from a nociplastic pain sensitisation and that her fear-avoidance behaviors were a critical aspect of the problems suffered.

The exercises, although intended to treat joint deficits and sensorimotor control deficits, were especially intended to serve as elements of gradual exposure. The main objective, therefore, was to reduce her fear of moving.

Another major aspect was to emphasize that the best way to recover was to resume daily activities and avoid social self-exclusion. Improving her cognition, self-efficacy and mood was just as important as fulfilling her functional needs of everyday life.

Clinical Reasoning Commentary:

General management and specific treatments need to have clear aims linked to patients' particular clinical presentations and personal goals. This is evident here in the specific impairments summarized from the examination and the overriding emphasis on management to facilitate restructuring of Monica's beliefs about her injury. A range of manual and exercise interventions was used to treat joint deficits and sensorimotor control deficits, not simply targeting the impairments themselves but with a broader objective of providing graded exposure to symptom-provoking stimuli to reduce fear of movement. This illustrates a more complex reasoned management plan that can still be seen as a hypothesis re-assessment of the impairments, and Monica's beliefs, fears and activities/participation guided the management progression.

REFERENCES

American Psychiatric Association, 2013. Diagnostic and Statistical Manual of Mental Disorders, fifth ed. American Psychiatric Association, Arlington, VA.

Burns, J.W., Glenn, B., Bruehl, S., Harden, R.N., Lofland, K., 2003. Cognitive factors influence outcome following multidisciplinary chronic pain treatment: a replication and extension of a cross-lagged panel analysis. Behav. Res. Ther. 41 (10), 1163–1182.

Carpenter, M.G., Frank, J.S., Silcher, C.P., Peysar, G.W., 2001. The influence of postural threat on the control of upright stance. Exp. Brain Res. 138 (2), 210–218.

Carroll, L.J., Holm, L.W., Ferrari, R., Ozegovic, D., Cassidy, J.D., 2009. Recovery in whiplash-associated disorders: do you get what you expect? J. Rheumatol. 36 (5), 1063–1070.

Comerford, M., Mottram, S., 2012. Kinetic Control. The Management of Uncontrolled Movement. Churchill Livingstone, Australia.

Field, S., Treleaven, J., Jull, G., 2008. Standing balance: a comparison between idiopathic and whiplash-induced neck pain. Man. Ther. 13 (3), 183–191.

Gagey, P.M., Toupet, M., 1991. Orthostatic postural control in vestibular neuritis: a stabilometric analysis. Ann. Otol. Rhinol. Laryngol. 100 (12), 971–975.

Glattacker, M., Heyduck, K., Meffert, C., 2013. Illness beliefs and treatment beliefs as predictors of short-term and medium-term outcome in chronic back pain. J. Rehabil. Med. 45 (3), 268–276.

Headache Classification Committee of the International Headache Society, 2013. The International Classification of Headache Disorders, 3rd edition (beta version). Cephalalgia 33 (9), 629–808.

Jull, G., Sterling, M., Falla, D., Treleaven, J., O'Leary, S., 2008. Whiplash, Headache, and Neck Pain: Research-Based Directions for Physical Therapies. Churchill Livingstone (Elsevier, Edinburgh.

Kahneman, D., 2011. Thinking, Fast and Slow. Allen Lane, London.

Leaver, A.M., Maher, C.G., McAuley, J.H., Jull, G., Latimer, J., Refshauge, K.M., 2013. People seeking treatment for a new episode of neck pain typically have rapid improvement in symptoms: an observational study. J Physiother 59 (1), 31–37.

Nijs, J., Torres-Cueco, R., van Wilgen, C.P., Girbes, E.L., Struyf, F., Roussel, N., et al., 2014. Applying modern pain neuroscience in clinical practice: criteria for the classification of central sensitization pain. Pain Physician 17 (5), 447–457.

Nijs, J., Van Geel, C., Van der Auwera, C., Van de Velde, B., 2006. Diagnostic value of five clinical tests in patellofemoral pain syndrome. Man. Ther. 11 (1), 69–77.

Nijs, J., Van Houdenhove, B., 2009. From acute musculoskeletal pain to chronic widespread pain and fibromyalgia: application of pain neurophysiology in manual therapy practice. Man. Ther. 14 (1), 3–12.

Sahrmann, S., 2011. Movement System Impairment Syndromes of the Extremities, Cervical and Thoracic Spines. Elsevier, St. Louis.

Sjaastad, O., Fredriksen, T.A., Pfaffenrath, V., 1998. Cervicogenic headache: diagnostic criteria. The Cervicogenic Headache International Study Group. Headache 38 (6), 442–445.

Treleaven, J., Jull, G., Lowchoy, N., 2005. Standing balance in persistent whiplash: a comparison between subjects with and without dizziness. J. Rehabil. Med. 37 (4), 224–229.

Vlaeyen, J., Morley, S.J., Linton, S.J., Boersma, K., De Jong, J., 2012. Pain-Related Fear. Exposure Treatment of Chronic Pain. IASP Press, Seattle.

World Health Organization, 2001. International Classification of Functioning, Disability and Health. World Health Organization, Washington, DC.

19

Orofacial, Nasal Respiratory and Lower-Quarter Symptoms in a Complex Presentation With Dental Malocclusion and Facial Scoliosis

Harry J. M. von Piekartz • Mariano Rocabado • Mark A. Jones

Subjective Examination
Personal Profile

Floor is a 27-year-old unemployed single woman who lives alone in Hamburg, Germany. She studied economics and earned a bachelor's degree 4 years ago; however, she has never been able to find work, largely related to her ongoing problems. She has one older sister who lives in the United States. Her parents have been divorced for 8 years, and she maintains a good relationship with both of them. Floor lives in her own apartment. Financially, she is partly supported by her mother and partly by an inheritance from her grandparents. Floor enjoys running, biking and swimming but has had to give these up due to her ongoing problems. She also enjoys listening to music, which for her serves as a form of relaxation.

Floor presented with a combination of head-region and lower-quarter complaints.

Orofacial and Head-Region Symptoms

Floor's main complaints were unilateral right tinnitus and bilateral headache (right more than left), as well as a pressure and a feeling of altered position in her tongue as though her 'tongue is being pulled out' (Fig. 19.1). She reported no decrease in the strength or coordination of her jaw when chewing and talking and no change in her taste.

Floor described that she would regularly experience two different occlusions (jaw alignments). During eating, talking and chewing, she felt that what she called her 'bad occlusion' (later determined to be a retracted mandible) would increase and influence these orofacial functions, in addition to her other symptoms. In particular, it increased the headache and the tinnitus and also the weird 'pressure' feeling of her tongue. She described her other occlusion as her 'relaxed occlusion' that appeared when she was relaxed, mostly in the supine-lying position (later determined to be a cross-bite and overbite position). A cross-bite is an abnormal relation of one or more teeth of one arch to the opposing tooth or teeth of the other arch, caused by deviation of tooth position or abnormal jaw position. An overbite is a malocclusion of the teeth in which the front upper incisor and canine teeth project over the lower (also called vertical overlap). Floor described her relaxed occlusion as follows; 'my jaw position is changed when lying down because my spine is more relaxed'. Floor's previous experience with dentists and orofacial surgeons provided her with a level of understanding to describe these as different occlusions.

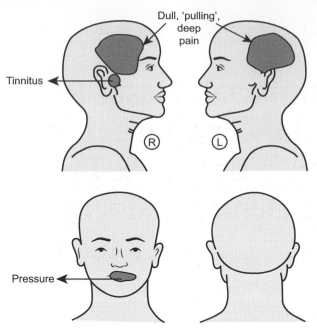

Fig. 19.1   Body chart of Floor's head-region symptoms.

Floor reported that her orofacial symptoms (headache, tinnitus, tongue pressure feeling and her bad occlusion feeling) all occurred together and increased during the day after just 10 minutes of talking or eating. The headache and tinnitus were worst, increasing up to a score of 7–8/10 on the visual analogue scale (VAS). She then had to stop the activities and rest or lie down. She also reported that sitting for longer than 60 minutes, either at the computer or watching TV, aggravated the headache and tinnitus. More physical activities, like running, biking and swimming, also increased all these symptoms, and consequently, she had stopped these physical activities about 6 years ago.

These same orofacial symptoms were all eased after 20 minutes of lying down or sleeping overnight and were also improved by manipulating the skin by squeezing her mandible, generally when she was lying supine in her 'relaxed occlusion' position. This was problematic, as her skin would then become red and start to bleed. This experience occurred at least three times per week. Floor understood the harm of this, which then made her angry but also ashamed. She reported she no longer liked to look at her own face and even avoided the mirror.

Spine, Hip and Knee-Area Symptoms

Floor further described a dull, deep low back pain (Fig. 19.2) that would often radiate into the right groin and deep anterior right hip. The right hip also felt stiff to movement in all directions. An anterior dull right knee pain also occurred in combination with the lumbar and hip-area pains. These lower-quarter complaints shared some relationship with the orofacial symptoms in that they would all generally only occur during the day. The lower back, hip and knee symptoms were mostly aggravated by standing and walking for longer than 20 minutes or 10 minutes of attempted jogging. When she stopped these activities, all three area pains decreased and were gone within 15 minutes, quicker if she would lie down. Any prolonged sitting left her feeling stiff through the lower spine and right hip for 5–10 minutes, which reduced with standing or walking, although this then provoked the lower-quarter pains. Floor also reported that the lumbar and hip pains became worse than usual (more easily aggravated) for 2 days premenstrual.

Screening for other lumbar, sacroiliac joint, hip and knee potential aggravating factors revealed no problems with specific low back movements in different directions (except sustained flexion when sitting), turning in bed, stairs (except if already standing too long) and hip or knee movements (including crossing legs, squatting and kneeling).

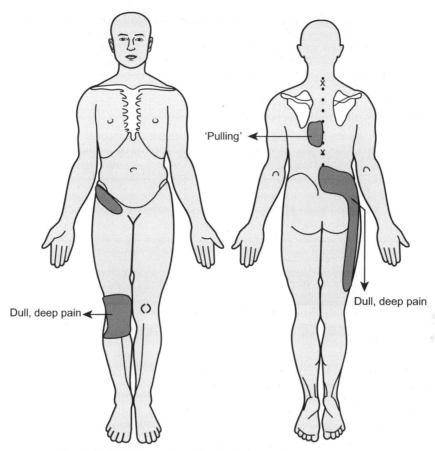

Fig. 19.2   Body chart of Floor's spine, hip and knee-area symptoms.

Floor did not report any areas of numbness or pins and needles or any weakness, potential cervical arterial dysfunction or any symptoms associated with spinal cord or cauda equina.

Patient Perspectives

When asked about her understanding of her orofacial symptoms, Floor felt strongly that all those symptoms were directly related to her dental occlusion, as were her lower-quarter symptoms.

Initial discussion around the influences her problems had on her life and how she coped elicited a clear theme of altered self-concept and social withdrawal. Floor volunteered feeling unattractive and embarrassed by her facial appearance. She disliked it because of the increased facial asymmetry. She did not like meeting other people in groups and consequently had significantly reduced her socializing. Whenever possible, she would present the left side of her face to others, which she described as the 'less ugly' side. She declared that she 'does not feel like a pretty young woman', and this, is in her opinion, was one reason why she had difficulties finding a partner. She was convinced that nobody was interested in a woman with these problems.

General Health Screening

Floor's general health was reported as being good. She had no systemic medical conditions, no visceral problems and no unexplained weight loss. Her blood tests had been negative, and she reported no allergies, otitis media, sinusitis or eye diseases. She had never had any trauma to her face, neck or lower quadrant and there was no history of cancer in her life or in her family. Her urogenital functions had always been normal, and she had no balance or walking disturbances suggestive of spinal cord involvement. Sleeping had never been a problem, and she reported sleeping 7–8 hours a night without complaints. She was not currently on any medications. From the age of 20–22, she took antidepressants (amitriptyline 50 mg per day) and paracetamol (50 mg) as needed according to her complaints. Neither of those provided any real help.

History

At the age of 11 years, Floor was prescribed an interocclusal splint for her overbite of more than 6 mm. After a few months she developed 'tinnitus' in her right ear, and her nasal respiration decreased such that she had to breathe more through her mouth. It was around that time that her mother first noticed Floor's increasing facial asymmetry. The orthodontics treatment continued until Floor was 17 years old. Although the orthodontist was 'satisfied' with the result, Floor and her mother completely disagreed, as by then she was suffering from constant tinnitus and regular headaches. Floor decided to consult a plastic surgeon, who reconstructed her nose and chin when she was 21 years old. Following this, the respiration did not improve, and her headaches increased. The weird 'pressure' feeling of her tongue started and slowly increased over a period of 5 years after the surgery. She saw different doctors, dentists and physical therapists for her complaints, but they could do nothing for her.

Floor's lumbar, hip and knee pains spontaneously started at the age of 22 years without any clear local predisposing factor and gradually worsened to their present level. She decided to consult an orthopaedic doctor and another physical therapist, and both diagnosed spinal scoliosis, which they explained could be responsible for her low back, hip and knee pains. She received manual therapy for her low back and exercises for her posture over a period of 6 months. Although these interventions would reduce her back, hip and knee pains, the relief would only last up to 2–3 days, and there was no improvement in her face complaints.

At the age of 23 years, a specialist temporomandibular joint (TMJ) surgeon diagnosed an extreme frontal dysgnathia (i.e. open-bite, where the front teeth, both upper and lower, are forced outward to such an extent that the teeth of the upper and the lower jaw do not touch each other, even when the mouth is closed) and a mandibular retrognathia (retracted mandible), with a left convex face scoliosis (an extreme maxillary rotation and mandible shift toward the right side). Between the ages of 23–25 years, Floor received preoperative orthodontic treatment to correct the asymmetry of the teeth arch and chin augmentation (surgical reconstruction of the chin by bone implant, providing a better balance to the facial features, in this case Floor's facial scoliosis). After 8 months, this was followed by a surgical bimaxillary osteotomy and a septo-rhinoplasty (surgical reconfiguration of nasal septum) to improve her nasal respiration. Following this surgery, Floor felt that her face symptoms (tinnitus, headache) and facial asymmetry were significantly improved. Also, her breathing pattern and her thoracic scoliosis were much better, and she felt 'free in her spine and her hips', with reduced lower-quarter pains as well.

Fourteen days after the bimaxillary osteotomy, two rubber bands were placed on the molars on her left and right maxilla and mandible to support correct mandibular movement. After 12 days, she opened her mouth a little bit too much, and due to the high external forces, the mandible retracted again. She immediately felt this repositioning of the mandible, and shortly after this her familiar face and lower-quarter symptoms returned. When consulting the maxillofacial surgeon and the orthodontist, she felt ignored, as they said there was nothing further they could do because there was no overt change to the surgical reconstructions. Slowly, her complaints all returned and worsened, especially the headaches, tinnitus and nasal breathing restriction.

During the last 2 years, she had consulted three specialist maxillofacial surgeons and two specialist orthodontists. Neither the surgeons nor the orthodontists believed her story of the relaxed 'cross-bite'. This relaxed 'cross-bite' in supine lying is also the position where the orthodontist wanted to correct her occlusion, first with a Michigan splint and then after 6 months with braces. Floor did not believe this was the solution, and they were unable to reach agreement. Eventually, she found a surgeon who would operate again with the aim of correcting her bite and restoring her normal nasal respiration. This initially

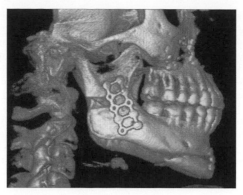

Fig. 19.3 Three-dimensional tomography taken 2 weeks after Floor's first bimaxillary osteotomy surgery at age 23. Note the surgery has created a forced protraction of the mandible, resulting in a 'head-bite' (direct contact of the incisors) and a bilateral open-bite (no teeth contact during habitual occlusion – in this case, the last three molars of the maxilla and mandible on the right).

required removing the screws in her mandible (Fig. 19.3) followed by preoperative ortho-dontics for a minimum of 1 year to reprogram the occlusion (retrain her neuromuscular system to the preferred occlusion).

Floor's goals for the second bimaxillary surgery were, firstly, a solution for her breathing problem and orofacial symptoms, especially the tinnitus and the 'weird' tongue feeling, and, secondly, to regain the symmetry of her face that was achieved after the first surgery. At present, her pre-surgical orthodontic treatment was planned in 3 or 4 months, although whether she proceeded or not depended on her financial status. She would have to sell her apartment to pay for these pre-orthodontic treatments and the planned bimaxillary reconstruction. In the meantime, she had decided to consult a specialist orofacial musculoskeletal physiotherapist (first author) who had been recommended to her by her local dentist.

Past History

Floor had a normal birth, normal progression of developmental milestones and normal childhood health, with no otitis media and no long-term sinusitis. She had never had problems before the initial orthodontic treatment. Her puberty commenced early (around 10 years), and her body subsequently underwent a quicker growth spurt than her maxil-lofacial skeleton. This was determined on the basis that her deciduous teeth had more caries because the mandible was shorter and abnormally retracted. According to the orthodontist, it was not hereditary, and the cause of her rapid growth was unknown.

Reasoning Question:

1. Would you please discuss the possible neurophysiological or structural mechanisms that may be responsible for Floor's development of tinnitus, impaired nasal respiration, headache, unusual tongue feeling and even the lower-quarter symptoms following the application of the interocclusal splint to correct her overbite?

Answer to Reasoning Question:

It is likely that there are different mechanisms involved with Floor's different symptoms. Potential mechanisms underpinning the relationship between tinnitus and occlusion discussed in the literature include anatomical connections between the TMJ and middle ear and altered neural processing. The discomalleolar ligament connects the malleus in the tympanic cavity and the articular disc and capsule of the TMJ. This anatomical relationship between the middle ear and the TMJ may enable altered occlusion to mechanically stress the malleus, resulting in aural symptoms associated with temporo-mandibular dysfunction (TMD) such as tinnitus (Cohen and Perzez, 2003; Hardell et al., 2003; Rowicki and Zakrzewska, 2006).

Continued on following page

Floor's persistent tinnitus, combined with her different maxillofacial surgeries with long-term nociception of local tissues (e.g. TMJ capsule, muscles and peripheral nervous tissue), also may have contributed to maladaptive central nervous system (CNS) processing, particularly at the brainstem level (Levine et al., 2003). Disinhibition of the ipsilateral dorsal cochlear nucleus in the brainstem is hypothesized to alter the perception of acoustic information in the brain, and this can be interpreted as tinnitus. Within this model, altered afferent input in the craniomandibular–cervical region has the potential to change the intensity and frequency of tinnitus (Abel and Levine, 2004; Kaltenbach et al., 2004).

Floor's impaired nasal respiration was likely related to the architecture of her maxilla facial structures, as her nasal respiration improved significantly following her bimaxillary osteotomy and a septo-rhinoplasty. Although the incident of opening her mouth too wide against the rubber bands with her ensuing perception that her occlusion had returned to its previous position should not have physically altered her reconstructions, it is possible that the added force of the rubber bands may have been sufficient to influence her nasal aerodynamics through the forces imparted on the maxilla–facial structures and associated nasal septum.

The localization of the bilateral but unilaterally dominant temporal headache fits with a cervicogenic headache (Vincent, 2010); however, there is nothing in the behaviour of the symptoms or history that supports upper cervical spine involvement. The headache is comorbid with the tinnitus, which together are related to oral activities. On this basis, we can hypothesize that TMJ intra- or peri-articular nociception may be associated with the headache.

The tongue is innervated by four cranial nerves and is the organ with the largest projection on the somatosensory cortex (Okayasu et al., 2014). Floor reported having normal taste and also seemed to have normal coordination of orofacial activities, suggesting normal function of the facial, glossopharyngeal and hypoglossal cranial nerves. The sensory function of the tongue is supplied by the mandibular nerve and the 3rd branch of the trigeminal nerve, which together also supply the structures of the middle ear. In Floor's case, her tinnitus, unilaterally dominant headache and the 'weird' feeling of her tongue are comorbid, which suggests that altered afferent input of the mandibular nerve into the CNS may have contributed to changes in her body perceptions (i.e. phantom experiences), including possibly the malposition and pressure feeling of her tongue (Avivi-Arber et al., 2010).

The improvement in Floor's lower-quarter symptoms following the application of the interocclusal splint to correct her overbite, and later return of symptoms when she felt her bite had returned to its retracted position, may relate to the recognized relationship between mandibular position and the spine. Previous studies have confirmed that patients with mandibular deviation with cross-bite often have morphological and positional changes of the cervical spine, and subgroups may present with functional scoliosis and trunk balance changes (Saccucci et al., 2011; Zhou et al., 2013). In Floor's case, the corrected central occlusion (which is not her habitual functional occlusion) may have strongly influenced her motor body reflex system, and this was expressed in her changed posture causing a nociceptive ischemic pain reaction in her trunk and hip areas.

Reasoning Question:

2. Would you please briefly discuss whether you feel Floor's facial scoliosis was a structural deformity requiring the surgery she had, or could it have been a functional consequence of her altered occlusion? Also, how would you explain Floor's relapse of symptoms from what appears to be an innocuous trigger of opening her mouth too wide against the rubber bands?

Answer to Reasoning Question:

The preoperative orthodontic treatment of 13 months and chin argumentation, together with the bimaxillary osteotomy and septo-rhinoplasty, improved the symmetry of Floor's face, which is still possible in younger adults (Proffit, 2006). The chin augmentation is done solely for cosmetic purposes. In Floor's situation, the dentist, orthodontist and maxillofacial surgeon had two principal aims they hoped to achieve:

- A maximal intercuspation: occlusal position of the mandible in which the cusps of the teeth of both arches fully interpose themselves with the cusps of the teeth of the opposing arch
- A centric occlusion: the occlusion of opposing teeth when the mandible is in a centric relation such that the head of the condyle is situated as far anteriorly and superiorly as it possibly can be within the mandibular glenoid fossa

Both these aims were probably reached after surgery. Although it is not possible to know for certain, the pulling forces of the rubber bands during (forced) mouth opening may have placed sufficient force on the maxilla–mandible alignment to result in a return to Floor's preoperative position that was strongly associated with her complaints (i.e. reduced nasal respiration, headache and lower-quarter symptoms).

Reasoning Question:

3. Based on your subjective examination, including the extent and behaviour of symptoms, history of facial and occlusal malalignment and Floor's altered self-concept and social withdrawal, what were your early impressions (hypotheses) regarding which 'pain type' (i.e. nociceptive, neuropathic and/or nociplastic) was dominant?

Answer to Reasoning Question:

At this stage there are clinical features of both nociceptive and nociplastic pain types (Okeson, 2014). In support of a nociceptive component for Floor's main complaints are the clear unilateral symptom distribution and predictable pattern of symptom behaviour related to orofacial and neck posture and movement (i.e. chewing, talking, cycling, swimming, etc.). However, in support of nociplastic driven symptoms, Floor's problem is clearly chronic, with her symptoms commencing at the age of 11 and spreading to her lower quarter without any specific trauma, clear overuse or overt trigger to account for those symptoms. Importantly, Floor openly discussed her negative self-image she associated with her facial asymmetry. Her persistent pain experience had also been quite negative, with failed interventions and conflict with some of the practitioners she had seen. These explicit negative cognitions and emotions would likely contribute to some level of maladaptive CNS sensitization (Maísa Soares and Rizzatti-Barbosa, 2015).

Clinical Reasoning Commentary:

Floor is a great example of how patient presentations often do not match clear diagnostic categorizations. In these situations, care is needed to avoid definitive cause-and-effect explanations and to keep the diagnostic causal reasoning as hypotheses. However, identification of potential causal mechanisms as occurs here is still important to clinical reasoning because established anatomical, biomechanical and neuromodulatory processes may enable quite unusual presentations to be better understood and assist logical exploration of novel assessment and management procedures.

   Also evident in the reasoning expressed in these answers is the need for musculoskeletal clinicians to constantly balance their pathology-/structural-based reasoning (e.g. Floor's confirmed malocclusions, surgical and orthodontic corrections) with their impairment-based reasoning emanating from the physical examination. Although the body has an impressive ability to adapt to pathology and structural dysfunction without consequent nociception, pathoanatomical change can also contribute to nociception. The clinical reasoning hypothesis categories of 'pain type', 'sources of symptoms' and 'pathology' (see Chapter 1) are an attempt to encourage understanding and recognition of clinical patterns related to these categories. Pain type is particularly important because nociplastic pain/symptoms can partially mimic specific pathology or tissue nociception and misdirect management if not understood. However, clinically, it is still not possible to definitively confirm pain type, and it is probable that combinations of different pain types can co-exist (see Chapter 2). Nevertheless, formulating such hypotheses (as occurs here) enables the physical examination to proceed to further 'test' both 'pain type' dominance and possible 'sources of symptoms' and 'pathology' and the relationship of each to specific physical impairments.

Physical Examination
Clinical Observation

Face

At first sight, a clear facial asymmetry (scoliosis) can be seen. The right side seems to be smaller, with the following abnormalities:

1. Deeper nasolabial fault (Fig. 19.4A)
2. Orbital width on the right smaller than on the left (Fig. 19.4A)
3. Nostril on the right side flatter than that on the left (Figs 19.4A and B)
4. No upper-to-lower-lip contact (Fig. 19.4A)
5. Mental fault (small impression of the skin of the chin) on the right less than on the left (Fig. 19.4A)
6. Skin changes (reddening) in the lower two-thirds of the face (Figs 19.4A and B).

   During execution of a small active upper cervical extension movement (20 degrees), the head is seen to deviate toward the left, and the changed nostril (passage) can be seen (Fig. 19.4B). In supine lying, a clear chin and nose bridge deviation is evident toward the left, and an asymmetry in the nose bridge (left flatter than right) is noted. The head is orientated in a small lateral flexion position toward the left.

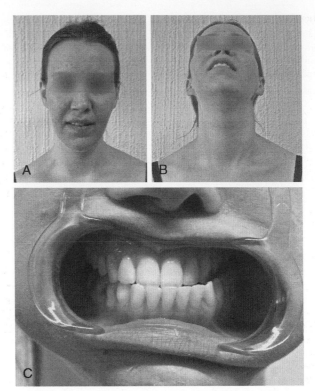

Fig. 19.4 (A) Frontal view illustrating the form of Floor's face (see case text for key features to note). (B) Cranial ventral view from supine position taken at a 30-degree angle from the horizontal line of the face. Note the deviation of the nose bridge in relation to the mandible. (C) Floor's habitual occlusion. Note the head-bite of the incisors and clear left laterotrusion of the mandible resulting in a cross-bite. Also note the possible open-bite left and right in the (pre)molar region and at the front.

Intraoral (Assessed in Supine Lying, Floor's Relaxed Habitual Occlusion Position)

An open-bite and a cross-bite toward the left can be observed, as described previously (Fig. 19.4C). A clear protrusion and laterotrusion position of the mandible toward the left is also evident, and if Floor corrects this to maximal intercuspidation (i.e. correction of the mandibular laterotrusion and protrusion so that upper teeth and lower teeth contact), she feels local discomfort, with an increase in the tinnitus and headache. There is no attrition (i.e. wear and tear of the teeth by parafunctional activities) observed (Fig. 19.4C).

Nasal Respiration

Floor was asked to inspire slowly as the therapist applied gentle pressure to block one nostril at a time. Inspiration through the left nostril (right trill blocked) was executed with a lower pitch and for longer duration (6 seconds) than the right side (left trill blocked), which produced a much higher pitch over a shorter duration (2.5 seconds), accompanied with a 'right ear pressure' (6/10 on the VAS) and right temporal pressure (4/10).

Spine

Floor had a flexion posture of the upper cervical spine. When asked to look up and correct the postural deviation, she experienced a heavy feeling in her neck and had difficulty holding it. The craniocervical angle, measured using a CRAFTA digital clinometric program version 1.06 (www.physioedu.com), was clearly reduced (45 degrees; normal = 51 degrees). Posterior observation revealed a position of minimal head rotation to the right, lateral flexion to the left, elevation of the left shoulder and increased pelvic height on the left (Fig. 19.5).

Fig. 19.5 Dorsal view of Floor's standing posture. Note the lateroflexion and rotation asymmetry of the head and neck and elevation of the left shoulder and pelvis.

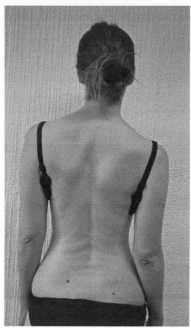

Centre of Gravity

Floor's centre of gravity (COG) was measured with a multifunctional force measuring plate (Zebris Medical GmbH, Germany). Relative to Floor's base of support, the COG assessment revealed a posterior (41 mm) and right shift (2.6 mm) which was accompanied by other changes in body-mass positioning (e.g. right foot pressure was 59% of her body weight, compared with 41% on the left).

TMJ Assessment

This was performed in the upright posture position of the mandible (UPPM), which is an active corrected upright position without teeth contact (von Piekartz, 2007).

TMJ Active Movement Assessment (Performed with the Mandible Passively Corrected to the UPPM)

There were no resting symptoms except tinnitus 2/10 on the VAS.

- Mouth opening (depression) was 46 mm (normal = 45–60 mm), with no symptoms until moderate overpressure was applied, causing a 'pulling' in the masticatory muscles, a 'pulling' (3/10 on the VAS) in the right ear and 'pressure' (3/10) in the right temporal region.
- Laterotrusion to the left was 10 mm (normal = 12 mm), with no symptoms until minimal overpressure was applied, causing a 'pulling' in the masticatory muscles.
- Laterotrusion to the right was 6 mm and provoked head pain (right > left, 3/10 on the VAS) and a pressure feeling in the right ear. Tinnitus increased up to 4/10. With slight overpressure, a steep increase in resistance was felt from onset to end range, with an accompanying further increase in the tinnitus (6/10).
- Protrusion was 5 mm (normal = 5 mm), with a click starting at 3 mm. There was provocation of 'stress' and 'local pain' in the right ear with a small shift of the mandible toward the right, and also a 'pulling in ear' feeling when the shift was corrected (2/10). Moderate overpressure produced a 'pulling' in the masticatory muscles and the 'pulling in the ear' increased to 5/10.
- Retrusion was 3–4 mm (normal = 3 mm), with no symptoms until moderate overpressure was applied, causing a local pressure feeling in the right ear and head pain (right > left, 3/10).

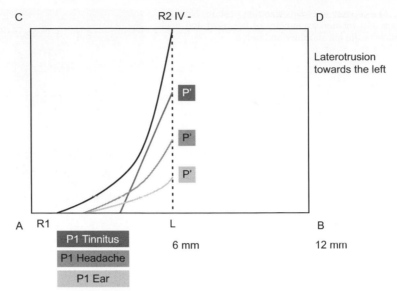

Fig. 19.6 Movement diagram illustrating the response to passive laterotrusion movement of the mandible toward the left. The AB line represents the average maximal range of passive laterotrusion movement (12 mm). The AC line represents the quality, nature or intensity of the factors being plotted (in this case, resistance, headache, ear pressure and tinnitus). R1 is the first resistance felt by the examiner during the passive movement. R2, in this case, is where movement was limited when the examiner reached a Grade IV – estimated to be 25% of the available resistance (6 mm). In this case, a decision was made not to perform a stronger movement because the headache increased to VAS 5/10, pressure in the ear to VAS 3/10 and the tinnitus to VAS 7/10. Note each symptom (headache, ear pressure, tinnitus) has a point through the passive movement where that symptom is first provoked (P1) and a level of intensity when the movement test is stopped (P'). Also note that all three increase somewhat proportionally to the increase in resistance, supporting the symptoms that are associated with the laterotrusion movement and also associated with the resistance to this movement.

TMJ Passive Physiological Movement Assessment

Because the laterotrusion toward the left reproduced the most musculoskeletal signs and symptoms, it was assessed and expressed in a 'movement diagram' (Hengeveld and Banks, 2014) (Fig. 19.6). Passive laterotrusion to the left provoked head pain and a pressure feeling in the right ear (2/10 on the VAS) at 4 mm. Tinnitus started at 6 mm. The 'limit' of the movement was determined at the onset of resistance (R2) and was stopped at 6 mm because the headache increased to 5/10, the pressure in the ear to 3/10 and the tinnitus to 7/10. In this case, the passive movement was not limited by a true R2 (i.e. no further passive movement available due to resistance) or P2 (i.e. passive movement stopped at patient's request due to pain); rather, the therapist elected to stop the movement due to the increase in symptoms and his judgement regarding the 'nature' of the problem – in this case, the irritability of the presentation and his decision not to let the symptoms increase any further.

Passive neurodynamic assessment challenging the cranioneural sensitivity of the mandibular nerve was undertaken by performing left laterotrusion in upper cervical flexion and latero-flexion toward the left (Geerse and von Piekartz, 2015; von Piekartz, 2007). There was no clear difference when compared with laterotrusion performed without this upper cervical pre-positioning.

TMJ Accessory Movement Assessment

- Passive transverse movements of the mandible medially and laterally were both subjectively judged to be more than 50% restricted on the right compared with the left side. The lateral transverse glide, in particular, changed the tinnitus to a lower tone and improved Floor's respiration through her right nostril for about 15 seconds.
- Passive distraction, antero-posterior translation and postero-anterior translation were each minimally restricted, with no symptom change.

Masticatory Muscles Assessment

The masticatory muscles were screened for tone, sensitivity or pain provocation and endurance:

- Palpation of the masseter, medial pterygoid, temporalis and sternocleidomastoid muscles revealed increased tone on the left compared with the right.
- Mechanical pain threshold was measured by a mechanical algometer (Wagner Instruments, Type FDK5, www.wagnerforce.com) in the most sensitive area compared with the left side:
  - Right masseter (0.4 kg/cm^2); left masseter (2.8 kg/cm^2)
  - Right anterior temporalis (0.2 kg/cm^2); left anterior temporalis (3.1 kg/cm^2)
  - Right upper clavicular part of sternocleidomastoid (1.2 kg/cm^2); left upper clavicular part of sternocleidomastoid (3.2 kg/cm^2)
  - Medial pterygoid palpation sensitivity was not assessed due to the poor reliability for testing this muscle (de Leeuw and Klasser, 2013).
- Endurance and coordination: during 10 repetitions of mouth opening and closing against minor manual resistance (less than 0.5 kg), there was no asymmetry of movement, there was no pain provocation, and the strength did not deteriorate.

Cervical Spine Assessment

Active Physiological Movements Assessment

Active movement was measured with a cervical range-of-motion measurement (Sammons Preston Basic CROM, www.rehabmart.com) instrument without overpressure (there were no symptoms at rest except for tinnitus of 2/10 on the VAS):

- Flexion was 65 degrees (less movement was observed in the C7–T4 region), no change in symptoms.
- Extension was 46 degrees (no upper cervical movement, increased midcervical movement), with a 'heavy feeling in the neck'.
- Left lateral flexion was 22 degrees, with no change in symptoms.
- Right lateral flexion was 9 degrees, provoking a 'pulling' sensation (3/10) in the lower right side of the neck.
- Left rotation was 78 degrees, with a 'pressure feeling' in the right side of the neck and right ear.
- Right rotation was 60 degrees, with no symptom change.

Flexion/Rotation Test

In supine lying with full cervical flexion, passive rotation to the left was 43 degrees, and rotation to the right was 28 degrees, as measured with a digital goniometer (HALO Medical Devices, Australia).

Passive Physiological Intervertebral Movement Assessment (PPIVM)

During palpation in supine lying, the transverse process of C1 was more prominent on the left compared with right, and the distance between the mastoid and the tip of C1 was greater compared with the right side. The spinous process of C2 was angled to the right.

- Occiput – C1
  - Lateral flexion to the left no movement; to the right 2–3 degrees
  - Rotation to the left no movement; to the right 2–3 degrees
  - Flexion 5 degrees
  - Extension < 5 degrees, sub-occipital neck pain
- C1 – C2
  - Flexion 4–5 degrees
  - Extension < 5 degrees
  - Lateral flexion left = right (2–3 degrees)
  - Rotation to the left 15 degrees; to the right 30 degrees

Passive Accessory Movement Assessment (PAM)

- The dominant impairment was the right unilateral postero-anterior movement at both C1 and C2 that reproduced local neck pain and was restricted by 50% compared with the left, with movement limited by resistance.
- Differentiation assessment between C1–C2 versus C2–C3 using the same PAM in 30 degrees rotation to the right supported a C1–C2 source for this pain.

Craniofacial Region

Neurocranium

During the standard craniofacial assessment by passive movements where the 'resistance rebounce' (i.e. reaction of the compliance qualities of the cranium) and the sensory response (i.e. the subjective perception of the patient) are tested, clear dysfunctions were found. This was most evident with the diagonal occiput right – frontal left, and the combined movement of temporal dorsal rotation around the transverse plane together with rotation of the occiput toward the right around the sagittal plane (Fig. 19.7). Each movement exhibited decreased resistance (rebounce) and provoked Floor's bilateral headache (6/10 on the VAS), right tinnitus (4/10) and minimal ear pain (2/10). The other standard movements (von Piekartz, 2007) were negative. After this passive craniofacial assessment, Floor noted that she could breathe better through her right nostril. Re-assessment of inspiration through the right nostril showed a short-term improvement reflected as a lower pitch for up to 3 seconds, accompanied by a reduced 'right ear pressure' (2/10) and complete relief of the right temporal pressure that had been present.

Viscerocranium

Floor had fear of any passive techniques being performed on her face (i.e. she was afraid that they might shift her maxilla even more in the wrong direction) and preferred not to have any manual assessment of her facial bones.

Neurodynamics of the Cranial Nervous System. The general impression of the mechano-sensitivity of the neuro-axis (longitudinally) following assessment by the cervical slump test (Butler, 2000) was normal, with full range of movement and no provocation of symptoms.

> **Reasoning Question:**
>
> 4. Based on your subjective and now these physical findings, please discuss your hypotheses and associated reasoning at this stage regarding:
>
>   a. What you consider are the most likely 'sources' of Floor's different symptoms, and
>
>   b. Your hypotheses regarding physical or non-physical factors you feel may have contributed to the development and/or maintenance of her problems.

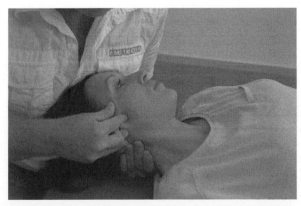

Fig. 19.7 An example of manual assessment of the neurocranium. A combination of posterior rotation of the right temporal bone around the transverse plane and a rotation of the occiput toward the right around the sagittal plane is illustrated. This manual procedure had increased resistance and decreased rebounce and was provocative to all three of Floor's symptoms.

Answer to Reasoning Question:

The consistent reproduction of Floor's tinnitus and headache by active and passive mandible excursion support a nociceptive component to these symptoms. The TMJ, along with associated tissues, would have to be considered as a structure that may be a nociceptive source for these symptoms. However, with respect to recognized patterns of TMD, Floor's physical signs do not support a clear intra-articular disc displacement or a clear neuropathic pattern. As mentioned in the answer to the previous reasoning question, stress to the discomalleolar (Pinto's) ligament from mandibular movements may precipitate both tinnitus and headache. Because the nasal respiration was improved by the assessment techniques performed on the neurocranium but not on the mandible, this would support the neurocranium's association with the quality of nasal respiration, which is also consistent with Floor's history.

Long-term facial symptoms may be comorbid with neurocranial and viscerocranial (i.e. facial skeleton) changes in alignment, with associated changes in TMJ mobility and face and masticatory muscle function (e.g. reduced endurance, coordination, increased muscle tone, etc.) (Joshi et al., 2014). It is not possible to know if the physical impairments are a consequence of Floor's long-term symptoms or whether they may have been part of a predisposing cause. Similarly, non-physical aspects of Floor's presentation, such as her reduced self-concept associated with her perception of feeling 'ugly', may also represent cognitive and emotional contributing factors to her ongoing symptoms and physical impairments. Again, it is not possible to know whether these perspectives precipitated or were a consequence of her current symptoms, but they are clearly now a significant part of her disability experience and as such require further assessment and consideration in management (Lumley et al., 2011). Therefore, screening of her emotional–cognitive status, body schema disruption and emotion recognition will assist in clarifying and confirming their involvement and the need for any associated management strategies.

Clinical Reasoning Commentary:

The hypothesis categories 'sources of symptoms', 'pathology' and 'contributing factors' are discussed in Chapter 1. Consistent with what is understood about the nociceptive 'pain type', repeatable reproduction of Floor's symptoms through active and passive assessment of the mandible support the TMJ and associated tissues as possible sources of nociception (headache, but also tinnitus). Although no discernible specific pathology (e.g. intra-articular disc displacement or neuropathic) is evident, local tissue stress or load may be sufficient to elicit nociception, especially when non-physical factors such as stress coexist. The recognition of Floor's negative perspective regarding her appearance signals the hypothesis that this may not simply be a consequence of her facial asymmetry but now may also represent a contributing factor to her persistent symptoms. In either case, it a real feature of her disability experience that requires more thorough assessment to understand and to determine the need for specific targeted management.

Lateralization and Emotion Recognition Assessment. This was undertaken using the Cranial Facial Therapy Academy (CRAFTA) Face Lateralization–Emotion Recognition Test (see www.physioedu.com or www.trainyourface.com).

Results:

- Lateralization: from the 48 pictures presented, Floor correctly identified 46 at an average speed of 3.6 seconds for left face pictures and 1.9 seconds for right face pictures, which represents normal interpretation but slower judgements involving right face recognition (average reference value speed is 2.60 seconds).
- Emotion recognition: Floor scored 100% for happiness, 86% for astonished and disgusted, and 17% for fear and sadness. In total, 32% were answered incorrectly, and 10% were not answered in time (decision > 5 seconds), with the average judgement speed being 3.92 seconds (reference value 3.60 seconds).

Questionnaires. Three questionnaires were chosen, an alexithymia assessment questionnaire, a functional status questionnaire and a depression assessment questionnaire:

- The Toronto Alexithymia Scale 26 (Kupfer et al., 2000) measures three key characteristics of alexithymia (i.e. emotional consciousness): difficulty identifying emotions (scale 1), difficulty describing emotions (scale 2), and externally oriented thinking style (i.e. the extent and manner of analytical thinking, scale 3). Floor's total score was 2.21, which represents minor alexithymia on scale 1 and marked alexithymia on scale 3.
- The Neck Disability Index (Vernon, 2008) is a functional status questionnaire. Floor scored 62 out of 100 possible points, which represents a moderate neck-associated disability, especially manifest during reading, concentrating when driving a car and free-time activities (response questions 4, 6, 8 and 10).

- The Beck Disability Index II (BDI; Beck et al., 1996) provides a measure of depression. Floor scored 21 out of a possible 63 on the 21-item assessment, which represents minimal to mild depression.

Reasoning Question:

5. What was your rationale for including the Face Lateralization–Emotion Recognition Test and the Toronto Alexithymia Scale 26 Questionnaire for Floor, and how do you envisage using this information in her case?

Answer to Reasoning Question:

Because of Floor's long-term negative self-concept and feelings about the appearance of her face, left/right lateralization and emotion recognition, assessments were conducted using the CRAFTA Face Lateralization–Emotion Recognition Test (Leake, H., 2012). Implicit motor imagery seems to be strongly related with left/right recognition tasks that are reduced in chronic pain states (Bray and Moseley, 2011). It has been reported that facial pain is underpinned, at least in part, by disruption of cortical motor processing (left/right recognition) rather than disruption of cortical emotion processing (von Piekartz et al., 2014). That is, just because a patient has a left/right recognition problem, we can't assume the patient will also have emotion-recognition problems, and therefore this needs to be assessed separately. Identifying these impairments in lateralization and emotion recognition also create an opportunity to specifically target these and Floor's alexithymia in management.

Reasoning Question:

6. Some would argue that assessment and management of depression is outside musculoskeletal clinicians' scope of practice. Would you discuss your views on using the BDI and whether you feel Floor's result representing 'minimal to mild depression' warrants referral to a psychologist?

Answer to Reasoning Question:

Research has demonstrated that patients with TMD and symptoms including face pain, headaches, tinnitus and hypoacusis (oversensitivity to certain frequency and volume ranges of sound) are strongly comorbid with higher levels of depression (Hilgenberg et al., 2012). Research criteria for the diagnosis of temporomandibular disorders advocate clinicians' assessment of depression and somatization (Dworkin and LeResche, 1992; Manfredini et al., 2010). Given Floor's long history of surgery with unsuccessful results, her negative feelings about herself and the results of the BDI, Floor will be advised to consult a psychologist.

Reasoning Question:

7. How has the additional information obtained in the physical examination, including the lateralization, emotion and depression assessments, supported or not supported your initial hypotheses regarding 'pain type' (nociceptive, neuropathic, maladaptive CNS sensitization)?

Answer to Reasoning Question:

Chronic (face) pain can adversely affect body image (reflected in part in lateralization) and influence motor responses (Berryman et al., 2014). This was also evident in Floor's clearly reduced unilateral accuracy and reaction time during the lateralization test and the low accuracy of the dominantly asymmetric (negative) emotions of sadness and fear. Long-term nociception may also change emotion status expressed in depression (Taylor and Corder 2014). Collectively, these may have contributed to Floor's pain and disability experiences and her quality of life.

Clinical Reasoning Commentary:

Use of specialized lateralization, emotion recognition and alexithymia assessments have provided further insight into the scope of Floor's presentation. Although musculoskeletal clinicians are historically well trained in physical assessment and physical diagnosis, cognitive and emotional assessment and management is arguably less well understood and less structured. Validated assessments such as these are important to objectively identify these impairments and inform reasoning regarding additional management strategies that may be helpful.

Consistent with the recommendations from Chapter 3, screening for depression and other 'orange flags' by a musculoskeletal clinician is not for the purpose of formally diagnosing depression; rather, the aim is to identify when depression may be present for consideration of consultation and referral back to the referring physician and/or a psychologist. These data also may be used for re-assessment.

As discussed in Chapters 1 and 2, clinical 'diagnosis' of 'pain type' is limited to identification of common features in both the subjective and physical presentations. Although impaired lateralization and emotion recognition on their own would not confirm a maladaptive CNS-sensitization 'pain type', when these impairments are considered alongside other features already highlighted (e.g. chronicity of symptoms, negative 'patient perspectives'), a growing picture emerges supporting maladaptive CNS sensitization.

First Appointment Treatment (Day 1)

Treatment commenced with an explanation of the main examination findings and discussion of short-term and long-term management goals. The relationships between the face, neck and lower quarter were broadly explained with respect to potential neurological, biomechanical and pain mechanism influences. Given Floor's history of symptoms, as well as the clear TMJ, cranium and neck signs and the improved tinnitus and respiration following assessment of accessory translation movements of the right TMJ, it was discussed and decided to start with a session of treatment directed to the right TMJ.

Passive transverse mobilization of the right TMJ directed laterally (grade IV⁻, proposed after Maitland no symptom provocation) was applied for about 90 seconds (Hengeveld and Banks, 2014). Re-assessment revealed the following changes:

- Observation:
  - Standing posture: reduced lateral flexion and rotation of the head and also reduced elevation of the left shoulder and left pelvis (Fig. 19.8)
  - Active protrusion: increased shift of mandible and cross-bite with complete cessation of 'pulling' feeling previously felt in the masticatory muscles during overpressure
- Improvement in active mandibular laterotrusion to the right to 10 mm (previously 6 mm), with the pressure feeling in the right ear unchanged but tinnitus reduced (2/10 on the VAS, previously 4/10). With slight overpressure, a normal resistance (previously felt as steep resistance) is felt in comparison with the other side, and Floor experienced no increased tinnitus.
- Improvement in passive TMJ lateral transverse gliding (decreased resistance)
- Nasal respiration unchanged
- Improvement in C1–C2 right unilateral postero-anterior PAM (decreased local pain and resistance)
- Improvement in the flexion/rotation test to the right from 28 degrees to 35 degrees
- No change to tone or pain thresholds on masticatory muscle palpation

Given the complexity of Floor's presentation, no self-management strategies were initiated at this stage. Because of the distance Floor had to travel (3 hours), the duration of the next session was planned for 60–90 minutes to ensure self-management strategies could be included.

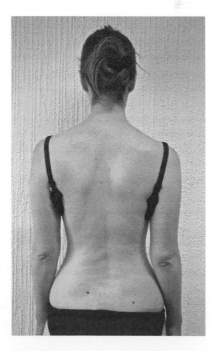

Fig. 19.8 Dorsal observation of Floor's posture after the first treatment. Note the clear change (improvement) in head and neck position and in shoulder and pelvic symmetry.

Second Appointment (8 Days Later)

Floor reported no treatment soreness and no change in her symptom pattern since her initial examination and treatment. The proposed plan for the appointment was discussed and agreed, including re-checking her main physical findings; further assessment of her spine, hips and knees; and treatment of a second potential source of her symptoms, her neurocranium, so as to determine its effect.

Physical Re-assessment

Re-assessment of the TMJ and upper cervical signs revealed no change in comparison to re-assessment after treatment on the first appointment.

Additional Screening of the Thoracic and Lumbar Spines, Hips and Knees

Thoracic spine PPIVM and PAM assessments revealed only minor stiffness of the T4–T8 segments in extension and postero-anterior directions, respectively. Examination of the lumbar spine, hips and knees revealed relatively normal ranges of movement, with no provocation of symptoms.

Treatment

Neurocranium mobilization was introduced. This consisted of passive mobilization of the sphenoid/temporal articulation into resistance, with minimal provocation of headache and no change to tinnitus for 5 minutes, in a rhythm of 7–10 seconds, essentially slowly increasing the mobilization pressure up to a grade IV and then slowly reducing the pressure. From clinical experience, a very slow rhythm is more effective at improving the compliance of the cranial tissues.

Re-assessment demonstrated the following:

- Improved active mandibular laterotrusion to the right (from 10 to 12 mm), with no pressure feeling in the right ear and no tinnitus to moderate overpressure
- Improved nasal respiration through the right nostril (lower noise and longer duration of 4 seconds) with less ear and temporal 'pressure' (4/10 on the VAS)
- No change in cervical signs
- Thoracic scoliosis and pelvic tilt minimally improved

Reasoning Question:

8. Please discuss your interpretation of the first two treatments. Because mobilization of the neurocranium will not be as familiar as mobilization elsewhere in the body, would you please also include a brief discussion of the aim of these procedures and a comment on the current state of evidence regarding their efficacy?

Answer to Reasoning Question:

There is clinical evidence that passive cranial mobilization can lead to a reduction of abnormal orofacial motor activity and may reduce pain (Chaitow, 2005; von Piekartz, 2007; Schueler et al., 2013).

There are many models explaining how cranial manipulative techniques can change signs and facial sensory responses like pain, tinnitus and vertigo (Schueler et al., 2013). The standard cranial mobilization procedures used with Floor are based on a pragmatic functional approach related to (clinical) evidence from orthodontics and cranial plastic surgery (Zöller, 2005; Proffit, 2006). Craniomandibular-facial dental dysfunctions, such as malocclusion, TMJ disc displacements and maxilla-facial deformity, can facilitate abnormal interactive bone tension (stress transduction). This phenomenon may facilitate (abnormal) craniofacial growth and cranial bone tension, which may influence the function of soft tissues, such as the masticatory and facial muscles, but also facial organ functions of the ears, eyes, nose and tongue with reciprocal influences from organs and soft tissue to bone (Linder-Aronson and Woodside, 2000; Oudhof, 2001; Joshi et al., 2014). Craniofacial imbalance can also contribute to abnormal afferent input and nociception (Proffit, 2006; Schueler et al., 2013).

In Floor's case, her craniofacial microsomia (i.e. a spectrum of abnormalities that primarily affect the development of the cranium and face before birth) was not directly related to a specific head organ dysfunction or macro trauma. Rather, as suggested by her orthodontist, it may have been genetic or possibly caused by her rapid prepubescent body growth (Heike and Hing, 2009). With Floor, this abnormal stress-transducer mechanism associated with her facial asymmetry and occlusal forces may be continuing to affect her facial and neurocranial bones and associated soft tissues contributing to her persistent tinnitus, reduced unilateral respiration (Kluemper and Spalding, 2001) and abnormal motor responses (e.g. increased muscle tone in sternocleidomastoid, masseter and temporalis muscles), which may explain her predominantly muscular headache (Palazzi et al., 1996).

Clinical Reasoning Commentary:

In the absence of research evidence, clinicians need to draw from critical theoretical propositions embedded in sound health practice (e.g. orthodontics and cranial plastic surgery). Such an 'abductive' inference or inference to the best explanation (also called abduction; see Chapter 1) is a creative explanation used when clear deductions are not available. Clinically, this is required when trying to account for what may initially present as disparate, unclear information or situations. It is essentially an unproven explanatory hypothesis that best explains the clinical findings, much like the detective who must entertain the best explanation that could account for the evidence surrounding a crime. Whereas uncritical acceptance of such explanations can lead to a confirmation bias error of reasoning, cautious abduction is a real part of all thinking that informs further 'testing', both clinically and empirically.

Third Appointment (2 Weeks Later, Day 21)

Floor reported the improved respiration lasted for 3 days. She also discovered that when her respiration is better, her tinnitus and headache, especially on the right side, are reduced (2/10 on the VAS).

Physical Re-assessment

There was no clear change in the main physical findings compared with the end of the second appointment except the sound (pitch) of Floor's nasal inspiration through the right nostril was lower and longer (5 seconds), along with minor ear pressure (3/10 on the VAS) and no temporal 'pressure'. Masticatory muscle tone and endurance were the same; however, mechanical pain threshold assessment had changed:

- Right masseter 2.1 kg/cm^2, previously 0.4 kg/cm^2
- Right anterior temporalis 1.7 kg/cm^2, previously 0.2 kg/cm^2
- Right upper clavicular part of sternocleidomastoid 2.7 kg/cm^2, previously 1.2 kg/cm^2

Treatment

Floor was provided with the explanation that abnormal stress in her skull was likely affecting her nasal respiration, and together they may be provoking her tinnitus and headache but also possibly her jaw and TMJ problems. On this basis, a plan for combined manual treatment of the neurocranium and the TMJ was discussed and agreed.

Passive mobilization of the right TMJ was performed in posterior rotation of the temporal bone around the transverse arches (due to its increased resistance, reduced rebounce and effect on reducing the tinnitus) for 5 minutes. Immediate re-assessment revealed the same pattern as after the second treatment, except:

- The cross-bite was again decreased (her relaxed position).
- The nasal respiration was clearly improved (inspiration sounds were equal between the left and right nostrils, with equal duration [6 seconds]) and only minimal ear pressure (2/10 on the VAS) and no temporal 'pressure'.

There was also a trial treatment of the right C1–C2 segment for 3 minutes using unilateral postero-anterior mobilization into stiffness (with 1 minute performed in 30 degrees rotation toward the right).

Re-assessment

- Increased TMJ active laterotrusion to the right (now 13 mm), with no provocation of tinnitus on moderate overpressure
- Elimination of the protrusion 'click'

- Reduced cross-bite
- Reduced thoracic scoliosis and pelvic tilt
- COG: posterior (from 41 mm to 5 mm) and right (from 26 mm to 16 mm) shifts clearly changed, as reflected in changes in body mass (right foot pressure reduced from 59% to 54%).
- Nasal respiration was unchanged.

Floor felt that the combination of the cranio-temporomandibular and neck treatments gave her the best change thus far, noting that even her low back and hip complaints were reduced.

Home exercises were then prescribed as follows:

- Laterotrusion exercise of the TMJ: Floor was instructed to place her left index finger against the left side of her chin and try to guide her mandible as she actively moves into right laterotrusion combined with a passive stretch through her right hand of the right temporal bone toward posterior rotation. She was asked to do 6–10 repetitions six times per day. She was also instructed in how to re-assess her own laterotrusion movement and her nasal respiration and to continue with the exercises unless her symptoms worsened.
- Respiration exercises: Floor was taught a modified Valsalva maneuver to train the air dynamics of the nasal–facial sinus–ear region. This involved Floor performing a slightly more forced exhalation against a closed airway. This is done by exhaling while closing the mouth and pinching the nose shut, as if one were trying to block a sneeze. If the pressure is built up slowly, the eustachian tube will open, and increased pressure may build up in the ears. If Floor felt a pressure deep in her ears, she was instructed to swallow with the mouth and nose closed, which causes an increased negative pressure in the inner ear and the eustachian tube. She was asked to perform this exercise three times per day for 2–3 minutes without increasing the symptoms or decreasing the quality of her nasal inspiration.

Fourth Appointment (2 Weeks Later, Day 34)
Subjective Re-assessment

Floor was very surprised that her tinnitus had reduced (2/10 on the VAS) since the last appointment and was now even completely absent for several hours a day. Also, her nasal inspiration was much better, and she was quite pleased with these improvements. Her temporal headache and even her lower-quarter symptoms had also reduced for the first 3 days post-treatment. Floor reported her tinnitus, headache and reduced nasal inspiration all returned after 8 days, but she felt each of these was still approximately 50% improved overall.

Physical Re-assessment

Home Exercises

- Floor reproduced the two home exercises perfectly and reported that both exercises improved her tinnitus and inspiration while performing them.

Nasal Respiration

- No change compared with the end of the third appointment
- TMJ
  - Further decrease in the difference of the right passive mandibular lateral transverse glide compared with left
  - Active laterotrusion to the right 12 mm, with no provocation of tinnitus on moderate overpressure

Neurocranium

- The diagonal occiput right – frontal left – temporal dorsal rotation around the transverse arches and the transverse rotation of the occiput to the left still provoked Floor's bilateral headache (2/10 on the VAS) and right tinnitus (2/10), but only after six repetitions of grade IV pressure, each sustained for 5–10 seconds.

Upper Cervical Spine

- Flexion/rotation test rotation to the right was 33 degrees (initially 28 degrees).
- Right unilateral postero-anterior accessory movement at C1–C2 still demonstrated 50% less movement than on the left, with local neck pain produced (5/10 on the VAS). When performed in 30 degrees right rotation, both stiffness and neck pain increased (7/10).
- Grade IV right unilateral postero-anterior accessory movement at C2 assessed concurrently with a TMJ laterotrusion position toward the left provoked the tinnitus (4/10 on the VAS).

Occlusal Kinaesthetic Sensitizing Test

This is an additional test performed when cervical spine and TMJ movement and symptom relationships exist, as suggested by the previous assessment (von Piekartz, 2007). A small piece of paper or foil (1 mm thick) is placed between the teeth, and the patient is asked to make gentle teeth-to-teeth contact without biting. The upper cervical spine active physiological and passive accessory movements are then re-assessed while this mandibular position is maintained. For Floor, these were as follows:

- Extension – normal head-on-neck movement (60 degrees, previously 46 degrees)
- Lateral flexion to the right – 15 degrees no 'pulling' (previously 9 degrees with a 3/10 'pulling' on the VAS)
- Rotation right – 76 degrees (previously 60 degrees)
- Flexion/rotation test – right rotation 42 degrees (previously 33 degrees)
- PAMs:
  - Right unilateral postero-anterior accessory movement at C1–C2 demonstrated a reduction of more than 50% in stiffness, and only minimal neck pain was reproduced when performed both in neutral (2/10 on the VAS) and in 30 degrees right rotation (3/10).
  - Right unilateral postero-anterior accessory movement at C1–C2 performed in maximal active left laterotrusion of the mandible did not provoke any tinnitus (previously 4/10 on the VAS).

Treatment

The neurophysiological connections between the orofacial region and the upper cervical spine were briefly explained as a possible mechanism for Floor's tinnitus and headache (discussed with respect to the findings of the passive unilateral pressure on C1–C2 performed in left laterotrusion of the mandible and the occlusal kinaesthetic test). The neurocranial techniques were proposed to decrease the nasal resistance, with the increase in airflow contributing to the decrease in tinnitus. As such, the following were performed:

- Right passive accessory unilateral postero-anterior mobilization at C1–C2 with the mandible at end of range active laterotrusion to the left
- Passive medial temporal mobilizations (grade IV) sustained for 5–8 seconds around the transverse arche for 8 minutes, without increasing face symptoms

Physical Re-assessment

Nasal Respiration

- Inspiration sounds were equal between right and left, with equal 5-second durations and no symptom provocation.

TMJ

- Active laterotrusion to the right was 13 mm, with no symptom provocation on overpressure.
- Passive laterotrusion to the right demonstrated no stiffness compared with the left and no provocation of symptoms.

Neurocranium

- The neurocranium was not re-assessed because of the intense treatment of the neurocranium and the minor signs and symptoms reproduced during the previous upper cervical spine assessment.
- The same pattern as found during the occlusal kinaesthetic test was present, only now the upper cervical movements had retained the improved range of movement without the teeth-to-teeth occlusal position being maintained.
- Passive right unilateral accessory movement at C1–C2 now demonstrated a 75% improvement in stiffness, with no provocation of local pain when performed in neutral and only slight pain (1/10 on the VAS) when performed in 30 degrees right rotation.
- At the end of the appointment, Floor was asked to continue both the laterotrusion and the respiration exercises at the same dosage but was to increase the time with each by 50% or more.

Fifth Appointment (2 Weeks Later, Day 47)

Subjective re-assessment

Floor reported only having one episode of headache and tinnitus (2/10 on the VAS) since the last appointment, and she associated that with a minor cold she had experienced for 2 days. Both the headache and tinnitus went away immediately after the cold resolved. She stated she was now less conscious of her cross-bite (which was still present) and was still happy with her improved nasal respiration, noting she could now get 'more air'. Floor also reported she had not experienced any of her lower-quarter pains in the last 14 days.

Floor discussed her thoughts about canceling the second bimaxillary surgery. Although she continued to worry about the cost and acknowledged the enormous reduction in her symptoms with the current treatment, she still found her face unattractive and therefore was still considering going ahead with surgery. She also added that her family had advised her to cancel the operation.

Physical Re-assessment

TMJ and Upper Cervical Spine

- Habitual occlusion – cross-bite toward left still present.
- Nasal respiration equal between the right and left sides
- Active and passive TMJ movements were now relatively equal and within the normal range of movement, with no provocation of symptoms.
- Upper cervical spine active and passive movement assessments were also now within a relatively normal range of movement, with no provocation of symptoms, except for passive right unilateral postero-anterior accessory movement at C1–C2 performed in mandible laterotrusion to the right, which still provoked local neck pain (3/10 on the VAS) with a grade IV pressure. The flexion/rotation test to the right was 40 degrees (previously 42 degrees after the fourth treatment).

Craniofacial Region

- The diagonal occiput right – frontal left – temporal dorsal rotation around the transverse arches and the transverse rotation of the occiput to the left no longer provoked Floor's headache and tinnitus. The resistance and the rebounce qualities of these movements were now the same as on the left side.
- The only abnormality found with the craniofacial assessments was a provocation of tinnitus (2/10 on the VAS) with a grade IV temporal–sphenoid accessory movement repeated five times for 5–8 seconds.

Spine and Posture

- The improvement in observation of posture and objective assessment of COG reported at the end of the third appointment was retained, with no further change.
- The craniocervical angle now measured 49 degrees (initially this was 45 degrees; normal is 51 degrees).

After this re-assessment, a systematic process of reflection with Floor was undertaken to assess her current understanding. The following were discussed:

- All her symptoms seemed to have resolved, and this was likely related to the improvements in her different physical dysfunctions (TMJ, upper cervical spine, neurocranium, lower quarter).
- The lower-quarter symptoms were probably due to compensations of her body for her face and neck problems.
- Some of the dysfunctions may have been due to stiffness in the tissues themselves, but it is likely a lot of the problems were due to patterns of neck and jaw movement she had acquired over her life and that these two areas have a neurophysiological connection.
- Because of these neurophysiological links, it is important to have a long-term management plan in order to minimize recurrence of her symptoms.
- It would also be a good idea to have further opinions and a multidisciplinary consensus about the value of the planned bimaxillary surgery.

Given the significant reduction in Floor's symptoms and signs, a retrospective assessment of the questionnaires and the Face Lateralization–Emotion Recognition Test were conducted, as follows
Questionnaires

- Toronto Alexithymia Scale 26 = 2.19 (previously 2.21), which is not indicative of a clear change.
- Neck Disability Index = 34 (previously 63), suggesting a clear change.
- Beck Disability Index II = 12 (previously 18), which represents a small reduction.

Lateralization and Emotion Recognition Assessment

- Lateralization: of the 48 pictures presented, Floor correctly identified 47 at an average speed of 2.8 seconds (previously 3.6) for left face pictures and 1.4 seconds (previously 1.9) for right face pictures. This shows that normal interpretation had been retained and that the speed of judgements involving right face recognition had improved, with an average of 2.2 seconds (previously 2.6).
- Emotion recognition: Floor again scored 100% for happiness, 86% for astonished and disgusted and 21% (previously 17%) for fear and sadness. The total percentage of incorrect answers was 26% (previously 32%), and 8% (previously 10%) were not answered in time (decision > 5 seconds), with the average judgement speed being 3.75 seconds (previously 3.92). Emotion recognition was still clearly below normal reference values. From this, it may be concluded that Floor still had a disturbed (face) body image that was likely contributing to her emotion recognition dysfunction, all of which was related to her negative personal self-image.

The proposed long-term management was multi-faceted, to include the following:

- Continued treatment (e.g. once every 4–6 weeks) to further reduce the minor neuro-musculoskeletal impairments and progress the home exercises
- A graded activity program challenging Floor's daily activities, including running, biking, swimming and possibly her work
- Daily facial motor imagery and face-emotion training on her home computer to improve her explicit, and eventually her implicit, image recognition and hopefully also her self-image
- Multidisciplinary consultations involving a psychologist regarding her cognitive and emotional status related to her personal self-image and with her maxillofacial surgeon to discuss the likelihood of surgery providing a symmetrical face, given this is her sole purpose for still considering the surgery

Treatment

Floor's treatment at this stage was predominantly 'hands off' because her neuromusculoskeletal impairments were now relatively minor.

Additional activities at home were prescribed:

- Neck exercise: The flexion/rotation test toward the right in supine lying was explained. Floor was asked to lay supine with both hands on the dorsal side of her head. From this position, she was asked to actively perform an upper cervical flexion nodding without teeth contact. Next, she was instructed to maintain this supported upper cervical flexion position and actively perform a cervical rotation to the right up to the end of her available movement. There should not be any provocation of facial symptoms; however, an upper cervical 'pulling' may be felt, and that is normal. The exercise should be done as 6–10 repetitions and added to the TMJ and face exercises she had already been doing.
- Graded activity program: In the past, Floor had enjoyed running. Although she liked to run daily for 45 minutes, more recently she had only been running 20 minutes because any longer would tend to aggravate both her headache and her restricted respiration. For graded activity of running, Floor was asked to reduce her daily runs to 15 minutes with a 20% reduction in her running effort. If after 7 days she felt well and had no aggravation of her symptoms, she could increase her time by 20% (about 2 minutes) up to 18 minutes and also try increasing her effort. After 3 weeks she could increase her duration again a further 20% up to 22 minutes. While implementing this program, Floor was asked to keep track of her daily reactions and to write these down in a diary that we could review at the next appointment.
- Lateralization training: Related to Floor's disrupted body (face) image, lateralization exercises were initiated with a special assessment and exercise computer program (CRAFTA Face Lateralization–Emotion Recognition Program; see www.physioedu .com or www.trainyourface.com). The program includes a total of 72 randomized face and neck pictures with a time setting of 3 seconds for each picture. Floor was asked to practice this for 10 minutes each day at a time that was convenient for her.

It was also suggested that Floor visit a clinical psychologist who specializes in post-traumatic surgery. Although Floor was initially surprised by this suggestion, indicating she didn't feel she had a 'psychological' problem, after further discussion about the negative feelings she had shared (particularly related to her appearance) and explanation of how emotions can significantly influence other body processes and function (e.g. pain but also tinnitus and respiration), she agreed it was worth trying.

Sixth Appointment (4 Weeks Later, Day 72)

Subjective Re-assessment

The unilateral right tinnitus had only been provoked twice since the last appointment (4/10 on the VAS each time) and only lasted about 30–45 minutes. On further questioning, Floor associated both episodes of tinnitus to minor stressful situations that she said were easy to control. She only had her headache premenstrually (2/10 on the VAS), with no headaches proved by oral activity (talking, eating) or posture/activity (sitting, running). Floor also reported her respiration was significantly improved, with only minor awareness still present with her running. She felt her open-bite and shift of her mandible were also improved, and she was aware of having better teeth contact (see also Fig. 19.8 habitual occlusion). Floor reported her exercises had been going well, including the new flexion/rotation test exercise added at the last appointment. She had been able to progress her running time to 45 minutes, five times per week, without any complaints. Although she did perform the lateralization exercises regularly for 3 weeks, she felt they were becoming too easy and could not see how they were helping now, and consequently, she was doing them less frequently.

Visit to the Psychologist

After two visits to the psychologist, Floor was diagnosed with a minor form of 'dysmorphophobia'. Dysmorphophobia is a body dysmorphic disorder (Buhlmann et al., 2013) characterized by a profound negative distortion of body image. In Floor's case, this was linked to her perceived craniofacial flaws and associated perception of imperfections in appearance. This can lead to compulsive checking of one's appearance in the mirror, intense self-consciousness, social avoidance, isolation and depression (Enander et al., 2014). Floor's score of 7 on the Body Dysmorphic Symptoms Inventory (Buhlmann et al., 2013) was minor. This inventory is a valid and reliable measurement for body dysmorphic disorder. It is an 18-item self-report inventory with total scores ranging from 0 to 64 (Buhlmann et al., 2013). The psychologist recommended that Floor continue the lateralization and emotion recognition training and did not feel additional cognitive-behavioural therapy was indicated.

Visit to the Maxillofacial Surgeon

Floor informed the surgeon that she did not want surgery at this stage given her improvement with physiotherapy. The surgeon agreed but could not explain why her habitual occlusion was now less of an open-bite with a reduced shift toward the left because she still had the same maxillofacial deformity as noted at the last visit 8 months ago. The surgeon supported her continued therapy but advised her to come back annually over 5 years for re-evaluation.

Physical Re-assessment

There was a clear difference in Floor's occlusion when compared with the first appointment (Fig. 19.9).

Re-assessment of the main physical impairments as assessed at the fifth appointment revealed no change. Re-assessment of home performance of home exercises illustrated Floor had good understanding and technique.

Lateralization Test

Floor correctly identified all 48 pictures at an average speed of 1.5 seconds (previously 3.6 seconds during the first treatment) for left face pictures and 1.3 seconds (previously 1.9) for right face pictures, with an average of 1.6 seconds per picture (previously 2.2 seconds).

Treatment

Lateralization and Emotion Recognition Training

Because emotion recognition and expression may be a reflection of a dysfunction in motor processes, the following lateralization exercises, emotion recognition and expression training were followed (von Piekartz et al., 2014):

- Lateralization exercises as described in the last treatment, with left–right face activities progressed for better accuracy and speed. Left neck and hand pictures were integrated because there was no left–right accuracy difference, and the speed was (nearly) the same (< 0.5-second difference). Floor was also asked to attend to the left versus right head

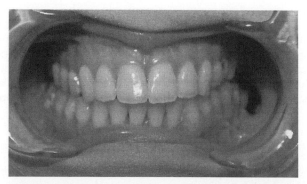

Fig. 19.9 Floor's habitual occlusion on day 72 compared to the first assessment (Fig. 19.4C). Note the reduced mandibular shift to the left and reduced open-bite occlusion.

rotation in any pictures she came across in articles or books, as described within the principles of Graded Motor Imagery (Moseley et al., 2012).

- Emotion recognition training was started with emotions that were easily recognized by Floor (happiness, astonished, disgusted) because the accuracy of the emotion recognition test was >95% and the average time was <0.5 seconds. Her training commenced with 75% of the pictures being of these easy-to-recognize emotions and the remaining 25% of the pictures being of emotions more difficult for Floor to recognize, like fear and sadness. The percentage of more difficult pictures can then be increased after a week. When all the emotions can be recognized with 90% accuracy, emotion imagination (implicit training) and emotion expression (explicit training) are introduced, together with face mirroring. Both of these are integrated in the CRAFTA face mirror program (von Piekartz and Mohr, 2014; Mohr et al., 2015).

The hypothesis guiding this management is that this training can improve perceptual dysfunction and alexithymia Glaros, A.G., Lumley, M.A., 2005, with potential to improve (chronic) pain and Floor's body dysmorphic disorder. Because Floor lived 300 km away, it was agreed that she would continue this face training program online (von Piekartz and Mohr, 2014).

Seventh (2 Months Later, Day 91) and Eighth (3 Months Later, Day 108) Appointments

Both of these appointments were conducted online, with a focus on assessing Floor's status and reviewing her home exercises, as well as her lateralization and emotion training.

At the eighth appointment the questionnaires and lateralization and emotion tests were re-assessed, and daily activities were discussed, with the following results:

Questionnaires (score compared with the first session)

- Neck Disability Index = 2 (64)
- Beck Disability Index II = 8 (21)
- Toronto Alexithymia Scale 26 = 1.28 (2.21).

Lateralization and emotion tests

- Online standard lateralization test accuracy 100% (left average of 1.0 seconds, right 1.3)
- Emotion recognition
  - Happiness 100% (was 100% at first appointment)
  - Astonished 100% (86%)
  - Disgusted 92% (86%)
  - Fear and sadness 92% (17%)

The total percentage of incorrect answers was just 4% (32%), none (0%) were not in time (10%) and average judgement speed was 1.3 seconds (3.92). Emotion recognition was now within normal reference values, reflecting that Floor's (face) body image and emotion recognition function were restored.

Daily activity: Floor was running three times per week, now for 45 minutes, without any complaints and was swimming twice a week, also without any problems. Floor had also commenced working at a bank the past 2 weeks for 20 hours per week and reported having no difficulties thus far. She also noted she no longer had any sleeping disturbances.

With these significant improvements in symptoms and function, it was agreed that no further appointments were required. Floor was advised she could discontinue her lateralization and emotion recognition training but should continue with her regular exercise. She was invited to get back in contact if she experienced any recurrence of symptoms.

REFERENCES

Abel, M.D., Levine, R.A., 2004. Muscle contractions and auditory perception in tinnitus patients and nonclinical subjects. Cranio. 22 (3), 81–191.

Avivi-Arber, L., et al., 2010. Neuroplasticity of face sensorimotor cortex and implications for control of orofacial movements. Jpn. Dent. Sci. Rev. 46–56.

Beck, A.T., Steer, R.A., Brown, G.K., 1996. Beck Depression Inventory: Manual, 2nd ed. Harcourt Brace, Boston.

Berryman, C., et al., 2014. Do people with chronic pain have impaired executive function? A meta-analytical review. Clin. Psychol. Rev. 34, 563–579.

Bray, H., Moseley, G., 2011. Disrupted working body schema of the trunk in people with back pain. Br. J. Sports Med. 45 (3), 168–173.

Buhlmann, U., Winter, A., Kathmann, N., 2013. Emotion recognition in body dysmorphic disorder: application of the Reading the Mind in the Eyes Task. Body Image 10 (2), 247–250.

Butler, D., 2000. The Sensitive Nervous System. Noigroup, Adelaide, Australia.

Chaitow, L.A., 2005. A brief historical perspective. In: Cranial Manipulation. Theory and Practice, 2nd ed. Elsevier, Edinburgh, pp. 1–13.

Cohen, D., Perez, R., 2003. Bilateral myoclonus of the tensor tympani: a case report. Otolaryngol. Head Neck Surg. 128, 441.

De Leeuw, R., Klasser, G., 2013. Orofacial Pain. Guidelines for Assessment, Diagnosis and Management, 5th ed. Quintessence, Chicago.

Dworkin, S.F., LeResche, L., 1992. Research diagnostic criteria for temporomandibular disorders: review, criteria examinations and specifications, critique. J. Craniomandib. Disord. 6, 301–355.

Enander, J., et al., 2014. Therapist-guided, Internet-based cognitive–behavioural therapy for body dysmorphic disorder (BDD-NET): a feasibility study. BMJ Open 4 (9), 1–11.

Geerse, W., Von Piekartz, H., 2015. Ear pain following temporomandibular surgery originating from the temporomandibular joint or the cranial nervous tissue? A case report. Man. Ther. 20 (1), 212–215.

Glaros, A.G., Lumley, M.A., 2005. Alexithymia and pain in temporomandibular disorder. J. Psychosom. Res. 59 (2), 85–88.

Hardell, L., et al., 2003. Vestibular schwannoma, tinnitus and cellular telephones. Neuroepidemiology 22 (2), 124–129.

Heike, C., Hing, A., 2009. Craniofacial Microsomia Overview. In: Pagon, R.A., et al. (Eds.), Gene Reviews. University of Washington, Seattle, pp. 1993–2014.

Hengeveld, E., Banks, K. (Eds.), 2014. Maitland's Peripheral Manipulation, 5th ed: Management of neuromusculoskeletal disorders, vol. 2. Churchill Livingstone, London, pp. 88–142.

Hilgenberg, P.B., et al., 2012. Temporomandibular disorders, otologic symptoms and depression levels in tinnitus patients. J. Oral. Rehabil. 39 (4), 239–244.

Joshi, N., Hamdan, A., Fakhour, W., 2014. Skeletal malocclusion: a developmental disorder with a life-long morbidity. J. Clin. Med. Res. 6 (6), 399–408.

Kaltenbach, J.A., et al., 2004. Activity in the dorsal cochlear nucleus of hamsters previously tested for tinnitus following intense tone exposure. Neurosci. Lett. 355 (1–2), 121–125.

Kluemper, G.T., Spalding, P.M., 2001. Realities of craniofacial growth modification. Atlas Oral Maxillofac. Surg. Clin. North Am. 9 (1), 23–51.

Kupfer, J., Brosig, B., Brähler, E., 2000. Testing and validation of the 26-Item Toronto Alexithymia Scale in a representative population sample. Z. Psychosom. Med. Psychother. 46 (4), 368–384.

Leake, H., 2012. Investigating cortical proprioceptive maps in people with neck pain: a left/right neck rotation judgment task [Honours]. University of South Australia.

Levine, R.A., Abel, M., Cheng, H., 2003. CNS somatosensory-auditory interactions elicit or modulate tinnitus. Exp. Brain Res. 153 (4), 643–648.

Linder-Aronson, S., Woodside, D., 2000. Excess face height malocclusion. Etiology 1–35.

Lumley, M.A., et al., 2011. Pain and emotion: a biopsychosocial review of recent research. J. Clin. Psychol. 67 (9), 942–968.

Maísa Soares, G., Rizzatti-Barbosa, C.M., 2015. Chronicity factors of temporomandibular disorders: a critical review of the literature. Braz. Oral Res. 29 (1).

Manfredini, D., et al., 2010. Chronic pain severity and depression/somatization levels in TMD patients. Int. J. Prosthodont. 23 (6), 529–534.

Mohr, G., Konnerth, V., Von Piekartz, H., 2015. von Piekartz, H. (Ed.), Lateralitätserkennung und (emotionale) Expressionen des Gesichts – Beurteilung und Behandlung in Kiefer, Gesichts - und Zervikalregion Neuromuskuloskeletale Untersuchung, Therapie und Mangagement. Thieme, Stuttgart, pp. 505–522.

Moseley, L., et al., 2012. The Graded Imagery Handbook. Noigroup Publications, Adelaide, Australia.

Okayasu, I., et al., 2014. Tactile sensory and pain thresholds in the face and tongue of subjects asymptomatic for oro-facial pain and headache. J. Oral Rehabil. 41 (12), 875–880.

Okeson, J., 2014. The Neurophysiology of Nociception. The Dorsal Horn in Oral and Facial Pain, 7th ed. Quintessence, Chicago, pp. 16–156.

Oudhof, H., 2001. Skull growth in relation with mechanical stimulation. Craniofacial Dysfunction 2001, 1–22.

Palazzi, C., et al., 1996. Body position effects on EMG activity of sternocleidomastoid and masseter muscle in patients with myogenic cranio-cervical-mandibular dysfunction. Cranio. 14, 200–207.

Proffit, W.R., Fields, H.W., Jr., Sarver, D.M., 2006. Contemporary Orthodontics. Elsevier Health Sciences, pp. 18–34.

Rowicki, T., Zakrzewska, J., 2006. A study of the discomalleolar ligament in the adult human. Folia Morphol. 65 (2), 121–125.

Saccucci, M., et al., 2011. Scoliosis and dental occlusion: a review of the literature. Scoliosis 6, 15.

Schueler, M., et al., 2013. Extracranial projections of meningeal afferents and their impact on meningeal nociception and headache. Pain 154 (9), 1622–1631.

Taylor, B.K., Corder, G., 2014. Endogenous analgesia, dependence, and latent pain sensitization. Curr. Top. Behav. Neurosci. 20, 283–325.

Vernon, H., 2008. The Neck Disability Index: state-of-the-art, 1991-2008. J. Manipulative Physiol. Ther. 31 (7), 491–502.

Vincent, M.B., 2010. Cervicogenic headache: a review comparison with migraine, tension-type headache, and whiplash. Curr. Pain Headache Rep. 14 (3), 238–243.

von Piekartz, H.J.M., 2007. von Piekartz, H. (Ed.), Craniomandibular region – clinical patterns and management. Craniofacial Pain: Neuromusculoskeletal Assessment, Treatment and Management, first ed. Elsevier, Edinburgh, pp. 214–243.

von Piekartz, H.J.M., et al., 2014. People with chronic facial pain perform worse than controls at a facial emotion recognition task; but it's not all about the emotion. J. Oral Rehabil. 1–7.

von Piekartz, H.J.M., Mohr, G., 2014. Reduction of head and face pain by challenging lateralization and basic emotions: a proposal for future assessment and rehabilitation strategies. J. Man. Manip. Ther. 22 (1), 24–35.

Zhou, S., et al., 2013. A correlational study of scoliosis and trunk balance in adult patients with mandibular deviation. PLoS ONE 8 (3), e59929.

Zöller, J.E., et al., 2005. Kraniosynosthosen in Kraniofaziale. Chirurgie. Diagnostik und therapie kraniofazialer Fehlbildung. Thieme Stuttgart 3–25.

20

Cervical Radiculopathy With Neurological Deficit

Helen Clare • Stephen May • Darren A. Rivett

History

Peter is a 55-year-old television news editor. His work requires him to be seated while viewing six television screens positioned around him and editing the film using a desktop computer. It is difficult for him to leave his desk apart from during his lunch break, and he is not able to adjust the height or position of the television monitors. When not at work, he spends between 2 and 3 hours each day on a laptop computer at home. He also spends 30 minutes in the car travelling to and from his work. Peter does no regular exercise but enjoys fishing and occasionally swimming in the summer.

Peter presented complaining of intermittent right-sided neck pain, which radiated into the posterior deltoid region, the posterior aspect of the forearm and into his hand. He constantly experienced tingling in the right thumb and index finger but reported no areas of decreased sensation (Fig. 20.1). Peter provided average ratings of the pain intensity on a numerical scale ranging from 0 (no pain) to 10 (worst pain imaginable) – he rated the neck and upper arm pain as 5/10 and the forearm pain as 8/10.

Peter woke 4 weeks ago with acute right-sided neck pain and limited neck movement. He could not recall any reason for this happening but had experienced similar episodes in the past, but these normally resolved over 2 or 3 days without any treatment. Specifically, he could not recall any changes in lifestyle or ergonomic setup that might have precipitated this episode or prolonged it beyond normal. Over the next 3 weeks, his symptoms worsened and radiated into the right arm, with tingling developing in his right hand 2 weeks ago. As the upper arm and forearm pain developed, the neck pain reduced in intensity, and his neck movement improved slightly.

Aggravating and Easing Activities and Postures

The symptoms worsened in Peter's arm when he was sitting, when using the mouse at his computer and when driving. His neck pain was worse when rotating his head to the right and when looking up. The arm pain was much worse by the end of the day, especially the days he worked. Generally, Peter's symptoms were better in the mornings and when he was moving. The pain in the right trapezius region and forearm woke him at night if he turned onto his left side or lay supine. Lying on his right side gave him relief. Peter reported that he used a contoured rubber pillow, which he has previously found comfortable. Having his arm hanging by his side when walking and standing aggravated his arm symptoms, which he relieved by supporting under his right elbow with his other arm. He was avoiding using his right arm for lifting and carrying, but he was unsure if those activities actually aggravated his symptoms.

Peter completed a Neck Disability Index functional questionnaire, on which he scored 28/50, which indicates a moderate level of perceived functional disability (Vernon and Mior, 1991; Vernon, 2000).

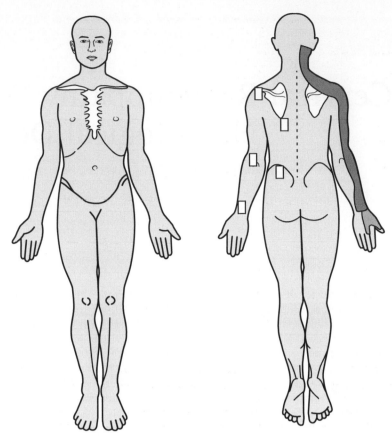

Fig. 20.1   Body chart depicting area of symptoms. Pain is indicated by dark grey shading and tingling by light grey shading.

General Health and Medical Management

Peter's general health was unremarkable, with no other comorbidities, and there was no reported weight loss. He had not experienced any dizziness, nausea or tinnitus. Nor had he noticed any alteration in his gait or clumsiness. He had not noticed any reduction in strength when using his right hand. His sleep was disturbed, but this related to the position of his neck, and he could reduce the pain and return to sleep by changing his neck position.

While Peter had remained at work, he had reduced the time he spent on his computer at home and tried to limit his driving time. He had consulted his general practitioner (GP), who had prescribed slow-release celecoxib tablets (anti-inflammatory medication), and he had been taking these regularly for 3 weeks but had not noticed any significant difference in his symptoms. Peter was also taking paracetamol (analgesic medication) two or three times per day for pain relief, primarily whilst he was at work. His GP had referred him for a magnetic resonance imaging (MRI) scan of his cervical spine, which revealed a right paracentral disc protrusion at C5/C6, narrowing the entry zone to the right neural foramen and compressing the right C6 nerve root (Fig. 20.2).

The GP had advised Peter that the cause of his symptoms was a disc impinging on a nerve in his neck, and if conservative treatment was not beneficial, she would refer him to a spinal surgeon. He commented that he definitely was not keen on surgery and was prepared to exhaust all forms of conservative treatment before considering surgery.

Reasoning Question:

1. What were your initial thoughts about Peter's presentation? In particular, did you entertain any hypotheses at this time relating to 'precautions and contraindications to physical examination and treatment' and also 'contributing factors' to the insidious onset?

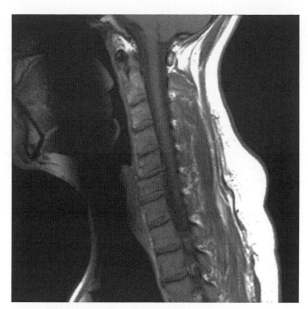

Fig. 20.2   Magnetic resonance imaging scan demonstrating right paracentral disc protrusion at C5/C6.

Answer to Reasoning Question:

There appeared to be no initial precautions or contraindications to conducting a physical examination. From the history, it was apparent that the symptoms were responsive to different postures and positions, being worse with long periods of sitting and better when he was moving, which was considered to be a positive sign that Peter might respond well to mechanical therapy (McKenzie and May, 2006). Hypothetically, the source of the symptoms could be related to a nerve root, but identifying the source of the symptoms (or contributing factors) was less clinically relevant in this case than determining whether the symptoms were responsive to mechanical therapy.

Reasoning Question:

2. Pain is clearly Peter's main complaint. What were your hypotheses at this stage regarding the dominant 'pain type' (nociceptive, peripheral neuropathic, nociplastic)? What evidence supported or negated your hypotheses?

Answer to Reasoning Question:

The clinical reasoning process undertaken in this case was not greatly focussed on identifying either the source of pain or the hypothesized 'pain type', whether it be nociceptive, peripheral neuropathic or nociplastic. However, from the clear mechanical nature of the presenting pain (i.e. linked to activities) and the lack of apparent psychological factors, it did not appear to be the latter, which has been defined as pain associated with maladaptive processes in the CNS (Wright, 2002) in which there is 'an amplification of neural signalling within the central nervous system that elicits pain hypersensitivity' (Woolf, 2010). The location of the symptoms and their consistent response to mechanical forces suggested that his pain was a mixture of nociceptive neck pain and peripheral neuropathic pain, with the referred arm symptoms and tingling in the hand originating from compromise of the peripheral nerve(s) or nerve root(s) (Wright, 2002). However, the clinical distinction between nerve root pain and musculoskeletal nociceptive pain is not straightforward: somatic structures can refer distally (Bogduk, 2002), and dermatomal pain patterns have been found not to be useful in the diagnosis of radicular pain (Murphy et al., 2009). Further testing of a neuropathic component would require a neurological examination.

Clinical Reasoning Commentary:

Although the 'hypothesis categories' framework presented in Chapter 1 is not integrated into all musculoskeletal approaches, these responses still reflect a clinical reasoning process guided by the McKenzie mechanical therapy approach. Patient cues (e.g. from the behaviour of symptoms) have elicited recognition of a mechanical pattern of aggravation and easing supportive of a nociceptive and/or peripheral neuropathic pain type and indicative of a favourable prognosis.

It is likely that the clinician did not undertake any procedures that peripheralized Peter's symptoms, partly because it is associated with a less successful outcome but also because it may be associated with further 'neural' irritation/compromise. In other words, the clinician is attending to the 'sources' of the symptoms. Further, the fact that the clinician is associating the arm symptoms with the neck

Continued on following page

symptoms, based on the pattern of behaviour, means it is also likely the judgement is being reached that the arm symptoms are arising from neck structures. This too represents consideration of 'sources'. This can be seen to reflect that while clinical reasoning language is not necessarily universal across musculoskeletal approaches, the actual processes of clinical reasoning and the actual hypothesis judgements made have a great deal of commonality.

This supports the supposition that hypotheses are generated as a normal or generic component of human thinking and problem solving, based on accessible knowledge derived from personal and direct clinical experiences, as well as empirical research and experiential professional craft knowledge. It is likely that whatever particular approach to musculoskeletal management that clinicians may typically prefer to adopt following their training, they will generally employ an underpinning clinical reasoning process similar to that of other clinicians providing they are not simply following pre-determined protocols on the basis of imaging rather that the patient's specific clinical presentation..

Physical Examination

Posture

During the history taking, Peter sat in a chair with a flexed lumbar and thoracic spine and a protruded head (Fig. 20.3A). When sitting in this position, he reported that he was experiencing right forearm pain which he verbally rated as 6/10. Correction of his sitting posture reduced the intensity of the forearm pain to a 3/10 but produced right scapula pain. Postural correction was undertaken by providing a support for the lumbar spine and manually facilitating an erect cervical spine, with Peter educated about the inter-relationship between these two spinal components (Fig. 20.3B).

Neurological Examination

A neurological examination was performed because of the radicular distribution of Peter's arm symptoms and because he reported constant tingling in his right thumb and index finger. There was only a minimal flicker with the right triceps reflex test, and the strength of the right triceps muscle was graded 2 out of 5 (movement possible, but not against gravity). There was decreased sensation to light touch over the right thumb and index finger.

Neurodynamics

A modified upper limb tension test was performed in sitting with the right arm abducted to 45 degrees, the elbow straight and forearm supinated; then, alternately, cervical spine

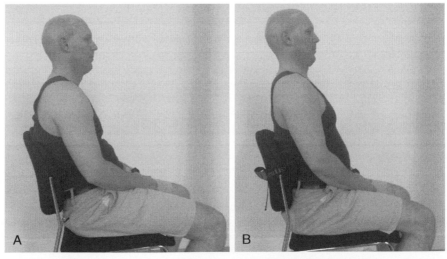

Fig. 20.3 (A) Habitual sitting posture. (B) Corrected sitting posture.

flexion and left lateral flexion were added. Neither of these cervical movements altered the symptoms that Peter had reported in his right arm.

Movement Testing

Cervical Spine

Peter demonstrated a major loss of cervical spine retraction and extension, with both movements causing right scapula area pain. He was able to flex so that his chin touched his sternum, but this produced pain in his right upper arm. Right rotation was limited to 35 degrees (producing right neck pain rated as 6/10) and left rotation to 45 degrees (producing left and right neck pain rated as 4/10). Peter had a major loss of right lateral flexion range of motion, which produced right upper arm pain, and a lesser loss of left lateral flexion, which produced only right-sided neck pain.

Right Shoulder

Peter's shoulder movements were next examined. On abduction of his right arm, he reported experiencing right deltoid area pain between 80 and 120 degrees. Forward elevation of his right arm produced pain in the deltoid region at 120 degrees, which increased as he moved further into range. External rotation at zero degrees of abduction performed with the elbow bent was limited to 50% of range (compared to the left arm) by right upper arm pain. Passively, there was full-range pain-free shoulder movement in all planes. On isometric resisted muscle testing, both abduction and external rotation of the right shoulder were painful and weak.

Repeated Movement Testing

A cervical spine repeated movement examination was performed in sitting. Prior to commencing, Peter reported a baseline level of right forearm pain of 4/10 and pins and needles in his right thumb and index finger. He performed cervical retraction 15 times. After five movements, his resting right forearm pain was abolished, pain in his right deltoid region was produced but was then abolished and strong right scapula pain was produced. Peter was encouraged to move further into range with each retraction movement as long as it did not increase his arm symptoms. Following the 15 repeated retraction movements, he reported a significant reduction in the pins and needles in his hand, the right forearm pain remained abolished, but he was now experiencing right scapula pain which he rated as 6/10. His cervical mobility was visually re-assessed, and there was an approximate 50% increase in the range of cervical rotation in both directions and also of cervical extension. On re-testing active right shoulder abduction, pain was not experienced until 120 degrees, and Peter commented that he was able to move his arm more freely. The other baseline measures, including the neurological deficit, were unaltered.

Reasoning Question:

3. What prompted you to examine repeated movements of the cervical spine, and what was your interpretation of the findings from that examination?

Answer to Reasoning Question:

Peter's symptoms demonstrated a directional preference in response to repeated retraction (which involves extension of the lower cervical spine and some flexion of the upper cervical spine). Initially, when his sitting posture was corrected, which positioned his head and neck in a retracted position, he reported a reduction in his forearm pain (which was his most distal) and production of right scapula pain (which was a more central location of pain than he had been experiencing). This response suggested a repeated cervical retraction movement examination might be useful. When Peter performed repeated retraction movements, both symptomatic and mechanical improvements were achieved. Centralization of his pain had occurred with his right forearm pain abolished and a more central scapula pain produced, and importantly, these changes remained after the retraction movements were ceased. On re-assessment of his mechanical (movement) baseline, an increase in cervical rotation had been achieved, and his active shoulder abduction range had increased before pain commenced.

Continued on following page

Thus, centralization of symptoms was achieved with repeated cervical retraction movements performed in sitting, and rapid changes were observed both in his symptoms and in his baseline mechanics. On interpretation, Peter had therefore demonstrated clinical criteria consistent with the classification of a 'derangement' under the McKenzie classification protocol (McKenzie and May, 2006). Derangement is operationally defined as follows:

- Centralization, abolition or decrease of symptoms in response to therapeutic loading
- Which is retained over time
- And accompanied by restoration of range of movement and function (McKenzie and May, 2006)

This centralization response also suggested repeated retraction movements were a potential option for treatment. In the lumbar spine, there is evidence that shows patients treated with exercises involving their directional preference have better outcomes than those treated with exercises involving the opposite direction to their directional preference or with generic exercise (Long et al., 2004, 2008; Browder et al., 2007; Fritz et al., 2003). The research support for the use of directional preference exercise is not as strong in the cervical spine, but it has been as commonly reported as for the lumbar spine in an observational study (Werneke et al., 1999), and clinical experience indicates that it has similar benefits.

Management Day 1

Management consisted of two components: an educational element and an exercise element.

Educational Element

Peter was informed that it was likely that mechanical loading of the right paracentral disc protrusion at C5/C6 was causing his neck pain, and at times, the exiting C6 nerve root was being irritated, and this was responsible for the arm pain and tingling in his hand. He was further informed it appeared that the problem was reversible, however, given that the symptoms were intermittent and were aggravated by certain activities and eased by others, that his management could utilise this apparent directional preference.

A key aspect of management was to educate Peter about how to avoid further aggravation of his symptoms. This involved education about trying to maintain a retracted head posture, especially when sitting at work, when driving and when using the computer at home. To assist in achieving this, the ergonomics of his workplace (desk, chair and computer relationship) was discussed. Peter advised that he was unable to adjust the height or position of the television monitors, but he was confident that he could alter his sitting posture and adjust the position of his computer. His sitting postures when driving and when working on his computer at home were also discussed.

Peter was provided with a lumbar support to use when sitting, as ensuring that the lumbar spine retains a lordosis makes it easier to keep the head retracted.

A cervical night roll was also provided for use at night, with the aim of maintaining a neutral position of the neck when sleeping. This was provided because Peter reported that his sleeping was disturbed, and he woke if he rolled onto his left side or back.

Exercise Element

For management, Peter was asked to perform cervical retraction exercises in sitting as often as required to minimize his right forearm symptoms. He was advised that when he was sitting at his computer, this may need to be as frequent as hourly. The number of repetitions he needed to perform depended on how many movements it took to abolish his forearm symptoms and produce right scapula pain – that is, to centralize his symptoms.

Guidelines for Daily Living

In the interim between appointments, Peter was asked to monitor both the location and intensity of his right arm symptoms. Using the concept of a 'traffic light' (green indicates go, red indicates stop, yellow indicates proceed with caution), Peter was advised that any activity that produced or increased his right forearm pain or pins and needles was a 'red light', and he needed to avoid or limit this position or activity. If he was experiencing scapula pain and minimal or no right arm symptoms, then this was a 'green light' and indicated that whatever position, movement or activity he was performing was appropriate. A 'yellow light' indicated movements or postures that did not appear to affect the symptoms, so it was not necessary to avoid these or to specifically perform them.

It was further explained to Peter that, ultimately, he was in control of how his symptoms behaved, but it was the clinician's responsibility to provide him with the education and knowledge so that he could self-manage his symptoms. It was stressed that it was important for him to perform the retraction exercises regularly and to limit or avoid his aggravating activities. At the conclusion, Peter was given the opportunity to ask any questions about his symptoms and about the information and instructions he had been given.

Reasoning Question:

4. Did you consider there to be any psychosocial factors influencing Peter's pain presentation?

Answer to Reasoning Question:

No, for the following reasons. In his history, Peter did not display any fear-avoidance behaviours to activities and movements. He had remained at work, despite it aggravating his symptoms, and he was taking sensible amounts of pain relief medication. His scoring on the Neck Disability Index also indicated a moderate but appropriate level of perceived functional disability. Given that Peter's presentation appeared to be mechanical in nature (based on the history), the physical examination was primarily aimed at determining a directional preference to repeated movements, and the findings supported the initial impression that psychosocial factors were not playing a significant (if, indeed, any) role. Nonetheless, and despite apparently having a straightforward mechanical presentation and response, Peter was questioned about whether he had any further concerns regarding his MRI scan and the GP's comments before he left the clinic, but he did not.

Reasoning Question:

5. Teaching as a reasoning strategy was clearly important in your management of Peter's problem and in enabling him to understand this. Can you please elaborate as to why you emphasized his education in your management of Peter, perhaps touching on your previous clinical experiences and any pertinent supportive literature?

Answer to Reasoning Question:

Education of patients about their problem and what they can do to assist their symptoms is central to management. It ensures that patients are 'on board' with their management and therefore likely to be compliant with instructions. Studies of patient satisfaction have shown that an explanation of the problem and their involvement with their management are key aspects of a satisfactory episode of physiotherapy (Hush et al., 2011). Specific to Peter's case, it was important to educate him about the role of postures, activities and exercises in aggravating, perpetuating and, most importantly, relieving his symptoms.

Clinical Reasoning Commentary:

Despite the focus on the mechanical examination and mechanical therapy/treatment thus far in this case, this does not occur in a vacuum devoid of psychological and social considerations relating to the clinical presentation and management. As discussed in Chapters 1, 3 and 4, musculoskeletal psychosocial assessment is often less formal and less structured than the physical assessment. Although caution is needed in assuming that information not volunteered is not relevant (hence the importance of 'screening', as discussed in Chapter 1), less formal consideration of psychosocial factors is clearly evident through cues such as no apparent fear avoidance, continued work, appropriate medication use and appropriate perceived disability.

The clear educative element to the clinical management and, more specifically, the emphasis on self-management, speak to the importance of engaging the patient as part of the therapeutic alliance and enabling them to at least share responsibility for their clinical outcome.

Second Appointment (24 Hours Later)

Peter was re-assessed 1 day after the initial assessment because this was important to confirm his classification. In addition, because there was a neurological deficit, frequent monitoring of his symptoms was essential.

Subjective Re-assessment

On review, Peter reported that there had been a significant reduction in the intensity and frequency of the pins and needles in his right hand and that the intensity and frequency of the pain in his right forearm were also considerably reduced. He reported the intensity of the forearm pain to now be 2 out of 10.

Physical Re-assessment

On examination, Peter's habitual sitting posture had improved, and he was attempting to maintain a retracted head posture. His cervical spine mobility had improved, with both active retraction and extension now being moderately limited and only reproducing local neck pain, not scapula pain. Active right rotation had increased to 40 degrees and left rotation to 50 degrees. Right lateral flexion had improved from demonstrating a major movement loss, to only a moderate loss now. Both shoulder mobility and strength had also improved.

On neurological testing, there was an increase in the strength of the triceps muscle, which was now graded as 4 out of 5 (movement possible against some resistance by the examiner). The sensation of light touch in the right thumb and index finger remained reduced, but the right triceps reflex now had a definite response.

No further physical examination was performed because the symptomatic and mechanical improvements supported the continuation of the same management approach.

Treatment

The same management was continued, with Peter being encouraged to move further to the end of range of retraction. He was taught how to self-apply 'overpressure' to retraction to ensure that he achieved end range with his exercises (Fig. 20.4). The prior education about posture correction and avoidance of aggravating postures was reinforced.

Third Appointment (2 Days After the Second Appointment)

Subjective Re-assessment

Peter reported that, overall, he was about 60% improved. He was now experiencing intermittent right-sided neck and scapula pain, the intensity of which he rated as 4 out of 10. He was only occasionally experiencing pins and needles in his right hand and pain

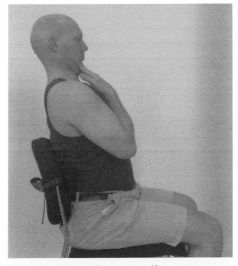

Fig. 20.4 Retraction with patient self-overpressure exercise.

in his right forearm. Whenever he became aware of these symptoms, he was able to abolish them by correcting his head posture.

Peter commented that he continued to experience pain mainly when he was sitting at work. He advised that he was finding it difficult to avoid protruding his head when he was working because of the position of the television monitors, which he was unable to adjust. Peter reported that he had spoken to the occupational health and safety representatives at his work, and they had agreed to perform an ergonomic workplace assessment of his workstation. He was confident his symptoms would be easier to control once this assessment was performed and the ergonomic changes to his workstation were implemented.

Since Peter had been placing the cervical neck roll inside his pillowcase, he was no longer waking at night and could sleep comfortably on both his left side and back. He no longer experienced pain on shoulder movements but did notice that his right arm was still not as strong as it used to be. Peter reported that he was using the lumbar roll in his car, and for the most part, his symptoms were now minimal when driving. He also commented that he had realized that he should not work on his laptop computer when sitting in front of the television at night because he found that within 5 minutes he experienced pins and needles in his right hand, as well as right arm pain.

Physical Re-assessment

On examination, Peter now sat habitually in an erect position with his head partially retracted. The strength of the right triceps muscle was graded as 4 out of 5, and the triceps reflex was 50% of that on the left. There was minimal difference in the sensation of light touch in the right thumb and index finger compared with the left.

There was a minimal loss of active cervical retraction and extension, with both movements causing local neck pain only. Cervical flexion was full range and only produced a stretch in the upper thoracic region. Active right rotation was 10 degrees less than left rotation, and Peter reported experiencing right-sided neck pain at the limit of range. Active right lateral flexion was now equal to left lateral flexion and was pain-free.

Peter's shoulder movements were re-examined. All active and passive movements of the right shoulder were now pain-free. Resisted right shoulder abduction at 45 degrees produced pain over the deltoid but was of equal strength to the left.

Treatment

Peter's technique of performing cervical retraction with self-overpressure was reviewed. His technique was appropriate, and he was able to produce central low cervical spine pain at the end of each movement. He was unable to abolish this end-range pain with two sets of 15 repetitions of cervical retraction. Overpressure was therefore applied by the clinician while Peter performed the retraction movement (Fig. 20.5), and this reduced the end-range pain he was experiencing, so the procedure was repeated.

On re-assessment, the pain previously felt with active cervical retraction had been abolished; however, there was still a loss of cervical extension and pain at the end range of this movement. Peter was then taught how to perform cervical extension from a mid-range retraction position. He was warned to watch for any peripheralization of symptoms into his right arm. However, if instead the movement produced central neck pain at end range, which improved with repetitions, then he had a 'green light' to continue.

Peter was instructed to continue with his self-management by performing cervical retraction exercises followed by retraction and extension exercises, with 10–15 repetitions completed every 2–3 hours or whenever required for relief of symptoms. He was also advised to continue to focus on maintaining an erect posture when sitting.

Reasoning Question:

6. Could you please discuss your evolving hypotheses after the third appointment regarding dominant 'pain type' (nociceptive, neuropathic, nociplastic), possible tissue sources of nociception, specific pathology and also prognosis? What particular findings from Peter's ongoing (re-)assessment support your reasoning?

Continued on following page

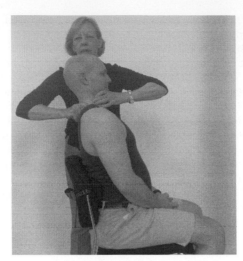

Fig. 20.5   Retraction with clinician-applied overpressure.

Answer to Reasoning Question:

The behaviour of Peter's symptoms suggested somatic nociceptive neck pain.

It is possible that the innervated outer layers of the annulus fibrosus could have been responsible for the neck pain (Bogduk, 2002). The arm symptoms were likely to be neuropathic, secondary to irritation of the C6 nerve root.

Interestingly, both shoulder mobility and strength had improved with treatment. This was re-assessed because, from clinical experience, it has been found that secondary consequences of spinal problems referred distally can frequently respond to management directed at the spine. Thus, this response suggested that the pain produced on shoulder movement and the weakness detected were likely secondary to cervical spine nociception and possibly pathology, rather than due to a primary shoulder problem.

The symptomatic and mechanical improvements achieved with the management supported the McKenzie provisional classification of a 'derangement' with a unilateral asymmetrical pain location below the elbow. Most importantly, Peter's symptoms displayed a directional preference for retraction and responded rapidly to the application of particular mechanical forces. The centralization of his symptoms and the improvement in the initial mechanical baseline measures supported the initial evaluation that his symptoms would be responsive to mechanical therapy, and it would be unlikely that he would require surgery.

Clinically, it is well understood that a decrease in peripheral symptoms can be accompanied by a temporary increase in central symptoms (McKenzie and May, 2003). However, centralization has been consistently associated with a good prognosis in multiple studies from different international sites (May and Aina, 2012), and in the lumbar spine, it is the only evidence-based physical examination predictor of outcome that is known (Chorti et al., 2009). This makes centralization an especially important clinical response to identify for determining the patient's prognosis, as well as for other clinical reasoning judgements.

Fourth Appointment (6 Days After the Third Appointment)

Subjective Re-assessment

Peter reported now being 80% improved. He completed a Neck Disability Index functional questionnaire for a second time and on this occasion scored 8/50, which was substantially lower than his initial score (28/50). He continued to experience intermittent central neck pain but no symptoms at all in his right arm. He was aware that his neck pain tended to recur toward the end of his workday, especially when he was tired and not watching his posture carefully. He had resumed all of his normal functional activities and felt that he had recovered his neck and shoulder mobility.

A workplace assessment had been performed, and it had been recommended that the height and position of the television monitors be adjusted to reduce the amount of cervical protrusion required. A new chair was to be provided which would accommodate the use of a lumbar support and allow Peter to be closer to the monitors.

Physical Re-assessment

On assessment, Peter had full pain-free range of active cervical spine movements. The neurological deficit that was present at the initial assessment had recovered, and he had full pain-free movement of his right shoulder.

At this point Peter was very confident that he could effectively self-manage any neck symptoms that he may experience. He further commented that he felt sure that once the ergonomic changes were made to his workplace, he would be able to control his symptoms more effectively during his days at work. He advised that the 'new' erect sitting posture no longer felt unusual and that he was in a regular routine with performing his neck exercises.

Treatment

It was recommended that Peter continue performing the cervical retraction with overpressure exercise and the retraction/extension exercise 4–5 times per day for another 4–6 weeks, or for as long as was required to manage any neck pain he may experience. To prevent recurrences, he was advised of the importance of continuing to be aware of his sitting posture, especially when he was sitting for lengthy periods as his work required. The importance of maintaining the mobility of his neck in the longer term by continuing to perform cervical retraction and extension exercises was also discussed. It was explained to Peter that the frequency of the exercises could be reduced once he was symptom-free, but because his lifestyle encouraged protruded postures, it was important he perform 'curve reversal' movements regularly.

Peter was then discharged but with instructions to return for further assistance if his self-management strategies were unsuccessful.

Reasoning Question:

7. Peter has made a reasonably rapid recovery from his symptoms considering his MRI findings, although some patients with similar problems are often not so responsive. Why do you think he responded so well to the self-management program you prescribed, and do you think he will maintain his improvement in the longer term? In coming to this prognostic hypothesis, what specific positive and negative prognostic factors did you consider?

Answer to Reasoning Question:

Peter presented with intermittent symptoms, which displayed a directional preference for mechanical loading. Both these findings are clinically associated with a positive response to mechanical therapy (McKenzie and May, 2003). On the other hand, there is a poor correlation between MRI findings and chosen interventions and clinical outcomes, which supports the need for a thorough mechanical evaluation despite positive radiological findings (You et al., 2012; Wassenaar et al., 2012).

Another important positive prognostic factor was that Peter was able to self-manage this episode because he was compliant with the instructions provided and was able and willing to make the necessary temporary lifestyle changes required. He did not display signs of fear avoidance and was keen to avoid surgery. Further motivation was provided during the assessment when it was demonstrated to Peter that changes in posture and the performance of neck movements resulted in a reduction in his symptoms and a change in their location. Most importantly, he could achieve these changes by himself rather than requiring a clinician to achieve them for him. This is a very powerful educational tool, which from clinical experience appears to encourage self-management.

The typical history of neck pain is that it is recurrent, with only 6% of an initial cohort reporting a single non-recurrent episode of neck pain (Picavet and Schouten, 2003). A positive association has been found between sitting, neck flexion and neck pain (Ariens et al., 2001), and because Peter's occupation involves both sitting and neck flexion, is it highly likely that he will experience intermittent neck symptoms. However, with his newfound knowledge of aggravating postures and the importance of regularly performing corrective exercises, he may be able to prevent future episodes. His experience in self-managing this episode should give him confidence in managing his neck pain if it does arise again.

Peter should generally be able to maintain his improvement in the long term and be pro-active in managing any future episodes of neck pain.

Continued on following page

Clinical Reasoning Commentary:

The role of the musculoskeletal clinician as a teacher is increasingly being recognized as being vital in the successful management of chronic or recurrent conditions. Despite the increasing accessibility of health advice from 'Dr Google', the educative role of the clinician has not diminished and, indeed, has gained in importance in relation to managing chronic or recurrent musculoskeletal problems.

In this case involving Peter, there are three distinct but inter-related aims of the clinician's teaching role:

1. To transfer relevant, personalized knowledge which *educates* and *empowers* the patient
2. To *motivate* the patient to take *control* and responsibility for his own management, thus lessening his reliance on the practitioner
3. To promote *confidence* in the patient that he will have a *positive* outcome if he complies and, where relevant, lessen fear (and other counterproductive emotions) regarding the outcome

Interestingly, all three aims were addressed in this case when it was '*demonstrated to Peter that changes in posture and the performance of neck movements resulted in a reduction in his symptoms and a change in their location*'. That is, the direct experience of patients feeling control over their pain and other symptoms (under the educative guidance of the practitioner) helps ensure their compliance with self-management of those conditions which may have a tendency to recur over the longer term.

REFERENCES

Ariens, G.A.M., Bongers, P.M., Douwes, M., Miedema, M.C., Hoogendoorn, W.E., van der Wal, G., et al., 2001. Are neck flexion, neck rotation, and sitting at work risk factors for neck pain? Results of a prospective cohort study. Occup. Environ. Med. 58, 200–207.

Bogduk, N., 2002. Innervation and pain patterns of the cervical spine. In: Grant, R. (Ed.), Physical Therapy of the Cervical and Thoracic spine, third ed. Churchill Livingstone, New York.

Browder, D.A., Childs, J.A., Cleland, J.D., Fritz, J., 2007. Effectiveness of an extension-oriented treatment approach in a subgroup of subjects with low back pain: a randomized clinical trial. Phys. Ther. 87, 1608–1618.

Chorti, A.G., Chortis, A.G., Strimpakos, N., McCarthy, C.J., Lamb, S.E., 2009. The prognostic value of symptom responses in the conservative management of spinal pain. A systematic review. Spine 34, 2686–2699.

Fritz, J.M., Delitto, A., Erhard, R.E., 2003. Comparison of classification-based approach to physical therapy with therapy based on clinical practice guidelines for patients with acute low back pain: a randomized clinical trial. Spine 28, 1363–1371.

Hush, J.M., Cameron, K., Mackey, M., 2011. Patient satisfaction with musculoskeletal physical therapy care: a systematic review. Phys. Ther. 91, 25–36.

Long, A., Donelson, R., Fung, T., 2004. Does it matter which exercise? A randomized control trial of exercise for low back pain. Spine 29 (23), 2593–2602.

Long, A., May, S., Fung, T., 2008. Specific directional exercises for patients with low back pain: a case series. Physiother. Can. 60 (4), 307–317.

May, S., Aina, A., 2012. Centralization and directional preference: a systematic review. Man. Ther. 17, 497–506.

McKenzie, R., May, S., 2003. The Lumbar Spine: Mechanical Diagnosis and Therapy. Spinal Publications Ltd, Waikanae, New Zealand.

McKenzie, R., May, S., 2006. The Cervical and Thoracic Spine: Mechanical Diagnosis and Therapy. Spinal Publications Ltd, Waikanae, New Zealand.

Murphy, D.R., Hurwitz, E.L., Gerrard, J.K., Clary, R., 2009. Pain patterns and descriptions in patients with radicular pain: does the pain necessarily follow a specific dermatome. Chiropr. Osteopat. 17, 9.

Picavet, H.S.J., Schouten, J.S.A.G., 2003. Musculoskeletal pain in the Netherlands: prevalence consequences and risk groups. Pain 102, 167–178.

Vernon, H., 2000. Assessment of self-reported disability, impairment and sincerity of effort in Whiplash-Associated - Disorders. J. Musculoskelet. Pain 8 (1–2), 155–167.

Vernon, H., Mior, S., 1991. The Neck Disability Index: A study of reliability and validity. J. Man. Manip. Ther. 14, 409–415.

Wassenaar, M., van Rijn, R.M., van Tulder, M.W., Verhagen, A.P., van der Windt, D.A.W.M., Koes, B.W., et al., 2012. Magnetic resonance imaging for diagnosing lumbar spinal pathology in adult patients with low back pain and sciatica: a diagnostic systematic review. Eur. Spine J. 21, 220–227.

Werneke, M., Hart, D.L., Cook, D., 1999. A descriptive study of the centralization phenomenon. Spine 24, 676–683.

Woolf, C.J., 2010. What is this thing called pain? J. Clin. Invest. 120, 3742–3744.

Wright, A., 2002. Neuropathic pain. In: Strong, J., Unruh, A.M., Wright, A. Baxter, G.D. (Eds.), Pain. A Textbook for Therapists. Churchill Livingstone, Edinburgh.

You, J.J., Bederman, S.S., Symons, S., Bell, C.M., Yun, L., Laupacis, A., et al., 2012. Patterns of care after magnetic resonance imaging of the spine in primary care. Spine 38, 51–59.

21

Incontinence in an International Hockey Player

Patricia Neumann • Judith Thompson • Mark A. Jones

Subjective Assessment
Personal Profile and Main Problem

Sarah was a 23-year-old international hockey player who had been involved in sport at an elite level since she was 15. When she first presented to physiotherapy with complaints of urinary incontinence (UI), she had two children who were 8 months and 30 months old. She became bothered by the leakage of urine after returning to training for her sport 5 months after the delivery of her second child. Sarah had managed the incontinence initially by wearing pads, thinking it would improve as she got fitter, but after a further 3 months, the problem was worsening. She complained of episodes of increasing wetness during hockey matches and training, such that she had to wear pads to contain the leakage. She was concerned about the worsening of her symptoms because her mother had developed a vaginal prolapse as a young woman and required surgery. Sarah was preparing for an international tournament and did not want to stop training.

At the first consultation, a comprehensive assessment was undertaken in accordance with the International Consultation on Incontinence (ICI) guidelines (Abrams et al., 2013).

History of Incontinence and Medical Details

Sarah had developed mild symptoms of incontinence associated with violent fits of sneezing after the delivery of her first baby, but physical exercise was not a trigger at that stage. Notably, her demanding training regimen and playing hockey at the highest level did not trigger any episodes of urinary incontinence. After the first baby, her bowel function was normal, and she had no symptoms of pelvic organ prolapse (POP), such as heaviness following sport or the feeling of a lump or bulge in the vagina (Jelovsek et al., 2007). Her pelvic floor muscles were not assessed by her obstetrician at her 6-week checkup, and she had not been back to the doctor about her UI because it was mild and did not impact on her sport. Sarah did not give it much thought because she had heard that it was normal after a baby.

In recent years, Sarah had gone to the toilet frequently for her bladder, but since the second pregnancy, she also had trouble with urinary urgency, 'going lots' and with occasional wetting on the way to the toilet (i.e. symptoms of urinary urgency [UU], frequency [F] and occasional episodes of urge urinary incontinence [UUI], complaint of involuntary loss of urine associated with urgency [Haylen et al., 2010]). She said that her fluid intake consisted mostly of water but also included juice, milk and some coffee (estimated intake 2 L of water plus 1 L of other fluids). She felt that she emptied completely and that her flow was strong and sustained. She was able to interrupt her urine stream. After the second baby, Sarah still had no sensation of vaginal heaviness or bulging of the vaginal walls, which would suggest a prolapse. She reported using her bowels daily with the passage of a soft stool without effort and with good control of flatus, suggestive of an intact anal sphincter.

Sarah had no childhood bladder problems such as nocturnal enuresis or recurrent urinary tract infections, and she reported no family history of bladder problems. She denied having any pelvic or other body area pains, nor was this a problem during her pregnancies. She had no gynaecological, neurological or vascular symptoms and described herself as 'very well' other than having mild asthma, which was well controlled.

Medications

Sarah was on the oral contraceptive pill and had regular, brief periods. She used an inhaled corticosteroid regularly and an inhaled bronchodilator as needed before training and matches.

Obstetric History

Sarah had a long first labour (30 hours first stage, 110 minutes second stage), epidural and forceps-assisted delivery of her son, Tom. His birth weight was 4080 g (about 9 pounds) with a head circumference in the 90th centile. An episiotomy had been performed, with extensive stitching. She described a protracted postnatal recovery with painful intercourse, which slowly resolved after about 12 weeks. She felt that the episiotomy had taken a long time to heal so that attempted vaginal penetration was uncomfortable, and the vagina felt dry. Sarah breastfed Tom fully for the first 3 months but then weaned him to resume training for competitive hockey when Tom was 5 months old. Eight months later, she became pregnant for the second time.

During Sarah's second pregnancy, she continued playing hockey and had no bladder problems until she was about 12 weeks pregnant, when she became 'quite wet' with sustained, high-intensity running and dodging. She was not unduly upset by the incontinence. She started using a pad and continued playing for the next 5 weeks of her pregnancy. She then stopped playing hockey but continued with swimming and pregnancy yoga until after the birth of this second baby, Olivia. The second delivery was a normal vaginal delivery with a 7-hour first stage and a 50-minute second stage with a small tear, which did not require suturing. Sarah breastfed Olivia for the first 3 months and then weaned her to be able to return to her training program, which involved going away to weekend training camps.

Previous Management

Sarah had been given a brochure about pelvic floor muscle (PFM) exercises after her first baby, but she had never had her pelvic floor muscles assessed internally. She had tried to do the exercises by squeezing her pelvic floor muscles, but she was not sure if she was doing the exercises correctly because she could not feel much happening. She said she felt she never really 'got it' and gave up.

After the onset of her exercise-induced UI, Sarah had consulted her previous physiotherapist, who had advised her to practice 'hanging on', that is, putting off the urge to go to the toilet, to improve her bladder control. She had also assessed her PFM with real-time transabdominal ultrasound (TAUS) performed in supine lying and had observed that she was apparently unable to contract her PFM, as there was no upward movement of her bladder base. She was informed that her pelvic floor was 'very weak'. Sarah had two sessions of biofeedback using TAUS but still felt unsure of what she was meant to do. At that time, she had joined the practice's Pilates class twice a week to help improve her pelvic floor and 'core' muscles. In addition, she was given instructions to practice 'stopping her flow'. Her urinary symptoms continued to worsen over the next 3 months, and at that point, she was referred on to a specialist Women's, Men's & Pelvic Health Physiotherapist (WMPH PT).

Sarah's goals were as follows:

1. To improve the incontinence ('mild' incontinence would be acceptable, that is, requiring a liner for occasional damp spots)
2. To continue training for selection for an international tournament in 3 months' time
3. To avoid surgical correction of her UI (She was mindful of her mother's gynaecological history and her advice to 'fix' the problem by having surgery, but she did not want to interrupt her training schedule.)

Urinalysis and Post-Void Residual Tests

The following tests were carried out according to International Consultation on Incontinence (ICI) guidelines (Abrams et al., 2013). First, a urinary tract infection, a potentially reversible cause of UI, was screened for, and incomplete bladder emptying, indicative of a voiding dysfunction, was investigated.

Screening tests included the following:

1. Urinalysis with dipstick: no leucocytes, nitrites or blood were detected, suggesting sterile urine (i.e. no abnormality detected).
2. Post-void residual test: the residual urine in the bladder after voiding was assessed with TAUS using the urological program setting for measurement of bladder volumes and was estimated at 0 ml.

A bladder diary and two questionnaires had been emailed to Sarah to complete and bring with her to the first appointment to facilitate a timely clinical diagnosis.

Bladder Diary

A 3-day bladder diary was used as a diagnostic tool to assess bladder function and included details of times of voids, voided volumes, leakage episodes, triggers for leakage, urinary urgency and fluid intake, both quantity and type of fluids. She was asked to complete the bladder diary on non-training days to facilitate adherence.

The bladder diary was evaluated and interpreted with Sarah: bladder capacity: 700 ml, mean voided volume: 450 ml, frequency: 8, nocturia: 1, total urine output per 24 hours: 4.00 L. The nocturnal void occurred after she had been woken by the baby. She recorded two episodes of UUI, both associated with urgency on the way to the toilet (Table 21.1).

Regarding fluid intake, objectively, Sarah consumed 2.2 L of water plus an additional 1.6 L of other fluids (sports drinks, milk and coffee) on the understanding that this was an appropriate amount of water for an elite athlete and that other fluids were not counted toward her intake. She drank more on training days. Her fluid intake had increased when breastfeeding Tom at a time when she had had difficulty with her milk supply. She also believed that a lot of water was good to flush out toxins and to prevent constipation.

Her body weight was 56 kg, giving an estimated appropriate fluid output per 24 hours of 1400 ml based on the formula [weight × 24 ml/kg body weight/24 hours], with polyuria defined by Haylen et al. (2010) as per the formula [>40 ml/kg/24 hours] (i.e. 2240 ml for Sarah).

TABLE 21.1

24-HOUR BLADDER DIARY

Time (* got up for the day/went to bed)	Voided Volume (ml)	Urine Loss (damp, wet, soaked)	Trigger (cough, sneeze, activity, urgency)	Fluid Type (times not specified)	Fluid Amount (ml)
*6.30 am	700			Water	450
9.00 am	400			Coffee/juice/milk	700
11.20 am	350	Damp	Urgency	Water	400
2.30 pm	480			Tea	250
4.45 pm	450			Water	450
6.30 pm	500	Damp	Urgency	Water	500
8.50 pm	460			Tea	300
*11.00 pm	350			Juice	300
3.15 am	310			Water	400
Total	4000			Total	3750

Patient-Reported Outcome Assessment

The following questionnaires were evaluated and discussed with Sarah:

1. The ICI Questionnaire for Urinary Incontinence – short form (ICIQ UISF) (Avery et al., 2004) was used to assess pelvic floor symptoms, symptom severity and impact on quality of life (QoL).

   Result: Total = 11/21, with a higher score denoting increased severity of symptoms. She rated herself at 7/10 for impact on QoL.

   Sarah had positive responses to the following questions suggestive of stress urinary incontinence (SUI; complaint of involuntary loss of urine on effort or physical exertion [e.g. sporting activities], or on sneezing or coughing [Haylen et al., 2010]):
   * Leaks when you cough or sneeze
   * Leaks when you are physically active/exercising and suggestive of overactive bladder syndrome
   * Leaks before you can get to the toilet

2. The Pelvic Floor (PF) Bother Questionnaire (Peterson et al., 2010), with a question about each of nine key aspects of PFM function, was administered; the results indicated no prolapse, pain or bowel symptoms, which corresponded with the subjective assessment. Question 9 asks whether the woman is sexually active and if yes, then whether she has pain with intercourse on a 4-point scale. Sarah's response indicated that she was sexually active and that intercourse was pain-free. PF Bother Questionnaire score = 4/9, where a higher score denotes more bother. Sarah scored 2/4 for urine loss with exertion (suggestive of SUI), 1/4 for urgency and 1/4 for loss of urine on the way to the toilet (both suggestive of overactive bladder syndrome).

Patient's Perspectives

In further exploring Sarah's understanding, she expressed concern regarding her worsening symptoms, particularly in light of her mother's history. Her beliefs about fluids needed to be challenged and ideally restructured to reflect the current evidence base, on the understanding that her current fluid intake may be negatively impacting her bladder control. Similarly, her goal regarding continued participation in sport would need to be considered against recommended management once her physical examination had been completed.

Reasoning Question:

1. Please discuss your rationale for specific information obtained and how that informs your differential diagnosis, identification of 'precautions/contraindications to physical examination and management' and your patient-specific 'management'.

Answer to Reasoning Question:

Sarah is a young, elite athlete in whom UI may at first seem surprising, but she has had two vaginal deliveries, which is a known risk factor for the development of UI (MacLennan et al., 2000). A high prevalence of UI has been reported among elite athletes performing high-intensity physical activities, including hockey (Bø, 2004; Bø and Borgen, 2001). Questions about her history of incontinence served to probe the function of her bladder and pelvic floor prior to pregnancy and childbirth, as childhood problems may persist into adulthood, suggesting more complex pathology (Feldman and Bauer, 2006). Her mother had a vaginal prolapse as a younger woman, suggesting a possible genetic link via a collagen deficiency (Chiaffarino et al., 1999).

Pregnancy is a time of great hormonal and musculoskeletal changes, which are commonly associated with pelvic floor dysfunction (Landon et al., 1990). These factors could explain the onset of more bothersome symptoms even before her second delivery, especially with a possibly compromised pelvic floor after the birth of baby Tom (DeLancey et al., 2008). Furthermore, her pregnancies were close together, which could contribute to incomplete resolution of any impairments after the first delivery.

Sarah's birth history provides a rationale for the development of pelvic floor dysfunction. Childbirth is a risk factor for the development of urinary incontinence (Persson et al., 2000) and POP (Hendrix et al., 2002). Vaginal childbirth and an instrumental delivery are each associated with an increased risk of anterior pelvic floor damage and POP development associated with avulsion of the pubovisceral muscle from the pubic symphysis and ramus, either unilaterally or bilaterally (Dietz and Simpson, 2008) (Fig. 21.1A and B).

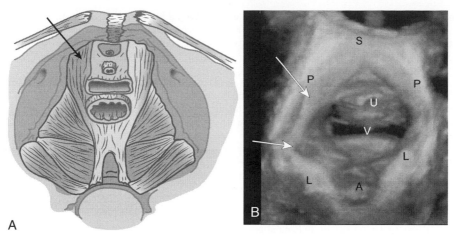

Fig. 21.1 (A) The levator ani, with the arrow indicating the area of trauma in an avulsion birth injury. The area of injury with muscle detachment from the posterior aspect of the pubic ramus is indicated on this diagram. (B) Typical right-sided avulsion injury in a rendered volume, axial plane. It is evident that the pelvic sidewall is blank, that is, that the morphological abnormality documented here is an 'avulsion' of the puborectalis muscle insertion. The top arrow indicates the site of avulsion on the inferior pubis ramus; the lower arrow indicates the margin of the retracted puborectalis muscle. *A,* Anus; *L,* levator ani; *P,* inferior pubic ramus; *S,* symphysis pubis; *U,* urethra; *V,* vagina. *(A, Redrawn with permission from Netter [2010]. B, Modified from Dietz [2009] with permission.)*

A forceps delivery also predisposes the mother to anal sphincter damage (Sultan, 1999), but Sarah had no symptoms of anal incontinence or urgency suggestive of this. Sarah initially reported typical symptoms of SUI (i.e. leakage with sneezing and exertion), but the second delivery precipitated the overt symptoms of exercise-induced SUI. In addition to her symptoms of SUI, her symptoms of UU and UUI are typical of overactive bladder syndrome (wet) (i.e. urgency that results in incontinence). This symptom may be associated with a urinary tract infection, which was excluded on the negative results of urinalysis, or with polydipsia (i.e. excessive fluid intake), a common female phenomenon in the 21st century due to erroneous beliefs about hydration (Valtin, 2002). Other differential diagnoses in a young woman include multiple sclerosis causing bladder-sphincter dyssynergia and a voiding dysfunction due to a hypotonic detrusor (bladder muscle), both leading to incomplete bladder emptying, which in Sarah's case had been excluded because she had no post-void residual on TAUS assessment. Multiple sclerosis was considered unlikely in a young woman performing sport at a high level without any neurological symptoms. A hypotonic detrusor may result from an episode of acute retention post-delivery, but this was not reported in Sarah's birth history, and absence of a residual following voiding also made this unlikely. Thus, no red flags were identified which would trigger a specialist referral.

The 3-day bladder diary provided objective evidence of fluid consumption and bladder function, which confirmed excessive total fluid intake over 24 hours and high bladder volumes. The reasons for Sarah's high fluid intake appeared to be benign, but polydipsia may be due to diabetes insipidus or diabetes mellitus. Persistent thirst, after normalizing fluid intake, should be investigated by a medical practitioner.

The PF Bother Questionnaire supported the subjective findings in that no other pelvic organ symptoms were present and that constipation with possible habitual straining was not contributing to the pressures on her pelvic floor. Question 9 confirmed that she was sexually active and that sexual pain was not present, as the presence of pain would have been a red flag for other possible pathology, such as an infectious or inflammatory condition or a sexually transmitted infection, triggering referral to her general practitioner for further investigation. Pain would not have been an absolute contraindication to internal examination but would have suggested a more cautious assessment. It is important for the clinician to exclude a history of sexual abuse, even in the absence of reports of pain, as it may make a vaginal examination traumatic and cause the patient to dissociate (i.e. relive the trauma during the examination) if it has not previously been identified. Sarah did report pain with intercourse postnatally, but this was consistent with the time taken for the episiotomy to heal and from the influence of postnatal hypooestrogenization causing vaginal dryness.

Sarah had previously been advised to stop her urine flow as a PFM exercise. This, however, is a test of urethral sphincter function, and although it should be possible, it is not advised as an exercise for the pelvic floor muscles because it may disturb the voiding reflexes responsible for the complex

Continued on following page

neurological interactions between bladder and urethra (Bø and Mørkved, 2015). The urethral sphincter has a separate nerve supply from the levator ani (pudendal nerve compared with direct branches from the S2–S4 nerve roots) so that action of one structure does not predict the activity of the other.

Sarah was also advised to 'hang on' to improve her bladder's ability to hold urine. This advice is appropriate in someone with urgency related to reduced bladder volumes because the practice may improve the bladder capacity. However, without a bladder diary, the physiotherapist could not know that the advice was inappropriate, and potentially harmful, because Sarah's bladder volumes were already at the upper end of the normal range (up to 700 ml), with the potential for damage to the detrusor muscle caused by overstretching.

A TAUS had been performed to assess her pelvic floor function (i.e. by visualizing movement of the bladder base), and this indicated no activity. Sarah was told that she had weak pelvic floor muscles, which motivated her to try harder to strengthen them. However, when using TAUS, the amount of movement of the bladder base does not reflect the force of the pelvic floor muscle contraction because other factors may be involved. It is therefore important to consider whether the pelvic floor muscles are able to completely relax (Dietz and Shek, 2008a; Messelink et al., 2005) and whether activity of the other muscles around the abdominal-pelvic cavity is increasing intra-abdominal pressure (Junginger et al., 2010; Neumann and Gill, 2002; Thompson et al., 2006a; Thompson et al., 2006b), mandating a digital vaginal assessment to confirm the hypothesis of a weak PFM.

Sarah had also been advised to do Pilates to improve her 'core' muscles and pelvic floor, but she had no awareness of her pelvic floor and was apparently unable to activate it functionally. Repetitive core abdominal work resulting in increased intra-abdominal pressure in the absence of a functional pelvic floor could exacerbate its dysfunction (Bø et al., 2009). Addressing the PFM dysfunction first would have been advisable in order to train the normal pattern of recruitment and neuromuscular control around the abdominopelvic cavity (Sapsford et al., 2001; Thompson et al., 2006b) (Fig. 21.2).

At this stage, the diagnosis of SUI was likely given her history of leakage during high levels of exertion and occasionally with extreme coughing and sneezing. This subjective finding could be supported by an objective stress test such as the Expanded Paper Towel Test (EPTT) (Neumann et al., 2004) performed with standardized bladder filling to demonstrate objective UI with a sudden rise in intra-abdominal pressure, for example, as occurs with coughing and jumping.

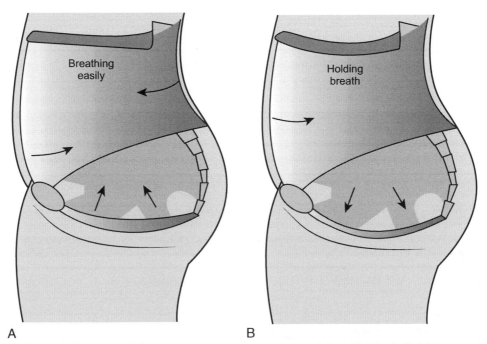

A   B

Fig. 21.2   (A) Correct pelvic floor muscle action with elevation, lower abdominal muscle co-activation and normal breathing. (B) Incorrect action with activation of the upper abdominals, bearing down on the pelvic floor and depression of the levator ani muscle. *(Redrawn with permission. Images courtesy of the Continence Foundation of Australia [continence.org.au].)*

The urinary urgency and frequency symptoms can be explained by the excessive fluid output of 4.0 L. The bladder chart confirms a normal bladder capacity and frequency appropriate for the volume of fluid intake.

Clinical Reasoning Commentary:

The systematic and thorough subjective assessment of Sarah has been used to ensure her complete symptom presentation is revealed and understood and so that potential causes and contributing factors are explored. This, combined with the necessary knowledge of clinical patterns potentially associated with Sarah's presentation, enables differential diagnoses to be considered and tested further. Revealing the complete symptom presentation is essential to thorough clinical reasoning because patients will often omit relevant information for a variety of reasons, including not appreciating its relevance, embarrassment or simply not remembering. 'Screening questions' to optimize thoroughness and minimize clinical assumptions (as presented in Chapter 1) include the following:

- Screening for additional symptoms or problems not spontaneously volunteered (e.g. as with the PF Bother Questionnaire for Sarah)
- Screening for additional activity and participation restrictions and capabilities not volunteered (e.g. screening Sarah for symptoms associated with sexual intercourse)
- Screening for 'patient perspectives' (i.e. psychosocial factors) and their relationship to the clinical presentation (e.g. screening Sarah's understanding, beliefs about fluids and her pelvic floor and her coping strategies regarding her problem)
- Screening for general health comorbidities and red flags

The activity profile; behavior of symptoms; and obstetric, bladder, pelvic floor, birth and family histories all assist identification of potential contributing factors or causes for Sarah's incontinence. Initial objective testing, for example, urinalysis and the bladder diary, provides essential information to be used alongside the physical assessment that follows for further differential diagnosis. A structured assessment with thorough screening enables formulation of diagnostic hypotheses that can then be tested further in the physical examination. For example, stress urinary incontinence subjectively associated with high levels of physical exertion can be tested further with the EPTT. The structured assessment may also reveal non-diagnostic hypotheses (e.g. patient perspectives) that may be contributing to the problem and require attention in management through education.

Education

Because Sarah had reported difficulty doing PFM exercises in the past, she was familiarized with the relevant anatomy. A model of the bony pelvis with a detachable PFM was used to show the structure and function of the levator ani as a support layer and as a mechanism to constrict the urethra, vagina and anal canal. Using palpation of her own bony landmarks to identify the ischial tuberosities laterally and pubic symphysis and coccyx anteriorly and posteriorly respectively, she could visualize the levator ani in its position from the perimeter of her pelvic outlet (Fig. 21.1A, Fig. 21.3). Education was provided before the physical examination to facilitate Sarah's understanding of her pelvic anatomy and how to correctly contract her PFM and to better integrate feedback from the examination.

Physical Assessment

Observation

Assessment of Sarah's abdominal wall in supine lying revealed moderate striae and no rectus diastasis.

Lumbar-Pelvic Deep Muscle Activation

On attempted straight leg raising, Sarah selectively recruited the upper rather than lower abdominal muscles, with bulging of the lower abdominal wall and breath holding. Initially in side-lying and then bent-knee supine lying, Sarah was taught to isolate and retract her lower abdominal wall. She was able to find and then maintain pelvic mid-position with relaxed diaphragmatic breathing and without movement of the pelvis while lifting the right foot 10 cm from the bed. The test was repeated satisfactorily with the left foot.

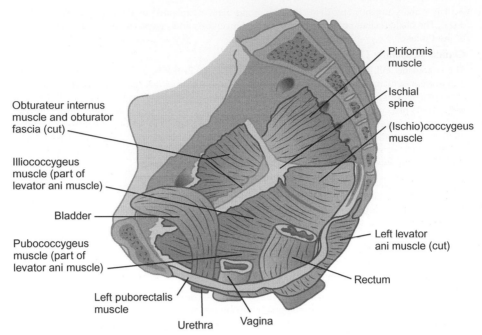

Fig. 21.3 Right side of levator ani originating from the obturator fascia on the right pelvic sidewall and joining in the midline.

Pelvic Floor Muscle Assessment

This part of the physical examination was performed with fully informed and written consent and with clear confirmation that she had not previously been the subject of sexual abuse. Sarah denied any allergy to latex gloves or lubricating gel.

External observation revealed that the vulval and vestibular skin was pink and appeared healthy. A right mediolateral scar deep into the right buttock was consistent with the reported trauma from the first instrumental delivery. On attempted PFM contraction, there was an incorrect activation pattern (a straining effort), with mild descent of the perineum, widening of the genital hiatus, excessive activation of the upper abdominal wall, bulging of the lower abdominal wall and breath holding.

With the labia separated and on request to cough strongly twice, urine loss was not demonstrated, but widening of the genital hiatus and mild descent of the anterior vaginal wall were observed. The same observation was replicated on straining forcefully (Valsalva manoeuvre).

On palpation, normal vulval sensation to light touch with a gloved finger was confirmed.

On internal vaginal examination, palpation of the left levator ani (Fig. 21.4) revealed overactivity (i.e. the levator plate was held in a shortened position) and weak reflex activity with a cough, but no voluntary activity on PFM cueing.

Sarah had poor proprioception and was unable to relax the levator ani on request. The instructions given to contract the PFM included 'squeeze and lift your vagina inward, tightening in your front and back passages as well'. She was then asked to 'relax as if passing urine or wind and to let the tummy go loose'. Attempted PFM contraction produced a strong contraction of the upper abdominal muscles in a straining effort, with low abdominal wall bulging, but not the desired elevation of the levator plate nor relaxation. On Valsalva straining, the bladder neck, that is, the point 3 cm proximal to the hymen on the anterior vaginal wall, descended.

The right levator was extensively avulsed from the pubic symphysis anteriorly (see Fig. 21.1A and B) so that no muscle attachment could be palpated along the right pubic ramus for 2–3 cm lateral to the urethra, nor was there any voluntary activity or reflex activity on coughing of the remaining levator ani (i.e. the right iliococcygeus).

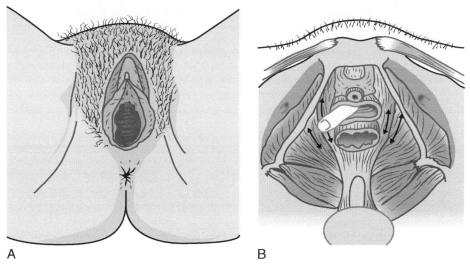

A   B

Fig. 21.4   Single-digit transvaginal palpation of the right levator ani to assess tone and voluntary activation. *(Reproduced with permission from Laycock [1994].)*

Attempted contraction produced a global straining effort with descent of the levator ani on this side.

Using transperineal ultrasound (TPUS) in bent-knee supine lying, descent of the bladder neck was evident on coughing and during the Valsalva manoeuvre. Sarah was unable to produce an elevation of the bladder neck despite the visual TPUS biofeedback.

Reasoning Question:
2. Please discuss your interpretation of your PFM assessment findings with respect to your previous differential diagnosis and 'management', 'precaution' and 'prognosis' hypotheses (particularly with respect to the avulsed right levator ani).

Answer to Reasoning Question:

Sarah's history of an instrumental delivery should alert the clinician to the possibility of levator ani trauma (Shek and Dietz, 2010), and this was indeed confirmed on physical examination. External observation of the vulva revealed perineal descent, associated with upper abdominal wall activation in a global pattern documented in women with PFM dysfunction who are unable to elevate the levator plate (Thompson et al., 2006b).

The internal assessment revealed a complex situation with respect to Sarah's pelvic floor muscles, with findings on each side of the levator ani requiring different and opposing interventions. One can only speculate as to why the left side of her pelvic floor musculature was overactive. Overactivity predating her first pregnancy is a possibility because she had never been able to perform pelvic floor exercises; however, she reported no symptoms of PFM dysfunction, such as difficulty emptying her bladder or bowel, or pain with intercourse. She is likely to have had a well-toned pelvic floor with her sporting background, and strong muscle development around the pelvis would be expected in an elite hockey player. Her habit of excessive drinking would likely upregulate external sphincter activity, and possibly also the pelvic floor muscles, as the bladder volume increases (Kamo et al., 2003).

TPUS, rather than TAUS, was chosen to assess her PFM activity because it provides direct visualization of all the organs and structures in the midline of the pelvis. TAUS, by contrast, provides only visualization of the bladder base, and its assumed position can be confounded by movement of the abdominal wall. TPUS is therefore more valid and the preferred method to provide unambiguous images for biofeedback and exact measurement from the bone of the pubic symphysis.

Assessment for levator ani trauma can be undertaken clinically with digital examination (Dietz & Shek 2008b), as in this instance, or with 3/4D TPUS (Dietz et al., 2012; Kruger et al., 2014; van Delft et al., 2015a). A complete avulsion of the insertion of the pubococcygeus muscle into the pubic ramus on the right side was found. The remaining lateral and posterior portions of the levator ani on the right had reduced muscle bulk and no palpable activity, consistent with muscle damage sustained during a difficult delivery. However, a dysfunctional global motor pattern could have been contributing to this lack of activity, with the potential for improved function with appropriate training.

Continued on following page

There is Level 1A evidence for pelvic floor muscle training (PFMT) for SUI, but with Sarah's complex presentation and poor muscle proprioception, it was not possible to start a PFMT strengthening program immediately.

At the end of the physical examination, the implications of continuing to play sport, with the generation of high intra-abdominal pressures without a functional pelvic floor, were discussed with Sarah because there was real potential to damage the pelvic connective tissue further in the absence of a protective muscle contraction. However, she was adamant that she was not going to stop training or playing under any circumstances.

Management

There were therefore several competing issues to consider with respect to clinical reasoning regarding management planning:

1. Sarah's wish to continue training to achieve adequate fitness for team selection versus the need to protect her pelvic tissues from forces which could precipitate POP and worsen her SUI due to the lack of muscular and connective tissue support
2. The need to provide relief of her urinary incontinence symptoms, both urgency-related and stress-related symptoms, despite continuing with high-impact sport
3. The goal of improving her PFM function in accordance with ICI guidelines but also the need to address the contrasting presentations of muscle dysfunction on each side of her pelvic floor

Currently, there are no guidelines for managing levator ani avulsions in the short or long term, so an emphasis on protecting the pelvic support structures was biologically the most plausible action. It has been shown that the presence of a levator ani avulsion injury is not a barrier to performing a PFMT program (Hilde et al., 2013). Strenuous exercise appears not to increase the risk of developing POP (Braekken et al., 2009), but the effects of the extreme physical demands of international level sport on POP development have not been investigated.

Appropriate counseling and advice about the possibility of POP development was considered important for Sarah because of her family history. The use of an intravaginal support device (i.e. a pessary) could be suggested for times of increased intra-abdominal pressure (e.g. with protracted coughing or high-impact sport) (Neumann, 2015). It was considered that a combined approach of a pessary with PFMT provided a biologically plausible rationale to prevent the onset of POP in Sarah's case.

On the basis of this reasoning, the following SMART (specific, measurable, achievable, reasonable, time-based) management objectives would be discussed with Sarah:

1. Reduce incontinence (measured on the Episodes of Incontinence Diary [EPTT]) over the next 6 months.
2. Normalize urine output (measured on the bladder diary).
3. Prevent progression of her pelvic floor dysfunction, particularly stretching of the connective tissue components (as measured by POP staging under Valsalva manoeuvre conditions).
4. Improve PFM function by normalizing PFM resting tone, teaching correct active elevating pelvic floor contraction with complete relaxation, and then by improving PFM strength and endurance as measured by digital vaginal examination (using International Continence Society [ICS] scales for PFM relaxation and strength) (Haylen et al., 2010).
5. Teach a voluntary contraction of the PFM just prior to a rise in intra-abdominal pressure, also known as 'the knack' (Miller et al., 1998), and incorporate a PFM pre-contraction into functional activities assessed using TAUS or TPUS.
6. Improve the abdominal wall recruitment pattern (i.e. preferential recruitment of lower abdominals before upper abdominals and their co-activation with the PFMs). Once the correct activation pattern is achieved, then abdominal muscle training is progressed.

In addition, exploring Sarah's beliefs about fluids would be important to understand the drivers of her behavior while also excluding possible metabolic disease.

Precautions

Ongoing fitness training without due consideration of the PFM dysfunction could worsen her symptoms and negatively impact on her response to physiotherapy. While physical exertion is known to raise intra-abdominal pressure, it is not known what the threshold of "damage" is for any individual (Tian et al., 2017). Nonetheless, liaison with her hockey fitness coach was deemed important to modify her training regimen with respect to the following:

- Avoid specific activities generating high intra-abdominal pressure, such as deep lunges or squats with weights (O'Dell et al., 2007).
- Stop strong upper abdominal exercises, such as head and shoulder curls (Simpson et al., 2016).
- Work on low-level deep abdominal muscle training until some PFM function is established.

Prognosis

Positive prognostic indicators for recovery included Sarah's motivation and the support of her hockey fitness coach. Negative prognostic indicators included (1) the extensive damage to the PFMs, with no established possibility for surgical repair (Dietz et al., 2013; Rostaminia et al., 2013) and thus potentially exposing Sarah to the risk of progressive PFM dysfunction as she ages; (2) the high intensity of her sport; and (3) her determination not to take time out for PFM rehabilitation. Rehabilitation of her pelvic floor muscles would be limited due to the muscle impairments, although recent research suggests the possibility of some spontaneous recovery between three and twelve months (van Delft et al., 2015b). An improvement in her urinary symptoms and prevention of a prolapse with the use of a support pessary in the short term were likely. In the long term, maintenance of optimal PFM function, general fitness and body mass would contribute to a better prognosis. Activities producing high levels of intra-abdominal pressure such as persistent coughing or trampolining, would negatively impact her prognosis.

Clinical Reasoning Commentary:

The physical assessment is used to 'test' diagnostic hypotheses formulated throughout the subjective assessment and to reveal specific pathology and impairments to address in management. Although evidence-informed practice (from research and experience) enables likely management strategies to be recognized from the description, behavior and history of symptoms, the varied and often complex presentations of physical impairments (e.g. Sarah's avulsed right levator ani and overactive left levator) highlight the balance in pathology- versus impairment-based reasoning needed to guide management. That is, although research may support particular management strategies for specific conditions (e.g. SUI), knowledge of each patient's unique presentation obtained through skilled subjective and physical assessment determines how research-supported management will be carried out.

Prognosis is a challenging judgement to make, and yet every patient wants and deserves to know their clinician's opinion of whether the clinician can help the patient or not. Examples of factors to consider when forming a hypothesis about 'prognosis' are highlighted in Chapter 1, and weighing of both positive and negative indicators, as occurs here, is an effective means to critically reach a decision. Later review of the initial prognosis and its rationale, particularly if shown to be inaccurate, facilitates learning from experience and improvement in future judgements.

Discussion of Findings and Management

In accordance with Sarah's goals, the following management plan was discussed with her:

1. Incontinence: immediate symptom management with a bladder neck support device for hockey matches and training (Fig. 21.5)
2. POP: use of the support device during activities involving high intra-abdominal pressures to prevent the development of POP
3. PFM re-education:
   a. Normalize the resting tone in the left levator ani using 'manual' technique (myofascial release) relaxation, and establish voluntary control using localization awareness and PFM down-training (using a prolonged relaxation phase after the PFM contraction, e.g., a 2-second contraction followed by a 6-second relaxation phase).
   b. After normalization of left levator ani tone, the aim is then to establish PFM voluntary activity in the right levator ani muscle. This is achieved by localization awareness of the right levator ani, 'manual' techniques such as quick stretch, vibration to increase tone/tension, then possibly electromyography (EMG) biofeedback and/or electrical stimulation.
   c. Subsequently train for strength, speed and function (Bø and Aschehoug, 2015).
4. Abdominal wall training:
   a. The focus is placed on lower/deep abdominal muscle recruitment and its co-activation with the PFM. Initially, assessment of deep abdominal co-activation during PFM contraction is undertaken in side-lying and standing, then progressed to graded abdominal muscle training with an emphasis on pre-contraction of the PFM and lower abdominal wall. This can be assessed by TAUS or TPUS, which can also be used for biofeedback. Subsequently, functional activities such as head or leg lifts can be introduced. Additional advanced training with upper and lower abdominal EMG could highlight the desired co-activation pattern if needed.

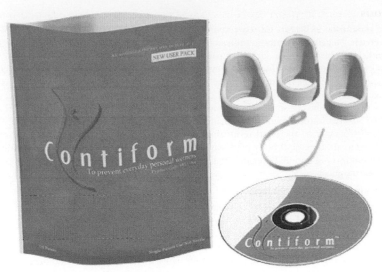

Fig. 21.5 Contiform bladder neck support device in three sizes with strap for removal.

5. Normalization of fluid intake and bladder volumes: education and advice to reduce fluids to achieve a urine output of no more than 2200 ml/24 hours to eliminate polyuria as a contributor to her urinary symptoms

Based on the bladder diary findings of polydipsia, Sarah's beliefs about fluids were challenged. Her excessive fluid intake may have been contributing to her incontinence and could potentially cause electrolyte loss, as well as also contributing to electrolyte imbalance. Excessive fluids and the resultant urgency may also have been contributing to the overactivity of her PFMs because Sarah needed to 'hold on' all the time. Education about the evidence base for adequate hydration was provided (Valtin, 2002), and a collaborative approach to reducing her fluids was explored. Sarah agreed to listen more to her body and respond to the physiological driver of thirst to trigger drinking, and not to force fluids. We further discussed the need to increase her intake as required to meet the demands for adequate hydration during matches and considering the ambient temperature. It was interesting to note that her extreme fluid intake had not been a recommendation of her hockey coach but was instead based on her perception of what was appropriate based on information obtained in the popular media.

Regarding a home program, Sarah agreed to modify her fluids in line with current evidence and to complete another 3 days and nights of a bladder diary with voided volumes, times and incontinent episodes. This would assist with re-assessing the impact of normalizing fluids on her symptoms before her next consultation.

In order to objectively test Sarah's bladder control under conditions of increased intra-abdominal pressure, she was asked to come next time prepared to perform the EPTT (Neumann et al., 2004), and accordingly, written instructions were provided. In preparation for this next visit, she was to empty her bladder 2 hours before her appointment, then drink 250 ml of water and not void before the appointment.

Second Consultation (2 Weeks Later)

Sarah had reduced her fluid intake, and her bladder diary demonstrated that she had achieved an output of between 1600 and 2200 ml per 24 hours. She was surprised that she hadn't felt thirsty. She had noted that the urgency had resolved almost immediately, and her incontinence was also less. There were no incontinent episodes associated with urgency since her last visit, and she had only had a damp pad at hockey training. She felt that this was a marked improvement, and she was motivated to continue with this drinking regimen.

The EPTT was performed in standing with a folded paper towel in the crotch of her underpants. She performed three coughs, three jumps with legs apart and five simultaneous coughs and jumps. The paper towel was examined visually, but no signs of urine loss were detected. This finding suggested that the reduced fluid intake had improved her functional bladder control and that more provocative activities were needed to potentially induce urine loss.

Because Sarah's symptoms were experienced in upright positions, assessment of Sarah's ability to perform a PFM contraction in standing was assessed. A visual assessment of the abdominopelvic cylinder activation was performed with Sarah's abdominal wall exposed and viewed in a full-length mirror while she attempted a PFM contraction. The upper abdominal muscles were excessively recruited, with bulging of the lower abdominal wall, which was similar to her recruitment pattern in supine lying. She was instructed in the desired pattern of relaxed upper abdominals with retraction of the lower abdominal wall, with cues to do what she would to stop her urine flow, while palpating her pubic symphysis. Assessment with TAUS in standing looked for a correctly elevating contraction without breath holding. The emphasis was on gentle specific recruitment for 2 seconds to avoid a global response, followed by complete relaxation of the abdominal wall and PFM over 10 seconds.

After discussion about the benefits and management of an intravaginal bladder neck support, Sarah was fitted with a bladder neck support device (see Fig. 21.5) in order to control her urine loss during sport. The device could also protect her pelvic connective tissue from potentially damaging stretching forces during high-impact activities. She was taught how to insert, remove and wash it herself. The plan was to trial it for fitness training and matches to allow her to be physically active without fear of leaking or of causing more damage to her pelvic support ligaments. A TPUS scan with the device in situ showed excellent support of her vaginal walls during forceful Valsalva manoevres and abdominal sit-up exercises. The TPUS scan was also used to view PFM activity and the idea of sucking the device up inside her vagina, while some traction was placed on the string provided for removal and while viewing PFM activity on the screen. Sarah was able to see some appropriate cranial activity of the anal sphincter on the screen.

Regarding home exercise, Sarah was to exercise her PFMs while sitting upright on a small roll of towel to increase the awareness of her perineum – she agreed to do this at least twice a day, concentrating on a sensation of lifting her perineum off the towel, with the idea of stopping her urine flow, and while palpating her upper abdominals (to reduce activity) and lower abdominals (to encourage gentle retraction). She also agreed to practice recruitment in standing twice a day in front of the bathroom mirror (i.e. two sets of five repetitions, held 2 seconds with 10 seconds of relaxation) and at other times when she was standing if she was confident she was doing it correctly.

For outcome measurement, Sarah was provided with a 12-week diary of incontinent episodes (Accident Diary) to record any episodes of urine loss, the severity (damp, wet or soaked) and the precipitating event (urgency, hockey, coughing, sneezing etc).

Reasoning Question:

3. Although the effectiveness of instructions for pelvic floor contraction must vary between patients, please discuss any research and your own experienced-based evidence regarding instructions that are usually effective and where caution with instructions is required to avoid eliciting incorrect patterns of activation.

Answer to Reasoning Question:

The aim of the first phase of PFMT is motor learning to establish a correct elevating PFM contraction and full relaxation. The emphasis is on establishing specific control over the pelvic floor muscles as distinct from the bigger and stronger outer pelvic muscles, such as the gluteals and adductors. These larger muscles tend to co-contract with, but may override, the much less obvious sensations of the pelvic floor. A model pelvis and palpation of a woman's own bony pelvis will help increase muscle awareness and proprioception. Postures and instructions need to facilitate awareness and control of the smaller and less obvious internal pelvic muscles. Pelvic tilting or pelvic lifts (bridging) are frequently confused with pelvic floor contractions, and PFM contraction during inhalation and breath holding is common and incorrect (Bø and Mørkved, 2015). Many women bear down and depress the levator plate when given written or simple verbal instructions (Bump et al., 1991; Thompson and O'Sullivan, 2003). This pattern has been observed in asymptomatic women but is more likely to occur in women with pelvic floor dysfunction (such as UI or POP) and results in a 'global' straining action with contraction of the

Continued on following page

upper abdominals, bulging of the lower abdominal wall and pelvic floor descent (Thompson et al., 2006b) (see Fig. 21.1). Thus, assessment and specific retraining of the PFMs and recruitment pattern must be addressed because ongoing practice of the wrong pattern leading to depression of the levator plate and the organs resting on it may accelerate the development of UI or POP.

The following cues and instructions may be helpful in the motor learning phase:

- Because the aim of instructions with a patient with UI is to recruit the striated urethral sphincter as well as the levator ani and puborectalis muscles, the instruction to 'tighten in your pelvic floor muscles as if you were stopping your flow of urine' is useful (Bø and Mørkved, 2015). As well as a squeezing in around the urethra, the patient should also be aware of the vagina and back passage contracting, with lower abdominal wall activity. Upper abdominal wall contraction or breath holding indicates a global rather than local strategy, usually associated with excessive effort.
- If she is still unable to feel a pelvic floor contraction, the patient could try actually stopping the flow of urine as an awareness exercise to get the feel of the correct action. This should *not* be done with every void, as it may disrupt the natural voiding pattern, which is to relax the pelvic floor until voiding is complete (Bø and Mørkved, 2015).
- Because the muscles around the vagina and anus are relatively larger and move further, and thus have greater proprioceptive potential, exploring instructions to contract each passage separately may be helpful initially, with progression to a whole PFM contraction when able.
- Viewing the perineum in a mirror to see an indrawing of the perineum in response to these instructions may provide powerful visual biofeedback about the correct direction of movement (i.e. in a cranial direction).
- Instructions to perform a very small localized contraction may facilitate an isolated contraction, separate from that of the adductors, gluteals and abdominals. Excessive effort in someone with poor proprioception of the PFMs may result in a global response, and the consequent downward strain on the pelvic floor is perceived as a contraction.
- Observation of the abdominal wall and breathing patterns will confirm if the woman is able to isolate a contraction to her pelvic floor and lower abdominal wall without breath holding. Proprioceptive cues include firmly touching the perineal area or the upper border of the pubic symphysis to which the puborectalis muscle is attached. Appropriate verbal cues such as limiting the contraction to the bottom of the abdominopelvic cylinder by 'lifting inside the pelvis' may be helpful, rather than simply 'lifting' or, erroneously, 'lifting to the belly button'.
- The idea of the 'elevator' exercise, with the lift going up, can be helpful, but the effort should be localized within the pelvis, with avoidance of excessive effort and unwanted co-contraction of the upper abdominal and chest muscles.

Clinical Reasoning Commentary:

Musculoskeletal management is informed by a combination of propositional research-informed knowledge and non-propositional craft knowledge that includes the 'how' of different interventions that typically have to be modified to individual patients' levels of understanding and impairment. 'Reasoning about teaching' is a clinical reasoning strategy described in Chapter 1 as follows:

Reasoning associated with the planning, execution and evaluation of individualized and context-sensitive teaching, including education for conceptual understanding (e.g. medical and musculoskeletal diagnosis, pain), education for physical performance (e.g. rehabilitative exercise, postural correction, sport technique enhancement) and education for behavioural change.

The variations in instructions and cues for pelvic floor training highlighted here are an example of craft knowledge related to teaching that requires reasoning to recognize when different cues are indicated and most likely to be effective for a given patient.

Third Consultation (2 Weeks Later)

Sarah reported that she had had no incontinent episodes as a result of wearing the bladder neck support for training. She was managing the bladder neck support device well, and it gave her confidence to play with energy. Her Accident Diary had been filled out daily and corroborated her reports.

After receiving consent, her PFMs were reviewed by vaginal examination. Management of her PFM impairment proceeded with down-training of the overactive left pubococcygeus and iliococcygeus muscles, using guided imagery to help Sarah to relax. Images of a lift going down to the basement or a trampoline sagging over 20 seconds were accompanied by gentle myofascial release performed with digital vaginal pressure on the cranial surface of the levator ani muscle (see Fig. 21.4) and accompanied by voluntary abdominal wall relaxation (bulging without force) to facilitate PFM relaxation.

Other verbal cues were given, such as letting go as if she were 'urinating or passing wind in a private place or letting a tampon go'. Quick stretch facilitation and lower abdominal wall retraction were used to facilitate contraction of the PFMs. Tactile stimulation to aid cortical localization of the activity was achieved by pressure of her fingers on the pubic symphysis. This training produced some reduction in the tone/tension and stimulated weak voluntary activity of the left side of the levator ani.

Dual-channel intravaginal and abdominal (external oblique) EMG biofeedback training was then used to provide intravaginal tactile stimulation (the EMG sensor) and visual feedback on the computer screen. Electrodes on the upper abdominals below the ribs bilaterally enabled their activity to be monitored and down-trained. A clear differentiation between the relaxation and contraction phases was emphasized, with the focus on performing the action gently, isolating it to the bottom of the abdominal 'barrel' and ensuring a long and complete relaxation phase.

Regarding home exercise, Sarah agreed to perform this exercise at home every evening on the floor once the children were in bed and when in bed herself before sleep. The focus was to be on complete relaxation and a gentle 2-second contraction for as many times as she could feel and coordinate it well, with her hands monitoring upper abdominal muscle activity or providing pubic symphysis pressure. She was also to practice in standing after voiding during the day, ideally in front of a mirror.

Fourth Consultation (2 Weeks Later)

After consent was given, vaginal examination demonstrated that the resting tone/tension of the left levator ani had reduced, although it was still higher than normal, and Sarah had established some weak voluntary activity on that side. The relaxation and myofascial release techniques were repeated, and a stronger contraction was elicited, which she could sustain for 3 seconds without breath holding. The aim was to produce a gentle, isolated contraction with quiet breathing. The emphasis was on the quality of the contraction. Stretch facilitation was performed digitally *per vaginum* with the aim of activating the right levator ani.

Some weak voluntary activity was elicited when Sarah focused on concomitant activation of the lower abdominal wall. This skill was then practiced in standing using a mirror to view her whole abdominal wall and localizing the contraction to her lower abdominals just above and lateral to the pubic symphysis, aided by proprioception from her palpating fingers. TAUS was used in standing to help her see an internal lifting action of her levator ani. It should be noted that if there had been reduced tone and weak voluntary activity bilaterally, use of an intravaginal muscle stimulator would have been the treatment of choice initially, but with overactivity on the left, this was not indicated in the early stages.

The next three sessions, each 2 weeks apart, focused on progressing her PFMT program as follows:

- PFM contractions were performed at low intensity initially to facilitate a localized action (i.e. the best effort that produced a correct contraction without upper abdominals and breath holding).
- EMG biofeedback was used to promote proprioception and isolated control without upper abdominal muscle activity.
- PFMT was progressed to incorporate maximal sustained contractions over 6 seconds with a longer relaxation phase of 10 seconds to facilitate complete relaxation, increasing to two sets of eight repetitions on alternate days (Bø and Aschehoug, 2015)
- In line with the PERFECT (power, endurance, repetitions, fast, elevation, co-contraction, timing [with cough]) system of PFM assessment (Bø and Sherburn, 2005), training addressed all these requirements for optimal PFM function, with an emphasis throughout on coordination.
- Once reliable voluntary control had been established, training was completed preferentially in standing as the most functional position.

- Training of a pre-contraction of the PFMs and lower abdominals before a rise in intra-abdominal pressure was taught in bent-knee supine lying, using TPUS with a cursor on the bladder neck, which had to be held in position during a small cough ('the knack'). Once this skill was mastered, the exercise was progressed to standing. Progressively, functional control was challenged, for example, pre-contracting before a small cough, a series of coughs, a small jump on the spot and then an increasing number of jumps while maintaining a PFM contraction.

Reasoning Question:

4. Would you highlight the research evidence related to PFM retraining for urinary incontinence generally and also with respect to specific procedures such as myofascial release? How do you typically integrate this research-based evidence with your clinical experiential evidence in your clinical reasoning?

Answer to Reasoning Question:

There are now a number of randomized controlled trials (RCTs) of excellent quality providing high-level evidence for the efficacy of PFMT for pelvic floor dysfunctions (PFDs), especially SUI and POP (Bø et al., 1999; Braekken et al., 2010; Dumoulin et al., 2004; Hagen et al., 2014). The mechanisms of PFMT appear to be primarily in developing muscle hypertrophy and increased stiffness (i.e. less distensibility) of the muscle and associated connective tissue (i.e. using a strength training protocol).

Before applying this evidence to train the PFM for strength, it is mandatory to ensure optimal PFM contraction technique for training to be effective (Bø and Mørkved, 2015, pp. 111–112).

After motor learning to perform the correct technique, the training program aims to develop hypertrophy by the performance of maximal contractions of the PFM, based on the known requirements for strength training of skeletal muscle (DiNubile, 1991). The training must target the correct muscles, that is, the PFM, and be performed regularly over a long enough time frame (i.e. 4–6 months) to effect changes in muscle morphology (e.g. increases in cross-sectional area, muscle tone and stiffness). The rationale for intensive strength training is that a stronger PFM would contribute to the structural support of the pelvic organs by positioning them higher inside the pelvis and by resisting descent caused by rises in intra-abdominal pressure. Indeed, an intensive PFMT program in women with POP was shown to significantly increase the thickness of the levator ani, reduce the area of the levator hiatus and elevate the pelvic organs within the pelvis (Braekken et al., 2010). Such PFMT is dependent on observing all of the usual principles of skeletal muscle strength training, such as dose–response issues, specificity, overload, duration and progression (Bø and Aschehoug, 2015).

It has also been shown in a small RCT that teaching women how to pre-contract the PFMs prior to rises in intra-abdominal pressure, specifically a cough, can reduce urine loss in women in 1 week (i.e. long before muscle hypertrophy could be achieved) (Miller et al., 1998). This has been dubbed 'the knack' or 'functional training', but there is not strong evidence to support such training as 'standalone' therapy to date (Bø, 2015). This functional training requires that the patient can contract her PFMs correctly with an elevating action that prevents descent of the bladder neck or other pelvic organs (rectum and uterus). Assessment by vaginal digital palpation or TPUS should confirm to the clinician that the action is correct and sufficient.

The evidence for PFM strength training cannot be applied immediately where PFM overactivity is encountered. In this case, the first step is to achieve lengthening and full relaxation of the muscle fibres, followed by contraction through full range. It is not appropriate to attempt to strengthen a stiff, shortened muscle, so specific techniques are needed to normalize this tension, such as myofascial release. It may simply in some cases be sufficient to make the woman aware of the overactivity and teach her to relax it, as in relaxing a clenched fist or a clenched jaw. Awareness of the interaction between the lower abdominals, gluteals, adductors and the pelvic floor and practice of specific relaxation of these outer pelvic muscles will aid in relaxation and 'resetting' of the tension of the PFMs. Internal techniques with gentle digital 'overpressure' to aid muscle lengthening and encourage full relaxation, or the use of visual biofeedback using vaginal EMG, may be helpful (Fitzgerald et al., 2012; Oyama et al., 2004).

The interactions between the pelvic floor and abdominal muscles have been documented in a number of studies (Bø et al., 2003; Madill and McLean, 2006, 2008; Neumann and Gill, 2002; Sapsford and Hodges, 2001; Thompson et al., 2006a), but the role that abdominal muscle training plays in women with PFD requires further rigorous study (Bø and Herbert, 2013). There is currently no strong evidence that alternative non-specific exercise programs such as training the pelvic floor via the abdominal muscles or Pilates are effective in reducing SUI in women (Bø and Herbert, 2013). Sapsford (2004) hypothesized that stress incontinence could be remediated by training the deep abdominal muscles relying on the co-activation patterns, and although this idea may have merit to facilitate a contraction of the pelvic floor, this type of training for SUI has not been subjected to a clinical trial. Dumoulin et al. (2004) found no benefit in continence outcomes with the addition of an abdominal muscle training program to PFMT for postnatal women with SUI, but the confidence intervals were wide, suggesting that subgroups of women may well have benefited. For example, it is possible that subgroups of women with dysfunctional coordination patterns will require specific abdominal muscle training to establish correct recruitment order to facilitate PFM activation. Hung et al. (2010), however, suggested some benefit from additional abdominal muscle training in all women with urinary incontinence. Clinically, a contraction of the lower abdominal wall may be used to facilitate a pelvic floor contraction in women with poor PFM awareness. In some women, there may be no co-contraction, and this must be individually assessed.

Clinical Reasoning Commentary:

As is often the case with musculoskeletal management, some aspects of management have better research evidence than others. There is strong evidence for the use of PFMT for SUI and POP, whereas the benefit of manual procedures to relax overactive muscles and the benefits of the addition of an abdominal muscle training program to improve pelvic floor function both require further research. Whether procedures used in a management program have research proven efficacy or not, clinical application, as demonstrated throughout this case, still requires careful re-assessment of the impairment targeted (e.g. PFM contraction, muscle overactivity) and the principal functional outcome (i.e. incontinence) to inform ongoing reasoning and management progression.

Abdominal Muscle Training

The literature provides insights into intra-abdominal pressure increases during different activities (Tian et al., 2017). Coughing and sneezing produce pressure rises in excess of most physical activities, except weight-lifting from a deep squat and heavy leg presses (O'Dell et al., 2007). Thus, in consultation with her fitness coach, Sarah's training regimen was modified to exclude these activities initially. Alternative abdominal exercises which promoted preferential activation of the PFMs and lower abdominal wall were implemented to address the imbalance between upper and lower abdominals. Consideration was also given to the lack of a protective reflex contraction of the pelvic floor found on assessment and the demonstrated maladaptive pattern of activation with excessive upper abdominal activation (Thompson et al., 2006b).

To address the muscle imbalance, Sarah's abdominal wall program focused on selectively recruiting the lower abdominal muscles before engaging the upper abdominal muscles and was progressed through the following stages:

- In four-point kneeling and also in a forward leaning position with the arms supported on a high counter, abdominal wall relaxation is followed by low-intensity PFM contraction, then by lower abdominal wall activation. Finally, full relaxation is emphasized. This same sequence of activation is also practiced on a fit ball.
- Pilates training with the bladder neck support device in situ. Liaison with Sarah's Pilates instructor emphasized the correct sequence of activation, starting with the PFMs, then co-activating the low abdominal wall prior to further abdominal wall activation. This was to promote the normal protective pre-contraction of the PFMs prior to rises in intra-abdominal pressure. Repetition of the correct pattern promotes motor learning. Training was initially undertaken at a low intensity to enable her to maintain relaxation of the upper abdominal wall but was then progressed to higher intensity. The importance of emphasizing, and allowing enough time for, complete PFM relaxation after each contraction was highlighted with the instructor.
- Sit-ups (or abdominal curls) and the 'plank' were not included in the early program with her trainer because these exercises selectively recruit the upper abdominals, with the potential for depression of the pelvic floor. Assessment with TPUS confirmed depression initially, but after 3 months of training Sarah's control had improved sufficiently to enable them to be gradually included in her program.

Sarah continued with all her other training activities, including running. Braekken et al. (2009) suggest that vigorous physical activity does not lead to a predisposition to POP, but there are no studies on the effect of extreme physical activities, such as international-level hockey, on the development of POP to help guide clinical practice. During training, Sarah wore the bladder neck support device in order to protect ligamentous and fascial supports of her bladder and to provide relief from her stress incontinence.

Outcomes

1. After 6 months, Sarah achieved her goal of returning to international-level hockey without UI, but she needed a bladder neck support device to be completely continent.
2. A repeat bladder diary showed that bladder volumes, voiding frequency and total urine output per 24 hours were within normal limits.
3. Regular use of the bladder neck support reduced the stress incontinence and also acted as a protective support for the vaginal connective tissue. No episodes of UI were noted on the Accident Diary over the last 3 months.
4. Sarah gained voluntary control of her PFMs, but an imbalance between the right and left sides persisted at 6 months. The right side remained weak (1/3 on the ICS scale) (Haylen et al., 2010), with ongoing mildly increased tone and a strong contraction (3/3) on the left. She was able to maintain an elevated position of her bladder neck with functional tasks (such as active straight leg raising and head lifts) on both digital and TAUS/TPUS assessment, but this skill may not have transferred to the hockey field.
5. Abdominal muscle tone improved, as did the order of recruitment and balance between the upper and lower abdominal walls. Recruitment was assessed visually in standing from the side, noting lower before upper abdominal wall retraction. Abdominal muscle strength had normalized, with good lower abdominal support even at rest.
6. Repeated administration of the ICIQ UISF: 0/21.
7. Patient Global Impression of Improvement: much better (2 on a 7-point scale from 'very much better (0)' to 'very much worse (7)'). However, her ongoing need to use the bladder neck support device was bothersome to her.

Ongoing Management

Sarah was given an ongoing PFMT program to maintain optimal bladder control and muscular support for her pelvic organs. She had no symptoms of POP, and her use of an intravaginal device for sport and acute episodes of coughing provided her with protection and the potential to avoid surgery. The persistent weakness of the right levator ani was likely to be a permanent muscle impairment, so ongoing self-management with the home exercise program, continuation of Pilates as part of her general fitness regimen and a clinical review in 3 months' time was planned. A follow-up assessment would determine that Sarah had no progression of her muscle impairment or signs of POP and that her symptoms of UI remained well controlled with an appropriate fluid intake. Her exercise regimen would be progressed in liaison with her Pilates instructor and hockey fitness coach.

REFERENCES

Abrams, P., Anderson, K.E., Artibani, W., Birder, L., Bliss, D., Cardozo, L., et al., 2013. Recommendations of the International Scientific Committee: Evaluation and treatment of urinary incontinence, pelvic organ prolapse and faecal incontinence. In: Abrams, P., Cardozo, L., Khoury, S.Wein, A. (Eds.), Incontinence. ICUD-EAU, Paris.

Avery, K., Donovan, J., Peters, T.J., Shaw, C., Gotoh, M., Abrams, P., 2004. ICIQ: A brief and robust measure for evaluating the symptoms and impact of urinary incontinence. Neurourol. Urodyn. 23 (4), 322–330.

Bø, K., 2004. Urinary incontinence, pelvic floor dysfunction, exercise and sport. Sports Medicine 34 (7), 451–464.

Bø, K., 2015. Pelvic floor muscle training for SUI. In: Bø, K., Berghmans, B., Mørkved, S., van Kampen, M. (Eds.), Evidence-Based Physical Therapy for the Pelvic Floor. Churchill Livingstone Elsevier, Edinburgh, pp. 162–178.

Bø, K., Aschehoug, A., 2015. Introduction to the concept of strength training for pelvic floor muscles. In: Bø, K., Berghmans, B., Mørkved, S., van Kampen, M. (Eds.), Evidence-Based Physical Therapy for the Pelvic Floor. Churchill Livingstone Elsevier, Edinburgh, pp. 117–130.

Bø, K., Borgen, J.S., 2001. Prevalence of stress and urge urinary incontinence in elite athletes and controls. Med. Sci. Sports Exerc. 33 (11), 1797–1802.

Bø, K., Braekken, I.H., Majida, M., 2009. Constriction of the levator hiatus during instruction of pelvic floor or transversus abdominis contraction: a 4D ultrasound study. Int. Urogynecol. J. Pelvic Floor Dysfunct. 20, 27–32.

Bø, K., Herbert, R., 2013. There is not yet strong evidence that exercise regimens other than pelvic floor muscle training can reduce stress urinary incontinence in women: a systematic review. J. Physiother. 59, 159–168.

Bø, K., Mørkved, S., 2015. Ability to contract the pelvic floor muscles. In: Bø, K., Berghmans, B., Mørkved, S., van Kampen, M. (Eds.), Evidence-Based Physical Therapy for the Pelvic Floor. Churchill Livingstone Elsevier, Edinburgh, pp. 111–117.

Bø, K., Mørkved, S., Frawley, H., Sherburn, M., 2009. Evidence for benefit of transversus abdominis training alone or in combination with pelvic floor muscle training to treat female urinary incontinence: a systematic review. Neurourol. Urodyn. 28 (5), 368–373.

Bø, K., Sherburn, M., 2005. Evaluation of female pelvic floor muscle function and strength. Phys. Ther. 85 (3), 269–282.

Bø, K., Sherburn, M., Allen, T., 2003. Transabdominal ultrasound measurement of pelvic floor muscle activity when activated directly or via transversus abdominal muscle contraction. Neurourol. Urodyn. 22 (6), 582–588.

Bø, K., Talseth, T., Holme, I., 1999. Single blind, randomised controlled trial of pelvic floor exercises, electrical stimulation, vaginal cones, and no treatment in management of genuine stress incontinence in women. Br. Med. J. 318, 487–493.

Braekken, I.H., Majida, M., Ellström Engh, M., Bo, K., 2010. Can pelvic floor muscle training reverse pelvic organ prolapse and reduce prolapse symptoms? An assessor-blinded, randomized, controlled trial. Am. J. Obstet. Gynecol. 203 (170), e1–e7. doi:10.1016/j.ajog.2010.02.037.

Braekken, I.H., Majida, M., Ellström Engh, M., Holme, I.M., Bø, K., 2009. Pelvic floor function is independently associated with pelvic organ prolapse. Br. J. Obstet. Gynaecol. 116, 1706–1714.

Bump, R.C., Hurt, W.G., Fantl, J.A., Wyman, J., 1991. Assessment of Kegel exercise performance after brief verbal instruction. Am. J. Obstet. Gynecol. 165, 322–329.

Chiaffarino, F., Chatenoud, L., Dindelli, M., Meschia, M., Buonaguidi, A., Amicarelli, F., et al., 1999. Reproductive factors, family history, occupation and risk of urogenital prolapse. Eur. J. Obstet. Gynecol. Reprod. Biol. 82 (1), 63–67.

Delancey, J.O.L., Kane Low, L., Miller, J.M., Patel, D.A., Tumbarello, J.A., 2008. Graphic integration of causal factors of pelvic floor disorders: an integrated life span model. Am. J. Obstet. Gynecol. 199, 610.e1–610.e5.

Dietz, H.P., 2009. Pelvic floor assessment: a review. Fetal Maternal Med. Rev. 20, 49–66.

Dietz, H.P., Moegni, F., Shek, K.L., 2012. Diagnosis of levator avulsion injury: a comparison of three methods. Ultrasound Obstet. Gynecol. 40, 693–698.

Dietz, H.P., Shek, K.L., 2008a. The quantification of levator muscle resting tone by digital assessment. Int. Urogynecol. J. Pelvic Floor Dysfunct. 19, 1489–1493.

Dietz, H.P., Shek, K.L., 2008b. Validity and reproducibility of the digital detection of levator trauma. Int. Urogynecol. J. Pelvic Floor Dysfunct. 19, 1097–1101.

Dietz, H.P., Shek, K.L., Daly, O., Korda, A., 2013. Can levator avulsion be repaired surgically? A prospective surgical pilot study. Int. Urogynecol. J. Pelvic Floor Dysfunct. 24, 1011–1015.

Dietz, H.P., Simpson, J., 2008. Levator trauma is associated with pelvic organ prolapse. Br. J. Obstet. Gynaecol. 115, 979–984.

DiNubile, N.A., 1991. Strength Training. Clinical Sports Medicine 10 (1), 33–62.

Dumoulin, C., Lemieux, M.C., Bourbonnais, D., Gravel, D., Bravo, G., Morin, M., 2004. Physiotherapy for persistent postnatal stress urinary incontinence: a randomized controlled trial. Obstet. Gynecol. 104, 504–510.

Feldman, A.S., Bauer, S.B., 2006. Diagnosis and management of dysfunctional voiding. Curr. Opin. Pediatr. 18 (2), 139–147.

FitzGerald, M.P., Payne, C.K., Lukacz, E.S., Yang, C.C., Peters, K.M., Chai, T.C., et al. for the Interstitial Cystitis Collaborative Research Network, 2012. Randomized multicenter clinical trial of myofascial physical therapy in women with interstitial cystitis/painful bladder syndrome and pelvic floor tenderness. J. Urol. 187, 2113–2118.

Hagen, S., Stark, D., Glazener, C., Dickson, S., Barry, S., Elders, A., et al., 2014. Individualised pelvic floor muscle training in women with pelvic organ prolapse (POPPY): a multicentre randomized controlled trial. Lancet 383 (9919), 796–806.

Haylen, B.T., de Ridder, D., Freeman, R.M., Swift, S.E., Berghmans, B., Lee, J., et al., 2010. An International Urogynecological Association (IUGA)/International Continence Society (ICS) Joint report on the terminology for female pelvic floor dysfunction. Neurourol. Urodyn. 29, 4–20.

Hendrix, S.L., Clark, A., Nygaard, I., Aragaki, A., Barnabei, V., McTiernan, A., 2002. Pelvic organ prolapse in the Women's Health Initiative: gravity and gravidity. Am. J. Obstet. Gynecol. 186, 1160–1166.

Hilde, G., Stær-Jensen, J., Siafarikas, F., Gjestland, K., Ellstrøm Engh, M., Bø, K., 2013. How well can pelvic floor muscles with major defects contract? A cross-sectional comparative study 6 weeks after delivery using transperineal 3D/4D ultrasound and manometer. Br. J. Obstet. Gynaecol. 120, 1423–1429.

Hung, H.C., Hsiao, S.M., Chih, S.Y., Lin, H.H., Tsauo, J.Y., 2010. An alternative intervention for urinary incontinence: retraining diaphragmatic, deep abdominal and pelvic floor muscle coordinated function. Man. Ther. 15 (3), 273–279.

Jelovsek, J.E., Maher, C., Marber, M.D., 2007. Pelvic organ prolapse. Lancet 369 (9566), 1027–1038.

Junginger, B., Baessler, K., Sapsford, R., Hodges, P.W., 2010. Effect of abdominal and pelvic floor tasks on muscle activity, abdominal pressure and bladder neck. Int. Urogynecol. J. Pelvic Floor Dysfunct. 21, 69–77.

Kamo, I., Torimoto, K., Chancellor, M.B., de Groat, W.C., Yoshimura, N., 2003. Urethral closure mechanisms under sneeze-induced stress condition in rats: a new animal model for evaluation of stress urinary incontinence. Am. J. Physiol. Regul. Integr. Comp. Physiol. 285, R356–R365.

Kruger, J.A., Dietz, H.P., Budgett, S.C., Dumoulin, C.L., 2014. Comparison between transperineal ultrasound and digital detection of levator trauma. Can we improve the odds? Neurourol. Urodyn. 33, 307–311.

Landon, C.R., Crofts, C.E., Smith, A.R.B., Trowbridge, E.A., 1990. Mechanical properties of fascia during pregnancy: a possible factor in the development of stress incontinence of urine. Contemp. Rev. Obstet. Gynaecol. 15 (2), 40–46.

Laycock, J., 1994. Chapter 2.2 Clinical evaluation of the pelvic floor. In: Schüssler, B., Laycock, J., Norton, P., Stanton, S. (Eds.), Pelvic Floor Re-Education, first ed. Springer Verlag, Berlin.

MacLennan, A., Taylor, A., Wilson, D.H., Wilson, D., 2000. The prevalence of pelvic floor disorders and their relationship to gender, age, parity and mode of delivery. Br. J. Obstet. Gynaecol. 107, 1460–1470.

Madill, S.J., McLean, L., 2006. Relationship between abdominal and pelvic floor muscle activation and intravaginal pressure during pelvic floor muscle contractions in healthy continent women. Neurourol. Urodyn. 25 (7), 722–730.

Madill, S.J., McLean, L., 2008. Quantification of abdominal and pelvic floor muscle synergies in response to voluntary pelvic floor muscle contractions. J. Electromyogr. Kinesiol. 18, 955–964.

Messelink, B., Benson, T., Berghmans, B., Bø, K., Corcos, J., Fowler, C., et al., 2005. Standardization of terminology of pelvic floor muscle function and dysfunction: report from the pelvic floor clinical assessment group of the International Continence Society. Neurourol. Urodyn. 24, 374–380.

Miller, J.M., Ashton-Miller, J.A., DeLancey, J.O.L., 1998. A pelvic muscle pre-contraction can reduce cough-related urine loss in selected women with mild SUI. J. Am. Geriatr. Soc. 46, 870–874.

Netter, F.H., 2010. Atlas of Human Anatomy, fifth ed. Elsevier Saunders, Philadelphia.

Neumann, P., 2015. Use of pessaries to prevent and treat pelvic organ prolapse. In: Bø, K., Berghmans, B., Mørkved, S., van Kampen, M. (Eds.), Evidence-Based Physical Therapy for the Pelvic Floor. Churchill Livingstone, Edinburgh, pp. 230–234.

Neumann, P., Blizzard, L., Grimmer, K., Grant, R., 2004. Expanded Paper Towel Test: an objective test of urine loss for stress incontinence. Neurourol. Urodyn. 23, 649–655.

Neumann, P., Gill, V., 2002. Pelvic floor and abdominal muscle interaction: EMG activity and intra-abdominal pressure. Int. Urogynecol. J. Pelvic Floor Dysfunct. 13, 125–132.

O'Dell, K.K., Morse, A.N., Crawford, S.L., Howard, A., 2007. Vaginal pressure during lifting, floor exercises, jogging, and use of hydraulic exercise machines. Int. Urogynecol. J. Pelvic Floor Dysfunct. 18, 1481–1489.

Oyama, I.A., Rejba, A., Lukban, J.C., Fletcher, E., Kellogg-Spadt, S., Holzberg, A.S., et al., 2004. Modified Thiele massage as therapeutic intervention for female patients with interstitial cystitis and high-tone pelvic floor dysfunction. Urology 64 (5), 862–865.

Persson, J., Wolner-Hanssen, P., Rydhstroem, H., 2000. Obstetric risk factors for stress urinary incontinence: a population-based study. Obstet. Gynecol. 96 (3), 440–445.

Peterson, T.V., Karp, D.R., Aguilar, V.C., Davila, G.W., 2010. Validation of a global pelvic floor symptom bother questionnaire. Int. Urogynecol. J. Pelvic Floor Dysfunct. 21, 1129–1135.

Rostaminia, G.1., Shobeiri, S.A., Quiroz, L.H., 2013. Surgical repair of bilateral levator ani muscles with ultrasound guidance. Int. Urogynecol. J. Pelvic Floor Dysfunct. 24 (7), 1237–1239.

Sapsford, R., 2004. Rehabilitation of pelvic floor muscles utilizing trunk stabilization. Man. Ther. 9, 3–12.

Sapsford, R., Hodges, P., 2001. Contraction of the pelvic floor muscles during abdominal maneuvers. Arch. Phys. Med. Rehabil. 82, 1081–1088.

Sapsford, R., Hodges, P., Richardson, C., Markwell, S., Jull, G., 2001. Co-activation of the abdominal and pelvic floor muscles during voluntary exercises. Neurourol. Urodyn. 20, 31–42.

Shek, K., Dietz, H., 2010. Intrapartum risk factors for levator trauma. Br. J. Obstet. Gynaecol. 117 (12), 1485–1492. doi:10.1111/j.1471-0528.2010.02704.x.

Simpson, S., Deeble, M., Thompson, J., Andrews, A., Briffa, K., 2016. Should women with incontinence and prolapse do abdominal curls? Int. Urogynecol. J. 27 (10), 1507–1512.

Sultan, A.H., 1999. Obstetric perineal injury and anal incontinence. Clinical Risk 5 (5), 193–196.

Thompson, J.A., O'Sullivan, P.B., 2003. Levator plate movement during voluntary pelvic floor muscle contraction in subjects with incontinence and prolapse: a cross-sectional study and review. Int. Urogynecol. J. Pelvic Floor Dysfunct. 14, 84–88.

Thompson, J.A., O'Sullivan, P.B., Briffa, N.K., Neumann, P.B., 2006a. Differences in muscle activation patterns during pelvic floor muscle contractions and Valsalva manoeuvre. Neurourol. Urodyn. 25, 148–155.

Thompson, J.A., O'Sullivan, P.B., Briffa, N.K., Neumann, P.B., 2006b. Altered muscle activation patterns in symptomatic women during pelvic floor muscle contraction and Valsalva manoeuvre. Neurourol. Urodyn. 25 (3), 268–276.

Tian, T., Budgett, S., Smalldridge, J., Hayward, L., Stinear, J., Kruger, J., 2017. Assessing exercises recommended for women at risk of pelvic floor disorders using multivariate statistical techniques. Int Urogynecol. J. doi:10.1007/s00192-017-3473-6.

Valtin, H., 2002. "Drink at least eight glasses of water a day." Really? Is there scientific evidence for "8 x 8"? Am. J. Physiol. Regul. Integr. Comp. Physiol. 283, R993–R1004.

van Delft, K.W.M., Sultan, A.H., Thakar, R., Shobeiri, S.A., Kluivers, K.B., 2015a. Agreement between palpation and transperineal and endovaginal ultrasound in the diagnosis of levator ani avulsion. Int. Urogynecol. J. Pelvic Floor Dysfunct. 26, 33–39.

van Delft, K.W.M., Thakar, R., Sultan, A.H., IntHout, J., Kluivers, K.B., 2015b. The natural history of levator avulsion one year following childbirth: a prospective study. BJOG 122, 1266–1273.

Neck and Upper Extremity Pain in a Female Office Assistant: Where Does the Problem Lie?

Jodi L. Young • Joshua A. Cleland • Darren A. Rivett • Mark A. Jones

History

Kelly is a 27-year-old female who was referred to physical therapy with a 3-month history of neck and left upper extremity pain. Her primary symptoms were in the left anterior shoulder, with radiation to the left lateral elbow described as achy and dull, and her neck pain was located on the left side of her cervical spine in the C5–C6 region with radiation into her left midscapular region during active cervical left rotation and side flexion (Fig. 22.1). The shoulder pain had an insidious onset 3 months ago, and the elbow symptoms also appeared insidiously within the last month. Her neck symptoms were originally only noticeable in the morning when Kelly woke up with reported stiffness, which she noted began about 5 months prior, with a recent progression to neck pain over the last few weeks. The neck stiffness subsided after an hour or two of Kelly moving around and doing her activities of daily living (ADLs), so she had paid little attention to her neck symptoms. However, she did note that the stiffness and neck pain, along with the shoulder pain, seemed to be getting worse over the past 3 weeks, and Kelly said that she had not done anything differently in her normal daily routine at work or home to exacerbate her symptoms. The shoulder and elbow pain were most prevalent when Kelly was using her arm, specifically at work and if doing activities such as cooking, cleaning or folding laundry at home. Kelly worked as an office assistant, so most of her 8-hour work day was spent sitting at a desk, typing, answering the phone, or working on the computer. At times she had to file charts, which required her to use her left arm extensively for a short duration of time. Recreationally, Kelly ran 3–4 days a week anywhere from 1 to 5 miles. Running provoked her shoulder and elbow pain after about a mile, but it would quickly subside with 15 minutes of rest. Of note is that Kelly was left-hand dominant.

Kelly's symptoms started with morning stiffness of the neck, as indicated previously, that subsided within 1–2 hours after waking. She indicated that there was originally not much pain in her neck but instead general stiffness, specifically with left cervical rotation and side flexion. The numeric pain rating scale (NPRS) was used to capture Kelly's level of pain. She was asked to indicate the intensity of current, best and worst levels of pain over the past 24 hours using an 11-point scale ranging from 0 ('no pain') to 10 ('worst pain imaginable'). The NPRS has been shown to exhibit a minimal clinically important difference of 2 points (Cleland et al., 2008b). Because of the recent worsening of her neck symptoms, she said that she was actually now beginning to have pain rated 4/10 on the NPRS when turning her head to the left while driving. Kelly stated that the pain in her left shoulder and elbow varied depending on her activity level. On weekends, when Kelly was not at work, her shoulder and elbow symptoms were much less noticeable (1/10) and only occurred if she was cooking, cleaning or folding laundry for more than an hour. If

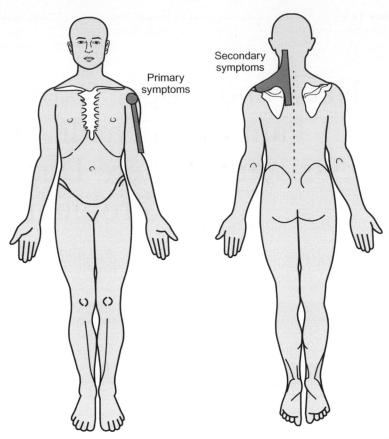

Primary symptoms

Secondary symptoms

Fig. 22.1 Kelly's body chart.

she did these activities for short periods of time, such as 30 minutes, there were no symptoms. She indicated that the pain level would reach a 4/10 on the NPRS if she performed these activities for more than an hour. If she stopped doing those activities, her pain would subside within 15–20 minutes. Kelly reported her work is what triggered her symptoms the most, and after 2 hours of sitting at her desk performing her normal work duties, her symptoms in the left shoulder and elbow would reach a 6/10 pain level, and her neck had begun to exhibit pain in the last few weeks reaching a 4/10. If Kelly were to stand up, walk around or rest her arm, the symptoms in her shoulder and elbow would decrease to a 2/10 pain level after approximately 15 minutes. Her neck pain would decrease within only a few minutes of getting up and moving around. We discussed an ergonomic assessment, and Kelly had already undergone this assessment through her employer, and changes had been made to her desk setup a month prior, but her symptoms had not changed.

Because Kelly was exhibiting both left upper extremity (UE) and neck symptoms, she was asked to complete two functional outcome measures: the Upper Extremity Functional Index (UEFI) and the Neck Disability Index (NDI). For the UEFI, patients are asked to rate the difficulty of performing 20 functional tasks on a Likert-type scale ranging from 0 (extremely difficult or unable to perform activity) to 4 (no difficulty). A total score out of 80 is calculated by summing each score. The answers provide a score between 0 and 80, with lower scores representing more disability. The reliability of the UEFI has been shown to be 0.95, and the minimal clinically important difference (MCID) has been identified at 9 points (Stratford et al., 2001).

The NDI is the most widely used condition-specific disability scale for patients with neck pain and consists of 10 items addressing different aspects of function, each scored from 0 to 5, with a maximum score of 50 points. The score is then doubled and interpreted as a percentage of the patient-perceived disability. Higher scores represent increased levels of disability. The NDI has been demonstrated to be a reliable and valid outcome measure for patients with neck pain (Hains et al., 1989; Riddle and Stratford 1998). The NDI has been shown to exhibit an MCID of 19 points (Cleland et al., 2008b). Kelly scored a 46/50 on the UEFI and a 56% on the NDI at the time of the initial visit.

Kelly also completed a modified Fear-Avoidance Beliefs Questionnaire to assess for any possible psychosocial involvement related to her symptoms. Kelly's overall score on the work and physical activity subscales did not indicate that her symptoms were related to a psychosocial component.

Kelly noted that she would continue to perform her work duties regardless of the pain level, trying to make modifications like standing up and walking around as often as possible. She also stated that there was no pattern of worsening pain or symptoms throughout the day; it solely depended on her overall activity level at work or home.

She woke up approximately three to four times per night with shoulder symptoms if she slept on her left side. However, Kelly stated that this was not much of a problem for her because she would fall asleep within a few minutes if she repositioned herself on her back or right side.

Kelly's past medical history was unremarkable for any significant illness, injury or hospitalizations, and her family history was also unremarkable. She denied any paresthesia in her upper extremities, reported no significant weakness in her upper or lower extremities and had no history of unexplained weight loss. She did not exhibit dizziness, diplopia, dysarthria, dysphagia, drop attacks, nystagmus, nausea or numbness that may be indicative of cervical arterial dysfunction (Sizer et al., 2007). Lastly, she did not report any dexterity loss or clumsiness during gait, ruling out cervical myelopathy (Cook et al., 2009).

Kelly had not been taking any medications until most recently when she was prescribed an anti-inflammatory by her physician for her current issue. However, she stated that she stopped taking it after a week because it did not seem to change any of her symptoms and resulted in gastrointestinal irritation.

At this point in time, it appeared that Kelly's symptoms in both her left shoulder and elbow were primarily originating from her shoulder, but because there seemed to be a recent, unexplained increase in neck and shoulder pain, the cervical spine was still considered the primary source of Kelly's symptoms.

Reasoning Question:

1. Please discuss your reasoning underpinning your analysis that Kelly's symptoms are originating from two sources, with the cervical spine being dominant.

Answer to Reasoning Question:

After working through the history with Kelly, it was apparent that there were a few possible pathologies to explore during the physical examination. The primary hypothesis was mechanical neck pain based on the behavior of Kelly's symptoms. Because Kelly's shoulder and elbow pain, as well as cervical spine pain and stiffness, had increased recently, it appeared these two symptom locations were related. Because there is evidence for dysfunction in the cervicothoracic region being related to lateral elbow pain (Berglund et al., 2008) and further evidence for positive outcomes for intervention directed toward the thoracic spine (Strunce et al., 2009) and cervicothoracic region in individuals with shoulder symptoms (Mintken et al., 2010), it was thought that the cervical spine was the primary source of Kelly's symptoms.

However, Kelly's shoulder and elbow presentation could not be neglected, as there could have also been local sources of nociception, for example, subacromial structures through a mechanism of subacromial impingement or symptomatic rotator cuff pathology. The presence of dull and achy anterior shoulder pain is common with rotator cuff pathology or subacromial impingement, and radiation to the lateral elbow may be seen in patients with these.

With the radiation of symptoms into Kelly's shoulder and elbow, cervical radiculopathy and a possible neurodynamic issue were also considered. Individuals with neck symptoms may have cervical radiculopathy or neurodynamic symptoms, but it is less common to have symptoms similar to Kelly's, and it would have been more likely to see symptoms originating in the neck, radiating to the anterior shoulder and lateral elbow, instead of neck symptoms that radiated to the midscapular region as Kelly described. Hence, although these were still on the hypotheses list to be examined, they were considered less likely.

Continued on following page

Reasoning Question:

2. What are your hypotheses in relation to the most likely 'pain type' (nociceptive, neuropathic, nociplastic) for the cervical and shoulder symptoms, and is it the same for both?

Answer to Reasoning Question:

Based on Kelly's description of pain in the cervical spine and left shoulder both at rest and during activity, a nociceptive pain type was hypothesized. She described her symptoms as a dull ache in the shoulder and elbow, and some somatic referral was present with her cervical symptoms; this description of symptoms is common in nociceptive pain. Kelly was able to describe specific activities that would increase her symptoms, specifically, active cervical left rotation and side flexion of the cervical spine and home and work duties for shoulder and elbow symptoms. She also described particular activities she could do to decrease or relieve the symptoms in both the cervical spine and upper extremity, which is also indicative of nociceptive pain (Smart et al., 2012a).

Kelly denied any numbness and tingling, which is often associated with peripheral neuropathic pain, and she also had never felt her pain was burning, shooting, sharp or similar to an electric shock. Kelly's symptom severity and irritability were relatively low or moderate, whereas individuals with neuropathic pain often have high severity and irritability (Smart et al., 2012b), so neuropathic pain was judged less likely.

As far as nociplastic pain, Kelly's history of symptoms was worsening over time, but she only had a 3-month history of neck and upper extremity symptoms, and it was not expected that her symptoms would be recovering more quickly at this time due to expected healing time frames. She did not describe constant, unremitting pain, and although she had some difficulty sleeping if she fell asleep on her left shoulder, this was not of concern for the presence of central sensitization. She had distinct locations of cervical, shoulder and elbow symptoms, not widespread pain locations or hypersensitivity as would be seen in patients with nociplastic pain. Most importantly, Kelly was very clear about which activities and positions provoked and decreased her symptoms. In those who have nociplastic pain, it is difficult to find clear aggravating and easing factors (Nijs et al., 2010). The only factor for nociplastic pain being present in Kelly's case is the possibility that her elbow symptoms were the result of a secondary hyperalgesia, although this will need to be tested in the physical examination.

Clinical Reasoning Commentary:

Clinical reasoning regarding potential 'sources of symptoms' can incorporate hypotheses regarding body areas (e.g. cervical spine versus shoulder complex) and specific structures (e.g. specific levels of whole cervical motion segments such as C4–C6, specific segmental cervical structures such as the posterior intervertebral joint, intervertebral disc, or shoulder subacromial tissues versus rotator cuff, subacromial bursa, biceps, etc.). Although symptoms can exist without overt pathology (e.g. postural strain precipitating nociception), hypotheses for symptomatic pathology can also be made through recognition of typical clinical patterns. However, because hypotheses regarding tissue 'sources' and symptomatic 'pathology' cannot usually be confirmed through the clinical examination, it is important to balance this diagnostic reasoning regarding source and pathology with impairment-focused reasoning (e.g. symptomatic restriction of shoulder flexion or symptomatic restriction of a specific cervical physiological or accessory movement).

At this stage, Kelly's presentation is hypothesized as being nociceptive dominant. As discussed in Chapter 1, clinical patterns exist in 'pain type' as they do in clinical syndromes and pathologies. Although the pain type cannot be confirmed clinically at present, typical clinical patterns have been described through expert consensus, enabling therapists to hypothesize regarding the dominant pain type or combination of pain types. This evolving focus of our reasoning is important because it has significant implications for other categories of clinical judgement, such as 'precautions', 'management' and 'prognosis'.

Reasoning Question:

3. Kelly mentioned that she thought her work was what triggered her symptoms most. Can you comment on whether you thought this was entirely from a physical perspective (e.g. posture) or whether you considered that there might be other psychosocial factors?

Answer to Reasoning Question:

When Kelly presented to physical therapy, she was given a modified Fear-Avoidance Beliefs Questionnaire for her neck symptoms, which is standard practice in this clinic. Although this questionnaire was developed by Waddell et al. (1993) for patients with low back pain, its psychometric properties for patients in neck pain has been studied in more recent years (Cleland et al., 2008a) and found to have substantial test-retest reliability and high internal consistency. The Fear-Avoidance Beliefs Questionnaire has two subscales, physical activity and work. Several questions are asked about patient beliefs in regard to how particular activities may increase their pain, and if overall scores are low in both of the subscales, it is less likely that psychosocial factors may impact the patient's overall symptoms and progress with physical therapy.

In the case of Kelly, she had a score of 4 out of 24 on the physical activity subscale and a score of 16 out of 42 on the work subscale (Waddell et al., 1993). Also, Kelly never discussed any stressful events in her life or in relation to her work that may have impacted her overall mental and physical health. Because of these reasons, it was felt that Kelly's cervical and upper extremity symptoms were solely from physical impairments, including poor posture and limited mobility of the cervicothoracic and shoulder joints.

Clinical Reasoning Commentary:

As with all assessment (interview, physical, outcome re-assessments), it is an error of reasoning to assume the absence of something without explicitly assessing it. Screening (for other symptoms and health comorbidities, for other aggravating and easing factors, for psychosocial factors) is discussed in Chapter 1 as a strategy that promotes thoroughness and minimizes errors of bias. Explicit screening for potential involvement of psychosocial factors in patients' pain and disability experiences, as occurs in this case, is essential to reason and practice in a biopsychosocial framework. Refer to Chapters 3 and 4 for theory underpinning the importance of psychosocial factor screening and discussion of questionnaires and suggested areas to question in the patient interview.

Physical Examination

Observation

Kelly presented with a slight forward head posture, and when cued to improve her posture, she was able to exhibit neutral posture. She noted that she attempted to remind herself at work to maintain good posture but that she often found herself with an increased forward head posture in order to 'get closer to the computer to see the screen better'. Her thoracic spine was slightly flexed from the cervicothoracic junction to T2. She had a relatively flat thoracic spine from T3 to T6.

Cervical Range of Motion

Active cervical flexion, right side flexion and rotation were all full and pain-free. Overpressure was performed on all full and pain-free movements, with no provocation of symptoms. Active extension, left side flexion and rotation were all stiff and provoked Kelly's most recent neck pain. Kelly had full cervical extension but noted feeling considerable stiffness and a pain level of 2/10 at end range. With left side flexion and rotation, Kelly experienced similar symptoms, but she was also restricted by approximately 20 degrees for each motion as measured by a bubble inclinometer (side flexion) and a universal goniometer (rotation). A passive quadrant test on the left side provoked Kelly's neck symptoms, with radiation into her left midscapular region. With left side flexion and rotation, Kelly noted increased anterior shoulder pain that radiated to the lateral elbow, similar to the symptoms that brought her to physical therapy.

Shoulder/Elbow Range of Motion

Kelly's right shoulder active range of motion and left shoulder extension and external rotation were full and painless, but she did have restricted left shoulder flexion to 140 degrees, left shoulder abduction to 120 degrees and internal rotation of 45 degrees when assessed at 60 degrees of abduction and functional internal rotation as measured with the hand behind the back, where Kelly was able to reach the L4 level. Each of these motions provoked Kelly's primary shoulder and elbow pain. When Kelly was cued to improve her posture prior to performing range of motion, her active range of motion improved by approximately 5 degrees with shoulder flexion and abduction, but she continued to have shoulder and elbow pain. Passively, Kelly had 155 degrees of left shoulder flexion, 130 degrees of shoulder abduction and 50 degrees of internal rotation when assessed at 60 degrees of abduction. Her right shoulder passive range of motion in all planes was full and painless, as expected, per the results of active range-of-motion assessment. Overpressure was performed on all full and painless active motions bilaterally, with no reproduction of symptoms. When overpressure was performed on left shoulder flexion and abduction after passive range of motion, Kelly reported provocation of her shoulder and elbow pain at end range.

Reasoning Question:

4. Could you comment on the scapula humeral kinematics and, in particular, any abnormal muscle activity/recruitment with the active shoulder movements?

Answer to Reasoning Question:

During active shoulder flexion and abduction, it did appear that Kelly had decreased upward rotation of the scapula (serratus/upper and lower trapezius) and instead appeared to be elevating her scapula through dominant use of her upper trapezius and levator scapulae. She also had delayed downward rotation and depression when returning to a neutral position from a flexed or abducted position actively.

Before even testing the strength of her musculature through scapular biomechanical observation, it appeared Kelly had a weak serratus anterior, rhomboid major/minor and middle and lower trapezius, all muscles that assist with upward rotation, downward rotation and depression of the scapula during shoulder motion (Ludewig and Braman, 2011).

These findings pointed further to the possibility of shoulder impingement (Ludewig and Braman, 2011), and as such, this disorder continued to be on the list of potential diagnoses. However, the idea of regional interdependence defined as 'the concept that seemingly unrelated impairments in a remote anatomical region may contribute to, or be associated with, the patient's primary complaint' (Wainner et al., 2007) was the primary reasoning at this point in time. Kelly had left shoulder and elbow symptoms that were increasing in nature, but so was her cervical pain and stiffness. It was still believed that the impairments from the shoulder and elbow were related to the cervical spine, consistent with the concept of regional interdependence.

Clinical Reasoning Commentary:

The recognition of impaired scapular humeral kinematics allows for inference of weakness in the muscle force couples responsible for scapular control and the possibility that poor scapular control may be a 'contributing factor' to a subacromial problem. Such hypotheses can then be tested through manual muscle and functional tests of strength and interventions that modify scapular kinematics to assess the effect on shoulder symptoms and movement impairments. The value of holding clinical judgements as hypotheses, particularly this early in the patient assessment, is that a range of possible explanations for a patient's disability can be abductively postulated and then 'tested' through the physical examination and the ongoing management–re-assessment process.

Joint Mobility

Joint mobility was assessed in the cervical spine, thoracic spine, shoulder and elbow. The elbow joint mobility was normal bilaterally, with no provocation of symptoms during left elbow joint mobility assessment. The sternoclavicular and acromioclavicular joints were assessed and determined to have normal mobility bilaterally. With a caudal and posterior glide of the glenohumeral joint on the left from a position of elevation short of pain, Kelly's primary shoulder and elbow symptoms were provoked. Along with the provocation of symptoms, there was also stiffness with these glides. Central posterior-anterior glides to the cervical spine exhibited stiffness at the C4–C6 region, along with provocation of Kelly's neck and shoulder symptoms. Unilateral posterior-anterior glides of the cervical spine in the C4–C6 region on the left side again provoked Kelly's neck and shoulder symptoms. Mobility of the cervicothoracic junction was hypomobile with central posterior-anterior glides, but there was no provocation of Kelly's primary symptoms. Thoracic spine mobility assessment revealed asymptomatic stiffness, both central and unilateral from T1–T7.

Reasoning Question:

5. Examination of both cervical and shoulder joint mobility reproduced shoulder pain. Can you comment on the significance of this finding and how it may relate to your initial hypothesis regarding the source of the pain?

Answer to Reasoning Question:

Initially, the hypotheses for Kelly's symptoms included mechanical neck pain but also local shoulder structures, for example, as involved in subacromial impingement or rotator cuff pathology. After seeing that Kelly had provocation of symptoms in her left shoulder and elbow with caudal and posterior glides of the glenohumeral joint, involvement of the shoulder was further supported, suggesting Kelly had both a cervical spine and shoulder component to her presentation. Yet the reproduction of the same symptoms with both cervical spine and shoulder joint mobility assessment was pointing toward a primary issue in the cervical spine.

After further thought, however, with the shoulder region being innervated by peripheral nerves emanating from C4–C6, it could still make sense that an individual with cervical spine pain and stiffness could have symptoms in the shoulder region that are actually from the cervical spine but mimic a shoulder pathology. Based on the discussion earlier regarding individuals with shoulder pain who respond well to interventions to the cervicothoracic region (Strunce et al., 2009; Mintken et al., 2010) and those who have cervical spine pathologies that present with elbow pain (Berglund et al., 2008), mechanical neck pain with subsequent shoulder and elbow symptoms was still the primary hypothesis. However, this hypothesis could only be confirmed with further objective information, as well as manual intervention.

Clinical Reasoning Commentary:

As previously commented, the physical examination provides the opportunity to screen the patient's physical status and to explicitly 'test' hypotheses formulated in the subjective examination (history). Here, physical impairments in shoulder movement associated with provocation of relevant symptoms are acknowledged as supporting a local shoulder component to the problem. The relationship between shoulder innervation and Kelly's demonstrated cervical impairment occurring at these same levels provides a mechanism for cervical somatic referral to the shoulder and/or sensitization of shoulder tissues. This highlights the importance of avoiding premature conclusions and the value of more open, hypothesis-oriented reasoning that considers physical findings as 'supporting' different components to a presentation. In this case, both cervical and shoulder components are acknowledged, even if one is judged more likely, keeping the reasoning open until further 'testing' is carried out through trial treatment interventions.

Strength Assessment

Because of the nature of involvement of the cervical spine, shoulder and elbow, specific muscles were manual muscle tested. Kelly exhibited strength of 4/5 in the shoulder external rotators and middle trapezius/rhomboids of her left shoulder, 3/5 in her lower trapezius bilaterally and 4/5 in her serratus anterior bilaterally.

The deep neck flexor endurance test was also assessed based on Kelly's forward head posture contributing to possible upper cross-postural syndrome, as well as cervical spine symptoms. Kelly was able to perform the deep neck flexor endurance test for only 18 seconds, whereas a normal finding has been reported to be greater than 38 seconds (Harris et al., 2005).

Neurological Assessment

To rule out any potential neurological involvement, upper extremity myotomes were assessed, with normal findings bilaterally. Dermatomal assessment with light touch and muscle stretch reflexes for the brachioradialis, biceps and triceps were also found to be normal bilaterally.

Other Tests

Although there was no reason to suspect that Kelly had upper cervical ligamentous instability or cervical arterial dysfunction from her history, because cervical spine manual therapy was a likely intervention for Kelly based on earlier findings, the Sharp-Purser, alar ligament stress, and anterior shear tests were assessed, with no movement impairment or reproduction of symptoms (Mintken, 2008). No specific special tests were performed to determine cervical arterial dysfunction due to the low sensitivity and specificity of these tests (Kerry and Taylor, 2009). Also, Kelly did not have any reports of dizziness, diplopia, dysarthria, dysphagia, drop attacks, nystagmus, nausea or numbness that may be indicative of cervical arterial dysfunction (Sizer et al., 2007). However, because manual therapy was likely to be implemented in Kelly's plan of care, sustained end-range cervical rotation to the left and right was performed, and Kelly had no provocation of any concerning symptoms, such as dizziness, nausea or nystagmus (Rivett et al., 2006).

In testing for subacromial impingement and rotator cuff pathology, it was difficult to obtain clear results because Kelly did not have the necessary flexion range of motion, actively or passively, to perform the Neer impingement test, which is included in two test-item clusters for subacromial impingement and full-thickness rotator cuff tears. To rule out subacromial impingement, the presence of a painful arc, weakness with external rotation and a negative Neer impingement test were assessed (Michener et al., 2009). Kelly did not exhibit a painful arc and was unable to move into the amount of passive shoulder elevation required for the Neer impingement test. She did have weakness and no pain with external rotation, but this finding occurred bilaterally, so this was not concerning and was thought to be general weakness in external rotation unrelated to any particular pathology. Based on all of the test-item cluster results from testing, subacromial impingement was ruled out. Kelly also did not exhibit a positive drop-arm sign, which allowed a full-thickness rotator cuff tear to be ruled out (Park et al., 2005).

To rule out cervical radiculopathy, the clinical prediction rule for cervical radiculopathy was utilized. This clinical prediction rule has four variables: the Spurling's test, the distraction test, upper limb tension test with a median nerve bias (ULTT A) and active cervical rotation. If the special tests are positive and the individual has active cervical rotation less than 60 degrees to the involved side, there is a positive likelihood ratio of 30.3 and a post-test probability of 90% that the individual has a diagnosis of cervical radiculopathy (Wainner et al., 2003). The Spurling's test was assessed by passively placing Kelly first into right side flexion, and then an axial load of up to 7 kg was provided from the examiner's hands. After performing this test on the right side with no provocation of symptoms, Kelly's head was positioned passively into left side flexion, and another axial load up to 7 kg was provided (Wainner et al., 2003). Kelly indicated there was discomfort in her midscapular region with only left side flexion, but there was no provocation of shoulder and elbow symptoms. To continue on with the cervical radiculopathy cluster, the distraction test was assessed in supine, with no change in symptoms.

The upper limb tension tests were assessed on Kelly due to the shoulder and elbow combination of symptoms to rule out any potential neurodynamic involvement, as well as finish assessing for the presence of cervical radiculopathy. It was thought that Kelly's description of anterior shoulder pain that radiated to the lateral elbow could be due to a radial nerve neurodynamic issue. The upper limb tension tests for median, radial and ulnar nerve biases were negative bilaterally.

Reasoning Question:

6. You indicate that you have ruled out subacromial impingement following your shoulder examination. Are you considering any other shoulder diagnoses given that glenohumeral joint mobilization reproduced shoulder and elbow symptoms?

Answer to Reasoning Question:

Following the shoulder examination, subacromial impingement and a full-thickness rotator cuff tear were ruled out. At this point, it appeared that the shoulder and elbow symptoms were a consequence of cervical involvement, but it was possible that Kelly had rotator cuff tendinopathy.

This was not a strong hypothesis, however, because subacromial impingement and rotator cuff tendinopathy are so intimately related because it is unclear which causes which (i.e. tendinopathy causing impingement or impingement causing tendinopathy). Because the test-item cluster for subacromial impingement was negative (Michener et al., 2009), rotator cuff tendinopathy was not suspected.

Other possible hypotheses that could create both shoulder and elbow symptoms are calcific tendinitis or subacromial bursitis, but without any imaging, it would be difficult to ascertain if these pathologies were present. A labral tear or glenohumeral joint instability was ruled out after the subjective examination because Kelly did not have clicking, popping or the sensation of the shoulder 'giving out' (Mazzocca et al., 2011; Dodson and Altchek, 2009). A last possible shoulder pathology would be glenohumeral arthritis, but Kelly did not fit the age group for this and had no prior history of trauma that could have led to early arthritis. Also, because Kelly indicated that the same shoulder and elbow symptoms were present with both shoulder and cervical spine joint mobility assessment, it was surmised that the cervical spine was the primary cause of her impairments and functional limitations.

Reasoning Question:

7. At the completion of your physical examination, did your hypotheses fit with your thoughts following the subjective examination?

Answer to Reasoning Question:

Subacromial impingement, rotator cuff pathology, cervical radiculopathy and neurodynamic issues were ruled out after the physical examination. Based on the findings from the examination and provocation of Kelly's primary and secondary symptoms, it was clear that the cervical spine, likely mechanical neck pain, was a source of Kelly's symptoms and that intervention should be directed toward the spine. However, the shoulder could not be ignored because limitations in range of motion and joint mobility also provoked similar symptoms. As discussed previously, there have been individuals with neck pain who have been found to have elbow symptoms, which would make sense based on the innervation that supplies the elbow region, C5–C6. Along with that, C4–C6 innervates the shoulder region. In this case, Kelly had provocation of symptoms with central posterior-anterior glides and unilateral posterior-anterior glides in the region of C4–C6. Because she had negative findings for specific shoulder and elbow pathologies, it remained most likely that the cervical spine was responsible for the shoulder and elbow findings. Regardless, Kelly had limited active and passive range of motion and stiffness with joint mobility assessment of the shoulder, so even if it was thought that the symptoms were originating from the cervical spine and mimicking a shoulder pathology, intervention was going to be directed at not only the cervical spine but also the shoulder complex.

Clinical Reasoning Commentary:

Medical 'diagnosis' typically refers to the categorization of disease, pathology or clinical syndrome. As discussed in the previous commentary, pathology-focused reasoning in musculoskeletal practice that relies on diagnostic categorization alone to guide management is fraught with error given the difficulty of confirming symptomatic pathology with a clinical examination and the poor correlation between pathology and disability. A broader view of 'diagnostic reasoning' was put forward in Chapter 1 as 'reasoning underpinning the formation of a musculoskeletal practice diagnosis related to functional limitation(s) and associated physical and movement impairments with consideration of pain type, tissue pathology and the broad scope of potential contributing factors'. This is consistent with the finding reported in this answer that shoulder and elbow symptoms were provoked and associated with restrictions in both cervical and shoulder assessments fulfilling an 'impairment' diagnosis, even when specific pathology cannot be identified.

Appointment 1

To address the cervical spine and the shoulder impairments, as well as thoracic impairments, thoracic manipulation was performed. A supine flexion manipulation targeting T3–T4 and a second targeting the cervicothoracic junction, also in a supine position, was used. When re-assessed, Kelly exhibited no change in active range of motion of either her left shoulder or her cervical extension, left side flexion or left rotation.

Because Kelly did not have a positive response to the thoracic manipulations, left glenohumeral posterior and caudal glides grades III and IV were utilized until a change in Kelly's symptoms occurred. After several bouts of glides, Kelly noted diminished stiffness and pain in the shoulder and elbow region, with an increase in left shoulder active flexion to 150 degrees, left shoulder active abduction to 140 degrees, left shoulder active internal rotation to 55 degrees and hand behind back measured with Kelly being able to reach the L2 region.

Kelly was instructed in a home exercise program for cervical flexor strengthening. She was to perform cervical flexor strengthening in a supine position, working on maintaining her head in a neutral position on a level surface while performing a chin tuck and holding for 5–10 seconds per repetition, working up to 10 repetitions one time per day. Correct form was emphasized on the first day. Based on the improvement in Kelly's range of motion and decreased pain from the glenohumeral joint mobilizations, she was also educated on how to perform self-mobilizations for glenohumeral caudal glides to maintain the motion that was achieved through the manual intervention. Lastly, Kelly was given a cross-body stretch to simulate the glenohumeral posterior glide.

Reasoning Question:

8. What was your reasoning behind starting with manipulation of the thoracic spine for your treatment? Were you surprised that it did not have an effect on the symptoms?

Answer to Reasoning Question:

Starting with a thoracic manipulation was guided by clinical experience and a plethora of research that has pointed toward the use of cervicothoracic joint thrust manipulation for those who have neck pain

Continued on following page

(Cleland et al., 2005, 2007, 2010; Dunning et al., 2012; Fernandez-de-las-Penas et al., 2009; Gonzalez-Iglesias et al., 2009) and those who have shoulder symptoms (Mintken et al., 2010; Strunce et al., 2009). Because of this, it was hoped that a thoracic manipulation would address both the cervical and shoulder symptoms that Kelly was having.

It was a surprise that the thoracic manipulation did not work because the hypothesis for the cervical spine being the primary cause of Kelly's symptoms was so strong, but research is also pointing toward the use of treatment directly at the cervical spine for those with neck pain (Puentedura et al., 2011; Puentedura et al., 2012; Boyles et al., 2010), so it is possible that Kelly is a patient who requires treatment directly at the source of her joint mobility limitations. Also, although Kelly agreed to a joint manipulation, she may not have expected that it would work, and this could have led to no change in her overall symptoms after the intervention, as it has been found that those who believe joint manipulation will work have greater success (Bishop et al., 2013). Kelly may have had the opposite expectation here, which led to no relief of her symptoms.

Reasoning Question:

9. How did the response to mobilization of the glenohumeral joint affect your initial hypotheses with respect to the overall involvement of the shoulder in the presentation?

Answer to Reasoning Question:

Kelly had many negative findings against the presence of subacromial impingement and a full-thickness rotator cuff tear, and all along, it was inferred that Kelly's shoulder and elbow symptoms were related to cervical spine involvement. Now that Kelly had a negative response to the thoracic spine manipulation directed toward the cervical and shoulder symptoms but had a positive response to an intervention directed locally at the glenohumeral joint, it led to the belief that perhaps Kelly's shoulder symptoms were truly from a glenohumeral joint issue, not just mimicking the appearance of a shoulder pathology and really a cervical spine issue. There is some evidence of shoulder impingement presenting as neck pain (Gorski and Schwartz, 2003), but could it be possible that individuals with cervical spine pathologies have symptoms that appear to be subacromial impingement also?

However, the overall hope with Kelly was still that by managing the cervical and thoracic spine with a different manual technique, Kelly's shoulder and elbow symptoms would dissipate due to the strength of the evidence for the use of a regional interdependence approach (Wainner et al., 2007).

Appointment 2 (2 Days Later)

Kelly returned to physical therapy 2 days after the initial examination/evaluation. Kelly reported that although she felt the left shoulder range of motion that was gained at the first visit was maintained, she only felt pain relief in her shoulder and elbow for approximately 2 hours after the first day of intervention. She was still experiencing similar pain levels throughout the day with all activities that were problematic the day of the examination/evaluation. Kelly confessed that she had only performed the self-mobilizations for her home exercise program because they 'were easy to do throughout the day', but she had not been compliant with the deep neck flexor strengthening exercise.

Because the glenohumeral caudal and posterior glides appeared to be working in regaining Kelly's range of motion, several bouts of grades III and IV glides were utilized in greater degrees of flexion and abduction than the first visit. When baseline range of motion was assessed at the beginning of the second visit, Kelly had 155 degrees of left active shoulder flexion, 145 degrees of left active shoulder abduction and 55 degrees of active internal rotation. She was able to reach L2 functionally in hand behind back. After mobilizing the glenohumeral joint, Kelly now exhibited 165 degrees of left active shoulder flexion, 155 degrees of left active shoulder abduction and 60 degrees of active internal rotation. Review of the home exercise program for self-mobilizations of the glenohumeral joint was performed, and Kelly was able to replicate the exercise accurately. It was believed that although Kelly's range of motion was maintained, she continued to have pain because the overall cause of her symptoms was not being fully addressed with the previous interventions. She had stiffness of the glenohumeral joint with joint mobility assessment that was related to the decrease in active and passive range of motion, but this did not seem to be related to the pain that Kelly was having because she showed good progress with range-of-motion gains with manual intervention to the glenohumeral joint but did not have an overall decrease in the pain in the region.

Not satisfied that Kelly's pain levels remained the same in the shoulder and elbow after the last appointment, treatment shifted back to the cervical and thoracic spine. Initially, Kelly was lacking 20 degrees in both left active side flexion and rotation of the cervical spine; these values remained the same on the second day of treatment, and Kelly continued to point to the left midscapular region as the area of pain during those active motions. To address the limited side flexion and rotation, grades III and IV unilateral posterior-anterior glides targeting the C4–C5 and C5–C6 segments were utilized with Kelly in a prone position. Upon re-assessment, Kelly was now only lacking 10 degrees in left active side flexion but still lacked 15 degrees in left active rotation; pain was a 4/10 on the NPRS when she came in, and it was now a 2/10 but still radiated to the midscapular region on the left side. Left active shoulder range of motion was re-assessed after the unilateral posterior-anterior glides, and Kelly exhibited the same amount of active motion, but she immediately noted that her pain was only a 1/10 on the NPRS.

It was apparent that the treatment directed at the cervical spine had an immediate positive impact on Kelly's cervical spine, shoulder and elbow symptoms. It would appear that the relationship of C4–C5 and C5–C6 to the shoulder and elbow impacted the symptoms when treated with manual therapy directed at the cervical spine. With limited time remaining in the session, Kelly was instructed on performing the deep neck flexor strengthening exercise in a seated position, if tolerated. Kelly agreed that performing the exercise in a seated position would more likely lead to her successfully completing the exercise more often than had been the case after the initial instruction.

Appointment 3 (1 Week Later)

Kelly had a 1-week lapse in intervention due to vacation, but when she returned, she relayed that she had been compliant in her home exercise program and especially felt that the glenohumeral self-mobilizations had been advantageous.

Upon re-assessing active range of motion, Kelly had maintained the cervical side flexion and rotation that was achieved on day 2. However, her pain level was still a 4/10 on the NPRS with driving and sitting for too long at her desk. Shoulder range of motion was also maintained from visit 2. In fact, Kelly indicated that she had an average pain level of 3/10 in her left shoulder while working, but she had felt no symptoms radiating to the elbow since the last visit.

Because unilateral posterior-anterior glides had been successful on day 2, they were utilized again. However, after several bouts of grades III and IV glides, there was no change in Kelly's cervical range of motion or pain. It was hypothesized that because Kelly was lacking the most cervical range of motion with left active rotation, she may benefit from transverse glides. Kelly was placed in a prone position and pre-positioned into approximately 45 degrees of left rotation. Grades III and IV transverse glides were performed from C4 to T2. Kelly had localized pain where therapist thumb pressure was, but she tolerated the mobilizations and had no other symptoms during the mobilizations. Upon re-assessment, Kelly gained 5 degrees of left active rotation and now had what was considered full active side flexion of the cervical spine. Of note was that Kelly had pain of only 1/10 on the NPRS with both active rotation and side flexion. Shoulder range of motion was assessed after the cervicothoracic interventions, and Kelly's range of motion only improved by 5 degrees with shoulder flexion, abduction and internal rotation, and functional hand-behind-back internal rotation was at the level of low thoracic spine after this intervention, but she reported no pain now with any of these active shoulder movements.

To try to increase the range of motion in Kelly's left shoulder, grade IV posterior and inferior mobilizations were utilized at Kelly's maximal range of flexion and abduction. Upon re-assessment, Kelly showed 175 degrees active flexion, 170 degrees active abduction, internal rotation measured goniometrically at 70 degrees and functional hand-behind-back internal rotation reaching the low thoracic spine. With overpressure, there was a pain level of 1/10 on the NPRS.

Because Kelly had shown progressive improvement with the manual interventions to this point, any therapeutic exercise was held until further sessions.

Reasoning Question:

10. The shoulder range of movement and pain seem to be changed by both cervical and glenohumeral mobilizations. Can you comment on this?

Answer to Reasoning Question:

Based on what had been theorized throughout the whole case, Kelly responded well in regard to pain and range of motion of both the cervical spine and shoulder when treatment was guided directly at the cervical spine. Yet, she also had some diminishing symptoms over the course of the physical therapy sessions with treatments aimed at the left glenohumeral joint.

It is possible that Kelly had an underlying shoulder pathology that was not caught during subjective and objective examination; however, the comprehensiveness of Kelly's examination ruled out many of the possible shoulder pathologies Kelly could have sustained. It is more likely that Kelly responded well to the regional interdependence approach (Wainner et al., 2007). There is a large amount of research that concludes that impairments in the cervical and/or thoracic spine may contribute to the intrinsic causes of shoulder issues (Mintken et al., 2010; Sobel et al., 1996), and in this case, it was believed that Kelly's shoulder and elbow issues were related to the presence of limited joint mobility in the cervical and thoracic regions.

Clinical Reasoning Commentary:

Whereas research evidence is available to assist selection of treatment, progression of treatment relies on thorough outcome re-assessment. As such, treatment progression can be challenging, particularly when there is support for more than one potential 'source of symptoms' and multiple potential 'contributing factors', as is often the case. Inter-relationships between impairments (neurologically, biomechanically, psychologically) underpin the changes that treating one impairment can have on others (as highlighted in the 'interdependence approach' referred to previously). Clinical reasoning regarding the contribution of potential components to a problem requires a systematic approach to progression of treatment, guided by comprehensive re-assessments that can reveal impairment relationships in nociceptive-dominant presentations. Active movement re-assessment alone can be misleading, with improvements not necessarily reflecting equivalent improvement in passive movement. Similarly, the more detail obtained regarding both active and passive movement impairments (e.g. onset of symptoms, quality of movement, relationship between symptoms and resistance to movement), the greater the ability to detect change. Although change in impairments must equate to change in function, detailed assessments reduce the risk of prematurely discarding effective interventions. Because many patient problems will have more than one component accounting for the patient's symptoms and disability, once an intervention has been demonstrated to positively change an impairment and function, it is often best to add an intervention to another potential component that has not been adequately improved by the first intervention.

Appointment 4 (2 Days Later)

Kelly's day 4 intervention was only 2 days after the third visit, and she noted that her work duties provoked a pain level of only 1/10 on the NPRS in her left shoulder and she did not have any radiating symptoms to the elbow while working. In fact, she noticed that she could partake in activities of daily living (ADLs) at home with no restrictions due to her left shoulder at this point, and she had noted zero elbow symptoms for a week. She also stated that she had woken up that morning and was sleeping on her left side. Lastly, she had returned to her normal recreational running routine and had zero symptoms.

Active shoulder range of motion was 180 degrees of shoulder flexion and 175 degrees of abduction, and Kelly now had functional hand-behind-back internal rotation reaching the low thoracic spine, and a goniometric measurement of active internal rotation was 75 degrees; she had no pain with any of these motions. It was clear that Kelly's active range of motion was improving with manual intervention and her self-mobilizations.

Kelly continued to be somewhat disappointed with her cervical spine symptoms. She indicated that the motion had improved and that overall pain had improved slightly from a baseline of 4/10 on the NPRS, but unlike her shoulder, she continued to have pain radiating to her left midscapular region that she rated as 2/10 while rotating her head during driving or any activity requiring side flexion. Along with that, the stiffness in the morning had not entirely abolished. She did feel that the stiffness resolved quicker and that working at her desk was easier on her cervical spine symptoms, but she was still disappointed in the overall improvement.

Although unilateral posterior-anterior glides and transverse glides to the midcervical and upper thoracic region had improved Kelly's symptoms within session, it did not appear that they were providing long-term improvement. Based on Kelly's initial posture of a flexed cervicothoracic junction to T2 and a flat thoracic spine from T3 to T7, this would be the targeted area of treatment for day 5. A supine manipulation targeting the cervicothoracic junction had not improved Kelly's symptoms on the first day of treatment, but it was hypothesized that using it now may have a positive impact because her shoulder and elbow symptoms appeared to be resolving well. A supine cervicothoracic junction manipulation was performed, but this time Kelly was asked to actively bridge while the manipulation was performed to provide optimal contact with the therapist's fulcrum and the cervicothoracic junction. Because Kelly had a flat thoracic spine, prone extension thoracic manipulations were performed, targeting the upper (T2–T3) and middle (T4–T5) thoracic spine (Fig. 22.2 A and B). After both the cervicothoracic junction and prone extension thoracic manipulations, Kelly's left cervical active side flexion and rotation were re-assessed. At the beginning of the visit, Kelly had painful, but full, side flexion and lacked 5 degrees of rotation, which was also painful. After the manipulations, Kelly had a pain level of 1/10 on the NPRS with side flexion and rotation. As well, Kelly's active left rotation was full after the manipulations.

Active mobility appeared to be key to Kelly's recovery, meaning that Kelly's personal input on her symptoms through self-mobilizations and active muscle contraction through strengthening was helpful in improving her overall condition. She had positive outcomes with manual interventions, and the symptoms in her shoulder and elbow were self-managed at this time, but the carryover in gains she saw for cervical spine manual interventions had not remained at this point. Kelly was instructed to tape two tennis balls together (Fig. 22.3), lie supine, placing the groove between the tennis balls over her spinous processes, and perform active dorsal glides to simulate the thoracic manipulations she had received during the day 5 intervention. While performing the dorsal glides over the tennis balls, she was instructed to rotate her head actively to the left at the same time. It was hoped that Kelly could maintain the motion she had gained at each of the visits, as well as decrease the pain over time, with her active participation on days she was not at physical therapy.

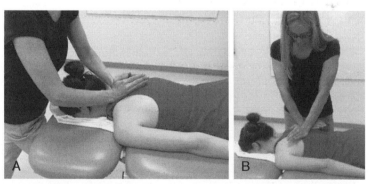

Fig. 22.2 Prone extension thoracic manipulations targeting the upper (T2–T3) thoracic spine (A) and the middle (T4–T5) thoracic spine (B).

Fig. 22.3 Dorsal glides were performed over two tennis balls taped together.

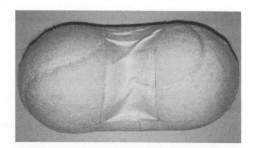

Appointment 5 (1 Week Later)

Kelly returned a week later and indicated that she was somewhat compliant with the active mobility exercises, similar to her compliance with the supine deep neck flexor strengthening activity. She was educated on the importance of her participation in her recovery, and she agreed. She stated that she would attempt to perform the exercises at least one time per day for deep neck flexor strengthening and the active dorsal glides.

She stated that her shoulder and elbow symptoms had resolved completely at this point. Her neck stiffness continued in the mornings, and pain was now rated 1/10 on the NPRS with any activity requiring active side flexion and rotation, so she continued to show gradual improvement. Active range of motion for left side flexion and rotation was now full, but end-range pain of 1/10 remained. The cervical quadrant test was re-assessed at the beginning of the visit, and it still provoked symptoms in the left midscapular region but again only caused 1/10 pain.

It was important that Kelly be given some strengthening exercises, not just manual interventions and active mobility exercises. Much of the session was focused on strengthening for the left shoulder external rotators, the bilateral middle trapezius/rhomboids, lower trapezius and serratus anterior. Kelly exhibited aberrant scapulohumeral rhythm with active left shoulder elevation (flexion and abduction), and the deviations that she had were related to weakness in the middle trapezius, rhomboid major/minor, lower trapezius and serratus anterior (Ludewig and Braman, 2011). Hence, focused strengthening exercises were developed to diminish the likelihood of future aberrant movements that could have contributed to her shoulder symptoms.

It was discussed with Kelly that she should work on the home exercise program, as well as the additional exercises from day 5, for a couple of weeks and return to physical therapy for follow-up. Kelly agreed that this plan was appropriate and that the manual interventions had worked well, but it appeared to her that she was going to have to put some work into strengthening and maintaining what gains she had earned at physical therapy.

Appointment 6 (2 Weeks Later)

Kelly returned to physical therapy 2 weeks after her day 5 intervention. She indicated that her compliance with her home exercise program had improved, and she was able to perform all of the exercises. Her symptoms in the left shoulder and elbow had continued to remain 100% improved, and she stated that she had far less stiffness in the mornings in her cervical spine. She indicated that she was able to actively rotate or side flex to the right, and she only had 1/10 on the NPRS half of the time; for the rest of the day, she would have zero pain with those activities. Also, she was able to work an 8-hour day without an onset of symptoms. The range of motion in her cervical spine had remained full in left side flexion and rotation since her last visit. Kelly indicated that she was independent with her home exercise program and felt she had returned to her prior level of function before physical therapy. Her NDI score at discharge was an 8%, and her UEFI score was a 12/50. Both of these scores exceeded the MCID for these outcome measures (Cleland et al., 2008b; Stratford et al., 2001). She was advised to contact the clinic with any further questions.

Outcome

Kelly initially presented with a myriad of symptoms that could have included the cervical spine, thoracic spine, shoulder and/or elbow. Based on a thorough assessment, it was hypothesized that Kelly's cervical and thoracic spine impairments were the most likely cause of her current status due to mechanical neck pain. Although specific manual interventions accelerated Kelly's final outcome, she ultimately realized that her individual involvement in her physical therapy intervention would lead to long-term improvement. With a combination of manual interventions that could be simulated through active mobility exercises, Kelly's recovery was excellent.

REFERENCES

Berglund, K.M., Persson, B.H., Denison, E., 2008. Prevalence of pain and dysfunction in the cervical and thoracic spine in persons with and without lateral elbow pain. Man. Ther. 13, 295–299.

Bishop, M.D., Mintken, P.E., Bialosky, J.E., Cleland, J.A., 2013. Patient expectations of benefit from interventions for neck pain and resulting influence on outcomes. Journal of Orthopaedic and Sports Physical Therapy 43, 457–465.

Boyles, R.E., Walker, M.J., Young, B.A., Strunce, J.B., Wainner, R.S., 2010. The addition of cervical thrust manipulations to a manual physical therapy approach in patients treated for mechanical neck pain: a secondary analysis. Journal of Orthopaedic and Sports Physical Therapy 40, 133–140.

Cleland, J.A., Childs, J.D., Fritz, J.M., Whitman, J.M., Eberhart, S.L., 2007. Development of a clinical prediction rule for guiding treatment of a subgroup of patients with neck pain: use of thoracic spine manipulation, exercise, and patient education. Phys. Ther. 87, 9–23.

Cleland, J.A., Childs, J.D., McRae, M., Palmer, J.A., Stowell, T., 2005. Immediate effects of thoracic manipulation in patients with neck pain: a randomized clinical trial. Man. Ther. 10, 127–135.

Cleland, J.A., Childs, J.D., Whitman, J.M., 2008a. Psychometric properties of the Neck Disability Index and Numeric Pain Rating Scale in patients with mechanical neck pain. Arch. Phys. Med. Rehabil. 89, 69–74.

Cleland, J.A., Fritz, J.M., Childs, J.D., 2008b. Psychometric properties of the Fear-Avoidance Beliefs Questionnaire and Tampa Scale of Kinesiophobia in patients with neck pain. Am. J. Phys. Med. Rehabil. 87, 109–117.

Cleland, J.A., Mintken, P.E., Carpenter, K., Fritz, J.M., Glynn, P., Whitman, J., et al., 2010. Examination of a clinical prediction rule to identify patients with neck pain likely to benefit from thoracic spine thrust manipulation and a general cervical range of motion exercise: multi-center randomized clinical trial. Phys. Ther. 90, 1239–1250.

Cook, C., Roman, M., Stewart, K.M., Leithe, L.G., Isaacs, R., 2009. Reliability and diagnostic accuracy of clinical special tests for myelopathy in patients seen for cervical dysfunction. Journal of Orthopaedic and Sports Physical Therapy 39, 172–178.

Dodson, C.C., Altchek, D.W., 2009. SLAP lesions: an update on recognition and treatment. Journal of Orthopaedic and Sports Physical Therapy 39, 71–80.

Dunning, J.R., Cleland, J.A., Waldrop, M.A., Arnot, C., Young, I., Turner, M., et al., 2012. Upper cervical and upper thoracic thrust manipulation versus nonthrust mobilization in patients with mechanical neck pain: a multicenter randomized clinical trial. Journal of Orthopaedic and Sports Physical Therapy 42, 5–18.

Fernandez-de-las-Penas, C., Cleland, J.A., Huijbregts, P., Palomeque-del-Cerro, L., Gonzalez-Iglesias, J., 2009. Repeated applications of thoracic spine thrust manipulation do not lead to tolerance in patients presenting with acute mechanical neck pain: a secondary analysis. Journal of Manual and Manipulative Therapy 17, 154–162.

Gonzalez-Iglesias, J., Fernandez-de-las-Penas, C., Cleland, J.A., Guiterrez-Vega, M.R., 2009. Thoracic spine manipulation for the management of patients with neck pain: a randomized clinical trial. Journal of Orthopaedic and Sports Physical Therapy 39, 20–27.

Gorski, J.M., Schwartz, L.H., 2003. Shoulder impingement presenting as neck pain. Journal of Bone and Joint Surgery 85_A, 635–638.

Hains, F., Waalen, J., Mior, S., 1989. Psychometric properties of the Neck Disability Index. J. Manipulative Physiol. Ther. 21, 75–80.

Harris, K.D., Heer, D.M., Roy, T.C., Santos, D.M., Whitman, J.M., Wainner, R.S., 2005. Reliability of a measurement of neck flexor muscle endurance. Phys. Ther. 85, 1349–1355.

Kerry, R., Taylor, A.J., 2009. Cervical arterial dysfunction: knowledge and reasoning for manual physical therapists. Journal of Orthopaedic and Sports Physical Therapy 39, 378–387.

Ludewig, P.M., Braman, J.P., 2011. Shoulder impingement: biomechanical considerations in rehabilitation. Man. Ther. 16, 33–39.

Mazzocca, A.D., Cote, M.P., Solovyova, O., Rizvi, S.H., Mostofi, A., Arciero, R.A., 2011. Traumatic shoulder instability involving anterior, inferior or posterior labral injury: a prospective clinical evaluation of arthroscopic repair of 270° labral tears. Am J Sports Med 39, 1687–1696.

Michener, L.A., Walsworth, M.K., Doukas, W.C., Murphy, K.P., 2009. Reliability and diagnostic accuracy of 5 physical examination tests and combination of tests for subacromial impingement. Arch. Phys. Med. Rehabil. 90, 1898–1903.

Mintken, P.E., 2008. Upper cervical ligament testing in a patient with os odontoideum presenting with headaches. Journal of Orthopaedic and Sports Physical Therapy 38, 465–475.

Mintken, P.E., Cleland, J.A., Carpenter, K.J., Bieniek, M.L., Keirns, M., Whitman, J.M., 2010. Some factors predict successful short-term outcomes in individuals with shoulder pain receiving cervicothoracic manipulation: a single-arm trial. Phys. Ther. 90, 26–42.

Nijs, J., Van Houdenhove, B., Oostendorp, R.A.B., 2010. Recognition of central sensitization in patients with musculoskeletal pain: application of pain neurophysiology in manual therapy practice. Man. Ther. 15, 135–141.

Park, H.B., Yokota, A., Gill, H.S., El Rassi, G., McFarland, E.G., 2005. Diagnostic accuracy of special tests for the different degrees of subacromial impingement syndrome. Journal of Bone and Joint Surgery 87_A, 1446–1455.

Puentedura, E.J., Cleland, J.A., Landers, M.R., Mintken, P., Louw, A., Fernandez-de-las-Penas, C., 2012. Development of a clinical prediction rule to identify patients with neck pain likely to benefit from thrust joint manipulation to the cervical spine. Journal of Orthopaedic and Sports Physical Therapy 42, 577–592.

Puentedura, E.J., Landers, M.R., Cleland, J.A., Mintken, P., Huijbregts, P., Fernandez-de-las-Penas, C., 2011. Thoracic spine thrust manipulation versus cervical spine thrust manipulation in patients with acute neck pain: a randomized clinical trial. Journal of Orthopaedic and Sports Physical Therapy 41, 208–220.

Riddle, D., Stratford, P., 1998. Use of generic versus region-specific functional status measures on patients with cervical spine disorders. Phys. Ther. 78, 951–963.

Rivett, D.A., Shirley, D., Magarey, M., Refshauge, K., 2006. Clinical Guidelines for Assessing Vertebrobasilar Insufficiency in the Management of Cervical Spine Disorders. Australian Physiotherapy Association, Camberwell, Australia.

Sizer, P.S., Brismée, J.M., Cook, C., 2007. Medical screening for red flags in the diagnosis and management of musculoskeletal spine pain. Pain Pract 7, 53–71.

Smart, K.M., Blake, C., Staines, A., Thacker, M., Doody, C., 2012a. Mechanisms-based classifications of musculoskeletal pain: Part 2 of 3: symptoms and signs of peripheral neuropathic pain in patients with low back (+leg) pain. Man. Ther. 17, 345–351.

Smart, K.M., Blake, C., Staines, A., Thacker, M., Doody, C., 2012b. Mechanisms-based classifications of musculoskeletal pain: Part 3 of 3: symptoms and signs of nociceptive pain in patients with low back (+ leg) pain. Man. Ther. 17, 352–357.

Sobel, J.S., Kremer, I., Winters, J.C., Arendzen, J.H., de Jong, B.M., 1996. The influence of the mobility in the cervicothoracic spine and the upper ribs (shoulder girdle) on the mobility of the scapulohumeral joint. J Manipulative Physiol Ther 19, 469–474.

Stratford, P.W., Binkley, J.M., Stratford, D.M., 2001. Development and initial validation of the Upper Extremity Functional Index. Physiotherapy Canada 53, 259–263.

Strunce, J.B., Walker, M.J., Boyles, R.E., Young, B.A., 2009. The immediate effects of thoracic spine and rib manipulation on subjects with primary complaints of shoulder pain. J Man Manip Ther 17, 230–236.

Waddell, G., Newton, M., Henderson, I., Somerville, D., Main, C.J., 1993. Fear-Avoidance Beliefs Questionnaire (FABQ) and the role of fear-avoidance beliefs in chronic low back pain and disability. Pain 52, 157–168.

Wainner, R.S., Fritz, J.M., Irrgang, J.J., Boninger, M.L., Delitto, A., Allison, S., 2003. Reliability and diagnostic accuracy of the clinical examination and patient self-report measures for cervical radiculopathy. Spine 28 (1), 52–62.

Wainner, R.S., Whitman, J.M., Cleland, J.A., Flynn, T.W., 2007. Regional interdependence: a musculoskeletal examination model whose time has come. J Orthop Sports Phys Ther 37, 658–660.

23

Managing a Chronic Whiplash Problem When the Patient Lives 900 Kilometres Away

Jochen Schomacher • Mark A. Jones

First Appointment

Current Complaints and Their History

Sabrina is a 29-year-old mother of a 3-year-old son. She is a musculoskeletal physiotherapist working part-time (27 hours per week) since the birth of her child. Living in another city 900 kilometres away, she was visiting to take a professional cervical spine examination and treatment course and took the opportunity to seek treatment by the first author, who was teaching in the course. Because Sabrina was in town for only 3 days, we agreed on initial daily appointments over 3 consecutive days, after which we would discuss how best to proceed.

Sabrina's primary complaint was a bilateral suboccipital pain (intensity on the Numeric Rating Scale [NRS] 3–4/10), which she described as feeling 'like something is locked, as if there is a screw inside' (Fig. 23.1). In addition, Sabrina described a constant low-intensity headache (NRS 1–2/10) located in the occipital region that was sometimes associated with the suboccipital pain. When her suboccipital pain was sufficiently aggravated, it would irradiate over the back of her head toward her forehead up to the eyes, worsening the constant headache. When this aggravation happened, usually about once a week, the field of vision was restricted, leaving only a kind of 'tunnel vision'. During these more severe attacks, her headache intensity reached NRS 8–9/10, with associated dizziness and nausea, which constrained Sabrina to bed rest in a dark room and to taking pain medication in the hope of being fit again the next morning. The dizziness was a kind of unsteadiness, as if she was 'drunk', but sometimes appeared as a brief but strong feeling of a '360-degree twisting', after which she felt fine again.

All of these complaints occurred for the first time 12 years ago after a rear-end whiplash trauma. Sabrina received physiotherapy elsewhere consisting of gentle manual therapy with manual traction and stabilizing exercises performed into pain. She reported being disappointed that it took 9 months of this treatment for all her symptoms to decrease. Unfortunately, 1 year after the first accident, Sabrina suffered a second rear-end whiplash trauma, causing the same combination of symptoms to return. She resumed the previous physiotherapy treatment, which again did not provide quick relief. She became increasingly frustrated with her lack of improvement and gave up on pursuing further treatment. Since that time, Sabrina had continued to experience the same symptoms intermittently at a high intensity (up to NRS 8–9/10 for the suboccipital pain and headache) about once a week, although with 'better and worse periods'. Overall, the symptoms had remained the same for about 11 years at the time of the initial appointment, during which her efforts to find alleviation with the help of various medical doctors (including medication) and other physiotherapists failed. Sabrina did not report any other neurological symptoms, such as numbness or pins and needles, nor any other potential cervical arterial dysfunction symptoms.

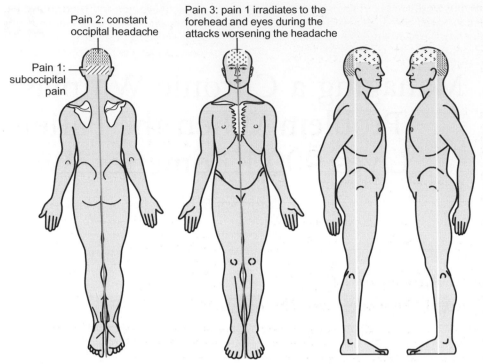

Fig. 23.1 Body chart illustrating Sabrina's three pains. *(Reproduced with permission from Schomacher [2014].)*

Behaviour of Current Symptoms

There was no specific movement that directly evoked Sabrina's complaints. Although her suboccipital 'locking pain' sometimes occurred following small casual movements of her head, it was more consistently associated with prolonged periods of sitting and being immobile and with high-intensity activities using her arms, like when carrying heavy objects. It was also precipitated by work stress. The locking pain increased during the day and was present many times during the week, although not every day. Aggravation of the headache was unpredictable, although it often started with the neck pain and following banal activities. Generally, her suboccipital neck pain and headache could be easily aggravated by different events as described previously. When asked about fitness activities, Sabrina reported she enjoyed exercise and used to complete 2-hour workouts at a fitness centre, but she had to abandon this, as well as her rock climbing, because all strengthening and group cardio exercise aggravated her symptoms. However, she was still able to jog, although only at moderate intensity, such as half an hour of slow running, because higher intensity or longer periods of running aggravated her symptoms. If kept to moderate intensity and shorter distances, her running provided some relief to her suboccipital neck pain. Intensive practice of cervical spine treatment techniques performed on her during a recent continuing education course also severely aggravated her symptoms later that evening. Her symptoms were generally less noticeable during holidays without stress.

General Health

Except for some low back pain that was not related to her neck pain and headache, Sabrina reported good health with no comorbidities. No red flags were present.

Patient Perspectives

Sabrina seemed resigned to living with her current symptoms and to making the best of her situation. Although she enjoyed her work as a physiotherapist, she acknowledged having work stress but added that she felt she was generally coping and tried to live her life as far as her complaints permitted. However, Sabrina was somewhat reserved in discussing her work and personal environment, and therefore this was not pursued further at this stage. Her goal for seeking assistance at this time was simply to improve as much as possible.

Reasoning Question:

1. Based on this initial information from your patient history, what were your early hypotheses and associated reasoning regarding (a) dominant 'pain type' (nociceptive, neuropathic, nociplastic) and (b) possible 'sources of symptoms' if you believed a nociceptive pain type might have been present?

Answer to Reasoning Question:

Dominant Pain Type

There were no features suggestive of a neuropathic pain (Tampin 2014). However, Sabrina's symptoms had become chronic, and her persistent pain and disability supported the presence of changes in her pain-modulating system (Chimenti et al. 2018). Her slow recovery during the 9 months after her first whiplash trauma might have been partially related to the painful exercises she had been given. Repeated evocation of pain might have created a sensitization of the pain-modulating system and even a 'pain memory' (Zusman, 2003). The localized nature of her suboccipital pain and consistent pattern of aggravation related to posture and movement supported a possible nociceptive component that may also have contributed to her ongoing symptoms (Giamberardino, 2003).

Sabrina had resigned herself to living with her symptoms, and her belief was that nobody could help her (but she was not happy with this situation and, accordingly, sought our assistance). This negative outlook could adversely affect her pain modulation because inappropriate emotions and cognitions can influence the descending pain-inhibitory mechanisms (Nijs et al., 2009). Her reserved attitude suggested she did not want to discuss this and limited further questioning.

Possible Sources of Symptoms

Specific structural sources of neck pain (nociception), such as the intervertebral disc or the zygapophyseal joint, cannot be clinically diagnosed (Bogduk and McGuirk, 2006). Furthermore, we do not have musculoskeletal treatment techniques specific to different spinal structures (Zusman, 2013). Consequently, as musculoskeletal clinicians, we should first look for dysfunctions in posture and movement as indicating possible sources of nociception (Jones and Rivett, 2004). Once a posture/movement dysfunction has been found, the clinician can then attempt to differentiate if it is caused or influenced by connective (joint), muscular or neural tissues, as the treatment techniques are different for these three tissues (Kaltenborn, 2012).

From a mechanical point of view, Sabrina's story pointed more to a hypermobility presentation than a hypomobility problem. If she had significant symptomatic restrictions in movement, they would be expected to evoke pain at the end of her cervical movements when tissues become tightened, stimulating mechanoreceptors and nociceptors. This pattern was not reflected in her reported behaviour of symptoms. Furthermore, the development of hypomobility requires a period of immobilization or of non-usage or a specific pathology such as ankylosing spondylitis, none of which were apparent in Sabrina's history. The variability of Sabrina's symptoms and the alleviation of her neck pain possibly through the movement associated with her moderate running were more consistent with a pattern of hypermobility. Intensive movements in a large range of motion or prolonged immobile postures in lying, sitting or standing usually aggravate hypermobility symptoms (Niere and Torney, 2004; Olson and Joder, 2001). This seems to fit with Sabrina's story.

The systematic physical examination will show whether Sabrina's symptoms are related to the neck and, if so, to which region or segment of the cervical spine. Although the information from the subjective examination supports a typical pattern of cervical hypermobility and a sensitized pain-modulating system, at this stage of the examination, specific hypotheses regarding potential nociceptive sources for her three major symptoms are not considered. Instead, a systematic structured physical examination for cervical problems is followed in order to generate specific hypotheses regarding the most likely tissues involved (e.g. connective tissue (joint), muscle, neural).

Reasoning Question:

2. What were your thoughts regarding 'precautions or contraindications to the patient's physical examination and initial treatment'?

The subjective examination did not reveal any 'red flags' suggestive of serious pathology or an acute and severe compression of the nervous system requiring medical intervention. Sabrina reported only two (dizziness and nausea) of the classic 5 D and 3 N symptoms associated with cervical arterial

Continued on following page

dysfunction (the others being diplopia, drop attacks, dysarthria, dysphagia; numbness, nystagmus). She also denied ataxia as the ninth 'classic sign' (Kerry and Taylor, 2006). This screening, however, is insufficient on its own to rule out this condition (Kerry and Taylor, 2006). Sabrina's dizziness, nausea and tunnel-vision symptoms represented a precaution and would need to be carefully monitored during the physical examination and treatment. Further screening would also need to be carried out in the physical examination prior to any orthopaedic manual therapy, including manipulation, mobilization and exercise (Rushton et al., 2014). In addition, the high irritability of her symptoms also warranted caution during the physical examination and treatment to avoid excessive aggravation.

At this point, without any evidence of serious pathology, Sabrina seemed to have what is called a 'simple mechanical dysfunction' (Waddell, 1998) with a possible sensitization of the pain-modulating system, including a 'pain memory'.

Clinical Reasoning Commentary:

As discussed in Chapters 1 and 2, it is important to hypothesize about 'pain type' because this influences the interpretation of physical findings, management decisions and prognosis. However, as highlighted here, even when features of a nociplastic pain type are present (e.g. sensitization of pain modulating system and pain memory) this does not discount a nociceptive component contributing to symptoms and sensitization. Physical examination will provide further clarification, as will initial treatments and re-assessments.

Clinical reasoning regarding potential 'sources of symptoms' (i.e. specific structures/tissues involved and pathology) is relevant to nociceptive- and/or neuropathic-dominant presentations and needs to be balanced with impairment-focussed reasoning. Although the validity of the clinical examination to differentiate specific sources of nociception and pathology is usually limited, these can still be hypothesized on the basis of common clinical patterns (involving area, behaviour and history of symptoms and later physical findings). We know pathology in general does not typically correlate well with the clinical presentation (i.e. pathology can be asymptomatic; pathology can have varied clinical presentations; symptoms can exist without overt pathology) – hence the importance of impairment-focussed assessment and management. However, despite these limitations, pathology should still be hypothesized because potential serious and sinister pathology has implications for safety (e.g. specific physical testing or referral for further investigation as with, for example, subjective features of craniovertebral instability, cervical arterial dysfunction, or neurological involvement). Potential 'sources of symptoms' and 'pathology' hypothesized from the subjective examination can then be correlated with symptomatic and asymptomatic impairments in posture, mobility, palpation and muscle control/strength from the physical examination to generate further hypotheses regarding joint, muscle, soft tissue, neural and vascular impairments that may require treatment.

Physical Examination

Inspection revealed a young woman in a relaxed sitting posture with general slight flexion of the lumbar and thoracic spines and typical protraction of the head.

Screening tests for upper cervical spine instability and cervical arterial dysfunction were unremarkable (i.e. traction C0–C1 and C1–C2, stability tests for alar ligaments and transverse ligament, active provocational positional tests for cervical arterial dysfunction).

Neurological tests for motor and sensory function of the upper extremities were unremarkable.

Active cervical movements (no resting symptoms) produced no symptoms.

- Flexion: although the range of movement was full, the quality was impaired, with a staccato movement performed – initially, craniocervical flexion, then followed by a sudden, quick flexion of the lower cervical spine as though her neck gave way.
- Extension: full range of movement with an accentuated lordotic curve in the lower cervical spine.
- Side bending: unremarkable.
- Rotation: less movement to the right (70°) compared with the left (80°).

General passive rotatory movement evaluation (Schomacher, 2014) in sitting was omitted in order to avoid symptom aggravation.

Regarding thoracic movements, active and passive extension movements of the whole thoracic spine were restricted but painless. All other thoracic spine movements demonstrated normal range of movement, with no provocation of symptoms. During the prior cervical active movements, no contribution of the thoracic spine was visible.

None of Sabrina's symptoms (including neck pain, headache, dizziness and nausea) was provoked during any of the active spinal movement tests. Sabrina could not demonstrate or even remember any specific aggravating cervical or thoracic movement. Consequently, symptom localization tests to differentiate the region or segment involved (Kaltenborn, 2012; Zahnd and Pfund, 2005) were not performed.

Specific rotatory-assisted segmental movements were as follows (Kaltenborn, 2012):

- Flexion of C0–C1 was surprisingly not limited; extension was also free.
- Side bending and rotation were limited to the right from C2–C3 to C4–C5 in sitting and in supine lying, with C2–C3 right side bending provoking Sabrina's suboccipital neck pain.
- Extension was markedly hypermobile in the lower cervical spine (C5–C6) but not provocative.

Translatoric passive movement testing was as follows (Kaltenborn, 2012)

- Traction at C0–C1 was limited on the right side more than on the left, but both were not unusually hypomobile compared with other healthy subjects.
- Traction at C1–C2 was unremarkable right and left.
- 'Joint play' of the motion segment was hypermobile in the lower cervical spine, most pronounced at C5–C6 (gliding from ventral to dorsal parallel to the disc plane).

(Note: All indications of segmental levels in this chapter are approximate ± 1 level due to poor validity of cervical spinous process palpation [Robinson et al., 2009]).

Neurodynamic tests for the median, radial and ulnar nerves, performed in sitting and with cervical flexion, were negative.

Muscle Testing

- Craniocervical flexion test (Jull et al., 2008): performed poorly, with an inability to isolate upper cervical nodding, instead revealing jerky movements down to the midcervical spine and excessive superficial flexor muscle activity.
- Cervical flexion endurance test (Grimmer, 1994; Grimmer and Trott, 1998): holding the head 1 cm above the treatment table in supine lying elicited trembling of muscles from about 30 seconds and interruption of the test due to fear of pain after 52 seconds.
- Isometric extensor muscle activation and strength test: revealed weakness at the C2–C3 level compared with the more caudal levels, which is opposite to that usually found (assessed subjectively by manual resistance over the vertebral arch in a ventral–cranial direction parallel to the treatment plane of the zygapophysial joints (Schomacher et al., 2012; Jull et al., 2008).

Muscle length was not assessed because active movements did not suggest muscle tightness. No further examination was carried out this day in order to avoid aggravation of symptoms.

Reasoning Question:

3. Please discuss how your reasoning regarding dominant 'pain type' and possible 'sources of symptoms' from the subjective examination has been supported or not supported by your physical examination findings.

Answer to Reasoning Question:

Fig. 23.2 presents an overview of the categories of problems considered and Sabrina's positive findings. Her physical examination revealed impairments in the mid- and upper cervical spine, which might activate the nociceptive system and/or stimulate the sensitized pain-modulating system. The major one was hypomobility at C2–C3 that was correlated with Sabrina's neck pain. In this segment, the gliding of the right inferior articular process of C2 in a dorsal–caudal direction seemed limited, possibly due to an articular capsular restriction. Furthermore, muscle activation in this segment seemed to be reduced, perhaps due to inhibition by nociception/pain (Lund et al., 1991; Arendt-Nielsen and Graven-Nielsen, 2008; Arendt-Nielsen and Falla, 2009).

Because Sabrina could not reproduce her headache and associated symptoms in any specific movement or position, it was not possible to correlate them through the specific symptom localization tests to

Continued on following page

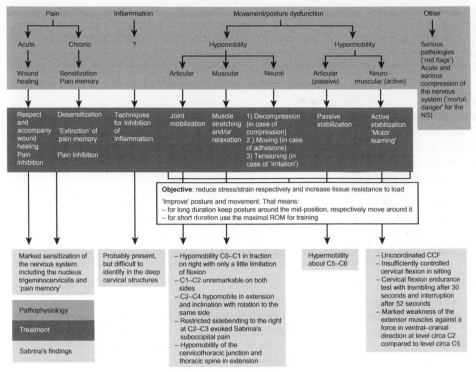

Fig. 23.2 Overview of the problem categories guiding musculoskeletal approach followed by Sabrina's positive findings. *CCF,* Craniocervical flexion; *NS,* nervous system; *ROM,* range of motion.

selected segments of the cervical spine. Therefore, it was unclear at this stage whether these impairments were related to her symptoms or not.

Theoretically, many structures can provoke headache and neck pain:

- The zygapophyseal joint of C2–C3 is often a structural cause of neck pain with headache, as confirmed by local anaesthesia in patients with idiopathic neck pain (Bogduk and Marsland, 1988) and with neck pain after whiplash injury (Lord et al., 1996).
- Headache activated by segment C2–C3 is often associated with headache and irradiating pain from segment C0–C1 (Watson and Drummond, 2012, 2014).
- The intervertebral discs from C2–C3 down to C6–C7 can cause cervicogenic headache and neck pain, as confirmed by discography (Slipman et al., 2005).

Thus, theoretically and based on the examination findings, possible involvement of dysfunction in the segments C2–C3, C0–C1 and C5–C6 had some support.

The differentiation between migraine, tension-type, cervicogenic or other types of headache is not an aim of our examination. Clinical tests for impairments, such as movement restrictions from C0 to C4 and motor control/strength impairments in the cranio-cervical flexion (CCF) test, allow differentiation of cervicogenic headache from migraine and tension-type headache with 100% sensitivity and 94% specificity (Jull et al., 2007). However, migraine and tension-type headaches can also be positively influenced by manual therapy of the cervical spine, similar to cervicogenic headache (Watson, 2014). Consequently, the usefulness of headache type differentiation can be questioned. All of Sabrina's physical impairments listed previously might therefore suggest musculoskeletal manual techniques could positively influence her symptoms.

However, because Sabrina's symptoms cannot be evoked with most physical assessments, it is unlikely she only has a simple nociceptive pain problem. A nociplastic pain type is further supported and might explain why afferent activity from these common impairments provokes the significant symptoms Sabrina has been suffering. This sensitization might affect her pain-modulating system, resulting in persistent pain, as well as her neurovegetative system, producing sensations of dizziness, nausea and tunnel vision. The contribution of each of Sabrina's impairments will be assessed further through a systematic process of manual trial treatments.

Reasoning Question:

4. Based on both the subjective and physical examination findings, do you have any hypotheses regarding possible 'contributing factors' to the development and/or maintenance of Sabrina's symptoms and disability?

Answer to Reasoning Question:

Contributing factors to the maintenance of pain and disability can be psychosocial, environmental and/or physical. However, Sabrina was reluctant to discuss her psychosocial status, and her story revealed no apparent relationship to environmental factors such as home or work ergonomics. Because Sabrina's symptoms were reported by her as being aggravated by certain movements/postures, including prolonged lying, sitting and standing, physical factors such as posture of the head and active or passive mobility dysfunctions might influence a nociceptive source of pain or a sensitization of the pain-modulating system, although physical dysfunctions were not exceptional in Sabrina's examination findings when compared with healthy subjects. The pain-provoking exercises prescribed by her initial physiotherapist, although unlikely to have caused any injury, may have contributed to creating or reinforcing a sensitization of the pain-modulating system, including a 'pain memory', potentially contributing to Sabrina's persistent pain and disability. Therefore, at this stage it was not clear whether her pain type was dominant nociceptive caused by one or more of the previously listed physical impairments or a nociplastic pain influenced by (some of) these impairments. Trial treatments of the mechanical impairments found during the physical examination will determine their relevance for a nociceptive pain type. If these trial treatments of the detected dysfunctions are not effective, management would then proceed with a trial treatment for nociplastic pain which will require more time and therefore is the second option.

Clinical Reasoning Commentary:

Clinical reasoning is not an exact science, and hence judgements are best considered as hypotheses. The complexity of interpreting patient information is evident in, for example, the influence judgements regarding dominant pain type have on judgements regarding potential sources of symptoms. As discussed in Chapter 1, nociplastic pain can create local false-positive provocation of symptoms suggestive of tissue nociception/pathology. As such, a challenge of interpreting physical findings is ensuring they are analyzed within the broader picture of the patient's full presentation and hypothesized dominant pain type. Whether the physical impairments should be treated initially as per the trial treatment planned here or whether other interventions more broadly addressing the pain-modulating system should be addressed first will elicit ongoing discussion and debate. However, from a reasoning perspective, what we feel is essential is that, as occurs here, whichever path clinicians take, they view their judgements regarding pain type and sources of symptoms as hypotheses and carefully monitor the effects of any intervention (passive, active, educational) on the patient's disability and symptoms, including the patient's activity and participation restrictions and capabilities, the patient's perspectives on his or her experience and key physical impairments.

First Trial Treatment

The findings of the initial examination were explained, and the recommendation for management was discussed and agreed on with Sabrina.

For the finding of hypomobility at C2–C3 with provocation of symptoms, intermittent traction grade I–II (i.e. performed before first resistance) (Schomacher, 2009) was applied to both right and left C2–C3 zygapophyseal joints because side bending was now also limited to the left, whereas it was initially only limited to the right. After about 2 minutes of gentle traction mobilization, Sabrina felt 'exhausted' on both sides of her neck. The technique was repeated after a short rest, but the feeling of exhaustion reappeared earlier than before, so the technique was stopped.

Upon re-assessment, active cervical flexion and rotation were 'easier', with improved quality (less staccato movement). No further treatment was carried out at this first appointment in order to assess Sabrina's reaction to the examination and trial treatment. She was asked to perform the cervical flexion endurance exercise in the evening, in supine lying, 10 times for 20 seconds each time (during the test, Sabrina started trembling after 30 seconds), with 20-second rest periods between each repetition. In addition, she was asked to practice the craniocervical flexion action without holding the position several times per day and while emphasizing the smoothness of the motion with relaxed breathing. Sabrina was asked to absolutely avoid pain during and after the exercises.

Reasoning Question:

5. Would you please briefly explain your use of a 'trial treatment' in the context of Sabrina's case?

Answer to Reasoning Question:

The summary of Sabrina's positive findings highlighted in Fig. 23.1 is categorized according to pain, inflammation and movement/posture dysfunction. The question is which finding in which category should be addressed first to most efficiently establish their relevance to her symptoms. Treatment directed to mechanical dysfunction has the potential to provide a relatively quick answer, whereas treatment directed to sensitization of the pain-modulating system in the form of progressive movement training would take considerably longer (e.g. several weeks). Because of the high irritability of Sabrina's symptoms, the mechanical treatment needed to be gentle and progressed slowly. A curious finding was the change in the direction of the hypomobility at C2–C3 from the right to the left side. This points more to a functional limitation instead of a structural restriction such as capsular tightness.

Traction of the zygapophyseal joint was chosen as a trial treatment because it is an effective technique for neck pain (Schomacher, 2009).

Second Appointment (Next Day)

Re-Assessment

After yesterday's initial examination and trial treatment, Sabrina's suboccipital pain became a bit worse, and she felt her neck was stiffer, with more limited movements. The headache along with dizziness and nausea were not aggravated. Two hours after the manual treatment yesterday, she performed the cervical flexion endurance exercise 10 times for 20 seconds, with a 20-second rest between repetitions. While holding her head for 20 seconds, she described it felt heavy 'like a flagstone'. This morning, her complaint of suboccipital pain was less compared to the previous evening's aggravation but still present.

Re-assessments of active cervical movements were unchanged except for flexion, which provoked tension on the right side of the neck and reproduced her typical 'locking pain', but not headache, dizziness or visual disturbance. Translatoric passive movement re-assessment of the C0–C1 segment revealed hypomobility right > left as per yesterday.

Second Trial Treatment

There were three stages to the manual treatment of C0–C1 on the right side:

1. C0–C1 intermittent traction grade I–II (i.e. before first resistance) on the right side for 2 minutes with a frequency of 0.5 Hz. Sabrina then reported an alleviation of her suboccipital pain and headache at rest and when performing both flexion and rotation movements.
2. Sustained traction grade III (i.e. beyond first resistance) with further relief and an easier movement sensation but less marked improvement compared with that following the intermittent traction immediately prior.
3. Repeat of intermittent traction grade II, which Sabrina stopped after about 1 minute, saying, 'It is enough now'.

Immediate re-assessment revealed a decrease in suboccipital pain and headache, and movement of the neck was easier and more pleasant. No further manual treatment was provided during this appointment, and her two home exercises were reviewed, corrected and kept the same.

For the rest of the day, Sabrina attended an upper cervical spine continuing education course, during which her symptoms became increasingly worse. It was unclear to her whether this was a reaction to the trial treatment this morning or to the intensive movements performed on her as a participant in the cervical spine course. Sabrina reported late in the afternoon about this latest aggravation of symptoms and was offered a further trial treatment.

Third Trial Treatment

Physical re-assessment revealed no change to the active cervical movements and continued to show hypomobility on traction of the right C0–C1 joint. Cervical arterial dysfunction testing and safety screening were still negative. A translatoric traction manipulation of C0–C1 on the right side was therefore performed. The technique was applied in sitting with little force, low amplitude, high velocity and in a mid-position where the greatest joint play was available (called the 'actual resting position' [Kaltenborn, 2008]). After this, active assisted movements in craniocervical flexion were alternated with intermittent C0–C1 traction grade II for 2–3 minutes.

On re-assessment, Sabrina reported a pleasant feeling with less headache, both at rest and with spontaneous movement of her head and neck.

Reasoning Question:

6. You indicated that the trial treatments directed at posture/movement dysfunction would be used to assess the contribution of these physical findings and the involvement of local tissue nociception in Sabrina's presentation. Would you please discuss how these trial treatments and the associated re-assessments have informed that reasoning?

Answer to Reasoning Question:

The initial trial treatment at C2–C3 worsened Sabrina's 'locking' neck pain that evening, potentially indicating a mechanical influence of this segment on her symptoms. It also reflected relatively high irritability of the tissues to this input. The lack of effect on her headache, dizziness and nausea also suggested those symptoms were not directly related to that segment.

The trial manipulation treatment of the C0–C1 segment produced immediate improvement in Sabrina's suboccipital pain and headache, with easier, more pleasant movement of the neck and positive neurovegetative signs (i.e. more fresh and vivid colour in her face).

Nociceptive afferent activity from the segments of the upper cervical spine arrive at the trigemino-cervical nucleus, where they might cause symptoms like headache, dizziness and nausea (Bogduk, 2004). This short-term relief indicated that the segment C0–C1 might provide an area where treatment could positively influence Sabrina's symptoms. However, her reaction to the treatment that evening and next day would need to be assessed prior to making such a decision.

Clinical Reasoning Commentary:

Traditional manual therapy may have interpreted upper cervical segmental hypomobility, associated with examination-elicited provocation of local pain, as sufficient evidence that the tissues of that segment are responsible for the pain (i.e. nociception). Although this is still reasonable when the pain type is nociceptive dominant, the greater the likelihood of nociplastic pain the more likely the segmental provocation of pain represents an allodynic mechanosensitivity, particularly if the hypomobility is minor and variable. As noted in the previous commentary, the debate about the place for manual therapy (even as trial treatments) versus hands-off interventions for chronic pain presentations is inevitable and important given our growing understanding of pain science (see Chapter 2) but also considering our lack of sufficient research to understand the benefits of differing and combined interventions for different pain types. All therapies will have CNS influences, and this is reflected in the previous interpretation that 'the segment C0–C1 might provide an area to positively influence Sabrina's symptoms', as opposed to claiming C0–C1 is the source of her pain and as such requires mobilization. Although there is growing evidence for pain neuroscience education and cognition-targeted exercise in the management of chronic nociplastic pain (Louw et al., 2018; Moseley and Butler, 2017; Nijs et al., 2014), manual therapy may also prove to be an additional adjunct to the desensitization of symptoms, provided it too is cognition-targeted and combined with appropriate education and activity promotion strategies.

Third Appointment (Next Day)
Result of the Third Trial Treatment

Sabrina reported feeling good 'in the joints' the previous evening after the traction manipulation, although she still had the suboccipital feeling of 'being in a screw clamp'. Then her headache returned, causing her to go to bed in search of alleviation. Avoiding movement of the neck this morning made Sabrina feel better, whereas movements of the upper cervical spine during the afternoon again worsened her symptoms. Consequently, Sabrina preferred not to have any passive treatment of her neck.

The likely reasons for this aggravation of symptoms were discussed with Sabrina, and together a decision was made to forego further mechanical treatments and instead to start treatment directed at the sensitization of her pain-modulating system.

Reasoning Question:

7. Would you briefly highlight the key features from the trial treatments and re-assessments that underpinned your judgement that treatment should now shift to the sensitization of her pain-modulating system?

Answer to Reasoning Question:

Even the initial positive effect of the C0–C1 traction manipulation was reversed during the evening, causing an aggravation of Sabrina's symptoms. Thus, no trial treatment of her cervical mechanical dysfunctions showed any lasting improvement. Sabrina seemed frustrated, understandably, and therefore I did not start a mechanical trial treatment of her lower cervical spine hypermobility or her thoracic spine hypomobility because it would require some weeks to train the muscles for hypermobility and to effectively mobilize a stiff thoracic spine (Schomacher, 1997; Kessler et al., 2005).

The negative late reaction to the C0–C1 treatment, however, confirmed the suspicion that Sabrina's symptoms might have been influenced by this segment. This is supported by clinical experience (Kaltenborn, 2008) and recent studies (Watson and Drummond, 2012, 2014). Sabrina's hypomobility at C0–C1 is not extraordinary, being frequently found in individuals without neck pain and headache. Nonetheless, it might have represented 'the straw that broke the camel's back' and thus contributed to a sensitization of the CNS causing Sabrina's neck pain. Sensitization, especially of the trigemino-cervical nucleus, might cause neurovegetative symptoms like Sabrina's headache, dizziness and nausea. Even fainting and tetany can be provoked as a neurovegetative reaction to gentle tests of the upper cervical spine (Christe and Balthazard, 2011; Schomacher, 2000).

Cognitive and emotional factors also might contribute to sensitization of the CNS (Zusman, 2010). Although Sabrina was not open to more detailed investigation of these aspects of her life, she was confident in her statement that she had been coping well, and less formal assessment of her beliefs and emotions over appointments thus far suggested these were not significant in her case. A certain amount of fear of motion is understandable considering Sabrina's pain experience and might explain her poor performance in the craniocervical flexion test. Fear of motion is a subjective measure that moderately correlates with range, velocity and smoothness of cervical motion (Sarig Bahat et al., 2014).

Nociception from Sabrina's other impairments in the lower cervical and the thoracic spine might simply have represented factors which increased the sensitization of the CNS (or the other load on the camel's back). It is important to distinguish between pain arising from dysfunctional processing of afferents in the nervous system and pain caused by stimulation of nociceptors and other receptors in the periphery because the treatment for each of these is different (Jones and O'Shaughnessy, 2014).

Treatment of Sabrina's mechanical dysfunctions consequently becomes secondary. The program for desensitization of the pain-modulating system should be done by Sabrina herself, with the therapist guiding and motivating her.

Fourth Trial Treatment

Sabrina received a home exercise program based on the physical examination findings of the first appointment (Figs 23.3–23.8), with a slow progression targeting desensitization of the pain-modulating and neurovegetative systems:

1. Cranio-cervical flexion (CCF): an exercise for activation and coordination of the deep craniocervical flexors (Fig. 23.3) as shown by electromyography (EMG; Falla et al., 2003, 2006). Sabrina was to perform the nodding movement repeatedly for improving coordination without using biofeedback by the air-filled pressure sensor as proposed for the training (Falla et al., 2012), simply because it was not available.

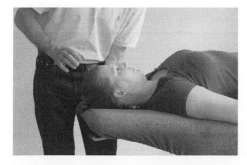

Fig. 23.3 Craniocervical flexion exercise. The patient lies supine, with the plane of the face horizontal, and is asked to perform a neck nodding movement. A pressure sensor placed under the upper cervical spine provides visual feedback (Jull et al., 2004; Sterling et al., 2001). In the absence of a pressure sensor, as in Sabrina's case, the clinician can place his or her fingers under the upper cervical spine to feel that movement occurs mainly in the craniocervical region.

Fig. 23.4   Cervical flexion endurance exercise. The patient lies supine, with the plane of the face horizontal, and is asked to lift the head about 1 cm off the plinth. The patient is then asked to hold the head in this position as the clinician measures the maximal holding time (Grimmer, 1994; Piper, 2009). For the exercise the patient takes about two-thirds of the maximal holding time.

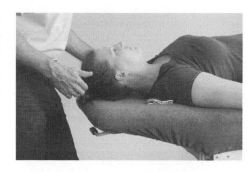

Fig. 23.5   Active self-mobilization at C2/C3 and midcervical spine. The clinician places the thumb and index finger of one hand at the level of the vertebral arch of C3 to provide fixation. The therapist's other hand guides the patient's head into left side-bending and rotation (and then to the right) and into extension so that the movement occurs above the fixating hand as far as possible (Schomacher and Learman, 2010). Once the patient has felt this movement, the clinician's index finger is replaced with the patient's index or middle finger, and the movement is repeated as a self-exercise.

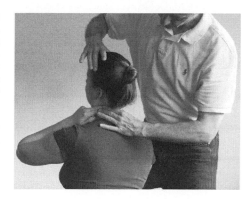

Fig. 23.6   Passive self-mobilization of the thoracic spine. The patient lies supine with a mobilization wedge placed under the thoracic spine so that the spine is stabilized caudal to the wedge. The patient is asked to hold this position, supporting the neck and head with one hand. Gravity forces the upper body dorsally and thus mobilizes the thoracic spine, mainly at the level of the edge of the wedge.

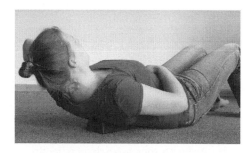

Fig. 23.7   Emphasized extension of the cervicothoracic junction. The patient stands in front of a table propped up on both forearms, with the head, neck and trunk aligned in the neutral position. The head is lowered maximally and then lifted up, extending the cervical spine. The patient is asked to fixate his or her gaze on a point between the elbows to ensure that extension mainly occurs in the lower cervical spine and cervicothoracic junction. The clinician can place his or her thumb and index finger on a vertebral arch in the lower cervical spine in order to emphasize extensor muscle activation in this region and to facilitate correct muscle activation for self-exercise (Schomacher et al., 2015).

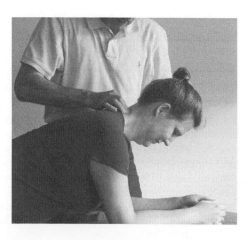

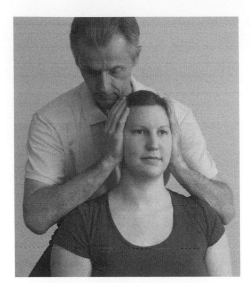

Fig. 23.8 Self-traction of the cervical spine. The clinician places the palms of his or her hands on the patient's occiput below the ears and gently lifts the head cranially (traction). The patient should aim to reproduce this feeling during self-exercise. For the self-exercise, the patient sits in front of a table, placing both of his or her hands where the clinician's hands were located. By propping on his or her elbows, the patient stabilizes the head while simultaneously lowering the body until the patient feels traction of the cervical spine, at which point the patient actively resists.

2. Cervical flexion (CF): an exercise for endurance training of the cervical flexors (Grimmer, 1994; Sterling et al., 2001; Piper, 2009). This exercise (Fig. 23.4) activates the longus colli and sternocleidomastoid muscles more compared with the CCF exercise, whereas the activity of longus capitis was found to be equal in the CF and CCF exercises in a muscle functional magnetic resonance imaging (MRI) study (Cagnie et al., 2008).

3. Repeated accentuated segmental movements in the midcervical spine with fixation of the caudal vertebral arch using the middle finger of the equilateral hand and active movement cranial to the fixation of ipsilateral side-bending and rotation with extension (Fig. 23.5). Using both hands for fixation on both sides of the neck, this exercise can also be done using pure extension.

4. Self-mobilization of the thoracic spine for extension while lying supine on a mobilization wedge (Fig. 23.6).

5. Activation of the lower cervical extensor muscles while standing and leaning on elbows on a table directly in front (Fig. 23.7). During this exercise, Sabrina had to pay attention to ensure she performed a rotatory extension movement and not a dorsal translation of the head.

6. General self-traction of the cervical spine sitting in front of a table and supporting the head with both hands placed below the ears, leaning backward with the body (Fig. 23.8). The aim of this exercise was just alleviation of pain and augmentation of well-being in order to increase Sabrina's feeling of self-efficacy in case of pain and flare-ups.

Pain education was commenced using the following analogy of hay fever to explain sensitization to Sabrina. The patient with hay fever is not suffering because he lives among too many flowers but because his system is sensitized to pollen. A single pollen grain is enough to trigger the allergic reaction. Similarly, Sabrina is not suffering because she moves too much or in a wrong way. She is simply extremely sensitive to movement (i.e. 'allergic to movement'). The hay fever patient cannot avoid every single pollen grain in the environment that elicits the allergic reaction, and similarly, Sabrina cannot avoid moving. The hay fever patient has two treatment options: first, the patient can suppress symptoms with antihistamine medication, and second, the patient can try to desensitize his or her system by gradually exposing it to increasing amounts of pollen. Sabrina has similar treatment options: first, she can suppress her symptoms by using painkillers and similar medication. Second, she can desensitize her system by moving clearly below the threshold of symptoms and by slowly increasing the intensity of movements, always without pain. Both treatment options have their advantages. Suppression of symptoms can be done quickly today with powerful medication, but it does not last, might have side-effects and needs continuous intake of drugs. Desensitization, on the other hand, has long-term effects without adverse reactions, but treatment takes time, usually months and even sometimes years.

Sabrina had already experienced the first option of symptom suppression by medication, without lasting success. Desensitization using repeated movements without pain and without tension, however, was new to her and therefore tempting. It was further explained to Sabrina that the hay fever patient does not have a structural lesion in his nose necessitating, for example, surgery; he is just sensitized. Analogous to this, it was explained that Sabrina's neck did not demonstrate any structural problem which a surgeon might solve. Even the movement dysfunctions we had found were common in healthy individuals and did not alone explain her symptoms. Her neck, therefore, might simply be sensitized.

For illustration, Sabrina was given the example of swinging the legs back and forth when sitting for several hours a day, which generally alleviates pain and improves movement in various pain conditions of the knee. To further help Sabrina understand, it was explained that small movements of the cervical spine occur (for instance) with walking and that, consequently, walking is recommended for the treatment of neck pain (Jull et al., 2008). Sabrina answered that she already knew this because when she got her headache attacks, she only had two possibilities for relief: either she went to bed in her completely dark room or she took a long walk.

The following principles to be applied to her home exercise program were discussed with Sabrina and also provided as handwritten notes:

1. Absolutely avoid pain and other symptoms.
2. Execution of the exercises:
   - Do each exercise as a test only once until symptoms appear.
   - Take about 60%–70% of this intensity (number of repetitions, duration, resistance, etc.) and perform the exercise at this level. Take sufficient breaks between the sets, that is, sufficient in order to be able to repeat the exercise at the same level for several times and always without symptom provocation.
   - Do the test to find the intensity of the exercise only once per week in order to avoid unnecessary pain provocation.

Sabrina also received the home exercises (see Figs 23.3–23.8) drawn as stick figures with the aforementioned principles highlighted.

Reasoning Question:

8. Literature regarding the facilitation of graded activity and exercise in patients with central sensitization (nociplastic pain) recommends that the activities and exercises are cognition targeted and time contingent. Would you discuss your rationale for advising that Sabrina absolutely avoid pain and other symptoms with her home exercises?

Answer to Reasoning Question:

Sabrina had received a detailed explanation about chronic pain with sensitization of the pain-modulating system and the concept of a 'pain memory'. Extinction of this memory is not possible when paying attention to the symptoms every day (Trojan and Diers, 2013).

Although time-contingent exercise is important for many patients who demonstrate maladaptive fear of exercise, this needs to be balanced with attempts to make exercise and graded activity as enjoyable as possible. For the brain, anticipation of pain is enough to change control of nociception even in the absence of pain (Nijs and Ickmans, 2014). Endogenous analgesia through exercise is dysfunctional in some chronic musculoskeletal pain conditions, and Nijs et al. (2012) recommend a range of measures that may facilitate activation of endogenous analgesia through exercise. Although these do include allowing exercise into pain, they also highlight that in the early stages, exercises should be individually tailored, with emphasis on prevention of symptom flares, and that exercises should be fun and not experienced as a burden (Nijs et al., 2012; Fordyce 1984; Sternbach 1978; Nielson et al., 2013). Sabrina had never displayed a maladaptive avoidance of pain. Rather, on the basis of previous exercise advice, she was more prone to exercising into pain. Consequently, Sabrina's exercises were 'cognition targeted' through education discussions regarding the meaning of pain, and a decision was made to individually tailor her exercises to be pain-free.

Clinical Reasoning Commentary:

Propositional knowledge (i.e. scholarly, research-based 'knowing that' knowledge; see Chapter 1) informing evidence-based practice is intended to be a guide, not a prescription (see Chapter 5). Consequently, recommendations such as cognition-targeted and time-contingent graded activity and exercise for patients with hypothesized sensitization of their pain-modulating system need to be tailored

Continued on following page

to patients' individual presentations, as occurred in this case with Sabrina. Importantly, however this is implemented, re-assessment of its effectiveness over time is essential to inform progression and, if necessary, change of treatment. Reasoning that assumes a particular intervention (e.g. to physical impairment or sensitization) that subsequently results in improvement is proof on its own that the hypothesized causal mechanism was correct represents a form of 'confirmation bias' (see Chapter 1), inductively reasonable but deductively wrong, as it presumes the intervention only affects the hypothesized cause. In reality, direct tissue treatments may have pain-modulating effects, and pain-modulating strategies can positively influence movement, activity and pain that have tissue effects. Although hypotheses regarding pain type and physical impairments that may be contributing to the persistence of symptoms and disability are encouraged because they promote systematic, reasoned management, ultimately, these are still just hypotheses when applied to individual patients. With an overall aim to positively change cognition (e.g. understanding), emotions (e.g. maladaptive fear) and behaviour (e.g. activity/function, coping strategies and life participation) and, when possible, to decrease or resolve pain, research recommendations should be followed and modified as required with regular, thorough and holistic outcome re-assessment to determine success and guide management revision.

Fourth Appointment (1 Week Later)

Re-Assessment

Sabrina reported that she felt better. Her headache attacks during the last week had reduced in intensity (from NRS 8–9 to 5/10). She described feeling confident about the approach and wanted to continue with the exercise program for desensitization. No physical re-assessment was performed because Sabrina's symptoms seemed to have decreased with the desensitization approach, which is not based on specific mechanical impairments.

Treatment – Prolonged Home Exercise Program

Time was spent discussing Sabrina's goals, which included resuming her sport activities without having pain afterward. She expressed her wish to eventually get back to her rock climbing, which was her favourite sport but which she had had to abandon due to her neck pain. The concept of first setting and then achieving short-term goals in order to eventually achieve these long-term goals was discussed, with the desensitization program being the first focus. It was agreed that the short-term goals of this program would be to increase, step by step, the resistance to stress of her locomotor system (i.e. neck and arms especially). Photos were taken of Sabrina performing each of the exercises and given to her together with a written description and a table for her to document her exercise progression.

The time to affect desensitization was discussed, and because Sabrina was not going to be able to return for the next 4 months, it was agreed that she would follow her home program over this time, with email contact every 2 to 3 weeks to assess her progress and adjust the program as required.

Sabrina was instructed to increase the intensity of self-exercises according to her feelings of effort/comfort and always to ensure the exercises were pain-free. She was advised to continue this schedule of exercises at the prescribed dosage until their execution became easy. Then she should slowly increase the dosage, for example, adding five more repetitions or increasing holding time by 5 seconds. Next, she should continue with this new intensity until execution again felt easy and continue this gradual progression. She was asked to re-evaluate her pain every 2 weeks by comparing it to the severity and frequency of symptoms 2 weeks prior rather than how it was that particular morning or the day before. As part of the ongoing discussion explaining pain and sensitization, the overattention to pain was highlighted as common but unhelpful because it can further contribute to the sensitization. The possibility of flare-ups was also discussed in the context of desensitization not being a linear process with continuous improvement but, rather, a longer-term approach with ups and downs and that amelioration will be perceived after some weeks or months.

First Email Contact: 8 Days Later

Sabrina reported via email that during the last week, she had experienced two suboccipital pain and headache attacks (NRS 8/10) necessitating the intake of pain medication. She was encouraged to consider this as 'normal' because various factors and stimuli can irritate the pain-modulating system. This is one reason why desensitization takes so long. Her compliance with the exercise program was positively acknowledged, and she was encouraged to remain patient and motivated and to continue regularly with her exercises, avoiding any pain and discomfort.

Second Email Contact: 2 Weeks Later

Sabrina answered via email that her last 2 weeks had been fine. She reported no major headache attacks with dizziness and nausea, only some with pain of a maximal intensity of NRS 4–5/10, despite some recent high job-related stress. Sabrina was reminded that her workload and stress in general could also influence her pain and her recovery. She indicated she understood this and repeated that she was coping fine with her work stress. She planned to increase the dosage of her exercises and was encouraged to do so and to always feel comfortable about progressing the exercises so long as she reached the agreed criteria for progression.

Third Email Contact: 3 Weeks Later

Sabrina was doing fine with the exercises, although she did not end up increasing the intensity of the exercises as much as she had planned (Table 23.1). Her headache reached a maximum pain intensity of NRS 6/10 without causing limitations in her daily activities. She had the feeling of 'single segments in the cervical spine causing trouble' without knowing if it was stiffness or too much stress. Overall, Sabrina had the feeling that she was coping better and able to continue with the exercise program.

Reasoning Question:
9. Although Sabrina reported on her suboccipital pain and headache in her first email and on her headache without dizziness and nausea in her second email, she has not commented on the locking feeling or tunnel vision. How do you balance a thorough re-assessment of symptoms to inform your advice regarding the progression of exercise with your previously stated aim of not encouraging Sabrina's overattention to symptoms?

Answer to Reasoning Question:
Because the reason for a relapse in cases of chronic neck pain is not usually a particular nociceptive input which requires treatment of specific peripheral impairments, it is unhelpful to look for the putative cause. Symptom flare-ups are often unavoidable when treating chronic neck pain (Nijs et al., 2012). Also, Sabrina had always been consistent in reporting on her symptoms without specific questioning of each, and the risk of symptom flare-ups was minimized by the encouragement that she should feel comfortable during and after her exercises and activities (Zusman, 2013). This also hopefully facilitated 're-training' of her cortical function (Wand and O'Connell, 2008). The current objective was to keep her motivated to follow the exercise program and to divert her attention from her symptoms. How this is achieved will be different for different patients and was implemented with Sabrina by not asking too many details about her individual symptoms.

Fourth Email Contact: 4 Weeks Later

Sabrina reported she was doing quite well overall. However, she admitted to not having been as diligent as she should have been. She had exercised less and not increased the dosage. She reported now perceiving more 'segmental complaints' and her locking pain, but she had not had the heavy attacks of headache with dizziness and nausea in spite of a high workload. The headache still occurred, but less intensely. Sabrina had reduced her use of pain medication significantly, and she was very happy about this.

Fifth Email Contact: 6 Weeks Later

Sabrina had resumed her normal work after her summer holiday. She was motivated now to put more effort into her exercise program. Her pain attacks had decreased considerably,

TABLE 23.1

LIST OF SABRINA'S HOME EXERCISES WITH THE PROGRESSIONS SHE ACHIEVED

Exercise	Outcome Measured	Test Result 3 Days After the First Appointment	60%	Dosage	Test Result 2 Weeks After the First Appointment	Test Result 6 Weeks After the First Appointment	Test Result 9 Weeks After the First Appointment
Cranio-cervical flexion exercise (Fig. 23.3)	Coordination and number of movements	83 controlled movements	50 controlled movements	50 repetitions in the evening Some sets of 10 repetitions during the day	55 repetitions in the evening Some sets of 10 repetitions during the day	60 repetitions in the evening No change during the day	Same
Cervical flexion endurance exercise (Fig. 23.4)	Time in seconds	33 seconds	20 seconds	10 repetitions 20-sec. hold with 15-sec. break	10 repetitions 20-sec. hold with 10- to 15-sec. break	10 repetitions 25-sec. hold with 15-sec. break	10 repetitions 2-sec. hold with 10-sec. break
Active self mobilization at C2/C3 and midcervical spine (Fig. 23.5)	Coordination and painless range of movement	50 repetitions	30 repetitions	30 repetitions per side 2–3 times a day	35 repetitions per side 2–3 times a day	Unchanged	40 repetitions per side 2 times a day
Passive self-mobilization of the thoracic spine (Fig. 23.6)	Time	Because there was no pain with this exercise, the usual time was suggested (i.e. 10–12 min once a day)		1–2 min per each thoracic segment (i.e. in total, about a quarter of an hour once a day)	Same	Same	Same
Emphasized extension of the cervico-thoracic junction (Fig. 23.7)	Number of movements leaning on elbows, each movement lasting about 2–3 seconds	50 repetitions	30 repetitions	30 repetitions once a day	Same	35 repetitions once a day	Same
Self-traction of the cervical spine (Fig. 23.8)	Time	Not tested because the aim was Sabrina's subjective well-being		Occasionally during the day	Same	Same	Same

Note: Jogging is not listed because we did not measure Sabrina's running time and distance, which she should dose according to her well-being and enjoyment.

both quantitatively and qualitatively (less intense, less bothersome). Although she still perceived stress in her daily life, she had learned to manage better her activities of daily living and pace of work so that the pain intensity did not exceed NRS 5–6/10, and she reported she could now go up to several days or even a few weeks without symptoms. She was also very pleased that she had been able to reduce her pain medication to a minimum. Although Sabrina had not progressed the dosage of her exercises, she had the feeling that the movement exercises had been effective in preventing provocation of symptoms if she did them when she started to feel stressed. She performed these unscheduled exercises as needed without counting or measuring anything. She described her current symptoms as mostly the suboccipital pain with less of the original locking feeling and said that the headache, dizziness and nausea were significantly reduced. Sabrina felt there was still a local restriction in her upper cervical spine, but overall, she considered that things were looking up, although she knew it would take a lot more work.

Sabrina was complimented on her efforts and encouraged to persist because there should be a progression. She was reminded that when exercises are enjoyable, with a focus on well-being rather than a strict program 'because you have to do it', they will be more effective for desensitization of the pain-modulating system (Nielson et al., 2013; Sternbach, 1978). This explanation was expanded to highlight that setting the dosage of exercise is not an exact science and the importance of her decision-making in this. Her best guide to adjusting the dosage of exercises will be that they are mostly pain-free and provide a positive feeling of well-being. A meeting was arranged for the next week for re-assessment and possible treatment of any mechanical dysfunctions Sabrina might perceive as still being present in her upper cervical spine.

Fourth Appointment (1 Week Later) (Because Sabrina Was Back for 4 Days Attending a Professional Development Course, We Agreed to Have at Least Three Appointments in This Time)

Sabrina was happy and feeling much better. She experienced fewer pain attacks, and their intensity had reduced since starting treatment 4 months ago from initially being NRS 8–9/10 with pain medication to NRS 5–6/10 without pain medication. She described her major problem now as being a feeling of stiffness and local upper cervical neck pain.

Physical re-assessment revealed hypomobility in traction at C0–C1 on the right and hypomobility in side bending and rotation at C2–C3 on the left. This was similar to the findings of the first examination four months ago.

Treatment consisted of traction in supine lying to the left zygapophyseal joint at C2–C3 at grade III (i.e. beyond first resistance) for about 3–4 minutes, which provided an immediate subjective feeling of less stiffness with easier and 'freer' movement. This was followed by grade III traction treatment at C0–C1 on the right for about 3–4 minutes. Again, Sabrina felt better afterward, with easier movement. Each of the two treatments was followed by a short functional massage for about 2 minutes. Sabrina was advised to continue with her established home exercise program and to emphasize repeated movements of the upper cervical spine, especially in flexion (nodding movement), within an absolutely pain-free range of motion.

Reasoning Question:

10. Given you had judged Sabrina's chronic pain as being dominantly a sensitization of her pain-modulating system what was your rationale for returning to segmental mobilization?

Answer to Reasoning Question:

Chronic pain patients might have impairments whose nociceptive activity maintains sensitization of the CNS, although these impairments are not visible by normal medical investigations (Giamberardino, 2003). Sabrina's functional impairments were still present and might send nociceptive afferences to the nervous system, thus maintaining its sensitization. When we started the treatment, this sensitization prevented any attempt to treat these dysfunctions. Now, however, the sensitization was less and seemed to allow their treatment. In addition, a placebo effect cannot be ruled out and is worth trying (Benedetti et al., 2011).

Appointments 5 and 6 (Next Day)

Sabrina reported feeling bad this morning, with local neck pain on the right side a bit below the occiput and a feeling of stiffness turning her head to the right. Yesterday, after the treatment and during the whole evening, however, she was fine. She related the exacerbation this morning to her 3-year old son crawling into bed with her last night. He apparently kicked Sabrina's head and manoeuvred himself very close, causing her to sleep with an awkward neck position. The pain, however, was local and only associated with the stiffness feeling, without any irradiation, headache, nausea or dizziness. Sabrina's account of her son's nocturnal manoeuvring was discussed as a good example of the inevitable stresses to which our bodies are subjected. She felt she was now better able to cope with these minor setbacks and understood her rehabilitation and recovery would have these hiccups, yet when looked at over time, would hopefully continue to progress favourably.

A quick manual examination showed increased traction mobility of the C0–C1 segment on the right compared to yesterday. Sabrina was asked to feel the motion herself with her right index finger, like she had done yesterday during the evaluation. She reported feeling increased mobility without knowing the therapist's evaluation.

Furthermore, there was stiffness in rotation and side bending at the C2–C3 zygapophyseal joint on the right – although yesterday the segment was limited to the left. Traction of the right C2–C3 joint at grade III was undertaken, but after about 3 minutes, Sabrina had 'had enough', and no further physical assessment or treatment was performed that morning. In order to optimize her time while she was in town, we agreed to have a second appointment later this same day.

When Sabrina returned in the afternoon, she reported having developed increased tenderness to self-palpation and that rotation and side bending to the right remained painful and limited. Due to the tenderness to self-palpation, it was decided not to apply any further mobilization that day. Sabrina was advised to perform the repeated movements of her exercise program within the pain-free range of motion as long as she felt better with these exercises. Again, reassuring explanations regarding her symptom exacerbation as being a normal reaction to the incident in the night with her son and related sleeping posture were given.

Appointment 7 (2 Days Later)

Today Sabrina had woken up, and her local neck pain was gone. Yesterday, however (2 days after her pain-provoking night with her son), she felt only a bit better in the morning, and the local upper cervical pain she had the day before was still present. Sabrina took a short walk of about 20 minutes at midday, which considerably diminished her neck pain and improved the freedom of her neck movements. This was discussed along with the possibility of local tissue irritation occurring when tissues are sustained in awkward positions, as occurred with her sleeping with her young son. This was also linked to the sensitization that has been discussed previously so that she could see that her tissues were likely even more sensitive than normal but that this did not reflect tissue damage. Sabrina was reminded that she only had minor mechanical dysfunctions, supported by the decrease in the C0–C1 segmental stiffness for more than 1 day after a single treatment. Also, the changing direction of her side bending stiffness at C2–C3 was discussed as reflecting functional changes, such as in muscle tone or joint lubrication, rather than a true structural joint restriction, which could be linked back to the maladaptive sensitization of her pain-modulating system. Although the sensitization was almost certainly a factor, a reduced physical load capacity of her tissues was also discussed and explained as likely related to the non-utilization, or less utilization, during the last 12 years when she had significantly reduced her activity levels (Torstensen, 2015).

Sabrina also reported that she was really pleased that she had started to read books again. Reading was always a major pleasure for her, but since her accidents 12 years ago and her related neck problems, she had given up reading because the associated sustained position aggravated her symptoms.

Next cervical flexion in supine lying through the whole range of motion was demonstrated in order to show Sabrina what is 'normal' for this movement. She became afraid that she might be asked to do this exercise, and we discussed her fear of exacerbation of symptoms, reviewing that aggravation of her pain was mostly reflective of a too-sensitive nervous system. The purpose of her exercise program and the need to gradually increase the dosage intensity to help desensitize her pain-modulating system were also reviewed. The importance of increasing her load and stress capacity was again emphasized, noting that this, together with her better understanding of pain, would help her to overcome her fear of movement (kinesiophobia) (Zusman, 2013). Various examples were presented to Sabrina within this discussion to assist her understanding and to facilitate her motivation to continue. Sabrina was very receptive to the overall approach, commenting that nobody had explained things in this way or taken this approach before. Patients often need repeated explanations and reassurance (Main and Watson, 1999).

Sabrina appeared more energetic, less anxious and even noted that her friends commented she seemed happier. When asked what she thought about her friends' impressions, she answered spontaneously: 'It is logical because if you are always afraid of these symptoms, you cannot be so happy.'

No mobilization treatment was performed at this appointment because there was no evidence of real joint stiffness. Instead, emphasis was placed on the previously described education and then cervical muscle activation and stabilization exercises. Specific segmental stabilization exercises were practiced, requiring Sabrina to isometrically resist various movement stimuli, including traction, compression, gliding for flexion and gliding for extension in relation to the treatment plane of the zygapophyseal joints, all performed in both supine lying and sitting (Schomacher, 2013). It was difficult for Sabrina to resist these specific stimuli. Similar to 4 months before, Sabrina had more difficulty resisting/stabilizing the segments around C2–C3 and less around C5–C6, which is the opposite of what is most frequently seen.

Sabrina reacted well to all the exercises performed this day. Because Sabrina was present during 4 consecutive days due to a continuing education course she attended in the city, we met briefly for review during a break in the morning and again after her course, and she reported no negative reaction. This suggested her pain-modulating system was less sensitized and supported the value and importance of her continued exercise in order to increase her load capacity. This concept was explained to Sabrina in detail, and she was quite motivated to follow the existing exercise program with minor variations, plus the addition of paced jogging/running. The principle of keeping all exercises relatively pain-free and starting new exercises at about 60% of the intensity which evoked her pain/symptoms was reviewed. This was particularly important for her resuming her jogging. Sabrina was told to initially test how many minutes or meters she could run until she felt exhausted or until fear of pain appeared, without waiting until the pain actually started. Then she should take about 60%–70% of this intensity for her running, walk during the breaks and restart running once she felt recovered and 'full of energy' again. Once confident, she should use this principle with any activity, for example, climbing. Sabrina seemed convinced now that this approach would continue to work and expressed clear motivation to continue. When Sabrina asked about prognosis and how long it would take for her symptoms to resolve, it was suggested that given the rate of progress thus far, another 4 months should be sufficient for her symptoms to be nearly gone or at least be 'under control'.

Lastly, new photos were taken of her exercises to update her previous exercise sheet. Although we had added only jogging to her program, it was hoped that a new exercise sheet with new pictures would assist Sabrina's motivation to continue with the exercise progression. It was agreed that we would continue our email contact and organize the next appointment for 5 months' time.

Reasoning Question:

11. On several occasions, Sabrina has alluded to her work stress. It appears you have elected not to pursue this with further questioning to explore whether there is any relationship of her stress to her pain experience. Would you please discuss your reasoning regarding this?

Answer to Reasoning Question:

Sabrina reported in the beginning that she had work stress which precipitated her complaints. This topic was raised several times, reminding her that workload and other kinds of stress in her life might also influence her pain management and her recovery. Sabrina always answered that she knew this and that she was generally coping well with these problems. The impression was that she did not want

Continued on following page

to discuss this further, and she appeared to be coping and emotionally fine, so it was decided to respect this and not pursue it further.

Clinical Reasoning Commentary:

Psychosocial factors can predispose and contribute to the development and the maintenance of pain and disability. In Chapter 1, this important area of clinical judgement is discussed within the hypothesis category framework as 'patient's perspectives on his or her experience'. It includes such things as the following:

- Patients' understanding of their problem (including attributions about the cause, beliefs about pain and associated cognitions)
- Response to stressors in their lives and any relationship these have with their clinical presentation
- Any effects the problem and stressors appear to have on their thoughts, feelings, coping strategies, motivation and self-efficacy to participate in management
- Goals and expectations for management

As discussed in Chapter 1, psychosocial assessment can be integrated into the clinician's routine examination, both within the patient interview and through using a combination of multidimensional measure and unidimensional measure questionnaires. In this case, Sabrina's perspectives on her experience are addressed in the education regarding sensitization and the 'desensitizing' exercises that also target her fear of movement. Musculoskeletal clinicians should be able to provide skilled therapeutic pain neuroscience education and facilitate the resumption of exercise and activity. However, it is also important through our psychosocial screening to recognize 'orange flags', or possible psychopathology, such as clinical depression (see Chapters 3 and 4), and when apparent sources of stress in patients' lives require assessment and management skills outside our scope of practice (e.g. relationship-driven stress). This sort of screening is analogous to screening for visceral disease in that the aim is not diagnosis of depression or relationship problems. Instead, reasoning that identifies aspects of patients' problems outside the clinician's scope of practice should elicit discussion with the patient regarding further consultation with the referring doctor and/or referral to another suitably qualified health professional (e.g. psychologist, counsellor). In this case, continuous informal assessment of Sabrina's psychosocial status, including any overt 'orange flags', suggested this was not a significant factor in her presentation.

Sixth Email Contact (6 Weeks Later)

Sabrina had received the updated sheet of her home exercise program a few days after our last meeting. In general, she was fine and doing well with the exercises, although she was suffering from headache the last few days. However, she knew the reason for the headache and felt able to control the pain with walking and gentle exercises. She stated that it was very valuable to know what to do in order to ease and control the symptoms. Sabrina was encouraged to continue with the exercise progression in order to achieve further improvement.

Seventh Email Contact (2 Months Later)

Sabrina reported feeling 'really fine'. She was 'enjoying her time without headache', which now only occurred occasionally and rarely required any medication, basically only when she did not have the time to do something else for relief. She no longer had the heavy pain attacks that used to constrain her to bed rest and hadn't had any episodes of dizziness, nausea or tunnel vision. Also, the 'locking feeling' was gone. She was doing her exercises when she had time during the day but not following a strict program, and she noted that they were gradually becoming easier. In addition, she was now back to full running and swimming, although she still hadn't tried rock climbing. She stated she was gradually increasing her running times and was not having any pain during or afterward. She had experienced nearly no pain after a heavy work week and was generally very satisfied.

When asked what she thought helped her most, Sabrina answered 'the new understanding; knowing what to do when the pain increases and the cautious increase in exercise'.

Eighth Email Contact (10 Months After First Appointment)

Although Sabrina had continued stress at work and at home and reported being weakened by a persistent influenza infection, she highlighted that she had otherwise been feeling fine, without any of her original symptoms. She noted that on the few occasions she felt they might reoccur, she did her exercises and felt fine again. Due to a lack of time, she had not resumed her sports intensively, but she reported that she was not having any problem with the bit of running and rock climbing she was doing. She was happy with the result.

Epilog

More than three years after the first appointment Sabrina still feels fine. She has become mother of a second child and experiences some headache and dizziness when she carries her little daughter a lot. However, she is dealing well with these minor symptoms. She continues doing a small home exercise program and is confident that time will restore everything.

REFERENCES

Arendt-Nielsen, L., Falla, D., 2009. Motor control adjustments in musculoskeletal pain and the implications for pain recurrence. Pain 142, 171–172.

Arendt-Nielsen, L., Graven-Nielsen, T., 2008. Muscle pain: sensory implications and interaction with motor control. Clin. J. Pain 24, 291–298.

Benedetti, F., Carlino, E., Pollo, A., 2011. How placebo change the patient's brain. Neuropsychopharmacology 36, 339–354.

Bogduk, N., 2004. The neck and headaches. Neurol. Clin. 22, 151–171.

Bogduk, N., Marsland, A., 1988. The cervical zygapophysial joints as a source of neck pain. Spine 13, 610–617.

Bogduk, N., McGuirk, B., 2006. Management of Acute and Chronic Neck Pain, an Evidence-Based Approach. Elsevier, Edinburgh.

Cagnie, B., Dickx, N., Peeters, I., Tuytens, J., Achten, E., Cambier, D., et al., 2008. The use of functional MRI to evaluate cervical flexor activity during different cervical flexion exercises. J. Appl. Physiol. 104, 230–235.

Chimenti, R.L., Frey-Law, L.A., Sluka, K., 2018. A mechanism-based approach to physical therapist managament of pain. Phys. Ther. 98 (5), 302–314.

Christe, G., Balthazar, D.P., 2011. Episode of fainting and tetany after an evaluation technique of the upper cervical region: a case report. Man. Ther. 16, 94–96.

Falla, D., Jull, G., Dall'alba, P., Rainoldi, A., Merletti, R., 2003. An electromyographic analysis of the deep cervical flexor muscles in performance of craniocervical flexion. Phys. Ther. 83, 899–906.

Falla, D., Jull, G., O'Leary, S., Dall'alba, P., 2006. Further evaluation of an EMG technique for assessment of the deep cervical flexor muscles. J. Electromyogr. Kinesiol. 16, 621–628.

Falla, D., O'Leary, S., Farina, D., Jull, G., 2012. The change in deep cervical flexor activity after training is associated with the degree of pain reduction in patients with chronic neck pain. Clin. J. Pain 28, 628–634.

Fordyce, W.F., 1984. Behavioural science and chronic pain. Postgrad. Med. J. 60, 865–868.

Giamberardino, M.A., 2003. Von den eingeweiden her übertragene hyperalgesie. In: Van Den Berg, F. (Ed.), Angewandte Physiologie, 4 Schmerz Verstehen und Beeinflussen. Georg Thieme Verlag, Stuttgart - New York.

Grimmer, K.A., 1994. Measuring the endurance capacity of the cervical short flexor muscle group. Aust. J. Physiother. 40, 251–254.

Grimmer, K.A., Trott, P., 1998. The association between cervical excursion angles and cervical short flexor muscle endurance. Aust. J. Physiother. 44, 201–207.

Jones, L.E., O'Shaughnessy, D.F.P., 2014. The Pain and Movement Reasoning Model: introduction to a simple tool for integrated pain assessment. Man. Ther. 19, 270–276.

Jones, M.A., Rivett, D.A., 2004. Clinical Reasoning for Manual Therapists. Butterworth Heinemann, Edinburgh.

Jull, G., Amiri, M., Bullock-Saxton, J., Darnell, R., Lander, C., 2007. Cervical musculoskeletal impairment in frequent intermittent headache. Part 1: subjects with single headaches. Cephalalgia 27, 793–802.

Jull, G., Falla, D., Treleaven, J., Sterling, M., O'Leary, S., 2004. A therapeutic exercise approach for cervical disorders. In: Boyling, J.D., Jull, G. (Eds.), Grieve's Modern Manual Therapy: The Vertebral Column, third ed. Elsevier, Edinburgh.

Jull, G., Sterling, M., Falla, D., Treleaven, J., O'Leary, S., 2008. Whiplash, Headache, and Neck Pain: Research-Based Directions for Physical Therapies: Research-Based Directions for Physical Therapies. Churchill Livingstone (Elsevier), Edinburgh.

Kaltenborn, F.M., 2008. Manual Mobilization of the Joints, Volume III: Traction-Manipulation of the Extremities and Spine, Basic Thrust Techniques, Oslo, Norli.

Kaltenborn, F.M., 2012. Manual Mobilization of the Joints, Joint Examination and Basic Treatment, Volume II, The Spine, Oslo, Norli.

Kerry, R., Taylor, A.J., 2006. Cervical arterial dysfunction assessment and manual therapy. Man. Ther. 11, 243–253.

Kessler, T.J., Brunner, F., Künzer, S., Crippa, M., Kissling, R., 2005. Auswirkungen einer manuellen Mobilisation nach Maitland auf die Brustwirbelsäule. Rehabilitation 44, 361–366.

Lord, S., Barnsley, L., Wallis, B.J., Bogduk, N., 1996. Chronic cervical zygapophysial joint pain after whiplash. Spine 21, 1737–1745.

Louw, A., Puentedura, E., Schmidt, S., Zimney, K., 2018. Pain Neuroscience Education, vol. 2. OPTP, Minneapolis, MN.

Louw, A., Diener, I., Butler, D.S., Puentedura, E., 2011. The effect of neuroscience education on pain, disability, anxiety, and stress in chronic musculoskeletal pain. Arch. Phys. Med. Rehabil. 92, 2041–2056.

Lund, J.P., Donga, R., Widmer, C.G., Stohler, C.S., 1991. The pain-adaptation model: a discussion of the relationship between musculoskeletal pain and motor activity. Can. J. Physiol. Pharmacol. 49, 683–694.

Main, C.J., Watson, P.J., 1999. Psychological aspects of pain. Man. Ther. 4, 203–215.

Moseley, G.L., Butler, D.S., 2017. Explain Pain Supercharged. Noigroup Publications, Adelaide.

Nielson, W.R., Mensen, M.P., Karsdorp, P.A., Vlaeyen, J.W.S., 2013. Activity pacing in chronic pain: concepts, evidence, and future directions. Clin. J. Pain 29 (5), 461–468.

Niere, K.R., Torney, S.K., 2004. Clinicians' perceptions of minor cervical instability. Man. Ther. 9, 144–150.

Nijs, J., Ickmans, K., 2014. Chronic whiplash-associated disorders: to exercise or not? Lancet 384, 109–111.

Nijs, J., Kosek, E., Oosterwijck, J.V., Meeus, M., 2012. Dysfunctional endogenous analgesia during exercise in patients with chronic pain: to exercise or not to exercise? Pain Physician 15, ES205–ES213.

Nijs, J., Meeus, M., Cagnie, B., Roussel, N.A., Dolphens, M., Van Oosterwijck, J., et al., 2014. A modern neuroscience approach to chronic spinal pain: combining pain neuroscience education with cognition-targeted motor control training. Phys. Ther. 94, 730–738.

Nijs, J., Van Oosterwijck, J., De Hertogh, W., 2009. Rehabilitation of chronic whiplash: treatment of cervical dysfunctions or chronic pain syndrome? Clin. Rheumatol. 28, 243–251.

Olson, K.A., Joder, D., 2001. Diagnosis and treatment of cervical spine clinical instability. J. Orthop. Sports Phy. Ther. 31, 194–206.

Piper, A., 2009. Vergleich der Ausdauerleistungsfähigkeit der vorwiegend tiefen Flexoren der Halswirbelsäule (HWS) zwischen Gesunden und Probanden mit HWS-Schmerz. Manuelle Therapie 13.

Robinson, R., Robinson, H.S., Bjørke, G., Kvale, A., 2009. Reliability and validity of a palpation technique for identifying the spinous processes of C7 and L5. Man. Ther. 14, 409–414.

Rushton, A., Rivet, D., Carlesso, L., Flynn, T., Hing, W., Kerry, R., 2014. International framework for examination of the cervical region for potential of Cervical Arterial Dysfunction prior to Orthopaedic Manual Therapy intervention. Man. Ther. 19.

Sarig Bahat, H., Weiss, P.L.T., Sprecher, E., Krasovsky, A., Laufer, Y., 2014. Do neck kinematics correlate with pain intensity, neck disability or with fear of motion? Man. Ther. 19, 252–258.

Schomacher, J., 1997. Mobilisation der Brustwirbelsäule, Vergleichende Studie zur Wirkung der translatorischen und rotatorischen Mobilisation der BWS im OMT Kaltenborn-Evjenth-Konzept®. Manuelle Therapie 1, 3–9.

Schomacher, J., 2000. Falsch positiver Stabilitätstest der Ligamenta alaria. Manuelle Therapie 4, 127–132.

Schomacher, J., 2009. The effect of an analgesic mobilization technique when applied at symptomatic or asymptomatic levels of the cervical spine in subjects with neck pain: a randomized controlled trial. J. Man. Manip. Ther. 17, 101–108.

Schomacher, J., 2013. Therapievorschlag 2: spezifisch stabilisieren und kontrolliert bewegen. Manuelle Therapie 17, 19–24.

Schomacher, J., 2014. Orthopedic Manual Therapy, Assessment and Management. Thieme, Stuttgart, New York.

Schomacher, J., Erlenwein, J., Dieterich, A., Petzke, F., Falla, D., 2015. Can neck exercises enhance the activation of the semispinalis cervicis relative to the splenius capitis at specific spinal levels? Man. Ther. 20 (5), 694–702.

Schomacher, J., Learman, K., 2010. Symptom localization tests in the cervical spine: a descriptive study using imaging verification. J. Man. Manip. Ther. 18, 97–101.

Schomacher, J., Petzke, F., Falla, D., 2012. Localised resistance selectively activates the semispinalis cervicis muscle in patients with neck pain. Man. Ther. 17, 544–548.

Slipman, C.W., Plastaras, C., Patel, R., Isaac, Z., Chow, D., Garavan, C., et al., 2005. Provocative cervical discography symptom mapping. Spine J. 5, 381–388.

Sterling, M., Jull, G., Wright, A., 2001. Cervical mobilisation: concurrent effects on pain, sympathetic nervous system activity and motor activity. Man. Ther. 6, 72–81.

Sternbach, R.A., 1978. Treatment of the chronic pain patient. J. Human Stress 4 (3), 11–15.

Tampin, B., 2014. Neuropathischer schmerz. Physioscience 10 (4), 161–168.

Torstensen, T.A., 2015. The Mirror Book. How to Understand and Deal With Pain and Stress Lidingö. Holten Institute AB, Sweden.

Trojan, J., Diers, M., 2013. Update: physiologie und psychologie des schmerzes. Manuelle Therapie 17, 153–161.

Waddell, G., 1998. The Back Pain Revolution. Churchill Livingstone, Edinburgh.

Wand, B.M., O'Connell, N.E., 2008. Chronic non-specific low back pain – sub-groups or a single mechanism? BMC Musculoskelet. Disord. 9, 1–15.

Watson, D.H., 2014. Zervikogene kopfschmerzen: diagnosekriterien im "praxistest". Manuelle Therapie 18, 166–170.

Watson, D.H., Drummond, P.D., 2012. Head pain referral during examination of the neck in migraine and tension-type headache. Headache 52, 1226–1235.

Watson, D.H., Drummond, P.D., 2014. Cervical referral of head pain in migraineurs: effects on the nociceptive blink reflex. Headache 54, 1035–1045.

Zahnd, F., Pfund, R., 2005. Differentiation, Examination and Treatment of Movement Disorders in Manual Therapy. Elsevier - Butterworth-Heinemann Ltd., Oxford.

Zusman, M., 2003. Gewebespezifischer Schmerz. In: Van Den Berg, F. (Ed.), Angewandte Physiologie, 4 Schmerz Verstehen und Beeinflussen. Georg Thieme Verlag, Stuttgart, New York.

Zusman, M., 2010. Das biopsychosoziale Modell als Leitfaden für die Behandlung von muskuloskelettalen Schmerzen und Behinderungen durch bewegungsbasierte Therapie. Physioscience 6, 112–120.

Zusman, M., 2013. Belief reinforcement: one reason why costs for low back pain have not decreased. J. Multidiscip. Healthc. 6, 197–204.

24

A Professional Football Career Lost: Chronic Low Back Pain in a 22 Year Old

Peter O'Sullivan • Darren A. Rivett

Subjective Examination

Jack is a 22-year-old man who presented with a 7-year history of progressively disabling chronic central low back pain. Jack's symptoms began gradually when he was 15 years of age while he was undergoing intensive football (soccer) training. He had tried to manage the pain by doing a lot of core stability exercises, as advised by his physiotherapist. However, 6 months after this time, when he was 16 years of age, he experienced a 'major' episode of pain at training, whereby his back 'spasmed' and he was carried off the field. He reported his pain was 10/10 and 'frightening'. At this time, he was playing at an elite level and was aiming for a professional contract.

Jack went to see his general practitioner, who referred him for a magnetic resonance imaging (MRI) scan, which he stated had found a number of 'damaged discs and bulges'. He was referred to an orthopaedic surgeon who, after reviewing the MRI, told him that he had the 'back of a 70-year-old'. He also told Jack that he would have to stop playing football and might need to have a spinal fusion, whereby they would have to 'operate through his stomach'. He was further told this operation could prevent him from having children in the future and 'all this [other] scary stuff'. As a young man of 16 years, Jack described how this frightened him and that he feared for his future. Jack denied any contextual life stressors around the time of this severe pain episode.

Based on this advice, Jack ceased playing football, left school and started a manual job. Since that major episode of pain, he reported that 'his back was never the same again – it is always tense and doesn't relax'. He further reported that over the subsequent years, his back pain had slowly become more intense and disabling. A year prior to the first consultation, Jack ceased doing manual work due to the high levels of pain he experienced and instead took a desk job. However, because his pain was aggravated by sitting, he had now been out of work for 3 months due to his back pain. He was currently spending his time at home, lying down or going for walks.

Jack had trialled various passive interventions (mobilization, manipulation, massage and acupuncture), which he reported only gave him short-term relief. He noted that having his girlfriend walk on his back with heels had given him the most relief, as had massage and heat. He had undertaken no self-management strategies.

Pain Characteristics

Jack stated that he experienced constant tension in his back which increased when he maintained upright postures, such as sitting and standing. He reported a deep, gnawing pain in his lower back that increased during the day, and he also reported a severe, sharp pain when he flexed, extended or rotated his back. He rated his gnawing pain as 9/10 and his sharp pain as 9/10 on a numerical pain rating scale. He described a positive relationship between the level of 'tension' in his back and his pain. That is, when one increased, so did the other. Jack denied any leg pain or neurological symptoms (see Fig. 24.1).

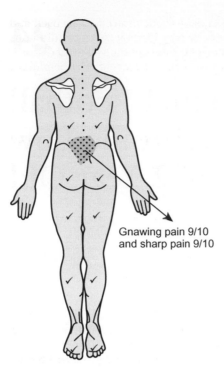

Fig. 24.1 Jack's body chart showing symptoms.

Gnawing pain 9/10
and sharp pain 9/10

Primary Aggravating Factors

Postures: sustained sitting, standing, lying
Activities: transferring load, bending, lifting, running, rolling in bed

Jack recounted that he consciously tensed his trunk muscles when undertaking these activities to help protect his back. He also said that he avoided bending and lifting due to pain.

Easing Factors

Jack only reported pain relief after a massage or applying heat to his back. He also repeatedly self-manipulated his back for relief. When his back muscles were relaxed, he also felt less pain.

Sleep

Jack reported that he experienced very disrupted sleep because he couldn't find a position of comfort and woke whenever he rolled over. He described that he was stiff in the morning and found it difficult to move, get out of bed and dress.

Activity Levels

Jack reported that he walked daily and that he enjoyed physical activity, but whenever he went to the gym or went for a run, it flared his back pain, and so he had stopped these activities. This made him feel sad and disabled.

Beliefs

Based on what he had been informed from the MRI, Jack believed that his back was damaged, and he had little hope this could change. He reported that he was fearful of doing further damage and believed that pain was a sign of damage. He felt that his back was going to 'snap'.

Jack further reported that he was constantly thinking about protecting his back and that he didn't believe that he would do manual work or play football again. He did hope he would return to a sitting job but was frightened that he would end up severely disabled and need a spinal fusion. Jack had no insight as to what treatment would be helpful for him and little expectation for symptomatic change.

Levels of Distress

Jack reported that he often felt down and that he also felt high levels of frustration and anger about his situation. He denied that his emotional state influenced his levels of pain, and he was very certain that these factors were a response to pain, as previously he had been a happy person.

Coping Strategies

The coping strategies Jack had adopted were avoidance of provocative activities, protective behaviours and passive treatments. Apart from walking, Jack reported no active coping strategies.

Protective Behaviours

Jack had become very protective of his back; he postured his back into a lordosis, used his hands to unload it and slowed all his movements down to control the pain. Because he feared his back would 'snap', he avoided doing activities that caused pain, such as bending and lifting.

Social Factors

Jack lived with his girlfriend and didn't socialize much due to his pain. Although he was not currently working, he indicated that he would like to return to work if he could control his pain better. He had supportive family and friends.

General Health and Comorbidities

There were no other reported health disorders; however, Jack felt run down and fatigued due to the pain and lack of sleep. Given there is evidence that low back pain and associated beliefs and behaviours are clustered in families (O'Sullivan et al., 2008), his family history was pursued. However, he reported there was no family history of back pain.

Medication

Jack had trialled various medications such as gabapentin (anti-epileptic medication used to treat neuropathic pain) and strong analgesics; however, he stopped them because he didn't like the side effects such as feeling tired and 'foggy'.

MRI Scans

MRI scans (Fig. 24.2) conducted when he was 16 and then repeated when he was 21 years of age confirmed his reports of multi-level disc degeneration in the lower lumbar spine. Disc bulges were noted at L4/L5 and L5/S1, and multiple levels of disc fissures and Schmorl's nodes were visible at T12 and L1. There was no sign of nerve compression.

Goals

Jack reported that he wanted to be able to control his pain, get back to work and return to light sport such as football. He didn't know if this was realistic or how to achieve these goals.

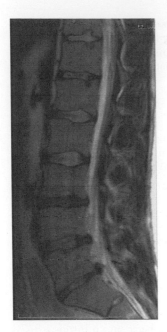

Fig. 24.2 Magnetic resonance imaging (MRI) of the lumbar spine.

Örebro Screening Questionnaire

The score recorded for the Örebro Screening Questionnaire was 132, indicating that Jack was at high risk for chronicity (Boersma and Linton, 2005; WorkSafe Victoria, 2016).

Of particular note were the high scores recorded for the following questions:

1. In the *past 3 months*, on average, how bad was your pain on a 0–10 scale? (10/10)
2. Based on all things you do to cope, or deal with your pain, on an average day, how much are you able to decrease it? (I can't decrease it at all, 10/10)
3. How tense or anxious have you felt in *the past week*? (as tense and anxious as I have felt, 8/10)
4. How much have you been bothered by feeling depressed in the *past week*? (extremely, 7/10)
5. In your view, how large is the risk that your current pain may become persistent? (high risk, 10/10)
6. In your estimation, what are the chances that you will be able to work *in 6 months*? (no chance, 1/10)
7. An increase in pain is an indication that I should stop what I'm doing until the pain decreases (completely, 9/10).

Reasoning Question:

1. Can you please briefly outline what you considered were the key findings and related hypotheses immediately following the subjective examination? In particular, can you comment on how you planned to test these hypotheses, especially in relation to the dominant 'pain types' you hypothesized?

Answer to Reasoning Question:

At the end of the interview, it was very clear to me that Jack was in big trouble. He was a young man who was reporting high levels of pain, and he was very disabled, distressed, fearful and pain-vigilant, with no active coping strategies to manage his pain. His distress levels appeared to be proportionate to his circumstances. He believed his back pain was due to his spine being damaged, as advised by the orthopaedic surgeon based on his MRI, and he held little hope for this to change.

Jack reported that his pain was relatively constant, with mechanical provocation on bending and twisting activities. He was highly guarded and protective of these movements. He had been out of work for 3 months, and he had minimal expectations of returning to work. He didn't know whether physiotherapy could help this time because it hadn't in the past, but he was desperate to try anything.

There was one clear discrepancy in his story. On the one hand, he reported that he was constantly protecting his back for fear of doing harm; however, on the other hand, the only thing that gave him relief was massage, self-manipulation and heat that relaxed his muscles. It was thus deemed important to investigate this relationship in the physical examination. Finally, based on the interview, it sounded like Jack had high levels of sensitization of local spinal structures, with pain amplification due to his lack of pain control and his high levels of vigilance, fear, distress and inactivity (O'Sullivan et al., 2014; Rabey et al., 2016).

Therefore, the aims of the physical examination were as follows:

1. Ascertain exactly where his symptoms were located.
2. Determine his level of tissue sensitivity to palpation and pain responses to movement.
3. Determine his levels of resting trunk muscle tension and body posture by observation and palpation in his pain-provocative postures (sitting, standing and lying).
4. Examine his movement-control strategies during provocative tasks (bending, lifting and rolling) and his thoughts and beliefs in relation to this.
5. Explore the relationship between Jack's muscle 'tension' and his protective behaviours in relation to his provocative postures (sitting and standing) and feared movements (load transfer, bending and rolling). This was deemed critical to determine whether his protective behaviours were provocative of his pain.
6. Conduct a series of postural and movement-guided behavioural experiments to determine the following:
   • Whether he could normalize his movement patterns
   • Whether his pain was influenced by his levels of muscle tension
   • Whether his pain was modifiable/controllable by doing so
7. Use these guided behavioural experiments to encourage Jack to reflect on the relationship between his beliefs, behaviours and pain experiences.

Reasoning Question:

2. Were you surprised that the onset of back pain at such an early age had such a dramatic effect on Jack's life given the apparent lack of external stressors?

Answer to Reasoning Question:

No – sadly, there are many cases such as Jack's where negative interactions with healthcare practitioners reinforce catastrophic beliefs and provocative behaviours that leave people with no control strategies and, consequently, disabled and distressed. This notion of the health system actually driving disability, largely due to the misinterpretation of imaging results and the reinforcement of avoidance and protective behaviours, has been reported previously in the literature (Lin et al., 2013).

Perhaps if Jack had taken a different clinical path that instead 'dethreatened' his pain, that is, provided him with an evidence-based understanding of his pain, as well as active pain-coping strategies, all with a view to Jack returning to his valued activities, he likely would have avoided years of unnecessary suffering.

Clinical Reasoning Commentary:

Two interesting aspects to the clinician's reasoning are apparent in these responses. First, the clinician has clearly encountered many similar cases previously and recognizes the 'pattern' encapsulating typical key clinical findings, particularly those indicating that the patient has adopted catastrophic beliefs and fear-based understandings of the pain largely borne of the structurally focussed biomedical approach to musculoskeletal diagnosis and management (see Chapter 2). Counterproductive guarded back postures and avoidant actions are the natural result of these maladaptive thoughts, as the patient seeks to protect the back structures and follow typical health professional advice accordingly. However, the clinician here, despite having seen this pattern many times previously, remains open-minded, which allows for the detection of the 'clear discrepancy' that the pain best responds to interventions designed to relax the back muscles (e.g. massage, heat) and move the spine (e.g. self-manipulation, walking). It is apparent how this 'discrepancy' has influenced the clinician's determination of the physical examination aims.

The other interesting aspect of the clinician's reasoning evident in these answers is how the list of seven aims flowing from the patient interview demonstrate the planning process, whereby hypotheses regarding movement patterns formulated in the patient interview will be tested through the physical examination. Elements of guided self-management, especially the 'correction' of counterproductive beliefs and understandings underpinning Jack's protective/guarded postures and movements, are planned to evaluate their effect and inform further management. The physical examination and management phases of the clinical session are essentially planned to be executed concurrently, albeit in a modifiable and individualized fashion if unexpected/atypical responses from the patient arise.

Physical Examination

During the interview, Jack had held his posture very erect and stiff, and he had appeared to attempt to unload his spine by taking the load on the back of the chair with his elbows and on the base of the chair with his hands. While he was seated, he reported his pain level to be 8/10. While he remained seated, palpation was undertaken through his clothes to determine the resting tension of his abdominal wall and back muscles. Both muscle regions were very tense at rest. He had a rapid apical breathing pattern (aim 3).

Jack was then asked to move from sitting to standing. He performed this by extending his spine, propping off his arms and holding his breath. The movement was performed very slowly, and he reported pain with the movement. When asked, he acknowledged that this was how he normally transferred off a chair (aims 4 and 5).

At this point, the *first guided behavioural experiment* was conducted. Jack was asked whether he could sit and relax his abdominal wall and back muscles, then sink back into the chair. He was then asked to focus on slow diaphragmatic breathing (belly breathing). He reported that this was difficult to do but that he felt less tension in the back (aims 5 and 6).

The *second guided behavioural experiment* was then conducted in sitting. Jack was asked to relax his spine from its erect position toward flexion, bending his trunk forward and pushing through his feet while breathing in and moving from sitting to standing, all without using his hands. This task was first demonstrated, and then Jack was asked to visualize doing this himself before actually doing it. He repeated this three times and reported that it felt 'strange' but that there was less pain with the movement. He was asked to reflect on what that might tell him about how he usually moved and its relationship to the pain (aims 5, 6 and 7).

Jack reflected that he was always holding his back in tension, and it appeared that this made his pain worse. He further reflected that when he relaxed his trunk muscles, he had less pain. When he was prompted as to why he held himself tensely, he responded that he had been doing this since he had his first major 'spasm' when he was 16 years of age and that he had maintained a tense stomach and upright posture because the previous physiotherapist had told him this was good for his back (aim 7).

Once in standing, palpation of the back and abdominal wall muscles was performed to determine the level of muscle tension and tissue sensitivity. As with standing from sitting, Jack was again very tense and reported moderate levels of hyperalgesia to firm palpation over the lower lumbar spine spinous processes and paraspinal muscles (aims 1 and 2). He was then asked to palpate his own back and abdominal wall. Upon questioning about what he felt, he responded that they felt hard and tense. Following this, he was next instructed to clench and relax his fist and to feel his forearm muscles, then reflect on the feeling in his forearm and how this may feel similar to his back and what his trunk muscles were doing (aim 7).

The *third guided behavioural experiment* was the pen-drop test. A pen was dropped on the floor, and Jack was asked to pick it up. It was noted that he first hesitated before bracing his left hand on his left thigh, maintaining his back erect with a lower lumbar lordosis, and then squatted to pick up the pen. Upon questioning, he admitted that he had held his breath during this task (aim 3).

In the *fourth guided behavioural experiment,* Jack was asked how it would be if he bent over to pick up the pen without bending his knees, and he reported that he didn't think he would be able to get back up. He was then requested to do this, and he forward bent while maintaining his spine in a lordosis, to the point where his fingertips reached mid-thigh, and then he stopped, reporting back pain. On a second attempt at this task, his abdominal wall was simultaneously palpated, and muscle bracing and breath holding were noted. Jack was asked to feel this himself, and he was told that it was not normal to brace the abdominal wall during forward bending (aim 7). It was like clenching a fist and then trying to move it. He was instructed to do this with his fist and to feel what it was like (aim 7).

Jack was then asked to lie supine. It was noted that his abdominal wall and back muscles were still tense on palpation, and he had difficulty relaxing them.

The *fifth guided behavioural experiment* involved Jack flexing his right hip. He moved to 90 degrees and then reported back pain. During this manoevre, both his back and abdominal wall were tense.

The *sixth guided behavioural experiment* required Jack to roll over as he would in bed. It was noted that he braced himself through the elbows on the bed, fixing his head and thorax, and then rolled over via the pelvis while reporting back pain.

The *seventh guided behavioural experiment* involved asking Jack to move into four-point kneeling and then flex back through his knees. Again, he stopped at 90 degrees of hip flexion while also reporting pain. It was also clear that he tensed his abdominal wall.

Jack was asked to reflect on his body's response in every functional task he had just performed where he had experienced pain. He reflected that he tensed up and held his breath. When asked if he thought this was helpful, he further reflected that he wasn't sure but that he didn't know any other way to move.

It was then explained to him that he would now be taught how to relax his abdominal wall and back muscles while flexing his trunk so that he could see whether his pain experience would be any different. It was explained to Jack that this was safe to do and that his levels of pain would be respected.

Jack was then taken back through the series of guided behavioral experiments, again starting in supine crook lying (the least threatening first), where he was taught diaphragmatic breathing (into his belly) and asked to focus on relaxing his back into the clinician's hand (which was under his back). He was next requested to flex a hip and bring it to his chest with his hand while his other hand rested on his abdomen to monitor his breathing patterns. He reported a reduction in pain.

He was then moved to four-point kneeling, where his abdominal wall muscle tension and breathing were monitored as he flexed his hips back toward his heels. Jack realized that if he relaxed his abdominal wall and continued to breathe, he had less pain. Following this, he was asked to roll over, leading from his head, while relaxing his trunk and breathing, and he again reported less pain.

Jack was next instructed to sit on the edge of the bed and relax his spinal posture, breathe into his belly and bend over toward the floor without tensing up. He reported a 'pulling feeling' but no sharp pain. Once this was repeated five times, he was asked to stand up without using his hands or tensing up, which he did without any pain.

Finally, Jack was directed to bend over while relaxing his back and abdominal wall muscles and pick up a dropped pen. He was stopped each time he tensed up and asked to repeat the task until he was successful in doing so. At the end of the session, he picked the pen up off the floor without tensing up and reported no pain at all.

Reasoning Question:

3. You conducted a number of 'guided behavioural experiments' rather than more traditionally assessing individual examination components, such as range of movement, muscle strength, passive accessory joint movement and so forth. What were the particular findings in the history that led you to select this approach to assessment in order to gain the necessary information to test key hypotheses from the subjective examination and to also provide direction for treatment?

Answer to Reasoning Question:

There is growing evidence that when pain becomes persistent and disabling, this is linked to a vicious cycle of catastrophic thoughts, fear, protective and avoidant behaviours, distress leading to pain amplification and disability (O'Sullivan et al., 2015; Vlaeyen et al., 2016). All of these factors became apparent from the interview. In this context, traditional assessments of range and strength and so on become redundant.

The examination process in this case focussed on Jack's pain beliefs and protective behaviours that had left him disabled. Using this behavioural learning process helped him realize that rather than being caused by structural damage, his pain and disability were being driven by modifiable processes such as fear, vigilance, protective guarding and avoidance. Rather than didactically telling him this, however, the reflective nature of the examination allowed him to experience this firsthand, thereby changing his mind-set (beliefs), reducing his fear and demonstrating to him that he had pain-control strategies that he could master. This examination approach therefore conveyed to Jack that his protective bracing behaviours may actually be provocative and maladaptive and also that he had the capacity to change them and exercise some control over his pain.

Reasoning Question:

4. What was your clinically reasoned interpretation of Jack's story in a nutshell? In particular, how was his back pain mediated and then maintained for 6 years?

Continued on following page

Answer to Reasoning Question:

The most likely interpretation of Jack's presentation was that he had developed a vicious cycle of pain sensitization and disability related to high levels of fear based on the belief he had the spine of a 70-year-old, related to what he had been told by health practitioners. This was associated with pain hypervigilance, fear, distress, protective muscle guarding and avoidance behaviours. Although his pain characteristics were largely mechanically provoked during load transfer and bending, his thresholds for provocation were very low, suggestive of central nervous system (CNS) factors related to pain amplification. His movement behaviours during these tasks were maladaptive (notably, he held his low back in a hyperlordotic posture, and any attempt to flex led to co-contraction of his back and abdominal wall muscles, which resulted in pain), directly reinforcing his beliefs that it was dangerous to bend. Over time, he had gradually lost the functional capacity to work, be active and socialize. This left him feeling depressed, frustrated and anxious.

This presentation reflected both a 'top-down' and 'bottom-up' process of pain sensitization, presumably involving both central sensitizing factors (related to fear, pain vigilance, anxiety and distress) (O'Sullivan et al., 2014; Rabey et al., 2016) and peripheral nociceptive processes (linked to protective muscle guarding and spinal loading; Dankaerts et al., 2009; O'Sullivan et al., 2015). Even though Jack had low pain self-efficacy and a loss of hope, during the examination (particularly the guided behavioural experiments), he demonstrated high levels of self-efficacy and adaptability. This was manifested by his ability to control and adapt the way he moved, change the way he responded to pain and exercise immediate control over his pain during provocative tasks. This provided Jack with a powerful new insight into his pain disorder which conflicted with his structural 'damage' beliefs and provided him with confidence, thus enhancing his self-efficacy to control his pain disorder.

A summary of the estimated various contributions of the factors explored during the examination to Jack's pain is provided in Fig. 24.3.

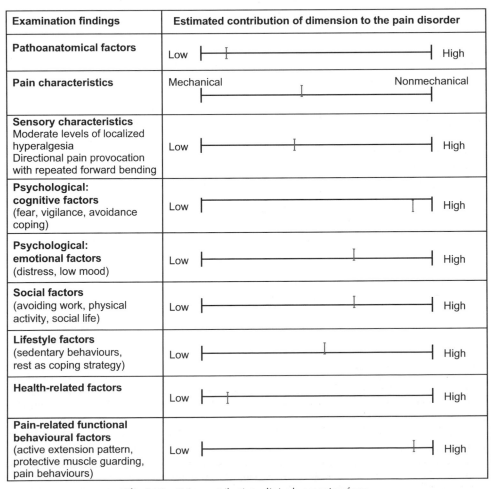

Fig. 24.3 Pain contribution clinical reasoning form.

Reasoning Question:

5. You comment that Jack's pain characteristics were largely mechanically provoked and that his movement behaviours during various tasks were maladaptive. Were these findings consistent with the clinical reasoning you entertained before you commenced the physical examination?

Answer to Reasoning Question:

Yes – Jack was clear about the activities that provoked his pain and that he avoided. These activities set the framework for the physical examination. It was also apparent when Jack sat during the interview that he held himself tense and erect and that he was unable to relax. Further, from the interview, he reported the common contradiction that he felt tense and stiff all the time and constantly braced his 'core' muscles, but he obtained relief from heat, relaxation and massage. This highlighted that in contrast to his coping strategies (to tense and protect his back), he was likely to gain relief from treatment involving relaxation and movement.

Clinical Reasoning Commentary:

The clinician has adopted a deliberate patient-reflective approach to the physical examination. Rather than the patient being passively examined and 'told' what is 'wrong' with him or her by the clinician, the patient is instead an active partner in the process of 'collaborative discovery' of the relationships between the patient's beliefs and understandings (mind) and his or her muscle activity and pain (body). This approach is potentially very powerful because the patient can immediately feel (in real time) the difference in pain levels during functional movements as the patient is challenged to change the way he or she moves by changing his or her beliefs about how he or she should move.

The insight that arises for Jack following skilful guidance in his reflection (via the guided behavioural experiments) is that he can control his pain level by not being fearful of damaging his back during movement and by consequently relaxing his 'core' muscles. Direct experience is a powerful teacher, and when coupled with a confident and attentive clinician who gently guides the reflective process, it can result in immediate and profound positive changes in self-efficacy. Hence the physical examination and the management phases are almost seamlessly intertwined and sequentially linked.

Cognitive Functional Therapy (CFT) Intervention
Making Sense of His Pain

Jack was asked to recount what he had learnt from the encounter thus far. He reported, 'I have learnt that I have been tense in all my postures and movements, and this hurts me, but when I relax and move, it doesn't'. He was then asked to reflect why he had been doing this, and he said, 'Because I have been frightened, and I have been told to do this'. When questioned which was the better way, he reflected, the 'new way'.

It was then outlined to Jack how his pain disorder had evolved – particularly, how his experience of pain, negative advice regarding his spine's structure, his high levels of fear and his protective behaviours led him into a vicious cycle of pain, avoidance and disability. He was informed that his changes on MRI were common and poorly predictive of back pain and disability and that athletes with similar findings (but who were active at a high level) had been seen in the clinic.

Upon being asked to reflect on this, Jack said it all made sense to him. He was then challenged to say how he might change this process. He reflected that he needed to change how he thought about his back, learn to relax and move and not be afraid to get his life back. This was agreed to as being very appropriate.

Exposure With Pain Control

An exercise sheet with all the movement experiments we had conducted in the session was provided to Jack: starting with hip flexion in supine lying, then four-point kneeling hip and spine flexion, rolling, sitting relaxed and moving from sitting to standing, and finally forward bending. He was prescribed 15–20 repetitions of each exercise, while being mindful of his breathing and muscle tension. He was then observed performing all the exercises.

Jack was asked to stop bracing his abdominal wall and self-manipulating and to instead replace this with 'belly breathing' and relaxing. He was also instructed to slouch into the chair when sitting, rather than sitting tall and tense. He was further advised that when he felt pain during the day, he was to be aware of his level of muscle tension and to respond to the pain by relaxing using belly breathing.

Lifestyle Aspects

Finally, Jack was recommended to keep up his walking but to ensure he relaxed his abdominal wall when he walked. With sleeping, he was instructed to perform some relaxed breathing and rolling in bed before going to sleep to help break the cycle of protective guarding in bed which he reported disrupted his sleep.

Session 2 (1 Day Later)

Jack was reviewed the next day. He reported that his back felt immediately better, with markedly less pain. He further reported that he was able to sit in traffic for an hour with little pain and that he had been thinking about 'relaxing his back all the time'. He experienced little pain with the exercises, and when he attended to his pain, he did so by relaxing and breathing. This positive response came as a huge surprise to Jack, as he didn't expect this.

CFT Intervention

Making Sense of Pain

Jack was asked about his thinking about his back pain following the previous session. He reported that it had 'blown his mind'. He felt he had a new way to think about his pain and control it. He felt very excited. He stated that he was constantly aware that his body's response to pain was to tense and hold his breath, but he was confident he could overcome this. He felt hopeful that he could take control of his back-pain problem and get his life back.

Exposure With Control

All his behavioural exercises were reviewed, and he was able to do these with minimal pain. His sitting posture and habitual movements, such as sitting to standing and undressing, were visibly easier, quicker and less tense. This was a dramatic change. The importance of integrating these new movements into activities of daily living, work and physical activity to help make them habitual was reinforced with Jack. He was then asked to run on the spot and lift a chair. From this re-assessment, a plan was mapped out to gradually build his confidence in returning to bending with speed, lifting, twisting and loading his spine.

Lifestyle

Linked to the aforementioned plan, a plan to gradually progress him toward his valued goals of returning to work, socializing and physical activity (football) was also outlined.

1-Year Follow-up

When Jack was reviewed 1 year later, he reported that since he had last attended the clinic, he had experienced very little pain and was fully active. He had set up his own business where he was putting in gas and water mains, which involved digging and manual work. He reported that he didn't really think about his back anymore and that he trusted it. He indicated he had received no treatment in the intervening year.

When asked what his reflections were on why he had changed, he stated, 'I thought my back was in pieces, and when you told me that these changes (on MRI) were normal and that you had seen these before in athletes, it gave me confidence'. Upon further interrogation, he indicated that the key things that had changed for him were as follows: 'my mind-set changed', 'realizing that when I was moving, I wasn't doing damage' and 'relaxing and moving, but the mind-set was the big thing'.

On examination, Jack moved freely, with no hesitation or pain. He was discharged.

Reasoning Question:

6. After 6 years of back pain, Jack seemed to grasp the concepts you were teaching him very quickly. In your experience, is that typical, or do most people take longer to understand and learn to apply CFT?

Answer to Reasoning Question:

Jack was a very fast learner. This was likely linked to the fact that he possessed many resilience factors, such as high levels of self-efficacy, an open mind-set, an adaptive learning ability, motivation to be in control, a strong desire to work and be active and a lack of historical mental health issues. The factors influencing the ability of an individual to change can be varied and complex and likely relate to all these resilience factors, as well as the therapeutic alliance itself. Establishing Jack's trust was very important in this regard.

Clinical experience has shown that most people possess an extraordinary ability to change. However, this can be hampered by factors such as their contextual social stressors, biomedical beliefs, comorbid mental and physical health conditions and a closed mind-set. In these instances, change may take some months, or in other cases, it may never occur. Sadly, we have cultural beliefs about pain and a healthcare system that reinforces that 'pain = damage' and that if you have pain, you need to strengthen your core muscles and avoid flexing the spine. Changing these beliefs can be very confronting to patients when they are heavily invested in them or where they have placed trust in the people who have told them this.

Reasoning Question:

7. Can you please briefly outline the main learning points from this case to assist the reader in recognizing and managing similar clinical patterns or presentations?

Answer to Reasoning Question:

Sadly, there are too many stories like Jack's that fill our waiting rooms. These are people for whom the health system has failed by reinforcing that pain means they are damaged, creating fear, and by reinforcing protective guarding and avoidance behaviours, commonly resulting in escalating distress and disability. This case demonstrates the multidimensional nature of chronic low back pain and its management in reinforcing pain and disability. It highlights the need for the clinician to possess an expanded skill set to effectively interview and examine pain disorders in a primary care setting. It also highlights the power of reflective questioning and use of behavioural learning to communicate to the patients that their backs can be trusted and that there is a pathway to participate in the activities in life that they value.

The nature of the underlying plasticity and adaptability of the nervous system and people's ability to change is extraordinary. Jack's case exemplifies this, and this can give encouragement and hope for change to people like Jack where the health system may have failed them. The potential role of CFT in the management of musculoskeletal pain is also demonstrated in Jack's case. This management approach is not complicated, but it does demand a change in mind-set from the treating clinician. This change in understandings includes the following: pain should not be feared, helping people make sense of their pain and providing hope for change is an intervention in and of itself and behavioural learning is a powerful way to assist people regain the things in life that they value. By doing so, we can reduce the burden of pain in our communities. Overall, this case highlights the changing role of manual therapy to apply integrated and individualized management approaches for disabling pain disorders.

Clinical Reasoning Commentary:

The management of patients with musculoskeletal pain has changed over many years and has more recently been shaped by our evolving understanding of the influence of psychosocial factors, alongside physical and environmental factors, in patients' pain and disability presentations. This case demonstrates clinical reasoning using a less conventional method of assessment and management, yet achieves an excellent and rapid outcome by virtue of recognizing and targeting the patient's beliefs, fears and behaviour (movement pattern, muscle tensing, breathing pattern) within meaningful functional activities. Clearly, significant clinical experience with similar patient presentations underpins this approach and associated reasoning. Presumably, had Jack not responded as anticipated, further assessment of relevant physical impairments potentially also contributing to his pain and disability would likely then have been undertaken. For example, if Jack had not demonstrated normal physiological movements with 'relaxation' of his trunk muscles, the clinician may have gone on to perform additional spinal movement tests.

Importantly, this case also highlights that education and training in manual therapy need to be sufficiently broad to encompass the burgeoning skill set that CFT demands of the clinician. Historically, manual therapy education programs have tended to focus significant time on technical 'hands-on' skills, usually within a framework driven by pathological or physical impairment. However, these

Continued on following page

programs have evolved within the last 10 or so years to become more biopsychosocially focussed, whereby both 'biomedical' and 'psychosocial' factors are equally considered.

Manual therapy clinicians have often also tended to practice within professional 'approaches', further limiting their ability to professionally grow and expand their skill set. When one operates within a busy clinical setting that requires high patient turnover, this can lead to two undesirable outcomes. First, there is typically little or no time for reflection on cases which may provide an opportunity for learning. Second, it becomes very easy to adopt the clinical routine in which you were originally trained for almost each and every patient. This is primarily driven by time pressures and the need for conservation of energy to enable clinicians to pace themselves through a full caseload day after day.

Improving clinical reasoning that is critical and not constrained by allegiance to one 'approach' and instead integrates assessment and management of the physical, the psychosocial and the environment, as appropriate to patients' unique presentations, is promoted through this book. Chapter 31 provides strategies that may be utilized in the busy clinic to facilitate improving clinical reasoning.

Jack's story can be viewed at https://www.youtube.com/watch?v=j4gmtpdwmrs.

REFERENCES

Boersma, K., Linton, S.J., 2005. Screening to identify patients at risk: profiles of psychological risk factors for early intervention. Clin. J. Pain 21 (1), 38–43.

Dankaerts, W., O'Sullivan, P.B., Burnett, A.F., Straker, L.M., 2009. Discriminating healthy controls and two clinical sub-groups of non-specific chronic low back pain patients using trunk muscle activation and lumbo-sacral kinematics of postures and movements - a statistical classification model. Spine 34 (15), 1610–1618.

Lin, I., O'Sullivan, P., Coffin, J., Mak, D., Toussaint, S., Straker, L., 2013. Disabling chronic low back pain as an iatrogenic disorder: a qualitative study in Aboriginal Australians. BMJ Open 3 (4), e002654.

O'Sullivan, P., Caniero, J.P., O'Keeffe, M., Smith, A., Dankaerts, W., Fersum, K., et al., 2018. Cognitive functional therapy: an integrated behavioral approach for the targeted management of disabling low back pain. Phys. Ther. 98 (5), 408–423. https://academic.oup.com/ptj/article/98/5/408/4925487.

O'Sullivan, P., Straker, L., Smith, A., Perry, M., et al., 2008. Carer experience of back pain is associated with adolescent back pain experience even when controlling for other carer and family factors. Clin. J. Pain 42 (3), 226–231.

O'Sullivan, P., Waller, R., Gardner, J., Johnston, R., Payne, C., Shannon, A., et al., 2014. Sensory characteristics of chronic non-specific low back pain: a subgroup investigation. Man. Ther. 19 (4), 311–318.

Rabey, M., Smith, A., Slater, S., Beales, D., O'Sullivan, P., 2016. Differing psychologically-derived clusters in people with chronic low back pain are associated with different multidimensional profiles. Clin. J. Pain 32 (12), 1015–1027.

Vlaeyen, J.W.S., Crombez, G., Linton, J., 2016. The fear-avoidance model of pain. Pain 157 (8), 1588–1589.

WorkSafe Victoria (2016). Outcome measures. http://www.worksafe.vic.gov.au/health-professionals/treating-injured-workers/outcome-measures.

Applying Contemporary Pain Neuroscience for a Patient With Maladaptive Central Sensitization Pain

Jo Nijs • Margot De Kooning •
Anneleen Malfliet • Mark A. Jones

A Brief Background of Pain Neuroscience

Despite extensive global research efforts, chronic 'unexplained' pain remains a challenging issue for clinicians and an emerging socioeconomic problem. Pain neuroscience has evolved, and musculoskeletal clinicians around the globe are at the front line for implementing contemporary pain neuroscience in clinical practice.

Contemporary pain neuroscience has advanced our understanding of pain. The initial paradigm was pain proportional to nociceptive input; the second was Wall and Melzak's gate theory (Wall and Melzack, 1994), and the most recent is pain as central sensitization (CS). Peripheral sensitization and, to some extent, also CS, occurs normally with acute pain but normally decreases soon after the inflammatory phase. Therefore, here we conceptualize the sensitization in chronic pain as 'maladaptive central sensitization' (referred to as nociplastic pain elsewhere in this book). For brevity reasons, maladaptive central sensitization in chronic pain is abbreviated throughout this chapter as CS pain. It is now well established that sensitization of the central nervous system (CNS) is an important feature in many patients with chronic pain, including those with whiplash (Van Oosterwijck et al., 2013b), shoulder impingement syndrome (Paul et al., 2012), chronic low back pain (Roussel et al., 2013), osteoarthritis (Lluch Girbes et al., 2013), headache (Ashina et al., 2005; Perrotta et al., 2010), fibromyalgia (Price et al., 2002), chronic fatigue syndrome (Nijs et al., 2012c), rheumatoid arthritis (Meeus et al., 2012), patellar tendinopathy (van Wilgen et al., 2011), and lateral epicondylalgia (Coombes et al., 2012; Fernandez-Carnero et al., 2009). Also, neuropathic pain may be characterized/accompanied by sensitization; peripheral and central (segmentally related) pain pathways can become hyperexcitable in patients with neuropathic pain.

CS has been defined as 'an amplification of neural signaling within the central nervous system that elicits pain hypersensitivity' (Woolf, 2011) or 'an augmentation of responsiveness of central neurons to input from unimodal and polymodal receptors' (Meyer et al., 1995). Such definitions originate from laboratory research, but the awareness that the concept of CS should be translated to the clinic is growing, which is illustrated by the present case report.

CS encompasses various related dysfunctions of the CNS, all contributing to an increased responsiveness to a variety of stimuli, such as mechanical pressure, chemical substances, light, sound, cold, heat, stress and electrical stimuli (Nijs et al., 2010). Such dysfunctions of the CNS include altered sensory processing in the brain (Staud et al., 2008), malfunctioning of descending anti-nociceptive mechanisms (Yarnitsky, 2010; Meeus et al., 2008), increased activity of pain facilitatory pathways and enhanced temporal summation of second pain or wind-up (Filatova et al., 2008; Raphael et al., 2009). In addition, the pain (neuro)matrix is overactive in CS and chronic pain, with increased brain activity in areas known to be involved in acute pain sensations (the insula, anterior cingulate cortex and the prefrontal cortex) as well as in regions not involved in acute pain sensations (various brainstem nuclei, dorsolateral frontal cortex and the parietal associated cortex) (Seifert and Maihofner, 2009).

Musculoskeletal practice has come a long way in terms of integrating the understanding of contemporary pain neuroscience. Pain neurophysiology has traditionally been one of the cornerstones of musculoskeletal practice, making it easier for us to understand new concepts like CS. Still, clinicians struggle with the treatment of CS pain. Given the complexity of the mechanisms behind CS pain and the lack of evidence-based treatment for CS pain, this comes as no surprise. Here we illustrate how musculoskeletal clinicians can apply contemporary pain neuroscience in a patient with chronic (neck) pain. The majority of the reasoning outlined herein applies to many chronic pain patients rather than being specific for (traumatic) neck pain only.

History

Anna is a 37-year-old female patient who suffered a traumatic neck injury due to a car accident 8 years before she entered our practice upon referral from a physician specialized in rehabilitation medicine. She was driving the car herself and was wearing a seatbelt. The day following her car accident, she went to work (full-time teaching at a university college) but experienced difficulties concentrating and suffered from a headache and increased sensitivity to bright light as well as sound. After work, she consulted her family physician, who referred her for x-rays of her cervical spine and prescribed sick leave. After 3 months of sick leave, she was obliged to return to work according to the local insurance system. Because she felt unable to resume work, she took her available holidays. In total, she didn't return to work until 2 years post-injury.

The initial imaging findings (x-rays and nuclear magnetic resonance [NMR] imaging of the cervical spine and the brain) were rather limited, showing nothing but slight degeneration of the C4–C5 facet joints and anterior bulging of the C5–C6 disc. The NMR re-assessment 3 years later showed similar findings without progression. A third NMR scan a few months before she entered our practice confirmed the lack of progression.

Since her car accident up to her first attendance in our practice, Anna had developed severe chronic whiplash-associated disorder (WAD), including shoulder and neck pain radiating to her arms, headache, concentration difficulties, fatigue, sleeping problems and hypersensitivity to bright light and sound. Anna described her shoulder, neck and arm pains as 'fatiguing and vague'. She sometimes experienced sensory loss in both arms (including the hands), but these symptoms would come and go. Anna did not report any other new-onset hypersensitivity symptoms such as increased sensitivity to smell and hot or cold sensations. She also had extensive previous screening for neurological and arterial symptoms, which were negative. Anna experienced difficulties (variable provocation of neck, shoulder, arm pains and headache) undressing, lifting, walking or standing for a long time, looking down and upward, and during household activities (especially repetitive overhead activities). She used to be good at coping with stress, but in the last couple of years, she had been very irritable, anxious and ineffective at coping with everyday stressors. At the time of the initial appointment, Anna was able to work full-time, but besides working, she had little energy left for other activities. Notably, her social activities, including catching up with friends, were at a very low level, much lower than she would like.

Anna is happily married with two lovely children of 3 and 6 years. Her husband is very supportive of her medical problems. Her symptoms have been fluctuating over time ever since her car accident.

Anna has no other health conditions (comorbidities) and has never been diagnosed with any other long-term illness. She has no history of unexplained weight loss or any other red flag.

In the early phase post-injury, she was advised by her treating physician to wear a collar and to continue wearing it whenever necessary. She tried physiotherapy several times, with mixed results and only small, non-lasting improvements in pain. Treatments included exercise therapy, massage, electrotherapy and heat therapy. At the moment, she is taking muscle relaxants and painkillers (acetaminophen) depending on pain severity, which offer some relief, but she indicates that they appear to work less effectively than they used to.

Questionnaires

The Pain Catastrophizing Scale (Sullivan et al., 1995) generated a total score of 30/52, with a normal score on the subscale of pain magnification (5/12) but high scores on the helplessness (15/24) and rumination (10/16) subscales. The brief Illness Perceptions Questionnaire (Broadbent et al., 2006) revealed that Anna thought that increased muscle tension and doing too much caused her sustained disability, did not understand her health problem, believed that her pain would last for a long time, worried a lot about her health problem and was unable to find a cure or way to self-control her pain. Finally, the Pain Vigilance and Awareness Questionnaire (Roelofs et al., 2003) clearly revealed pain hypervigilance.

Reasoning Question:

1. Would you comment on your choice of questionnaires and your use of the information obtained? Also, were there issues regarding Anna's 'perspectives on her experience' that emerged in her questionnaire responses and/or her interview/history that you noted for returning to at later appointments to explore further with Anna?

Answer to Reasoning Question:

There are so many questionnaires we can use. Although they generate very useful information for clinicians, patients generally don't like filling them out, and considerable time is required for interpreting them. Hence, it is important to be selective in the choice of questionnaires. A classic mistake clinicians make is using questionnaires to decide which type of pain they are faced with. Unless you are willing to use a diagnostic neuropathic pain questionnaire, this is not advised. In fact, maladaptive pain cognitions can be present in any patient, regardless of whether patients have nociceptive, neuropathic or CS pain. It is important to realize that we do not use these questionnaires for diagnostic purposes but, rather, for identifying treatment goals and informing our client-centred pain neuroscience education. Indeed, pain neuroscience education should always try to address the maladaptive pain cognitions and illness perceptions (van Wilgen et al., 2014). While the Pain Catastrophizing Scale and Pain Vigilance and Awareness Questionnaire often generate clear findings from scoring the answers and computing the results, the brief Illness Perceptions Questionnaire often identifies patient perceptions that require further, more thorough exploration. This is, in fact, an enjoyable part of the history taking, as you often hear amazing stories from patients who have adopted strange illness perceptions from family members, friends, neighbours or even other healthcare providers!

Regarding ongoing assessment of Anna's perspectives through later appointments, we continuously assessed them through questioning Anna's perceptions about changes in pain severity throughout the treatment period (i.e. the fluctuating nature of her pain), as well as her perceptions about (anticipated) pain increases following exercises and daily activities.

Clinical Reasoning Commentary:

Here an important distinction is highlighted regarding obtaining patient information to diagnose or categorize versus obtaining patient information to inform understanding and management and to monitor change. In the 'hypothesis categories' framework presented in Chapter 1, we encouraged a balance in reasoning between 'pathology' and 'impairment'. A similar balance is needed between categorizing the type of pain and understanding the patient's perspectives. They both have direct implications for management and prognosis, and hence both are important. But as emphasized in this answer, questionnaires on their own mostly will not provide a diagnosis of pain type. Their primary value is what they reveal regarding patient perspectives. This is highlighted in the point made about exploring patients' responses to the brief Illness Perceptions Questionnaire further. Three patients may tick the same questionnaire box, provide the same score to a stated perspective or provide the same written illness perception, but for quite different reasons. Although the questionnaire can be re-administered to assess change, for this information to be most useful in informing management, the clinician needs to clarify apparent maladaptive/unhelpful responses to better understand the basis of those responses.

Assessment to inform clinical reasoning is never completed in a single appointment. This is particularly the case for the continued assessment of patient perspectives (i.e. psychosocial status) that the authors highlight throughout the ongoing management.

Clinical Examination

On examining her posture in standing and sitting, no major issues were identified. Anna's passive physiological and accessory cervical joint mobility was normal (full range of motion at all levels and in all directions with no provocation of symptoms), but active cervical mobility in sitting was restricted toward flexion, and combined neck extension and rotation to the left and the right was painful and restricted. She indicated she was afraid to hurt her neck when performing the active movements. The examination of her shoulder complex was negative. Her breathing pattern was normal, including the coordinated action of the thoracic cage with the abdomen. Anna tested positive on the craniocervical flexion test, showing impaired deep cervical neuromuscular control, with clear overshooting of the requested movements (Jull et al., 2008). Anna had moderately increased cervical muscle tone limited to the cervical muscles (trapezius, scaleni and upper cervical muscles) but no active trigger points. As is often the case in patients with chronic WAD, the outcome of the examination of neurodynamic tests (previously known as brachial plexus tests or upper limb tension tests) was rather vague and did not generate a consistent picture of restricted mobility or symptom provocation consistent with any of the major upper limb nerves (median, ulnar, radial).

In addition, we used a hand-held analogue Fisher algometer (Force Dial model FDK 40 Push Pull Force Gage, Wagner Instruments, P.O.B. 1217, Greenwich CT 06836) for assessing pressure pain thresholds at three anatomical locations: the right trapezius belly (midway between the spinous process of T1 and lateral part of the acromion), her right hand (midpoint of the first metacarpal) and the midpoint of her right calf. In order to determine pressure pain thresholds at each location, pressure was gradually increased at a rate of 1 kg/s until she reported the first onset of pain (at which point Anna said 'stop').

Next, for assessing the functioning of brain-orchestrated endogenous analgesia, conditioned pain modulation was induced by inflating an occlusion cuff (conditioning stimulus) around Anna's left arm (midway of her upper arm) to a painful intensity (Daenen et al., 2013b). The occlusion cuff was inflated at a rate of 20 mmHg/s until 'the first sensation of pain' was reported. This cuff inflation was maintained for 30 seconds. Afterward, Anna was asked to rate the pain intensity, as a result of cuff inflation around the left arm, on a numerical rating scale (0 = no pain to 10 = worst possible pain). Next, the cuff inflation was increased or decreased until pain intensity at the left arm was rated as 3/10 on the verbal rating scale. Then the previously described pressure pain thresholds were repeated during maintenance of the cuff inflation and relaxation of the left arm. This way of assessing conditioned pain modulation has revealed impaired endogenous analgesia in patients with chronic WAD (Daenen et al., 2013b) and allows performance in a clinical setting. Anna's results at the baseline pain threshold measurements and the change during conditioned pain modulation indicated dysfunctional endogenous analgesia in the lower limb (from 6.8 kg/s at baseline to 7.2 during cuff inflation) and the neck (from 2.0 kg/s to 2.6), but not at the hand (7.2 kg/s to 13.4).

Contrary to her ability to activate pain inhibition at rest, Anna was able to activate endogenous analgesia in response to a short, low-intensity, graded bicycle test (4 minutes of stationary cycling starting from 50 watts increasing by 25 watts per minute). This was shown by the increases in manually assessed pressure pain threshold at the right hand (increase from 8.25 kg/s at baseline to 9.20 immediately post-exercise) and right lower limb (6.8 kg/s to 10.6). The small increase in pressure pain threshold at the right hand should not be interpreted as an important change, but the fact that it did not decrease as is often seen in chronic pain patients (Nijs et al., 2012), together with the observed increased pain threshold at her right lower limb, supports a physiological activation of endogenous analgesia during exercise.

Reasoning Question:

2. In your opening background on pain neuroscience, you explained what maladaptive CS is and discussed its contribution to chronic 'unexplained' pain. Would you discuss how you differentiate neuropathic, nociceptive and CS pain and highlight the key features from Anna's history and clinical examination that support or refute a dominant CS pain mechanism? Also, would you presume that

Anna initially had some level of soft tissue injuries, and if so, can you identify any likely factors in her history that may account for her progression to CS and chronic pain?

Answer to Reasoning Question:

Any pain complaint can be either nociceptive, neuropathic or CS in nature, and combinations are also possible (e.g. neuropathic and CS pain). We used the information from Anna's history, and later her clinical examination, for differentiating nociceptive, neuropathic and CS pain. For that, diagnosing or excluding neuropathic pain is often the first step in musculoskeletal practice. Indeed, although recent guidelines have been published for classification of neuropathic pain (Treede et al., 2008; Haanpää M, 2010), the criteria specify that a lesion or disease of the nervous system is identifiable and that pain is limited to a 'neuroanatomically plausible' distribution. These criteria, however, preclude the use of the term 'neuropathic pain' for people with widespread pain and nervous system sensitization (i.e. CS pain).

We used the five questions that follow to examine the odds of a neuropathic cause for Anna's pain (Treede et al., 2008; Haanpää, 2010). It is important to note the issue of sensory dysfunction for the differential diagnosis between neuropathic and CS pain. Sensory testing is of prime importance for the diagnosis of neuropathic pain (Treede et al., 2008; Haanpää, 2010). This includes testing of the function of sensory fibers with simple tools (e.g. a tuning fork for vibration, a soft brush for touch, and cold/warm objects for temperature), which typically assesses the relationship between the stimulus and the perceived sensation (Haanpää, 2010). Several options arise here, all suggestive of neuropathic pain: hyperesthesia[1], hypoesthesia[2], hyperalgesia[3], hypoalgesia[4], allodynia[5], aftersensations and so forth. Whereas in neuropathic pain the location of the sensory dysfunction should be neuroanatomically logical, in CS pain it should be spread in non-segmentally related areas of the body. Clinical examination in CS pain typically reveals increased sensitivity at sites segmentally unrelated to the primary source of nociception (Sterling et al., 2004; Nijs et al., 2010).

1. *Is there a history of a lesion or disease of the nervous system, either central or peripheral nervous system?* No, there was not in this case. Unless the traumatic event resulted in damage to the nervous system, which would preclude diagnosing WADs grade I to III (Spitzer et al., 1995), this is rarely the case in such patients. There was no evidence from Anna's diagnostic investigations to reveal an abnormality of the nervous system or post-traumatic damage to the nervous system (not in the spinal cord, peripheral nerves or brain).

2. *Does the patient present with comorbidities often related to neuropathic pain (e.g. cancer, stroke, diabetes, herpes or neurodegenerative disease)?* No, Anna does not present with such comorbidities.

3. *Is the pain distribution neuroanatomically logical?* No, the pain distribution is neuroanatomically illogical. Anna presents with neck pain combined with headache and pain in both shoulders, sometimes radiating to both arms/hands.

4. *Does the patient describe the pain as burning, shooting, or pricking?* No, instead Anna described the pain as fatiguing and vague.

5. *Is the location of the sensory dysfunction neuroanatomically logical?* Again no: Anna sometimes experiences sensory loss in both arms (including the hands), but these symptoms come and go.

From the reasoning evident in the answers to these questions, it becomes clear that Anna does not have neuropathic pain. In cases of neuropathic pain, these questions should be answered positively. This leaves us with three options: nociceptive, CS pain or both.

For differentiating nociceptive and CS pain, clinicians can use the algorithm presented in Fig. 25.1. The algorithm guides the clinician through the screening of three major differential criteria, each of which is explained in the following subsections with reference to Anna's case. The criteria are taken from a recently published international proposal for the classification of CS pain, which is based on a body of evidence from original research papers and expert opinion from 18 pain experts from seven different countries (Nijs, 2014). Although an increasing number of musculoskeletal clinicians have been trained in using these criteria in clinical practice, studies examining the validity of these criteria are currently unavailable (however, they are ongoing).

Criterion 1: Pain Experience Disproportionate to the Nature and Extent of Injury or Pathology (Nijs, 2014)

This first criterion is obligatory and implies that the severity of pain and related reported or perceived disability (e.g. restriction and intolerance to daily life activities, to stress, etc.) are disproportionate to the nature and extent of injury or pathology (i.e. tissue damage or structural impairments). This is in

Continued on following page

---

[1]Hyperesthesia is increased sensitivity to sensory stimuli.
[2]Hypoesthesia is decreased sensitivity to sensory stimuli.
[3]Hyperalgesia is increased sensitivity to nociceptive stimuli.
[4]Hypoalgesia is decreased sensitivity to nociceptive stimuli.
[5]Allodynia is feeling pain in response to non-nociceptive stimuli.

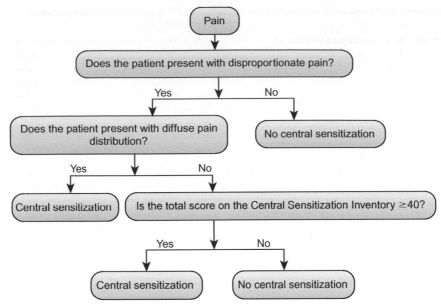

Fig. 25.1   Algorithm for the differential diagnosis of nociceptive versus central sensitization pain. *(Modified from Nijs et al. [2014].)*

contradiction to nociceptive pain, where the severity of pain and perceived disability are proportionate to the nature and extent of injury or pathology and physical impairments.

For screening of this first criterion, we initially considered the degree of Anna's injury and pathology against her reported pain and disability. Several imaging techniques were used to identify such nociceptive sources, but neither initial imaging (x-ray and NMR of the cervical region and the brain) or follow-up imaging 9 years post-injury (NMR of the cervical region and the brain) were positive. The increased muscle tension was limited in severity and restricted to the cervical muscles (trapezius, scaleni and upper cervical muscles). In addition, the clinical examination revealed dysfunctional neuromuscular control of the deep cervical flexors, as often seen in patients with chronic WAD (Elliott et al., 2010; Sterling et al., 2003b).

Next, we weighted the degree of injury, pathology and physical signs against her reported pain, disability and tolerance to activities of daily living for the likelihood of a dominant nociceptive input being responsible for her pain experience. We asked ourselves: Are Anna's evidence of injury, pathology and physical signs sufficient to account for her pattern of symptom behaviour as expected for a dominant nociceptive source? It was concluded that the functional difficulties Anna's was having were associated with too variable a pattern of symptom provocation to support a hypothesis of nociceptive pain. It was concluded that the limited muscle tension was neither able to explain the complexity of her symptoms and other signs nor capable of explaining her pain experience. After all, she had tried hands-on myofascial treatment before, with very limited benefits. In addition, research has taught us that the dysfunctional neuromuscular control of the deep cervical flexors in patients with chronic WAD is of limited clinical importance (Daenen et al., 2013a). Therefore, and in addition to our conclusion regarding the increased cervical muscle tone, it was decided that the dysfunctional neuromuscular control of the deep cervical flexors was also unable to explain the pain experienced by Anna. Hence, it was reasoned that she suffered from disproportionate pain.

Criterion 2: Diffuse Pain Distribution (Nijs, 2014)

For screening this criterion, a thorough assessment and interpretation of the patient's self-reported pain distribution are required. Examples of patterns of pain distribution that fulfill this criterion are bilateral pain/mirror pain (i.e. a symmetrical pain pattern), pain varying in (anatomical) location, large pain areas with a non-segmental (i.e. neuroanatomically illogical) distribution, widespread pain and/or allodynia/hyperalgesia outside the segmental area of (presumed) primary nociception (Nijs, 2014).

As explained previously, Anna had a pattern of pain distribution that complies with this criterion; she showed evidence of diffuse pain distribution (i.e. pain varying in location and large pain areas with a non-segmental distribution). Thus, the first two criteria are met, which is sufficient for classifying her pain as CS pain (Fig. 25.1). For comprehensiveness, the screening of criterion 3 is explained as well.

Criterion 3: Hypersensitivity of Senses Unrelated to the Musculoskeletal System (Nijs, 2014)

CS may manifest as much more than generalized hypersensitivity to pain: it may be characterized by an increased responsiveness to a variety of stimuli in addition to mechanical pressure, namely, chemical substances, cold, heat, electrical stimuli, stress and emotions. It is therefore recommended to question patients with suspected CS for new-onset hypersensitivity to bright light, sound, smell and hot or cold sensations. In this case, Anna reported suffering from hypersensitivity to light and sound. The screening for criterion 3 can be done using part A of the Central Sensitization Inventory (Mayer et al., 2012), which assesses symptoms common to CS, with total scores ranging from 0 to 100 and a recommended cutoff score of 40 (Neblett et al., 2013). At the time we assessed Anna, the Central Sensitization Inventory was not yet available.

Taken together, Anna fulfilled all three criteria for classifying her pain as CS pain. This does not imply that there is no (relevant) nociception contribution (for instance, in her cervical muscles); it only implies that central mechanisms rather than peripheral factors are dominating her clinical picture. The fact that Anna's signs and symptoms are dominated by CS comes as no surprise. There is consistent evidence for CS pain in patients with traumatic neck pain (i.e. chronic WAD), as shown by two independent systematic literature reviews (Van Oosterwijck et al., 2013b; Stone et al., 2013). Both reviews concluded that CS should be considered in the management of chronic WAD. The fact that during clinical examination her brain-orchestrated endogenous analgesia (conditioned pain modulation) at rest was deemed dysfunctional further supports the presence of CS pain.

Clinical Reasoning Commentary:

Diagnostic 'differentiation' classically refers to consideration of 'pathologies' or possible 'sources of symptoms (e.g. nociception) responsible for a patient's pain and physical signs. Here the authors apply the concept of differential diagnosis to the type of pain. 'Pain type' is an essential 'hypothesis category' (see Chapters 1 and 2) that must be reasoned alongside traditional structure/tissue/pathology differentiation when, for example, a hypothesis of a dominant CS pain moderates the clinician's interpretations of traditional physical tests for sources of nociception that may be false positives, that is, provocative due to CS and not local tissue 'injury'. Although the reasoning reflected in this answer supports that patient information was interpreted as it emerged, first-appointment hypotheses are not concluded until the examination is completed. Judgements are deduced on the basis of best available evidence, drawing from the congruity and proportionality of findings within and between the history/subjective examination (e.g. area of symptoms, behaviour of symptoms, nature and extent of injury or pathology, relevant comorbidities) and the clinical/physical examination (e.g. physical impairments, sensory testing). That is, when possible, reasoning judgements should be transparently linked to the synthesis of specific assessment findings.

Treatment

Initial treatment focussed on a combination of pain neuroscience education, stress management, graded activity and exercise therapy (Nijs et al., 2009). Each of the treatment components is detailed in the discussion that follows.

Reasoning Question:

3. What options do we have for treating CS pain, and should we target Anna's treatment using 'bottom-up' or 'top-down' interventions or perhaps a combination of both? Please discuss the rationale behind the selection of interventions you used for Anna and what others also may be available for the treatment of CS but were perhaps ruled out for Anna.

Answer to Reasoning Question:

Various treatment strategies specifically target pathophysiological mechanisms known to be involved in CS pain; that is, they hold – at least theoretically – the capacity to desensitize the CNS. Such treatments include pharmacological options (Nijs et al., 2011a), electrotherapy targeting the brain (i.e. transcranial magnetic stimulation) (Nijs et al., 2011a), manual therapy (Nijs et al., 2011a), virtual reality (Nijs et al., 2011a), stress management/neurofeedback training (Nijs et al., 2011a), transcutaneous electrical nerve stimulation (Nijs et al., 2011a), cranial electrotherapy stimulation (Nijs et al., 2011a), pain neuroscience education (Nijs et al., 2014a), exercise therapy (Nijs et al., 2012) and cognitive-behavioural therapy (Nijs et al., 2014a).

Most of these treatment options, when used for CS, have their effects through CNS modulation, that is, by targeting the brain (top-down approach) rather than peripheral nociceptive input (bottom-up approach). This appears to be a rational choice, especially if one considers CS to be the dominant feature in the patient with chronic pain. However, as is the case with Anna, the clinical picture of

Continued on following page

patients with chronic pain is often mixed, with some evidence of (in this case limited) peripheral nociceptive input combined with evidence of CS. For these patients, the question of whether successful treatment of peripheral input will diminish (or even resolve) CS as well arises.

Most often in patients with chronic WAD, specific changes in the cervical spine or the surrounding tissues cannot be revealed using magnetic resonance imaging (Anderson et al., 2012). This is likely the case for Anna as well. Still, posterior intervertebral joints (i.e. cervical facet joints) might be an active source of peripheral nociception in patients with chronic pain following whiplash injury (Curatolo et al., 2011), a view supported by animal studies (Dong et al., 2012) and studies that addressed the post-mortem features and biomechanics of injury to the cervical facet joints (Bogduk, 2011). In addition, recent work in humans suggests that cervical facet joints might play a role in (sustaining) CS in some patients with chronic WAD (Smith et al., 2013, 2014). In an uncontrolled observational study, cervical radiofrequency neurotomy attenuated CS in patients with chronic pain following whiplash injury up to 3 months post-treatment (Smith et al., 2014). Still, these findings apply to responders of cervical radiofrequency neurotomy, and a substantial number of patients with chronic WAD do not respond to such a treatment (Smith et al., 2013). It is concluded that musculoskeletal clinicians should keep in mind the possibility of local cervical nociception (e.g. posterior intervertebral joint nociception) in patients with chronic WAD. Given the outcome of Anna's cervical joint examination, the role of ongoing cervical joint nociception seems very limited.

This leaves us with the option of decreasing muscle tone in Anna's cervical muscles. The pain associated with myofascial trigger points is thought to arise from a hypersensitive nodule in a taut band of the skeletal muscle (Nijs and Van Houdenhove, 2009), and related activation of muscle nociceptors (Shah and Gilliams, 2008). Upon sustained noxious stimulation, myofascial trigger points might contribute to or initiate CS pain (Cagnie et al., 2013). Indeed, the vicinity of myofascial trigger points differs from normal muscle tissue by its lower pH levels (i.e. more acid), increased levels of substance P, calcitonin gene-related peptide, tumour necrosis factor-α and interleukine-1β, each of which has its role in increasing pain sensitivity (Shah et al., 2008). Sensitized muscle nociceptors are more easily activated and may respond to normally innocuous and weak stimuli such as light pressure and muscle movement (Shah et al., 2008; Shah and Gilliams, 2008).

Hence, if present, it seems rational to target myofascial trigger points for the treatment of nociceptive pain and even CS pain. A recent randomized trial reported that a single session of trigger point dry needling decreases widespread pressure sensitivity in patients with acute mechanical neck pain (Mejuto-Vazquez et al., 2014). However, Anna has limited increased cervical muscle tone and no active trigger points.

Similar to the reasoning regarding the increased cervical muscle tone, one might consider focussing Anna's treatment on improving the neuromuscular control of her deep cervical flexors. However, this is unlikely to benefit patients with chronic WAD as a sole treatment (Jull et al., 2007). Hence, we chose not to focus on retraining neuromuscular control of her deep cervical flexors in the early stages of the treatment, but we did include it later in our rehabilitation integrated into a cognition-targeted approach to exercise therapy (see later discussion).

From the available literature, it is concluded that limited evidence in selected chronic pain patients supports treatment strategies that eliminate peripheral nociceptive input for the effective management of CS pain (Nijs et al., 2014a). Hence, the focus of the treatment of CS pain in general should be targeted at the brain (i.e. top-down strategies). This is also supported by the previous treatment for Anna in which manual therapy generally had achieved little in improving her health status.

Clinical Reasoning Commentary:

Anna is hypothesized to have a dominant CS pain presentation supporting top-down therapeutic interventions, including pain neuroscience education, stress management, graded activity and exercise therapy. However, this answer highlights that peripheral nociceptive input (e.g. from spinal joints, muscles) may co-exist with CS and thereby contribute to some patients' pain presentations. These potential 'sources of symptoms' were considered, assessed and judged to be unsupported in Anna's clinical findings, resulting in a treatment plan targeting pathophysiological mechanisms of CS but tailored to the patient's individual presentation.

Pain Neuroscience Education

During her initial consultation, Anna demonstrated maladaptive illness beliefs and pain cognitions, including pain catastrophizing (rumination and helplessness rather than magnification) and pain hypervigilance. They should be addressed prior to initiating exercise and activity interventions. Therefore, considerable therapy time was invested in pain neuroscience education.

It was explained to Anna that the presence of CS implies that the brain produces pain and other 'warning signs' even when there is limited or no tissue damage or nociception. It is cardinal for the patient to understand this, which was done by in-depth patient education about pain neuroscience, a strategy known as pain neuroscience education.

Reasoning Question:

4. Would you comment on the research evidence regarding the efficacy of pain neuroscience education generally and also specifically for WAD patients?

Answer to Reasoning Question:

Research findings have repeatedly shown that such pain neuroscience education is therapeutic on its own, with level A evidence (based on meta-analysis or systematic review of available randomized controlled trials) supporting its use for changing pain beliefs and improving health status in patients with CS pain (Louw et al., 2011). None of the published trials focussed on chronic WAD patients, though, but positive results were reported in an uncontrolled study of pain neuroscience education with chronic WAD patients (Van Oosterwijck et al., 2011).

Reasoning Question:

5. Are there any practice guidelines addressing pain neuroscience education? Also, can you briefly discuss the main aim of this education and its potential benefits?

Answer to Reasoning Question:

Practice guidelines for therapeutic pain neuroscience education are available (Nijs et al., 2011b). Detailed pain neuroscience education is required to reconceptualize pain and to convince the patient that hypersensitivity of the CNS rather than local tissue damage may be the cause of their presenting symptoms. Hence, therapeutic pain neuroscience education is changing pain beliefs through the reconceptualization of pain (Louw et al. 2018; Moseley, 2003, 2004; Moseley and Butler, 2017; Meeus et al., 2010a; Van Oosterwijck et al., 2011). Inappropriate pain beliefs and cognitions, such as pain catastrophizing, anxiety, hypervigilance and kinesiophobia, have been shown to contribute to sensitization of the dorsal horn spinal cord neurons (through inhibition of descending tracks in the central nervous system) (Zusman, 2002; Burgmer et al., 2011; Gracely et al., 2004; Sjors et al., 2011). By changing these maladaptive pain beliefs and cognitions, therapeutic pain neuroscience education might be able to 'treat' core features of CS, namely, descending nociceptive facilitation, the overactive pain neuromatrix and dysfunctional endogenous analgesia. This notion is supported by the findings of a recent randomized controlled clinical trial showing that therapeutic pain neuroscience education resulted in improved endogenous analgesia in patients with fibromyalgia at 3 months post-treatment (Van Oosterwijck et al., 2013a).

How We Provided Pain Neuroscience Education to Anna

We provided Anna with three sessions of pain neuroscience education spread over 4 weeks. Her husband accompanied her to nearly all treatment sessions, and without taking over the communication from Anna, he was very supportive throughout. We felt it was very important that both Anna and her husband were able to understand contemporary pain neuroscience and how it explained her ongoing symptoms. Nociception, the role of descending inhibition, the pain matrix and the differences between acute and chronic pain mechanisms (i.e. central sensitization) were illustrated using PowerPoint slides (freely available from the Pain in Motion [2016a] website) and an information leaflet to read at home (freely available in French and Italian [Pain in Motion, 2016b]; for English-speaking patients, one can use parts of 'Explain Pain' [Butler and Moseley, 2003]). We made use of the test results from her clinical examination (i.e. her dysfunctional endogenous analgesia – conditioned pain modulation supporting the presence of CS pain) to prove to her that her pain mechanisms are no longer working properly.

Anna was very open-minded to the information provided. She was keen to learn and had many questions, especially during the second and third pain neuroscience education sessions (i.e. after having had the chance to reflect on the information provided and after having read and reread the information leaflet). This facilitated the communication between patient and clinician and resulted in rapid changes in reduced catastrophic illness beliefs, rumination and pain hypervigilance. However, pain neuroscience in and of itself did not provide her with sufficient skills for controlling her pain and/or related disability, explaining why her helplessness remained high. Therefore, stress management and activity self-management were initiated immediately following pain neuroscience education.

Reasoning Question:

6. Anna had clearly changed her conceptualizations of pain and of her problem. Although you note that this alone was insufficient in Anna's case, would you discuss what you believe are essential requirements for effective pain neuroscience education?

Answer to Reasoning Question:

Level A evidence supports the use of therapeutic pain neuroscience education for patients with chronic musculoskeletal pain. Three requirements are essential to effective pain neuroscience education (based on Siemonsma et al. [2008, 2010, 2013] and reproduced with permission from Pain in Motion [2016c]). However, when using it in clinical practice, not all patients reconceptualize their pain so easily as Anna.

Requirement 1: Only Patients Dissatisfied With Their Current Perceptions About Pain Are Open to Reconceptualization of Pain

The first requirement implies that clinicians should question the patient's pain perceptions thoroughly prior to commencing pain neuroscience education. Even though their pain perceptions lack medical and scientific validity, patients are often satisfied with them. In such cases, it is necessary to question whether the patient can think of other reasons/underlying mechanisms for his or her pain rather than just simply lecturing about pain mechanisms. Before initiating pain neuroscience education, the clinician should lead the patient toward a situation whereby the patient doubts his or her current pain perceptions. The following questions may assist clinicians in achieving this:

- 'Can you think of other reasons why you are still having neck pain?'
- 'I guess up to now, searching for the magic bullet to "cure" the damaged disc in your lower spine wasn't such a big success, was it?'

Requirement 2: Any New Perception Must Be Intelligible to the Patient

If the content of the pain neuroscience education is individually tailored (to the patient's ability to comprehend, etc.), then this should not be a problem. Still, it is essential to re-assess whether the patient has understood the pain neuroscience education. To achieve this, use the neurophysiology of pain test (Moseley, 2003), (re)question the patient's pain perception, or ask the patient to explain to you why he or she is in pain.

Requirement 3: A New Perception Must Appear Plausible and Beneficial to the Patient

Even though the content of pain neuroscience education is strongly supported by a body of scientific literature, it should apply to the patient's individual situation/pain. For instance, if you include the mechanism of central sensitization in your pain neuroscience education for a particular patient, then you want to be 100% certain that this patient is having a clinical picture dominated by central sensitization. If not, the patient might not recognize his or her own situation in the explanation, making it unlikely that the patient will reconceptualize his or her pain.

More detailed information on how pain neuroscience education was provided can be found in Nijs et al. (2011b).

Clinical Reasoning Commentary:

Although musculoskeletal clinicians utilize numerous treatment interventions, we are arguably teachers first and foremost, as virtually all management incorporates education. This is very evident in Anna's management and the answer here. In Chapter 1 we defined the reasoning strategy 'reasoning about teaching' as the *'reasoning associated with the planning, execution and evaluation of individualized and context-sensitive teaching, including education for conceptual understanding (e.g. diagnosis, pain) and education for physical performance (e.g. exercise, posture, sport technique correction)'*. The aim of the therapeutic pain neuroscience education here was to assist Anna to reconceptualize her pain. When helping patients construct new conceptualizations of their pain (and disability), we are effectively trying to promote deep learning that leads to personal change, as opposed to superficial understanding. The three requirements for effective pain neuroscience education discussed here each contribute to optimizing deep learning. Deep learning, and hopefully change, is facilitated when the learner has to process information. This is the basis of good university education in musculoskeletal clinical reasoning that strategically uses questions and discussion and is equally evident in the description of Anna's pain neuroscience education providing an opportunity for questions (i.e. processing of information) and explicit re-assessment of pain perceptions. The requirement that education must be plausible and beneficial underscores the importance of patient-specific education. Although there are excellent established resources on pain education, consistent with the 'reasoning about teaching' strategy, as highlighted in this answer, these need to be delivered in the context of the patient's story or circumstances for it to be meaningful to that patient.

Stress Management

Many patients with chronic WAD, including Anna, have major issues with handling everyday stressors. This comes as no surprise given the dysfunctional physiological stress response systems in patients with chronic WAD (Radanov et al., 1991; Radanov et al., 1993; Sterling et al., 2003a; Sterling and Kenardy, 2006; McLean, 2011; Gaab et al., 2005), including both the short- (i.e. sympathetic nervous system) and long-term stress response systems (i.e. hypothalamus–pituitary–adrenal axis). Hence, we defined improving Anna's capacity to cope with stress as a treatment goal of prime importance.

In total, Anna visited our clinic 15 times: the first time for assessment and 14 times for physiotherapy/manual therapy spread over 6 months. Of those 14 sessions, 7 were partly dedicated to initiating or following up the stress management module, comprising an explanation of the basic biology of the stress response systems and their interactions with central pain mechanisms and CS, teaching her stress management skills (Nijs et al., 2011a) and coaching her to apply them gradually in daily life.

Graded Activity and Exercise Therapy

The pain neuroscience education prepared Anna for a time-contingent, cognition-targeted approach to daily (physical) activity and exercise therapy. Pain neuroscience education was a continuous process commenced during Anna's initial consultations and continued during her activity and exercise-based longer-term rehabilitation (Nijs et al., 2011b). This required taking time to discuss the application of Anna's new understanding of (the meaning of) pain during her daily activities and exercises. Understanding contemporary pain neuroscience implies deep learning, whereas applying pain neuroscience during daily life implies a profound behavioural change by the patient. It is our job as musculoskeletal clinicians to guide the patient through this behavioural process. This is, in fact, a very exciting journey and one that is different every time with each new patient.

Graded activity was applied by first selecting activities with Anna based on her goals. The initial grading was determined based on her monitoring of her own performance during 2 'baseline' weeks. We asked her to perform the selected activities (e.g. walking) at least three times during the following 2 weeks and to monitor how long she was able to perform them. We instructed her to perform the activities as long as they were 'fun' for her (abandoning a symptom-contingent approach to performing activities). Anna returned 2 weeks later, informing us that she had walked four times over the past 2 weeks, and the duration varied substantially (10 minutes, 7 minutes, 27 minutes and 19 minutes). Her baseline was determined as the mean of the 4 numbers (i.e. 18 minutes), and she was asked to indicate how long she would like to walk ('A 3-hour walk is what my husband and I used to do quite often') and when she wants to obtain that goal ('Within 3 months'). With this information, we explained to Anna how she could design her grading program to achieve this goal within the preferred time period. She had 3 months to increase her walking duration from 18 minutes to 180 minutes, implying a grading of $180 - 18 = 162$ minutes spread over 12 weeks or 13.5 minutes grading per week, or 27 minutes per 2 weeks.

In addition to grading her daily activities, we applied exercise therapy. However, specific exercise therapy for training her neuromuscular control of her deep cervical flexors was not initiated before the seventh treatment session (2.5 months after initiating the treatment). This was so that neuromuscular control training was not initiated before Anna had adopted adaptive pain beliefs. Exercise therapy for improving Anna's cervical neuromuscular control was provided as cognition-targeted exercise, as described in detail elsewhere (Nijs et al., 2014b). This includes introducing new exercises using motor imagery and integrating them with increasing complexity using a time-contingent progression and practiced in different environments and contexts in order to maximize transfer to daily situations (Nijs et al., 2014b).

'Cognition-targeted' does not only imply time-contingent exercises; it also included addressing Anna's cognitions about her problems during exercises so that she had positive perceptions regarding the effects of the exercises on her pain and treatment outcome. Therefore, we regularly sat down with Anna and discussed her perceptions about each exercise, including the anticipated consequences of the exercises (e.g. pain increase, further damage to the spine), while challenging Anna's cognitions in relation to the exercises. This type of ongoing communication facilitates the application of the principles learned during the preparatory phase of therapeutic pain neuroscience education during actual exercise interventions (Nijs et al., 2014b).

For highly feared activities like using her full range of cervical motion (e.g. looking upward while walking), Anna's exercise therapy addressed movement-related pain memories by applying the 'exposure without danger' principle (Nijs et al., 2015). That is, by addressing Anna's perceptions about exercises, the anticipated danger (threat level) of the exercises was reduced by challenging the nature of and reasoning behind her fears, assuring the safety of the exercises and increasing her confidence in a successful accomplishment of the exercise. Examples of how we discussed Anna's perceptions about exercises before performing them for the first time and how we discussed her experience with the exercises (follow-up of the exercises) are available online (Nijs, 2014), and more information on retraining pain memories using exercise therapy in manual therapy practice is available elsewhere (Nijs et al., 2015).

Reasoning Question:

7. Although the graded activity and exercise therapy delivered with attention to both cognitions and emotions will hopefully enable Anna to increase her activity level and in turn, ideally, also her life participation levels, would you discuss the neurophysiological theory underpinning the cognitive behavioural application of graded activity and exercise therapy potential to influence CS?

Answer to Reasoning Question:

Many studies have shown associations between maladaptive pain cognitions (pain catastrophizing, anxiety, depression and anticipation of pain) and measures of CS (Burgmer et al., 2011; Gracely et al., 2004; Sjors et al., 2011; Vase et al., 2011). To address the cognitive-emotional sensitization, interventions such as cognitive-behavioural therapy target maladaptive pain cognitions. Pain neuroscience education motivates patients in applying cognitive-behavioural strategies to cope with their pain. For instance, we explained to Anna that she has little chance of controlling (the limited) peripheral nociceptive input but may exert volitional control over top-down mechanisms. Indeed, we applied cognitive-behavioural therapy (including graded activity) for Anna's chronic neck pain to help increase her self-control over the cognitive and affective responses to her pain.

This was done in order to deactivate brain-orchestrated top-down pain-facilitatory pathways, as evidenced by reduced CNS hyperexcitability (Ang et al., 2010) and an increase in prefrontal cortical volume (de Lange et al., 2008) following cognitive-behavioural therapy in patients with chronic pain. Still, more research is required to examine the real value of cognitive-behavioural therapy for the treatment of CS pain.

In addition to its potential effects on cognitive-emotional sensitization, exercise therapy in general (including grading physical activity levels) has the capacity to activate brain-orchestrated endogenous analgesia in patients with chronic pain (Nijs et al., 2012). In healthy people and some patients with chronic pain (including chronic low back pain (Hoffman et al., 2005; Meeus et al. 2010b), shoulder myalgia (Lannersten and Kosek, 2010) and rheumatoid arthritis (Meeus et al., 2014), exercise activates descending pain-inhibitory action referred to as exercise-induced endogenous analgesia (Koltyn, 2000). However, some patients with CS pain, including those with chronic WADs (Van Oosterwijck et al., 2012), chronic fatigue syndrome (Van Oosterwijck et al., 2010) and fibromyalgia (Lannersten and Kosek, 2010), are unable to activate endogenous analgesia following exercise (Nijs et al., 2012). Although Anna was diagnosed with chronic WAD, she was able to activate her endogenous analgesia in response to a short, low-intensity, graded bicycle test (see 'Physical examination' earlier in the chapter), which supported our use of grading physical activity levels and exercise therapy for Anna's treatment.

Clinical Reasoning Commentary:

Both assessment and management reasoning need to be grounded in theory and ideally supported by high-level evidence. Physiotherapy clinical identification and management of maladaptive central sensitization are still relatively new and, as cautioned here, require further validation. Having already outlined the theory and research-supported reasoning for diagnosing CS pain in Anna's presentation, the supporting evidence for the neurophysiological theory underpinning cognitive-behavioural application of graded activity and exercise therapy to influence CS, including innovative clinical assessment of Anna's ability to activate her endogenous analgesia, is put forward.

Outcome and Conclusions

Although the early sessions were slow and rather difficult, Anna responded well to the treatment. Her health status improved significantly, to the extent that we had to address her 'fear of relapse' midway through the treatment. The most spectacular progression was not made in terms of pain severity, even though her neck pain decreased throughout the treatment and is still low 3 years after having completed the treatment, but in terms of functional improvement. Her ability to perform household activities, enjoy leisure time with her family and friends, enjoy her work and so forth improved significantly.

The crucial part of the treatment may have been the change in her pain cognitions and beliefs. Without her understanding that nothing was wrong with her neck and that it was perfectly safe to use/move her neck, it would have been impossible to grade her exercise and activity levels as we did. The pain neuroscience education and the resulting reconceptualization of pain was not an end point but a starting point for the more active parts of the treatment, including not only the exercise and activity interventions but also the stress management module. Still, not all patients respond so positively to this type of treatment. Conservative treatment of chronic WAD remains a delicate issue of ongoing debate (Michaleff et al., 2014; Nijs and Ickmans, 2014), but progress has been made thanks to the implementation of contemporary neuroscience in manual therapy practice.

ACKNOWLEDGMENTS

Anneleen Malfliet is a PhD research fellow of the Agency for Innovation by Science and Technology (IWT) – Applied Biomedical Research Program (TBM), Belgium. Jo Nijs is holder of a chair funded by the European College for Decongestive Lymphatic Therapy, the Netherlands.

REFERENCES

Anderson, S.E., Boesch, C., Zimmermann, H., Busato, A., Hodler, J., Bingisser, R., et al., 2012. Are there cervical spine findings at MR imaging that are specific to acute symptomatic whiplash injury? A prospective controlled study with four experienced blinded readers. Radiology 262, 567–575.

Ang, D.C., Chakr, R., Mazzuca, S., France, C.R., Steiner, J., Stump, T., 2010. Cognitive-behavioral therapy attenuates nociceptive responding in patients with fibromyalgia: a pilot study. Arthritis Care Res (Hoboken) 62, 618–623.

Ashina, S., Bendtsen, L., Ashina, M., 2005. Pathophysiology of tension-type headache. Curr. Pain Headache Rep. 9, 415–422.

Bogduk, N., 2011. On cervical zygapophysial joint pain after whiplash. Spine 36, S194–S199.

Broadbent, E., Petrie, K.J., Main, J., Weinman, J., 2006. The brief illness perception questionnaire. J. Psychosom. Res. 60, 631–637.

Burgmer, M., Petzke, F., Giesecke, T., Gaubitz, M., Heuft, G., Pfleiderer, B., 2011. Cerebral activation and catastrophizing during pain anticipation in patients with fibromyalgia. Psychosom. Med. 73, 751–759.

Butler, D., Moseley, G.L., 2003. Explain pain. NOI Group Publishing, Adelaide.

Cagnie, B., Dewitte, V., Barbe, T., Timmermans, F., Delrue, N., Meeus, M., 2013. Physiologic effects of dry needling. Curr. Pain Headache Rep. 17, 348.

Coombes, B.K., Bisset, L., Vicenzino, B., 2012. Thermal hyperalgesia distinguishes those with severe pain and disability in unilateral lateral epicondylalgia. Clin. J. Pain 28, 595–601.

Curatolo, M., Bogduk, N., Ivancic, P.C., McLean, S.A., Siegmund, G.P., Winkelstein, B.A., 2011. The role of tissue damage in whiplash-associated disorders: discussion paper 1. Spine 36, S309–S315.

Daenen, L., Nijs, J., Raadsen, B., Roussel, N., Cras, P., Dankaerts, W., 2013a. Cervical motor dysfunction and its predictive value for long-term recovery in patients with acute whiplash-associated disorders: a systematic review. J. Rehabil. Med. 45, 113–122.

Daenen, L., Nijs, J., Roussel, N., Wouters, K., Van Loo, M., Cras, P., 2013b. Dysfunctional pain inhibition in patients with chronic whiplash-associated disorders: an experimental study. Clin. Rheumatol. 32, 23–31.

De Lange, F.P., Koers, A., Kalkman, J.S., Bleijenberg, G., Hagoort, P., Van Der Meer, J.W., et al., 2008. Increase in prefrontal cortical volume following cognitive behavioural therapy in patients with chronic fatigue syndrome. Brain 131, 2172–2180.

Dong, L., Quindlen, J.C., Lipschutz, D.E., Winkelstein, B.A., 2012. Whiplash-like facet joint loading initiates glutamatergic responses in the DRG and spinal cord associated with behavioral hypersensitivity. Brain Res. 1461, 51–63.

Elliott, J.M., O'Leary, S., Sterling, M., Hendrikz, J., Pedler, A., Jull, G., 2010. Magnetic resonance imaging findings of fatty infiltrate in the cervical flexors in chronic whiplash. Spine 35, 948–954.

Fernandez-Carnero, J., Fernandez-De-Las-Penas, C., De La Llave-Rincon, A.I., Ge, H.Y., Arendt-Nielsen, L., 2009. Widespread mechanical pain hypersensitivity as sign of central sensitization in unilateral epicondylalgia: a blinded, controlled study. Clin. J. Pain 25, 555–561.

Filatova, E., Latysheva, N., Kurenkov, A., 2008. Evidence of persistent central sensitization in chronic headaches: a multi-method study. J. Headache Pain 9, 295–300.

Gaab, J., Baumann, S., Budnoik, A., Gmunder, H., Hottinger, N., Ehlert, U., 2005. Reduced reactivity and enhanced negative feedback sensitivity of the hypothalamus-pituitary-adrenal axis in chronic whiplash-associated disorder. Pain 119, 219–224.

Gracely, R.H., Geisser, M.E., Giesecke, T., Grant, M.A., Petzke, F., Williams, D.A., et al., 2004. Pain catastrophizing and neural responses to pain among persons with fibromyalgia. Brain 127, 835–843.

Haanpää, M., Treede, R., 2010. Diagnosis and classification of neuropathic pain. Pain Clinical Updates XVII (7).

Hoffman, M.D., Shepanski, M.A., Mackenzie, S.P., Clifford, P.S., 2005. Experimentally induced pain perception is acutely reduced by aerobic exercise in people with chronic low back pain. J. Rehabil. Res. Dev. 42, 183–190.

Jull, G., Sterling, M., Kenardy, J., Beller, E., 2007. Does the presence of sensory hypersensitivity influence outcomes of physical rehabilitation for chronic whiplash? A preliminary RCT. Pain 129, 28–34.

Jull, G.A., O'Leary, S.P., Falla, D.L., 2008. Clinical assessment of the deep cervical flexor muscles: the craniocervical flexion test. J. Manipulative Physiol. Ther. 31, 525–533.

Koltyn, K.F., 2000. Analgesia following exercise: a review. Sports Med. 29, 85–98.

Lannersten, L., Kosek, E., 2010. Dysfunction of endogenous pain inhibition during exercise with painful muscles in patients with shoulder myalgia and fibromyalgia. Pain 151, 77–86.

Lluch Girbes, E., Nijs, J., Torres-Cueco, R., Lopez Cubas, C., 2013. Pain treatment for patients with osteoarthritis and central sensitization. Phys. Ther. 93, 842–851.

Louw, A., Diener, I., Butler, D.S., Puentedura, E.J., 2011. The effect of neuroscience education on pain, disability, anxiety, and stress in chronic musculoskeletal pain. Arch. Phys. Med. Rehabil. 92, 2041–2056.

Louw, A., Puentedura, E., Schmidt, S., Zimney, K., 2018. Pain Neuroscience Education, vol. 2. OPTP, Minneapolis, MN.

Mayer, T.G., Neblett, R., Cohen, H., Howard, K.J., Choi, Y.H., Williams, M.J., et al., 2012. The development and psychometric validation of the central sensitization inventory. Pain Pract. 12, 276–285.

McLean, S.A., 2011. The potential contribution of stress systems to the transition to chronic whiplash-associated disorders. Spine 36, S226–S232.

Meeus, M., Hermans, L., Ickmans, K., Struyf, F., Van Cauwenbergh, D., Bronckaerts, L., et al., 2014. Endogenous pain modulation in response to exercise in patients with rheumatoid arthritis, patients with chronic fatigue syndrome and comorbid fibromyalgia, and healthy controls: a double-blind randomized controlled trial. Pain Pract. 15 (2), 98–106.

Meeus, M., Nijs, J., Van De Wauwer, N., Toeback, L., Truijen, S., 2008. Diffuse noxious inhibitory control is delayed in chronic fatigue syndrome: an experimental study. Pain 139, 439–448.

Meeus, M., Nijs, J., Van Oosterwijck, J., Van Alsenoy, V., Truijen, S., 2010a. Pain physiology education improves pain beliefs in patients with chronic fatigue syndrome compared with pacing and self-management education: a double-blind randomized controlled trial. Arch. Phys. Med. Rehabil. 91, 1153–1159.

Meeus, M., Roussel, N.A., Truijen, S., Nijs, J., 2010b. Reduced pressure pain thresholds in response to exercise in chronic fatigue syndrome but not in chronic low back pain: an experimental study. J. Rehabil. Med. 42, 884–890.

Meeus, M., Vervisch, S., De Clerck, L.S., Moorkens, G., Hans, G., Nijs, J., 2012. Central sensitization in patients with rheumatoid arthritis: a systematic literature review. Semin. Arthritis Rheum. 41, 556–567.

Mejuto-Vazquez, M.J., Salom-Moreno, J., Ortega-Santiago, R., Truyols-Dominguez, S., Fernandez-De-Las-Penas, C., 2014. Short-term changes in neck pain, widespread pressure pain sensitivity, and cervical range of motion after the application of trigger point dry needling in patients with acute mechanical neck pain: a randomized clinical trial. J. Orthop. Sports Phys. Ther. 44 (4), 252–260.

Meyer, R.A., Campbell, I.T., Raja, S.N., 1995. Peripheral neural mechanisms of nociception. In: Wall, P.D., Melzack, R. (Eds.), Textbook of pain, third ed. Churchill Livingstone, Edinburgh.

Michaleff, Z.A., Maher, C.G., Lin, C.W., Rebbeck, T., Jull, G., Latimer, J., et al., 2014. Comprehensive physiotherapy exercise programme or advice for chronic whiplash (PROMISE): a pragmatic randomised controlled trial. Lancet 384, 133–141.

Moseley, G.L., 2003. Unraveling the barriers to reconceptualization of the problem in chronic pain: the actual and perceived ability of patients and health professionals to understand the neurophysiology. J. Pain 4, 184–189.

Moseley, G.L., 2004. Evidence for a direct relationship between cognitive and physical change during an education intervention in people with chronic low back pain. Eur. J. Pain 8, 39–45.

Moseley, G.L., Butler, D.S., 2017. Explain Pain Supercharged. The Clinician's Handbook. Noigroup publishing, Adelaide, Australia.

Neblett, R., Cohen, H., Choi, Y., Hartzell, M.M., Williams, M., Mayer, T.G., et al., 2013. The Central Sensitization Inventory (CSI): establishing clinically significant values for identifying central sensitivity syndromes in an outpatient chronic pain sample. J. Pain 14, 438–445.

Nijs, J., 2014. Retraining pain memories in chronic pain patients: the next generation of exercise therapy. Pain in Motion. Available at: http://www.paininmotion.be/EN/RetrainingPainMemoriesEnglish.html. (Accessed 8 November 2017).

Nijs, J., Ickmans, K., 2014. Chronic whiplash-associated disorders: to exercise or not? Lancet 384, 109–111.

Nijs, J., Kosek, E., Van Oosterwijck, J., Meeus, M., 2012. Dysfunctional endogenous analgesia during exercise in patients with chronic pain: to exercise or not to exercise? Pain Physician 15, ES205–ES213.

Nijs, J., Lluch Girbés, E., Lundberg, M., Malfliet, A., Sterling, M., 2015. Exercise therapy for chronic musculoskeletal pain: innovation by altering pain memories. Man. Ther. 20 (1), 216–220.

Nijs, J., Malfliet, A., Ickmans, K., Baert, I., Meeus, M., 2014a. Treatment of central sensitization in patients with 'unexplained' chronic pain: an update. Expert Opin. Pharmacother. 1–13.

Nijs, J., Meeus, M., Cagnie, B., Roussel, N.A., Dolphens, M., Van Oosterwijck, J., et al., 2014b. A modern neuroscience approach to chronic spinal pain: combining pain neuroscience education with cognition-targeted motor control training. Phys. Ther. 94, 730–738.

Nijs, J., Meeus, M., Van Oosterwijck, J., Ickmans, K., Moorkens, G., Hans, G., et al., 2012c. In the mind or in the brain? Scientific evidence for central sensitisation in chronic fatigue syndrome. Eur. J. Clin. Invest. 42, 203–212.

Nijs, J., Meeus, M., Van Oosterwijck, J., Roussel, N., De Kooning, M., Ickmans, K., et al., 2011a. Treatment of central sensitization in patients with 'unexplained' chronic pain: what options do we have? Expert Opin. Pharmacother. 12, 1087–1098.

Nijs, J., Paul Van Wilgen, C., Van Oosterwijck, J., Van Ittersum, M., Meeus, M., 2011b. How to explain central sensitization to patients with 'unexplained' chronic musculoskeletal pain: practice guidelines. Man. Ther. 16, 413–418.

Nijs, J., Torres-Cueco, R., van Wilgen, C.P., Girbes, E.L., Struyf, F., Roussel, N., et al., 2014a. Applying modern pain neuroscience in clinical practice: criteria for the classification of central sensitization pain. Pain Physician 17, 447–457.

Nijs, J., Van Houdenhove, B., 2009. From acute musculoskeletal pain to chronic widespread pain and fibromyalgia: application of pain neurophysiology in manual therapy practice. Man. Ther. 14 (1), 3–12.

Nijs, J., Van Houdenhove, B., Oostendorp, R.A., 2010. Recognition of central sensitization in patients with musculoskeletal pain: application of pain neurophysiology in manual therapy practice. Man. Ther. 15, 135–141.

Nijs, J., Van Oosterwijck, J., De Hertogh, W., 2009. Rehabilitation of chronic whiplash: treatment of cervical dysfunctions or chronic pain syndrome? Clin. Rheumatol. 28, 243–251.

Pain in Motion. 2016a. Pain neuroscience education: slides for supporting/illustrating your explanation (English version). Available at: http://www.paininmotion.be/EN/sem-PainPhysiologyEducationEnglish.pdf. (Accessed 8 November 2017).

Pain in Motion. 2016b. Information leaflet to read at home available in French and Italian. Available at http://www.paininmotion.be/education/tools-for-clinical-practice. (Accessed 8 November 2017).

Pain in Motion. 2016c. www.paininmotion.be. (Accessed 8 November 2017).

Paul, T.M., Soo Hoo, J., Chae, J., Wilson, R.D., 2012. Central hypersensitivity in patients with subacromial impingement syndrome. Arch. Phys. Med. Rehabil. 93, 2206–2209.

Perrotta, A., Serrao, M., Sandrini, G., Burstein, R., Sances, G., Rossi, P., et al., 2010. Sensitisation of spinal cord pain processing in medication overuse headache involves supraspinal pain control. Cephalalgia 30, 272–284.

Price, D.D., Staud, R., Robinson, M.E., Mauderli, A.P., Cannon, R., Vierck, C.J., 2002. Enhanced temporal summation of second pain and its central modulation in fibromyalgia patients. Pain 99, 49–59.

Radanov, B.P., Di Stefano, G., Schnidrig, A., Ballinari, P., 1991. Role of psychosocial stress in recovery from common whiplash [see comment]. Lancet 338, 712–715.

Radanov, B.P., Di Stefano, G., Schnidrig, A., Sturzenegger, M., 1993. Psychosocial stress, cognitive performance and disability after common whiplash. J. Psychosom. Res. 37, 1–10.

Raphael, K.G., Janal, M.N., Anathan, S., Cook, D.B., Staud, R., 2009. Temporal summation of heat pain in temporomandibular disorder patients. J. Orofac. Pain 23, 54–64.

Roelofs, J., Peters, M.L., McCracken, L., Vlaeyen, J.W., 2003. The pain vigilance and awareness questionnaire (PVAQ): further psychometric evaluation in fibromyalgia and other chronic pain syndromes. Pain 101, 299–306.

Roussel, N.A., Nijs, J., Meeus, M., Mylius, V., Fayt, C., Oostendorp, R., 2013. Central sensitization and altered central pain processing in chronic low back pain: fact or myth? Clin. J. Pain 29, 625–638.

Seifert, F., Maihofner, C., 2009. Central mechanisms of experimental and chronic neuropathic pain: findings from functional imaging studies. Cell. Mol. Life Sci. 66, 375–390.

Shah, J.P., Danoff, J.V., Desai, M.J., Parikh, S., Nakamura, L.Y., Phillips, T.M., et al., 2008. Biochemicals associated with pain and inflammation are elevated in sites near to and remote from active myofascial trigger points. Arch. Phys. Med. Rehabil. 89, 16–23.

Shah, J.P., Gilliams, E.A., 2008. Uncovering the biochemical milieu of myofascial trigger points using in vivo microdialysis: an application of muscle pain concepts to myofascial pain syndrome. J Bodyw Mov Ther 12, 371–384.

Siemonsma, P.C., Schroder, C.D., Dekker, J.H., Lettinga, A.T., 2008. The benefits of theory for clinical practice: cognitive treatment for chronic low back pain patients as an illustrative example. Disabil. Rehabil. 30, 1309–1317.

Siemonsma, P.C., Schroder, C.D., Roorda, L.D., Lettinga, A.T., 2010. Benefits of treatment theory in the design of explanatory trials: cognitive treatment of illness perception in chronic low back pain rehabilitation as an illustrative example. J. Rehabil. Med. 42, 111–116.

Siemonsma, P.C., Stuive, I., Roorda, L.D., Vollebregt, J.A., Walker, M.F., Lankhorst, G.J., et al., 2013. Cognitive treatment of illness perceptions in patients with chronic low back pain: a randomized controlled trial. Phys. Ther. 93, 435–448.

Sjors, A., Larsson, B., Persson, A.L., Gerdle, B., 2011. An increased response to experimental muscle pain is related to psychological status in women with chronic non-traumatic neck-shoulder pain. BMC Musculoskelet. Disord. 12, 230.

Smith, A.D., Jull, G., Schneider, G., Frizzell, B., Hooper, R.A., Sterling, M., 2013. A comparison of physical and psychological features of responders and non-responders to cervical facet blocks in chronic whiplash. BMC Musculoskelet. Disord. 14, 313.

Smith, A.D., Jull, G., Schneider, G., Frizzell, B., Hooper, R.A., Sterling, M., 2014. Cervical radiofrequency neurotomy reduces central hyperexcitability and improves neck movement in individuals with chronic whiplash. Pain Med. 15, 128–141.

Spitzer, W.O., Skovron, M.L., Salmi, L.R., Cassidy, J.D., Duranceau, J., Suissa, S., et al., 1995. Scientific monograph of the Quebec Task Force on Whiplash-Associated Disorders: redefining "whiplash" and its management. Spine 20, 1S–73S.

Staud, R., Craggs, J.G., Perlstein, W.M., Robinson, M.E., Price, D.D., 2008. Brain activity associated with slow temporal summation of C-fiber evoked pain in fibromyalgia patients and healthy controls. Eur. J. Pain 12, 1078–1089.

Sterling, M., Jull, G., Vicenzino, B., Kenardy, J., 2003a. Sensory hypersensitivity occurs soon after whiplash injury and is associated with poor recovery. Pain 104, 509–517.

Sterling, M., Jull, G., Vicenzino, B., Kenardy, J., 2004. Characterization of acute whiplash-associated disorders. Spine 29, 182–188.

Sterling, M., Jull, G., Vicenzino, B., Kenardy, J., Darnell, R., 2003b. Development of motor system dysfunction following whiplash injury. Pain 103, 65–73.

Sterling, M., Kenardy, J., 2006. The relationship between sensory and sympathetic nervous system changes and posttraumatic stress reaction following whiplash injury–a prospective study. J. Psychosom. Res. 60, 387–393.

Stone, A.M., Vicenzino, B., Lim, E.C., Sterling, M., 2013. Measures of central hyperexcitability in chronic whiplash associated disorder–a systematic review and meta-analysis. Man. Ther. 18, 111–117.

Sullivan, M.J.L., Bishop, S.R., Pivik, J., 1995. The pain catastrophizing scale: development and validation. Psychol Asses 7, 524–532.

Treede, R.D., Jensen, T.S., Campbell, J.N., Cruccu, G., Dostrovsky, J.O., Griffin, J.W., et al., 2008. Neuropathic pain: redefinition and a grading system for clinical and research purposes. Neurology 70, 1630–1635.

Van Oosterwijck, J., Meeus, M., Paul, L., De Schryver, M., Pascal, A., Lambrecht, L., et al., 2013a. Pain physiology education improves health status and endogenous pain inhibition in fibromyalgia: a double-blind randomized controlled trial. Clin. J. Pain 29 (10), 873–882.

Van Oosterwijck, J., Nijs, J., Meeus, M., Lefever, I., Huybrechts, L., Lambrecht, L., et al., 2010. Pain inhibition and postexertional malaise in myalgic encephalomyelitis/chronic fatigue syndrome: an experimental study. J. Intern. Med. 268, 265–278.

Van Oosterwijck, J., Nijs, J., Meeus, M., Paul, L., 2013b. Evidence for central sensitization in chronic whiplash: a systematic literature review. Eur. J. Pain 17, 299–312.

Van Oosterwijck, J., Nijs, J., Meeus, M., Truijen, S., Craps, J., Van De Keybus, N., et al., 2011. Pain neurophysiology education improves cognitions, pain thresholds and movement performance in people with chronic whiplash: a pilot study. J. Rehabil. Res. Dev. 48, 43–58.

Van Oosterwijck, J., Nijs, J., Meeus, M., Van Loo, M., Paul, L., 2012. Lack of endogenous pain inhibition during exercise in people with chronic whiplash associated disorders: an experimental study. J. Pain 13 (3), 242–254.

Van Wilgen, C.P., Konopka, K.H., Keizer, D., Zwerver, J., Dekker, R., 2011. Do patients with chronic patellar tendinopathy have an altered somatosensory profile? - A Quantitative Sensory Testing (QST) study. Scand. J. Med. Sci. Sports 23 (2), 149–155.

Van Wilgen, P., Beetsma, A., Neels, H., Roussel, N., Nijs, J., 2014. Physical therapists should integrate illness perceptions in their assessment in patients with chronic musculoskeletal pain; a qualitative analysis. Man. Ther. 19, 229–234.

Vase, L., Nikolajsen, L., Christensen, B., Egsgaard, L.L., Arendt-Nielsen, L., Svensson, P., et al., 2011. Cognitive-emotional sensitization contributes to wind-up-like pain in phantom limb pain patients. Pain 152, 157–162.

Wall, B., Melzack, R., 1994. Textbook of pain. Elsevier, London.

Woolf, C.J., 2011. Central sensitization: implications for the diagnosis and treatment of pain. Pain 152, S2–S15.

Yarnitsky, D., 2010. Conditioned pain modulation (the diffuse noxious inhibitory control-like effect): its relevance for acute and chronic pain states. Curr. Opin. Anaesthesiol. 23, 611–615.

Zusman, M., 2002. Forebrain-mediated sensitization of central pain pathways: 'non-specific' pain and a new image for MT. Man. Ther. 7, 80–88.

26

Thoracic Spine Pain in a Soccer Player: A Combined Movement Theory Approach

Christopher McCarthy • Darren A. Rivett

This case study uses the principles of combined movement theory (CMT) to underpin the clinical reasoning approach. CMT is a progression of the 'combined movements' concept developed by Brian Edwards (1992) as an approach to the application of passive joint movement and as a corollary of the Maitland concept of manual therapy (Maitland, 1986).

History of Present Complaint

Rohan is a 21-year-old semi-professional soccer (football) player who plays on the left wing. This position involves a considerable amount of running whilst the thoracic and cervical spines are rotated to the right, as the player watches the flight of the approaching ball. Rohan had developed right-sided, mid-thoracic pain over a period of a month, 6 months prior to his presentation for examination. He reported the pain as being 5/10 on a numerical pain scale (in which 0/10 is no pain, and 10/10 is the worst pain imaginable) when it was at its worst, usually an hour or so after the game finished. At other times, he felt local stiffness with a low-grade ache (3/10). He denied any features suggestive of neurodynamic sensitivity and had no symptoms indicative of lumbar spine, shoulder or cervical spine dysfunction. Rohan trained for, or played soccer, typically for 2–3 hours a day and undertook weight-training and aerobic exercise classes, supervised by the club physiotherapists.

Behaviour of Symptoms

Rohan reported that his pain developed slowly with prolonged standing of about 30 minutes and following unsupported sitting for an hour. He demonstrated how his pain was provoked with a movement combining extension and right rotation of his thorax, as occurred during gameplay. The pain did not alter with deep inhalation. Temporary relief was obtained with heat and by stretching into flexion and then rotating to the left. Notably, Rohan indicated he now found gently touching the affected region painful (allodynia), both locally and across the left and right sides of his mid-thoracic spine.

Previous Management

Previously, Rohan had undergone local spinal mobilization treatment from the club physiotherapist, with a short-term reduction in pain experienced for a day before returning to previous levels. The treatment had consisted of unilateral posterior-anterior (PA) manual pressures on the T7/T8 and T8/T9 zygapophyseal (facet) joints performed in prone lying in a neutral position, and a PA high-velocity thrust manipulation directed at this region. Because the symptoms were not improving and were returning after every game, Rohan underwent magnetic resonance imaging (MRI), which was normal. A 4-week course of non-steroidal anti-inflammatory medication had also not helped.

General Health

There were no symptoms reported indicative of radiculopathy or myelopathy, nor any red flags for spinal cancer, fracture or infection (specifically, no history of night pain, night sweats, weight loss, or neurological deficit in the trunk or limbs). There had been no significant thoracic spine stiffness in the morning suggestive of inflammatory disease. Rohan had no prior episodes of thoracic pain, but he recounted a previous history of right-sided anterior knee pain, which resulted in a physiotherapist-directed stretching programme (that he was not currently doing) to address "tight", right gluteus medius/maximus, external hip rotator and tensor fascia latae muscles.

Rohan had experienced some minor anxiety about why his pain persisted but had been reassured by the negative MRI scan result. He displayed no obvious psychosocial barriers to recovery.

Reasoning Question:

1. Can you please explain the theoretical underpinnings of the CMT approach? Briefly, by what mechanisms may it achieve improvement in a patient's pain with movement?

Answer to Reasoning Question:

In essence, CMT emphasizes the importance of consideration of the starting position for passive or active mobilization treatment and advocates a clinical reasoning process that incorporates changes in the starting position as part of progression and regression of treatment (Edwards, 1999; McCarthy, 2010). This approach appears to be most efficacious with patients who have a 'nociceptive pattern' to their dysfunction, a directional sensitivity to movement, commonly referred to as a 'mechanical presentation'. Typically, a mechanical presentation involves a combination of movements that reproduce local and referred pain and an opposite set of movements that reduce symptoms. Similar to most manual therapy approaches, it is generally not as useful when other pain types are dominant, such as peripheral neuropathic or nociplastic pain (McCarthy, 2010).

The CMT approach advocates the positioning of patients in severe pain in the opposite position to that in which they experience their symptoms. Here, the use of passively applied or patient-generated movement can be effective in decreasing pain, theoretically through afferent mechanoreceptor stimulation that evokes a (sympathetico-excitatory) rapid-responding, descending inhibitory pain mechanism. Thus, the perception of nociceptive pain can be rapidly reduced in this way; however, the analgesic effect of this approach will tend to plateau with repetition as the patient habituates to the repetitive stimulus. At this juncture, treatment progression involving a graded exposure to the provocative direction of movement is required. This is produced by altering the starting position in which treatment occurs to habituate or desensitize the patient to the painful or sensitive movement. In essence, the patient undergoing CMT is thus guided through a process of graded exposure to the specific directions of movement that are sensitized.

Conversely, in cases in which the pain is not severe the starting position used with CMT tends to be toward the end of the range of motion rather than being in a more midline or neutral position. In this manner, CMT deliberately aims to provoke the patient's symptoms, theoretically by eliciting afferent signals from high-threshold mechanoreceptors (type III/IV). These receptors normally remain silent unless significant tension is applied to them but can fire with lower levels of stimulation when sensitized by local inflammation (Pickar, 2002). The descending inhibitory pain mechanism moderated by the dorsal periaqueductal gray area of the brainstem is particularly sensitive to this type of mechanical afferent stimulation, which can be evoked with deep pressure and strong stretches (Kaufman et al., 2002).

The box diagram in Fig. 26.1 shows an example of classical CMT treatment progression. This diagram depicts the combination of movements that reproduces the symptoms (prime combination) and also the direction of movement in which the patient is most sensitive (prime movement). Around the outer boundary of the box is the direction that treatment could be progressed to provide a graded exposure to the sensitive movements. The anticlockwise direction of progression around the box ensures that the most sensitive movement is introduced toward the end of the progression, when the patient is less sensitive (i.e. not in severe pain). Thus, phase 1 of the CMT approach requires the patient to be positioned away from the pain and involves evocation of the descending inhibitory pain mechanism. Phase 2 involves habituation to sensitive movement, with a gradual increase in stimulus via changes in the starting position for treatment. Finally, phase 3 employs mobilization treatment to facilitate motion into the range of impaired movement, thereby stimulating and lengthening passive tissues that may be causing impairment. This, supported by the provision of a home stretch programme, will continue tissue remodelling over many weeks. With a non-severe clinical presentation, assessment and treatment would simply occur in the prime combination.

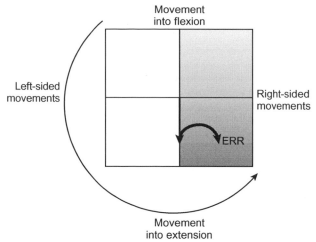

Fig. 26.1 Box diagram representing the directional sensitivity of the patient: the order and combination of active movements reproducing pain. An active-movement examination is depicted, including the prime movement and the prime combination, and the typical progression of treatment in combined movement theory (CMT). The shading represents the side of the pain. The thick black arrow arcing to the right represents the most painful movement – the prime movement of right rotation – with the thinner black arrow representing extension. These arrows indicate that the prime combination (position of most complete pain reproduction) is extension followed by right rotation. With a severely painful impairment, treatment would therefore commence in flexion/left rotation (i.e. the opposite quadrant of the box). As indicated by the large arrow around the box, progression of treatment would involve moving into extension followed by right rotation (i.e. toward the painful quadrant) to gradually expose (habituate) the patient to the painful movements, with the most sensitive movement last. *ERR,* Extension right rotation.

Reasoning Question:

2. What were your initial thoughts regarding the source of Rohan's symptoms, the persistence of the problem and his short-term response to previous treatment?

Answer to Reasoning Question:

The initial impression formed was that Rohan had developed some direction-specific sensitivity to movement, leading to localized pain in the right, mid-thoracic spinal region. It was clear that particular movements changed the symptoms in a reliable, repeatable manner. The sensitized patterns of movement matched patterns of motion that typically create tension in certain tissues of the vertebral column and potentially provided information on which to base the direction and location of applied passive-movement treatment. Previously, local passive movements had been applied to the sensitized area, resulting in short-term reductions in pain typical of those reported in the literature following the application of therapeutic movement and exercise (Koes et al., 1991; Martinez-Segura et al., 2012; O'Leary et al., 2007). Despite these repeated episodes of pain reduction, there had been no permanent reduction in the directional sensitivity to movement. This suggested that the movement impairment(s) remained and that normal motion had not yet been regained or, alternatively, that the resolution of the impairment(s) had been temporary and that the functional demands of playing were continuing to induce sensitivity.

In addition to providing a mechano-sensory afferent stimulus to evoke descending pain inhibition, therapeutic movement can be delivered in a localized manner that provides an upgrading of exposure in the sensitized direction. The impression formed of previous manual treatment was that essentially the same techniques, performed in a neutral spinal position, were repeated at each session and that there was no provision of graded exposure to movement in the specific direction of sensitivity. Combined movement theory affords a framework to introduce this approach to physical examination and management. This suggested that a biomechanical analysis of the sensitized patterns of movement would at least provide a guide for a treatment approach to influencing the perception of pain.

Reasoning Question:

3. Psychosocial factors are often an important part of a patient's presentation where pain persists and function is impacted. Can you comment on your psychosocial considerations in this case?

Continued on following page

Answer to Reasoning Question:

During the course of the initial interview of the patient, careful consideration of the psychosocial context of Rohan's presentation was undertaken. It is common for athletes to have psychological barriers to returning to play, ranging from hypervigilance to team politics (Clement et al., 2013); however, these were not evident during the interview. A sense of anxiety regarding 'the diagnosis' was evident, to some degree, but the patient felt that this had reduced since the return of his normal MRI scan results. Moreover, Rohan's view was that his problem was of a mechanical nature, and thus it was considered that approaching management from a mechanical paradigm would be well accepted by him and likely meet his expectations.

Reasoning Question:

4. What are your thoughts about the described allodynia and why this might occur? How might manual therapy be of benefit?

Answer to Reasoning Question:

Persistent nociceptive afferent stimulation of the pain neuromatrix will commonly lead to alterations in neurotransmitter levels, responsiveness of first- and second-order neurones, inhibitory pain mechanisms and processing within the pain neuromatrix and immune system (Iannetti and Mouraux, 2010). The duration of his persistent symptoms would have been sufficient for these physiological adaptations to have occurred, albeit the region of allodynia had apparently not expanded to beyond a few centimetres from the midline.

There is some evidence to suggest manual therapy can reduce the degree of temporal summation (or wind-up) in the dorsal horn of the spinal cord (Bialosky et al., 2009) and thus might have a role in preventing the development of clinical symptoms of chronic pain, such as allodynia or hyperpathia (typically considered features of peripheral neuropathic and nociplastic pain states [Bialosky et al., 2009]). However, with severe chronic pain states, where these features are already present, ongoing pain can reduce the level of the inhibitory neurotransmitter gamma-aminobutyric acid and lead to a relatively overactive hypothalamus–pituitary–adrenal (HPA) axis (Pickar, 2002). Manual therapy's influence on the HPA axis is overwhelmingly sympathetico-excitatory (Kovanur Sampath et al., 2015), and thus caution is needed in using manual therapy in such cases because further stimulating an amplified system can be counterproductive.

Planning the Physical Examination

After the patient interview, a planning sheet for the physical examination was completed to facilitate clarification of the key clinical reasoning issues to be considered before conducting the physical examination (Fig. 26.2). This helps to ensure appropriate clinical data are collected and to test hypotheses regarding the relative effectiveness of likely treatments.

Reasoning Question:

5. What were your key hypotheses following completion of the planning sheet?

Answer to Reasoning Question:

The reported pain-provocation pattern was suggestive of a directional sensitivity to movement. This was suggestive of an impairment of segmental motion of the superior vertebrae of the motion segment into extension and ipsilateral rotation. This degree of directional sensitivity would suggest a degree of sensitivity to mechano-receptive afferent information, typical of that experienced when nociceptive afferents are evoked (Zusman, 1986). The severity of pain produced in this combination of movements was likely not so severe as to make treatment in this position unacceptable to the patient. Thus, the choice of starting position for the physical assessment, including a test or 'mini-treatment' during the examination, as well as probably the full-duration treatment, was to be a combination of extension and right rotation. There would likely be no need to place the patient in the opposite quadrant of the box diagram (Fig. 26.1) – that is, to provide more of an 'analgesic' treatment (i.e. the provision of afferent stimulation that will evoke a brain-orchestrated inhibitory pain mechanism) – before progressing into the painful quadrant; the plan was to start in the painful quadrant immediately.

It is important to remember that diagnostic and treatment hypotheses first need to be tested and supported in the physical examination, and treatment ultimately will be based on the combined findings of the patient history and physical examination. Mobility testing may reveal restricted, normal or increased mobility at the involved motion segment. However, if a restriction is found, then in the patient's prime combination of extension/right rotation (E, RR; painful quadrant of the box diagram),

Continued on following page

1. Two main hypotheses for the nature of the condition

   A. *Mid-thoracic 'arthrogenic' impairment of ERR*

   B. *Mid-thoracic impairment of posterior rib rotation*

2. Weight these components?

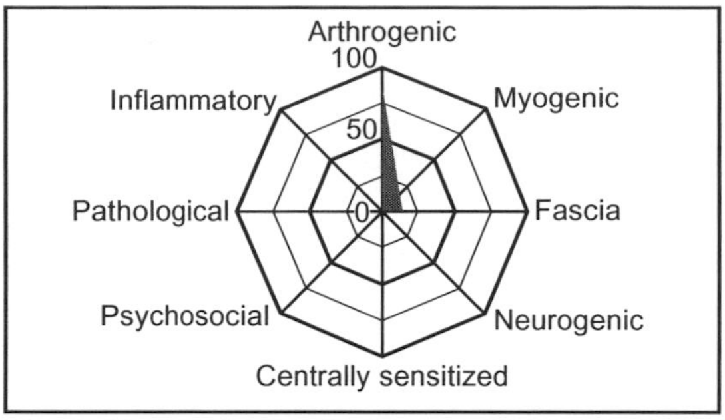

3. Severe?   Yes ☐   No ■
4. Irritable?   Yes ☐   No ■
5. Dominant pain mechanism?

   Nociceptive   ■
   Peripheral neurogenic   ☐
   Central   ☐
   Affective   ☐

6. Neurological exam today?

   None required   ■
   Lower motor neurone, upper motor   ☐
   neurone, limbs
   Lower motor neurone, upper motor   ☐
   neurone, limbs and cranial

---

7. To what point will you allow movement?

   To onset of pain   ☐
   To maximum extent of impairment   ■

8. Functional demonstration/retest marker?

   Mid-thoracic extension and right rotation

9. Starting position for passive assessment/treatment

   In their prime combination (PC)   ■
   In opposite quadrant to the prime combination   ☐

10. Treatments likely to reduce impairment

   A. *In ERR, right unilateral, caudal accessory glide of superior vertebrae*
   B. *In ERR, right rotation of superior vertebrae*
   C. *In ERR, right posterior rib rotation*

11. Likely treatments to be tested against each other this session?
   A versus B ■   A versus C ■   B versus C ■

12. Likely home programme and 'take-home messages'

   In ERR, lower thoracic spine fixed against back of chair – active RR

13. Comments

   Non-severe – expect rapid improvement with manual therapy

Fig. 26.2 The completed planning sheet clarifying the key issues before conducting the physical examination. Question 2 consists of a radar plot allowing a pictorial representation of the relative weighting of the components of the presentation. *ERR*, Extension right rotation; *RR*, right rotation.

restoration of movement and reduction of pain would more likely be achieved with one or more of the following passive movements:

- Passive accessory glides (unilateral PA pressure with caudal inclination of the superior vertebral level on the inferior level)
- Passive physiological rotation
- Passive posterior rotation of the ipsilateral rib (lifting the distal rib up – needed to gain full mid-thoracic rotation)

The plan was to undertake tests or mini-treatments of these three 'likely to be effective' passive movements in the patient's prime combination and to then treat with the movement that had reduced the impairment most significantly. This reasoning was based on the assumption that there was a limitation of movement into the direction of the prime combination and that the functional demand to look over his right shoulder while playing soccer on the left wing was painful for Rohan because segmental movement in the thoracic spine was restricted. Consequently, the restricted tissues were being repeatedly irritated and painfully provoked, possibly associated with local inflammation.

It was hypothesized that CMT would likely be of benefit because the rationale of CMT involves inducing movement in positions where tissue resistance is perceived by the clinician in order that the tissues are moved in ranges where higher-threshold mechanoreceptors are stimulated. This 'high-dose' stimulation evokes brain-orchestrated, inhibitory, descending pain mechanisms which are sympathetico-excitatory; thus, because Rohan's history suggested a normal HPA axis and a directional sensitivity to motion, the CMT approach to management appeared to be suited to him.

Clinical Reasoning Commentary:

The planned use of 'mini-treatments', at first impression, may seem an unusual strategy. We tend to think of treatment as being the final stage of a linear, sequential process comprising the initial patient encounter. As in this particular case, and putting aside jargon or labels employed in particular manual therapy approaches/philosophies, careful dissection of the clinical reasoning of expert clinicians often demonstrates that the patient encounter is indeed not strictly sequential and that the 'classical' stages of an initial consultation – history/interview followed by a physical/objective examination and concluding with the treatment/management – are often intermingled to varying degrees at particular junctures in the reasoning process. That is, expert practitioners do not limit the ways in which a certain piece of clinical data may inform their decision-making across various hypothesis categories.

So it could be argued that the 'mini-treatments' planned in Rohan's case may actually inform the clinician's reasoning judgements in relation to physical impairments and associated structures/tissues, in addition to indicating the treatment most likely to be of initial benefit (at least compared with two alternatives). The responses to the mini-treatments would probably also have some value in informing the clinician's thinking regarding the prognosis for Rohan. So in effect, it could further be argued that the strategy of 'mini-treatments' is potentially an efficient mechanism that expeditiously maximizes the collection of highly relevant information used to help make several key clinical decisions.

Physical Examination

Observation

Rohan appeared to be of low adiposity and with well-developed musculature. He walked and stood with out-turned feet (right > left). His pelvic level appeared symmetrical; however, he had a minor thoracic scoliosis concave to the right and rotated to the right. This gave him the appearance of having enlarged paraspinal muscles on the right. He also had an exaggerated low lumbar lordotic posture, but no excessive thoracic kyphosis.

Active Movements

Rohan's pain was reproduced with active thoracic spine right rotation (5/10) and extension (4/10). The prime movement combination for provocation of his pain was confirmed as being extension/right rotation (E, RR; as per the example in Fig. 26.1). Right and left active thoracic lateral flexion, flexion and left rotation all produced only a mild 'tightness' (1/10). Active movements, when localized to the mid-thoracic region, were equally limited in all movement planes but were only painful for those movements toward the painful quadrant. Deep inspiration, undertaken whilst being positioned in extension/right rotation, did not alter the pain or range response, suggesting that posterior rib rotation was not a significant component of the impairment. It was noted that the observed scoliosis reduced with flexion, indicating a postural rather than fixed scoliosis.

There was no sign of aberrant control of scapular or trunk muscles with movements of the upper limbs or neck. The external rotator muscles of the right hip were tight, resulting in reduced internal rotation of the right hip (25% less than the left hip).

Palpation and Passive Movement Testing

Soft tissue palpation performed in prone lying (neutral) revealed hypertonicity of the paraspinal muscles over the right mid-thoracic spine. These muscles and the transverse processes and rib angles of the right T6–T8 region felt more pronounced to palpation than those on the left.

In the patient's prime-combination position of extension/right rotation, unilateral PA with caudal inclination passive accessory glides applied to the transverse processes and rib angles revealed a severe restriction of movement when gliding T7 down on T8, with 5/10 pain reproduced. A 'mini-treatment' of approximately 1 minute resulted in a reduction in the perceived resistance to the passive accessory movement and a decrease in the pain level reported during the mobilization. However, after the mini-treatment, a review of the prime-combination movement revealed only a 10% reduction in pain and no change in the range of the prime-combination movement.

Next, an assessment of the relative effect of a passive physiological rotation 'mini-treatment' of T7 on T8 on the impairment was undertaken. In the extension/right rotation position, right rotation of T7 on T8 reproduced pain (5/10) very early in the range of passive motion. Mobilization for approximately 1 minute again produced only a 10% reduction in pain and no change in the range of the prime combination movement. Similarly, a mini-treatment mobilizing the right seventh and eighth ribs up into posterior rotation did not change the pain or range of movement of the prime combination by more than 10%.

Straight leg raise and slump testing revealed no symptom reproduction and normal mobility.

Positional Asymmetry

To test for a positional right rotation asymmetry of T7 on T8, passive physiological rotation in the mid-flexion/extension position and in the patient's primary combination (E, RR) was compared. Right rotation was found to be equally restricted in the two positions (by 50%). This was somewhat surprising because one would normally expect a greater range of right rotation when starting the movement from a neutral position rather than from a position of combined extension and right rotation. Interestingly, passive physiological left rotation was also equally limited at T7/T8 when performed in neutral and in flexion.

Reasoning Question:

6. What prompted you to consider that a 'positional asymmetry' of the T7/T8 segment may be of relevance in Rohan's presentation? What clinical significance did you attach to the findings in this regard, and in particular, were there any implications for management?

Answer to Reasoning Question:

The combination of the appearance of a right rotational asymmetry of T7 on T8 (prominent right T7/T8 transverse processes and rib angles), limited passive accessory intervertebral movement and the severely restricted passive physiological right rotation movement suggested the need to consider that there might be a 'static' positional asymmetry, clinically relevant to the patient's impairment. This consideration was approached with some caution because the measurement error associated with passive palpation of segmental symmetry has been shown to be of a magnitude that questions the validity of the tests (Najm et al., 2003). Passive-motion and pain-provocation testing also have levels of measurement error that suggest that inter-rater assessments are only just better than chance agreement (Seffinger et al., 2003; Stovall and Kumar, 2010). Intra-rater measurement error levels are, however, lower (Degenhardt et al., 2010; Potter et al., 2006), and combinations of these tests may provide a more valid platform on which treatment decisions can be based.

Because there was mounting evidence that T7 did indeed appear to be statically rotated to the right in relation to T8 and that it had limited passive capacity to be moved from this position, a shift in clinical reasoning was required. The classic CMT reasoning process assumes that the motion segment is 'resting' in a relatively neutral position but has developed an impaired motion, associated with pain

Continued on following page

on movement. In this typical scenario, it seems reasonable to expect a reduction in pain and an improvement in movement following passive mobilization into the impaired motion direction. This approach would likely provide pain relief, desensitize the specific movement and re-educate the sensorimotor system to recover the pain-free memories associated with this specific movement (Flor, 2002). However, because this usual CMT approach had not reduced the impairment in Rohan's case, further consideration as to how a potential segmental positional asymmetry might be improved was now required.

The initial plan for treatment was therefore discarded, and a new set of hypotheses was generated. It was possible that Rohan was experiencing pain in E, RR because the T7/T8 motion segment was in fact already in terminal E, RR when further E, RR was demanded during the soccer game. If the segment did not in fact have a restriction of E, RR but was instead "held" in this position, further mobilization into E, RR would simply evoke the descending inhibitory pain mechanism, providing temporary pain relief, but would be unlikely to reduce the amount of E, RR the segment was resting in.

Thus, the new hypotheses to be tested in the remainder of the initial physical examination were that pain associated with E, RR, due to the motion segment being 'held' in E, RR, would be rapidly improved if the following were undertaken in a starting position of flexion/left rotation (F, LR):

- Unilateral PA cephalad accessory glides applied to the superior level, 'pushing' the superior level away from its asymmetrical resting position
- Passive physiological left rotation movement of the superior level, 'pushing' the superior level away from its asymmetrical resting position
- Mobilization of the right-sided seventh and eighth ribs were mobilised down into anterior rotation, 'pulling' the superior level away from its asymmetrical resting position

Using the new 'mini-treatments' (applied in F, LR) to test the relative effectiveness of each of these hypotheses, a ranking of effectiveness was established. Cephalad accessory glides of the right T7 transverse process reduced the pain by 50% on re-assessment of the prime combination, whilst physiological intervertebral and rib rotation movements each only produced a 10% improvement. It was planned to undertake further accessory gliding movement testing at the next session.

Home Programme and Take-Home Message

An explanation of the clinical findings, including why the pain had changed so dramatically following the unilateral cephalad accessory glides of T7 in F, LR, was provided to Rohan, along with a home stretch to mimic this treatment (Fig. 26.3). It was reinforced that the pain was associated with a mechanical dysfunction and could be improved with a simple home stretch. By ensuring that the locus of control was with Rohan and that the treatment approach was not passive, the take-home message was that the clinician was not 'fixing' him. Simply showing Rohan what he could do himself helped encourage his active participation in the therapeutic encounter (Bronfort et al., 2014). Patients are more likely to adhere to prescribed behavioural advice (e.g. postures, stretches) if they see some immediate reward from it (Navratilova and Porreca, 2014). Thus, encouraging Rohan to test his primary combination before stretching and then again post-stretching should both guide him in terms of the number and vigour of the stretches and also provide him with an immediate incentive to comply with the stretching.

Second Session (1 Week Later)

Rohan reported significantly less pain experienced after soccer games (2/10) and virtually no pain during the game itself. The pain developed 1 hour after a game and was eased significantly by heat. The home stretches were being performed once per day, with an improvement in pain noted with each stretching session.

Physical Re-Examination

There was a reduction in the apparent size of the paraspinal muscles and the degree of postural right rotation observed in standing.

Fig. 26.3 T7/T8 flexion/left rotation home stretch. In sitting, the patient actively moves into flexion and left rotation whilst pulling on the towel with the right hand, thus encouraging T7 to move cephalad on T8. The movement is undertaken slowly and within a pain-free range of movement. However, a stretch sensation should be felt by the patient.

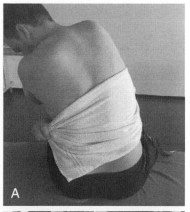

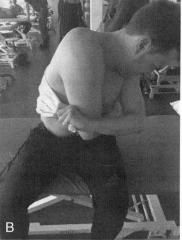

On thoracic spine active combined movement testing, there was less pain and greater range of movement (50%) in E, RR and F, LR than the week before.

On palpation, there was reduced hypertonicity in the right, mid-thoracic paraspinal muscles, but they were still more hypertonic than on the left side. Whilst passive movement had increased at T7/T8, 'mini-treatments' in F, LR applying accessory movement (unilateral PA cephalad glide of the superior level) and then passive physiological movement (left rotation of T7 on T8) provided only small, equivocal improvements in pain (20%) on re-assessment of the prime-movement combination. Paraspinal muscle hypertonicity was unchanged.

Because the impaired movement had improved but not completely resolved, alternative hypotheses for the maintenance of the impairment were required. To test these new hypotheses, 'mini-treatments' were again used in this session to determine their effect on the pain produced by E, RR. The mini-treatments were applied in F, LR as follows:

- Unilateral cephalad accessory glides applied to the superior level, 'pushing' the superior level away from its asymmetrical resting position
- Brief isometric contraction of the segmental extensors to evoke post-isometric relaxation (PIR) to reduce the hypertonicity
- Brief isometric contraction of the multisegmental extensor muscles (quadratus lumborum [QL], latissimus dorsi [LD]) to evoke PIR to reduce the hypertonicity.

PIR of the superficial muscles (QL, LD) provided complete relief of pain when E, RR was performed, whilst the more local segmental treatments each only reduced the pain by 10%. Rohan was then taught how to perform a home PIR technique (Fig. 26.4), and an explanation as to why the treatment had worked was given. In addition, because the overactivity (hypertonicity) of the thoracic right rotators may have been associated with a

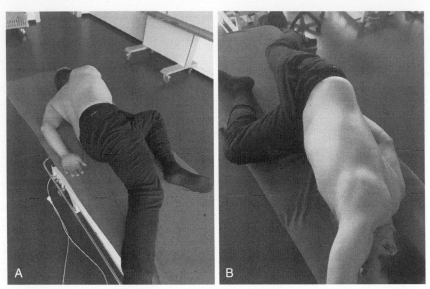

Fig. 26.4 Home post-isometric (PIR) technique. In left side-lying, the patient positions himself or herself in thoracic left rotation, lateral flexion and flexion, with the right shoulder in flexion and right hip in extension and adduction. This position tensions the lateral fascia, quadratus lumborum, latissimus dorsi and tensor fasciae latae.

compensatory demand during gameplay due to the lack of internal rotation of the right hip, an internal rotation PIR exercise was also taught to Rohan. The patient now had one F, LR stretch and two muscle PIR techniques to undertake daily and also pre- and post-game (Day and Nitz, 2012; Smith and Fryer, 2008).

Outcome

Rohan was discharged from treatment at this point. His pain did not return, and the club physiotherapist helped him to maintain his range of movement and symmetry of muscle tone in the thoracic paraspinal muscles for the following few months. This involved including sessions of active movement into thoracic flexion, thoracic left rotation and right hip internal rotation before games, as part of Rohan's warm-up and cool-down routines.

Reasoning Question:

7. You used a PIR technique as part of your management, which appeared to be quite effective. Can you offer an explanation as to the mechanism that may have produced this effect?

Answer to Reasoning Question:

The mechanism by which autogenic inhibition or PIR is purported to contribute to lengthening of muscle is unclear; however, increases in hamstring muscle length and spinal mobility have been reported following its application (Smith and Fryer, 2008). Theoretically, the voluntary static contraction performed against resistance places the musculotendinous unit on stretch, resulting in an increased firing of tension-sensing mechanoreceptors (Golgi tendon organs) within the same muscle. Increased inhibition from Ib-inhibitory interneurones, as a result of the amplified Golgi tendon organ input, leads to reduced excitability of the muscle, thereby facilitating additional stretch (Sharman et al., 2006). However, the evidence for significant change in this spinal reflex is very limited, and it is at best very short-lived (Sharman et al., 2006); thus, it can be hypothesized that the observed improvements are more likely to be mediated supra-spinally and may relate to benefits from a graded exposure to muscle contraction/relaxation in the impaired region. That is, these techniques typically use contractions at low levels of maximum voluntary contraction and may provide the patient with a 'no threat' (i.e. painless) message that muscle contraction and relaxation are possible without pain and are therefore non-threatening.

Reasoning Question:

8. You comment that the home programme placed the 'locus of control' with Rohan and thus that the treatment approach was not passive. Given the importance you ascribe to this part of the overall management, and noting the compliance demonstrated by Rohan, did you consider at all how you

may have dealt with the situation if he had been less willing to accept the prescribed active treatment?

Answer to Reasoning Question:

Patients have certain expectations of the interaction they will experience with a clinician. In my experience, those expectations usually include that they will receive an explanation as to why they are in pain, a discussion of a plan of treatment, including timescales for goals of treatment to be achieved, and the development of equal responsibility for the therapeutic encounter. If the process of meeting these expectations is undertaken early in the therapeutic encounter, discord between the locus of control and adherence to treatment plans can be addressed in an open and collaborative manner. As musculoskeletal practitioners, we often educate our patients through a period of their lives during which they have a physical impairment. We have the ability to include 'physical education' within our management strategies, and there is an expectation from many patients that they will undertake some form of physical intervention when seeing a musculoskeletal practitioner. Thus, clinical experience indicates that most patients respond well to the concept that movement impairment requires physical intervention. Most will readily develop an understanding that whilst passive movements applied to them may provide a 'shortcut' to pain relief, the techniques can often be self-administered as part of a functional rehabilitation programme.

Reasoning Question:

9. In retrospect, what do you consider were the key learnings from Rohan's case?

Answer to Reasoning Question:

The patient presented with a classic mechanical dysfunction, or 'specific direction sensitivity', a not-uncommon presentation. The predominant pain mechanism (nociceptive) was therefore likely to respond to manual therapy techniques (anti-nociceptive). The prime-movement combination of thoracic spine extension and ipsilateral rotation suggested an impairment of the superior spinal level moving 'back and down' on the inferior level, something that would typically respond to being passively moved in this direction. However, whilst this may typically be the case, Rohan's presentation nonetheless required an adaption of classic CMT reasoning.

Observation of static standing posture and palpation of local paraspinal muscle activity, as well as passive accessory and passive physiological segmental motion information, provided an accumulation of evidence to suggest that there was a local positional asymmetry at T7/T8. Specifically, T7 appeared to be held in a position of terminal right rotation on T8. This hypothesis was tested by 'mini-treatments' that moved the superior segment into right rotation compared with those moving the segment away from this position. Passively mobilizing the segment away from right rotation reduced the pain and movement impairment with E, RR. When the benefit of this approach had plateaued, reducing hypertonicity in the extensor and right rotator muscles using PIR became the more effective treatment.

Finally, the aetiology of the impairment was addressed by correcting the relative amount of rotation being shared between the hips and the thoracic spine during the functional task of playing soccer. Throughout the interaction with Rohan, emphasis was placed on ensuring the process was active for the patient, with the locus of control for managing his impairment residing with him. Thus, he should have felt he was correcting his problem with guidance from the clinician, rather than simply thinking the clinician 'fixed me'.

This case highlights that even with the most apparently straightforward presentation, clinical reasoning associated with manual therapy approaches such as CMT need to always be responsive to the individual patient's clinical findings. With CMT, the importance of testing likely hypotheses against each other using 'mini-treatments', both during assessment and treatment, helps to ensure that the practitioner is employing that specific treatment which is likely to make the most difference.

Clinical Reasoning Commentary:

The need to continually re-assess and challenge one's thinking if hypotheses are not supported by the clinical response is critical to successful clinical practice and to development along the continuum of clinical expertise. In this case, the practitioner has specifically referred to a 'shift in clinical reasoning' (Answer to Reasoning Question 5) and the importance of one's clinical reasoning being 'responsive to the individual patient's clinical findings'. There are several requisites required for this to occur. First, regular and meticulous re-assessment throughout the physical examination and management provides the clinician with the essentially real-time information required to help test the accuracy of hypotheses across the various categories. Second, it helps to avoid common reasoning errors, such as confirmation bias, which may be evident through focussing too much on a favourite hypothesis, overemphasizing those features of a presentation that support a favourite hypothesis or neglecting negating features.

An element of 'adaptive expertise' (Cutrer et al., 2017) is recognition and adjustment when an existing approach is found to be inadequate, as occurred here. It is important that the clinician should retain a degree of flexibility in his or her thinking at all stages of the patient encounter to enable responsiveness to new emerging information in clinical reasoning. Blinkered or biased reasoning, or

Continued on following page

not considering or testing competing hypotheses, can lead to suboptimal patient care and stunted development of clinical expertise. In this case, it is apparent that the clinician has reacted nimbly to an unexpected response to the initial manual therapy intervention, which challenged the diagnostic/impairment working hypothesis but, through a consequential change or 'shift' in reasoning, led to optimization of the treatment outcome.

ACKNOWLEDGMENTS FROM CHRISTOPHER MCCARTHY

With grateful thanks to Dr Brian Edwards, who taught me combined movement theory, and to Mr Peter Terry, who taught me the Maitland concept.

REFERENCES

Bialosky, J.E., Bishop, M.D., Price, D.D., Robinson, M.E., George, S.Z., 2009. The mechanisms of manual therapy in the treatment of musculoskeletal pain: a comprehensive model. Man. Ther. 14, 531–538.

Bronfort, G., Hondras, M.A., Schulz, C.A., Evans, R.L., Long, C.R., Grimm, R., 2014. Spinal manipulation and home exercise with advice for subacute and chronic back-related leg pain: a trial with adaptive allocation. Ann. Intern. Med. 161, 381–391.

Clement, D., Granquist, M.D., Arvinen-Barrow, M.M., 2013. Psychosocial aspects of athletic injuries as perceived by athletic trainers. J. Athl. Train. 48, 512–521.

Cutrer, W.B., Miller, B., Pusic, M., et al., 2017. Fostering the development of master adaptive learners: a conceptual model to guide skill acquisition in medical education. Acad. Med. 92, 70–75.

Day, J.M., Nitz, A.J., 2012. The effect of muscle energy techniques on disability and pain scores in individuals with low back pain. J. Sport Rehabil. 21, 194–198.

Degenhardt, B.F., Johnson, J.C., Snider, K.T., Snider, E.J., 2010. Maintenance and improvement of interobserver reliability of osteopathic palpatory tests over a 4-month period. J. Am. Osteopath. Assoc. 110, 579–586.

Edwards, B.C., 1992. Manual of Combined Movements, first ed. Churchill Livingstone, Edinburgh.

Edwards, B.C., 1999. Manual of Combined Movements: Their Use in the Examination and Treatment of Mechanical Vertebral Column Disorders. Churchill Livingstone, Perth.

Flor, H., 2002. Painful memories. Can we train chronic pain patients to 'forget' their pain? EMBO Rep. 3, 288–291.

Iannetti, G.D., Mouraux, A., 2010. From the neuromatrix to the pain matrix (and back). Exp. Brain Res. 205, 1–12.

Kaufman, M.P., Hayes, S.G., Adreani, C.M., Pickar, J.G., 2002. Discharge properties of group III and IV muscle afferents. Adv. Exp. Med. Biol. 508, 25–32.

Koes, B.W., Assendelft, W.J., van der Heijden, G.J., Bouter, L.M., Knipschild, P.G., 1991. Spinal manipulation and mobilisation for back and neck pain: a blinded review. BMJ 303, 1298–1303.

Kovanur Sampath, K., Mani, R., Cotter, J.D., Tumilty, S., 2015. Measureable changes in the neuro-endocrinal mechanism following spinal manipulation. Med. Hypotheses 85, 819–824.

Martinez-Segura, R., De-la-Llave-Rincon, A.I., Ortega-Santiago, R., Cleland, J.A., Fernandez-de-Las-Penas, C., 2012. Immediate changes in widespread pressure pain sensitivity, neck pain, and cervical range of motion after cervical or thoracic thrust manipulation in patients with bilateral chronic mechanical neck pain: a randomized clinical trial. J. Orthop. Sports Phys. Ther. 42, 806–814.

Maitland, G.D., 1986. Vertebral Manipulation, fifth ed. Churchill Livingstone, Sydney.

McCarthy, C.J., 2010. Combined Movement Theory: Rational Mobilization and Manipulation of the Vertebral Column. Elsevier Healthsciences, Oxford.

Najm, W.I., Seffinger, M.A., Mishra, S.I., Dickerson, V.M., Adams, A., Reinsch, S., et al., 2003. Content validity of manual spinal palpatory exams - A systematic review. BMC Complement. Altern. Med. 3, 1.

Navratilova, E., Porreca, F., 2014. Reward and motivation in pain and pain relief. Nat. Neurosci. 17, 1304–1312.

O'Leary, S., Falla, D., Hodges, P.W., Jull, G., Vicenzino, B., 2007. Specific therapeutic exercise of the neck induces immediate local hypoalgesia. J. Pain 8, 832–839.

Pickar, J.G., 2002. Neurophysiological effects of spinal manipulation. Spine J. 2, 357–371.

Potter, L., McCarthy, C., Oldham, J., 2006. Intraexaminer reliability of identifying a dysfunctional segment in the thoracic and lumbar spine. J. Manipulative Physiol. Ther. 29, 203–207.

Seffinger, M., Adams, A., Najm, W., Dickerson, V., Mishra, S., Reinsch, S., et al., 2003. Spinal palpatory diagnostic procedures utilized by practitioners of spinal manipulation: annotated bibliography of reliability studies. J. Can. Chiropr. Assoc. 47.

Sharman, M.J., Cresswell, A.G., Riek, S., 2006. Proprioceptive neuromuscular facilitation stretching: mechanisms and clinical implications. Sports Med. 36, 929–939.

Smith, M., Fryer, G., 2008. A comparison of two muscle energy techniques for increasing flexibility of the hamstring muscle group. J. Bodyw. Mov. Ther. 12, 312–317.

Stovall, B.A., Kumar, S., 2010. Reliability of bony anatomic landmark asymmetry assessment in the lumbopelvic region: application to osteopathic medical education. J. Am. Osteopath. Assoc. 110, 667–674.

Zusman, M., 1986. Spinal manipulative therapy: review of some proposed mechanisms, and a new hypothesis. Aust. J. Physiother. 32, 89–99.

27

Incorporating Biomechanical Data in the Analysis of a University Student With Shoulder Pain and Scapula Dyskinesis

Ricardo Matias • Mark A. Jones

Subjective Examination

Hugo is a Caucasian 23-year-old student undertaking a bachelor's degree in electronic engineering. He has an active lifestyle and is of average weight for his height (80 kg and 1.80 m tall). Hugo is the youngest of three sons and currently lives at home while he studies. He presented without a medical referral with pain in his left shoulder. His pain arose suddenly 1 week ago without incident during a strength-training gym session while lifting a greater weight of 70 kg on a barbell bench press (usual weight 60–64 kg). He could not identify any other predisposing factor to the onset of his shoulder pain. He is right-hand dominant.

Initially, Hugo was not concerned because the pain was only momentary during the bench press and did not limit the rest of his workout or participation in daily activities. However, after a week of continued pain with these two gym exercises and the development of pain in overhead activities at home, Hugo came to physiotherapy.

As illustrated in the body chart (Fig. 27.1), Hugo reported pain in the anterolateral aspect of his left shoulder. Screening for other potential symptoms was negative, including numbness, pins and needles, vascular-associated symptoms and joint noises or sensations (e.g. feelings of instability). Hugo also reported no symptoms in other body areas (e.g. spine and other peripheral joints). At the initial physiotherapy appointment, he rated his shoulder pain as 0/10 at rest on a verbal numeric rating scale (VNRS) and 5/10 VNRS when his symptoms were at their worst.

Hugo's shoulder pain was provoked with arm movements into elevation. Movements below 90 degrees and hand behind back were not a problem. The pain was elicited immediately with elevation and went as soon as he lowered his arm. He had no problem sleeping, including lying on either side, and reported no morning stiffness or progression of pain through the day. There was no change in the area or pattern of his pain provocation since the initial onset except for the development of pain on elevation starting to affect his daily activities both at home and in laboratory tasks within his engineering classes.

Hugo is a keen gym participant who regularly dedicates 90 minutes, three times per week, of his time to strength training. He is devoted to his third-year bachelor studies and highly motivated to continue his laboratory activities and to studying to maintain his 75th percentile grades. Hugo reported having no previous musculoskeletal injuries or problems, including no previous shoulder or spinal pain.

His general health is excellent, with no known medical conditions. He had not had any imaging of his shoulder or attempted any management other than discontinuing the bench press in his workout. He has not required any pain medication, and the only medication he takes is Symbicort for asthma.

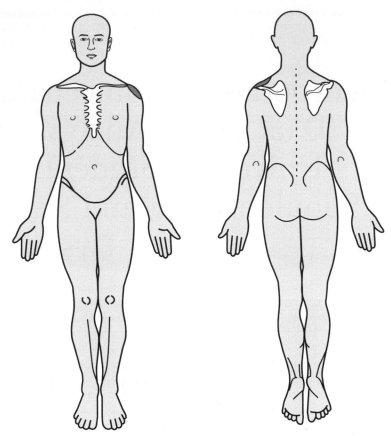

Fig. 27.1 Body chart illustrating area of Hugo's symptoms. No symptoms were reported in any other body areas.

When asked about his understanding of his problem, he reported having 'no idea' but assumed he must have strained something when adding extra weight to his bench press. He was not overly concerned or distressed by his problem, although he was keen to resume his full workout and a bit worried about the shoulder pain compromising his engineering lab activities. Hugo's goals were simply to get back to full activities without pain, and he was keen to follow any advice and exercise that was recommended, adding that, if possible, he would like to continue as much of his gym program as allowed while undergoing rehab.

Reasoning Question:

1. Please discuss your hypotheses regarding 'pain type' (nociceptive, neuropathic, nociplastic), possible 'sources of symptoms' and 'pathology', and potential 'contributing factors', including the basis for your reasoning.

Answer to Reasoning Question:

From the current subjective examination, there is no evidence of neurological symptoms or relevant history that would support a 'neuropathic pain' and no evidence of maladaptive cognitions, fears or behaviours that would support a nociplatic pain. Hugo's pain was reported as being localized in the anterolateral aspect of his left shoulder, with a consistent, predictable pattern of symptom behaviour that supports a nociceptive-dominant pain type (Smart et al., 2012).

Potential sources of nociception considered most likely would include local somatic tissues such as subcromial tissues (bursa, rotator cuff, long head of biceps), glenohumeral capsule and ligaments, labrum and acromioclavicular joint (ACJ), as well as referral from cervical spine somatic structures and viscera, although neither of those is considered likely given his lack of cervical symptoms and good general health. There is no macro trauma to suggest a specific pathology. Instead, the mechanism of onset supports a tissue nociception associated with strain during his bench press (e.g. a subcromial or intra-articular tissue but less likely ACJ or capsule).

The most likely contributing factor is inadequate scapular and glenohumeral control and strength for the increased bench-press load attempted. Error in bench-press technique is also possible, although considered less likely given his gym experience. He could also have a pre-existing capsular laxity (e.g. congenital, generalized hypermobility), and that will be screened for in the physical examination.

Clinical Reasoning Commentary:

Although musculoskeletal clinicians' diagnosis of 'pain type' can only be a hypothesis based on dominant features in the clinical presentation (see Chapters 1 and 2), it is nevertheless still an important hypothesis to consider up front because the greater the likelihood of a nociplastic pain type, the greater the caution required later in interpreting patient responses in the physical examination, where provocation of symptoms may be related to increased sensitization rather than local tissue strain or pathology. As discussed in Chapter 4, it is important to explicitly screen for potential psychosocial factors, initially through the patient interview, and if necessary also through questionnaire.

Similarly, although pathology cannot be validated through the shoulder clinical examination (interview or physical), the likelihood and nature of pathology, or in this case, tissue nociception, can be hypothesized based on the history and clinical presentation. Consideration of potential 'contributing factors' is particularly important with a spontaneous mechanism of onset such as this because both resolution of symptoms and prevention of recurrence require assessment and management of contributing factors.

Physical Examination

Physical examination procedures were intended to identify movement-related dysfunction and contributing factors that could support and direct clinical management decisions. Visual observation and physical clinical tests were used, along with three-dimensional kinematics and electromyographic analysis. Motion of the thorax, scapula and humerus was collected (with a sample rate of 120 Hz) using electromagnetic skin-mounted trakSTAR sensors (Ascension Technology, Burlington, Vermont) that were attached to the anterior face of sternal manubrium, to the flat surface on the superior acromion, and to the lateral side of the humerus, respectively. Motion data were reconstructed according to the International Society of Biomechanics recommendations for reporting upper extremity joint motion (Wu et al., 2005), providing a three-dimensional image that was then displayed for both Hugo and the therapist. All kinematic data were processed with The MotionMonitor software (Innovative Sports Training, Chicago, Illinois).

Muscle electromyographic activity was recorded (with a sample rate of 1000 Hz) using surface electrodes placed according to standard anatomic references (Ekstrom et al., 2003) over the bellies of the anterior deltoid, upper and lower trapezius, and serratus anterior muscles, in line with their fibre orientation. All electromyographic data were processed using a Physioplux system (PLUX Wireless Biosignals, Lisbon). Both Innovative Sports Training and PLUX software provided real-time biofeedback information using 'The MotionMonitor Toolbox' and the 'Dynamic Shoulder Stability' applications, respectively.

Posture and Alignment (No Symptoms at Rest)

In the standing position, observation demonstrated that Hugo did not present with any apparent shoulder girdle muscle asymmetry. At rest with the arms at 0 degrees of flexion, both his glenohumeral joints were anterior relative to an imaginary plumb line commencing from the base of support just anterior to the lateral malleolus of the ankle. When comparing both scapula orientations relative to the thorax by observation, the left scapula medial border and inferior angle were detached, representing an increased internal rotation or 'winging' dyskinesis.

When comparing the left scapula, three-dimensional orientation values at rest (45.3 degrees of internal rotation, 9.3 degrees of upward rotation and 11.9 degrees of anterior tilt) against data from impaired and non-impaired subjects (Lawrence et al., 2014), it can be concluded that Hugo had an increase of scapula internal rotation and upward rotation of 4.2 degrees and 3.9 degrees, respectively, and a minor difference in anterior tilt when compared with mean values of non-impaired subjects. Although the standard deviation of three-dimensional scapula orientation values from impaired and non-impaired subjects overlap, Hugo's rest position was closer to the impaired subjects' mean, supporting a clinical judgement of left scapula positional impairment at rest.

Active Shoulder Movement Testing

- Flexion – full range of movement with pain provoked at end range; no abnormal or excessive humeral head translation was observed; scapulothoracic motion revealed an increase in scapula internal rotation, a decrease in scapula upward rotation and a slight decrease in scapulae posterior tilt when compared to mean published values of non-impaired subjects (Lawrence et al., 2014).
- Abduction – full range of movement with pain provoked at end range; inferior humeral head translation appeared reduced. During abduction, the only deviation from the expected motion was the scapula's upward rotation, which was reduced.

Note: Manual assistance to left scapula lateral rotation and posterior tilt (analogous to the 'Scapular Assistance Test' [Burkhart et al., 2000] and 'Shoulder Symptom Modification Procedure' [Lewis, 2009]) during active flexion and abduction decreased end-of-range shoulder pain.

- Extension – painless full range of movement
- Internal and external rotation (at 0 degrees elevation and at 90 degrees abduction) – painless full range of movement
- Horizontal flexion and horizontal extension (at 90 degrees abduction) – painless full range of movement
- Hand behind back – painless full range of movement

Impingement Tests

- Hawkins-Kennedy Impingement Test (Hawkins and Kennedy, 1980) – positive, with provocation of pain as soon as glenohumeral internal rotation was added at 90 degrees flexion.
- Neer Impingement Test (Neer and Welsh, 1977) – positive, with provocation of pain at approximately ¾ of the expected range of elevation.

Note: Manual assistance to left scapula lateral rotation and posterior tilt during the Hawkins-Kennedy and Neer Impingement Tests decreased Hugo's pain.

Shoulder Passive-Movement Testing

All active-movement tests repeated as passive-movement assessments were full range of movement with no pain provocation except for passive flexion and abduction, where range of movement was within normal limits but provoked his shoulder pain at the limit. Passive accessory movements at the glenohumeral, acromioclavicular and sternoclavicular joints were judged to have normal movement and end-feel, with no pain provocation. Passive glenohumeral stability tests (e.g. anterior, posterior, inferior and antero-inferior) and labral tests (e.g. 'Active Compression Test [O'Brien et al., 1998], 'Bicep Load II Test [Kim et al., 2001] and 'Crank Test [Lui et al., 1996], plus variations) were negative, with no abnormal laxity detected and no provocation of pain, respectively.

Shoulder Palpation

No swelling, altered tissue texture or areas of tenderness were identified around the acromion, acromioclavicular joint, subcoracoid space or tissues overlying the humeral head.

Awareness and Dissociation of Thoracic Segmental Movement

While standing against the wall, Hugo was asked to focus on flexing and extending his thoracic spine, as if he had to curl every vertebra of his spinal column away (flexion) and roll back against the wall (extension). Although he was able to achieve this task after several trials, Hugo clearly demonstrated a lack of thoracic motion dissociation and awareness, as he constantly moved his thoracic spine as a block despite having good segmental mobility.

Still with Hugo standing against the wall, it was observed that the posterior borders of the acromion of both his left and right scapulae were notably spaced from the wall. If asked to modify his scapulae position in such a way that this space could be reduced, Hugo was able to correct the shoulder girdle posture without feeling any increase in tension in the pectoralis-minor area.

Active Cervical and Thoracic Movement Testing

All active cervical and thoracic movements were judged to have full range of movement with no provocation of symptoms.

Dynamic Rotary Stability Test (Magarey and Jones, 2003; Magarey and Jones, 2003a)

Gentle resistance was applied to isotonic internal and then external rotation performed at varying angles between 90 degrees and full elevation in the sagittal, frontal and scapular planes. Simultaneously, the therapist assessed at the anterior and posterior glenohumeral joint lines for any abnormal glenohumeral translation, as well as for pain provocation, weakness, reproduction of joint clicks and so forth. No abnormal translation was evident, and no pain or joint click was reproduced. External rotation strength was subjectively reduced (as judged by therapist and patient) when assessed toward full elevation compared to the same position of the left side. When repeated with scapular stabilization (i.e. 'Scapular Retraction/Repositioning Test' [Burkhart et al., 2000]), Hugo's external rotation 'weakness' was significantly improved.

Muscle Activation Pattern (Assessed With Surface Electromyography [EMG])

During upper extremity movements, it is expected that the activation of the scapulothoracic muscles will occur in advance of the arm motion for preparing the scapula for the perturbation resulting from the implicit joint moments. This activation is referred to as 'feedforward' if it occurs prior or shortly after (<50 ms) the primer mobilizer (e.g. anterior fibres of the deltoid during flexion) because it cannot be initiated by feedback from the limb movement (Aruin and Latash, 1995). The temporal recruitment analysis of the lower trapezius and serratus anterior in relation to the onset of the anterior deltoid showed a feedforward pattern of both muscles in active shoulder flexion and abduction with the exception of a feedback pattern of the serratus anterior during arm abduction.

Manual Muscle Testing (Kendall et al., 1993)

- Upper trapezius 5/5
- Lower trapezius 4+/5
- Serratus anterior 4/5
- Shoulder flexion (at 30 degrees and 90 degrees elevation) 4/5 with no pain provocation
- Shoulder abduction (at 0 degrees elevation) 5/5 with no pain provocation; (at 90 degrees elevation) 4/5 with no pain provocation
- Shoulder internal rotation (at 0 degrees elevation) 5/5 with no pain provocation
- Shoulder external rotation (at 0 degrees elevation) 4+/5 with no pain provocation
- Lift-off test (Gerber and Krushell, 1991), belly-press test (Scheibel et al., 2005) and bear-hug test (Barth et al., 2006) all 5/5 with no pain provocation

Questionnaire Assessment of Disability

To assess physical function and symptoms over time, two self-administered questionnaires were used:

- Disabilities of the Arm, Shoulder and Hand (DASH; Santos and Gonçalves, 2006) – disability/symptom score 28.33/100; work score 0/100; sport score 56.25/100
- Shoulder Pain and Disability Index (SPADI; Leal and Cavalheiro, 2001) – overall score 19.5/100

Reasoning Question:

2. Please discuss your analysis of the physical findings with respect to your previous hypotheses regarding 'pain type', potential 'source of symptoms', 'pathology' and 'contributing factors'. Also, on the basis of these findings, please highlight your plans for management.

Answer to Reasoning Question:

The physical examination findings were consistent with the previous hypothesis following the subjective examination that the pain type was nociceptive dominant. Pain was only provoked with a few tests, and it was repeatable and proportional to the behaviour of Hugo's symptoms as he previously described. There was no widespread tenderness, as is commonly found with nociplastic pain, and no verbal or non-verbal behaviour during either the subjective or physical examination suggestive of hypervigilance or catastrophizing.

No specific pathology was incriminated by the physical examination findings. Pain was only provoked at the end range of active and passive elevation, with normal range of movement and no pain provocation on palpation, resisted isometric tests or labral tests. Although it is not possible to clinically confirm the source of nociception, collectively, the examination supports a subacromial source of nociception, such as a minor bursitis or reactive tendinopathy.

Scapular muscle impairments (dyskinesis, timing of activation and strength) are the most significant findings in Hugo's physical examination. Although these can be a consequence of shoulder pain via 'pain inhibition', they also are potential contributing factors that may have predisposed to his 'strain' during his bench-press onset of pain. Regardless, they now are demonstrated in Hugo's physical examination to be contributing to his current pain and weakness (i.e. improved with scapular assistance) and therefore will become the focus of management.

Reasoning Question:

3. Use of three-dimensional kinematic analysis would not be common in most musculoskeletal clinics. Would you discuss the validity of the system you use and the clinical value you believe it offers?

Answer to Reasoning Question:

The study of the shoulder complex has been a great challenge for all those who have been interested in it. The challenge is even greater when a clinician uses simple visual observation to perceive and analyze scapula movements. Electromagnetic systems have been extensively used to measure three-dimensional scapular kinematics during shoulder movements in impaired and non-impaired individuals (e.g. Haik et al., 2014; Ludewig and Cook, 2000). To track the thorax, scapula and humerus motion, sensors are normally attached with double-sided tape to the anterior face of sternal manubrium, to the flat surface on the superior acromion and to the lateral aspect of the humerus. This skin-mounted sensor method has proven to be valid for the measurement of scapula kinematics (Karduna et al., 2001) and reliable for both within- and in-between-day assessments (Haik et al., 2014). During Hugo's treatment, an electromagnetic system was used to accurately and reliably reconstruct scapula kinematics, generating information important to both our physical examination and to our management decisions by providing a source of real-time kinematic biofeedback.

The study of individual muscles' roles in controlling and stabilizing the scapula has been primarily based on muscle anatomy and activity measured via EMG. Musculoskeletal models provide the opportunity to infer muscle function from the internal mechanics of the scapula in response to muscle forces. A new model capable of reproducing scapulothoracic joint physiological movements in response to applied forces to accurately track scapula kinematics has been recently published and is freely available for download (Seth et al., 2016). This model shows great promise for revealing the interactions of complex skeletal and muscle dynamics that are involved in producing healthy and dysfunctional shoulder movements.

Although electromagnetic systems (along with other systems such as the optoelectronic systems and inertial measurement units) are undoubtedly of great value for accurate human motion reconstruction, computational modeling and simulation of the musculoskeletal system will bring new insights regarding movement dynamics. With the observed price reduction of the motion-capture systems, the increased efficiency of modern computers and freely available modeling and simulation software platforms such as the OpenSim Project (Delp et al., 2007), an unprecedented opportunity arises to reduce the gap between human motion analysis and its use in clinical practice. A complementary approach that merges clinical and biomechanical information will help therapists better understand and manage patients with movement-related impairments like the scapula dyskinesis present in Hugo's shoulder-elevation movements.

Clinical Reasoning Commentary:

The answer to Reasoning Question 2 illustrates how hypotheses formulated through the subjective examination are not fixed; rather, they are 'tested' against findings from the physical examination to build an evolving understanding of the patient and their problem. Because physical impairment in posture symmetry and scapular dyskinesis can exist without symptoms or pathology, the relevance of Hugo's dyskinesis impairments is specifically tested. Having established their likely relevance in contributing to his current pain and weakness, they then become a focus of treatment, where later re-assessments will further test both the effectiveness of the treatment and the hypothesis that these scapular muscle impairments are relevant to Hugo's symptoms and activity restrictions.

The inclusion of the three-dimensional kinematic analysis is an impressive and exciting means of objectively establishing and measuring scapular dyskinesis impairment. Musculoskeletal examination relies considerably on clinicians' skills of observation and feel. Although procedural skill, including communicative proficiency, is a recognized attribute of expert clinicians, the subjective nature of many musculoskeletal examination judgements will always be a limiting factor to their validity and a challenge to less experienced clinicians. As highlighted in Chapter 1, clinical reasoning is only as good as the information on which it is based. As such, any means to improve the clinical objectivity and validity of our assessments should reduce our perceptual errors and, in turn, better inform our clinical reasoning.

Management

A scapula-focused intervention was used based on the sequential cognitive, associative and autonomous stages of motor relearning (Shumway-Cook and Woolacott, 2001) as a framework while promoting the integration of local and global muscle function (Comerford and Mottram, 2001) tailored to Hugo's clinical presentation. Three-dimensional kinematics and an EMG system were used both for outcomes assessment and as a real-time source of biofeedback. The MotionMonitor software allowed quick clinical setup of Hugo with three electromagnetic sensors that accurately reconstructed his left scapula motion with respect to the thorax, in Euclidean three-dimensional space, according to the Euler angle sequence: retraction/protraction, lateral/medial rotation and anterior/posterior scapula tilt. The Physioplux system was simultaneously used to record muscles' onset and activity (normalized with respect to maximum voluntary isometric contraction) during the therapeutic exercises. Both software packages permitted modeling the graphical representation of both motion variables and, specifically, which parameters would be displayed in real time.

First-Appointment Treatment

The main goal of Hugo's management program was to restore his functioning levels, abolish pain and restore scapula neuromuscular control and strength. Based on the most recent research findings on the association of scapula dyskinesis and glenohumeral joint pathologies (e.g. Kibler et al., 2013; Ludewig and Reynolds, 2009), management commenced with an explanation of the main physical findings and recommendation for therapy. This education commenced with an explanation of Hugo's movement-related impairments and the likely associated biomechanical mechanisms and daily activities that could be contributing to his movement impairments. Understanding was facilitated with the use of a skeleton and a dynamic video of normal scapulohumeral movement ('shoulder decide'). During this process, Hugo was encouraged to share and discuss his own ideas and thoughts regarding his shoulder problem. After this, the most appropriate management for his presentation was outlined based on emerging evidence and personal experience, with emphasis on the use of therapeutic exercise to reduce imbalances in neuromuscular activity and motor control (e.g. Başkurt et al., 2011; Struyf et al., 2013). As I explained how we could merge therapeutic motor-relearning exercises with real-time EMG and three-dimensional kinematic biofeedback, it was clear that these motion technologies sparked Hugo's curiosity and motivation. Hugo was enthusiastic about the proposed management plan.

Pain and function were set as primary outcomes: the VNRS cutoff point defined to distinguish the presence or absence of dysfunction was zero. A reported minimal clinically important difference of 10.2 points and ranging from 8 to 13 points for the DASH and SPADI questionnaires, respectively, was used to determine the clinical significance of the results (Roy et al., 2009). Their cutoff points were set to 2.67/100 for DASH and 3.66/100 for SPADI (MacDermid et al., 2007). Scapula alignment and kinematic control were defined as normal when scapulothoracic angles at rest fell within 41.1 degrees (±6.24) of internal rotation, 5.4 degrees (±3.12) of upward rotation and 13.5 degrees (±5.54) of anterior tilt and with published mean values of non-impaired subjects at 30 degrees and 90 degrees of humerothoracic flexion and abduction, respectively (Lawrence et al., 2014). 'Good' scapula neuromuscular control was defined as Hugo being able to integrate scapula stabilizer activity (feedforward pattern measured with EMG) while correctly performing scapula-focused exercises throughout the three stages of motor relearning. For each stage, three-dimensional scapula kinematic values and tolerance errors were defined and monitored with an electromagnetic three-dimensional kinematic system. In order to achieve these outcomes, a weekly 1-hour session was used, and home-based exercises were prescribed. Outcome results are summarized in Table 27.1.

Scapula cognitive-stage exercises commenced with instruction and practice of awareness and dynamic control of the scapulothoracic neutral zone through its stabilizers' (lower trapezius and serratus anterior) co-activation, with a minimum participation of the upper trapezius (or other scapulothoracic and glenohumeral muscles).

- Exercise 1: Scapula proprioceptive neuromuscular facilitation diagonals – Scapula motion awareness, particularly combining depression and retraction movements, was facilitated by using side-lying scapula proprioceptive neuromuscular facilitation diagonals (Magarey and Jones, 2003b). This started by passively moving Hugo's scapula through a diagonal from elevation with slight protraction to depression with retraction, providing verbal feedback on the movement and tactile cues on the direction. Next, Hugo was asked to assist, and the diagonal was continued as an active assisted movement, again with verbal and tactile feedback. Hugo was then asked to perform the diagonal movement against low-intensity resistance and finally to perform the movement independently without any verbal or tactile feedback. No source of biofeedback was used besides tactile and verbal information to reinforce the use of internal feedback loops.
- Once attached with both surface electrodes and electromagnetic sensors, the scapulothoracic neutral zone was determined in a sitting position according to Mottram (1997), and its values were recorded.

TABLE 27.1

PRIMARY AND SECONDARY OUTCOME AND SPECIAL TEST RESULTS ASSESSED AT FIRST APPOINTMENT (WEEK 1)

	Pain	Function			Scapula Alignment	Scapula Neuromuscular Control		Scapula Kinematics		Muscle Strength		Special Tests	
	Worst	*DASH Overall*	*DASH Sport*	*SPADI*	*Dif*	*Feedback*	*Feedforward*	*Abduction Dif*	*Flexion Dif*	*Scapulothoracic*	*Glenohumeral*	*Hawkins*	*Neer*
Week 1	5/10	28.3/ 100	56.2/ 100	19.5	3.2	SA	LT	3,5/ 3,7	4,9/ 4,7	4+/4	4/5/ 4+	+	+

DASH, Disabilities of the Arm, Shoulder and Hand; *Dif*, mean difference between Hugo's scapulothoracic values and normative from non-impaired subjects (in degrees) at 30 degrees/90 degrees humerothoracic elevation; *LT*, lower trapezius; *SA*, serratus anterior; *SPADI*, Shoulder Pain and Disability Index.

- Exercise 2 (Fig. 27.2): Scapula V-slide in prone – Lying prone with both arms supported along his trunk, Hugo was asked to slide both scapulae in a 'V' form (combining depression and retraction movements) toward the defined scapulothoracic neutral zone. The electromyographic system was used to facilitate Hugo's awareness of the upper and lower trapezius' activity during scapulothoracic neutral zone exercises. With the Physioplux tablet on the floor, Hugo was able to see (from the table face hole) the tablet screen depicting his muscles' activity while performing the exercise (Fig. 27.3). The program was set to illustrate when the normalized activity of the upper trapezius was less than 15% and that of the lower trapezius was greater than 20%. A success score was defined as the highest number of correct executed repetitions achieved in the three sets (Hugo achieved 8/10).
- Exercise 3: Scapula V-slide in sitting – In a sitting position with both arms along the trunk and hands over his thighs, Hugo was asked to slide both his scapula in the same 'V' form as on the previous exercise. To facilitate Hugo's awareness of the target position, this time, The MotionMonitor biofeedback module was used (Fig. 27.4). To reach the target position, Hugo was encouraged to use this V-slide representation of scapula depression and retraction movement in such a way that the yellow cross representing real-time scapulothoracic two-dimensional orientation should fall into the static red square on the monitor feedback image. The center of the square was defined by the scapulothoracic neutral zone values, and the dimensions for the magnitude of accepted error were set to 5 degrees for both scapula retraction/protraction (abscissa) and lateral/medial rotation (ordinate) values. When the square target was reached, Hugo was asked to maintain that position for 10 seconds. Hugo achieved a success score of 7/10.

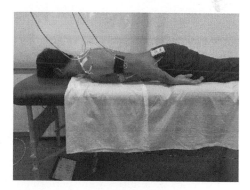

Fig. 27.2 Illustrating Exercise 2, scapula V-slide in prone, with Physioplux interface to focus Hugo's awareness on upper and lower trapezius activity during scapulothoracic neutral-zone exercises.

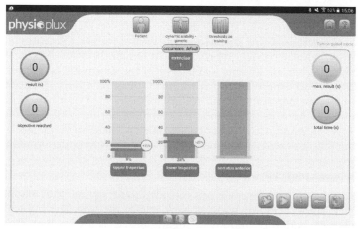

Fig. 27.3 Physioplux screen, as seen by Hugo, providing biofeedback as he aims to achieve and maintain the optimal levels of upper trapezius and lower trapezius activation during the scapula V-slide exercise. The program was set to illustrate when upper trapezius normalized activity was less than 15% and lower trapezius was greater than 20%. A success score was defined as the highest number of correctly executed repetitions achieved in the three sets (Hugo achieved 8/10). *(Screen used with the permission of Physioplux.)*

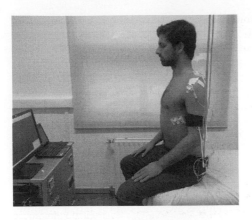

Fig. 27.4 Sitting scapular V-slide exercise while using The MotionMonitor kinematic biofeedback module to facilitate Hugo's awareness of the target position.

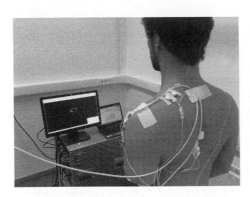

Fig. 27.5 Scapular V-slide exercise illustrating Hugo practicing correct awareness of scapulothoracic neutral zone via The MotionMonitor kinematic biofeedback and correct upper trapezius (normalized activity less than 15%) and lower trapezius (normalized activity greater than 20%) muscle activation.

- Exercise 4: To further facilitate Hugo's awareness of upper and lower trapezius activity during scapulothoracic neutral zone exercises, the Physioplux system was added (Fig. 27.5). Now Hugo was asked to perform the Exercise 3 goals but simultaneously recruit and maintain his upper trapezius and lower trapezius activity at the same levels as in Exercise 2. With this, Hugo achieved a success score of 7/10.

Exercises 2, 3 and 4 were performed throughout three series of 10 repetitions of 10 seconds each, with a minimum rest period between repetitions and a maximum of 30 seconds of rest between series.

With the purpose of assessing Hugo's dynamic control of scapulothoracic neutral zone on this first day, Exercise 4 was repeated at the end of the session without letting Hugo have access to visual biofeedback information. Although the level of muscle activity was being correctly achieved, he was not as efficient in the kinematic behaviour, resulting in a success score of 5/10. Hugo's correct recruitment of scapula muscles may be due to his short-term muscle memory rather than full motor relearning of a new skill because the EMG is 'saying' that he is using his muscles correctly, but the kinematics 'says' it is not good enough. When asked, Hugo reported a 'somewhat-hard' to 'hard' rating of perceived exertion during this last exercise, and most of the repetitions were performed while holding his breath.

The home-based program was as follows:

- Roll down on the wall: this exercise was intended to help Hugo gain mobility awareness of his thoracic spine. Standing with his back against the wall, feet hip-width apart and off the wall, with both hips and knees slightly flexed as if on a high stool, Hugo was instructed to drop his chin onto his chest and allow the weight of his head make him roll downward, feeling each spine level moving away from the wall until he reaches his lumbar spine. With both arms hanging relaxed, he was then instructed to segmentally slowly roll his thoracic spine back up to the wall. This exercise should be executed at least once a day, 3 series × 10 repetitions.

- Scapula V-slide in prone and sitting: To promote integration of the dynamic control of scapulothoracic neutral zone, Hugo was encouraged to performe Exercises 2 and 3 at least once a day, 3 series × 10 repetitions × 10 seconds.
- Hugo was asked to pay special attention to his shoulder girdle posture (e.g. while sitting for long periods of time) and to correct it whenever possible using the V-slide scapulae movement.
- Gym activity: Hugo was asked to restrict his gym activity for the next week to cardio training, with no upper extremity involvement. This could be done three times per week to maintain his regularity.

Reasoning Question:

4. Please discuss your rationale for the specific exercises selected, their dosage and the supporting evidence for the patterns of muscle activation you aimed to promote. Also, please comment on the efficacy of using the kinematic motion monitor and EMG as biofeedback for facilitating improved neuromuscular control.

Answer to Reasoning Question:

Over the last years, some studies have focused their intervention on muscle control and strength in patients with shoulder dysfunctions (e.g. Bae et al., 2011; Struyf et al., 2013; Worsley et al., 2013; doi: 0.1136/bjsports-2015-095460), resulting generally in better patient-rated outcomes but less consistent muscle activation and control results assessed through direct measures. The assumption that alterations in scapulothoracic muscle activation and control are related to scapular dyskinesis is being consolidated with the gradual accumulation of new insights in shoulder dysfunctions (Kibler et al., 2013). Hugo's rehabilitation aimed to promote the integration of local and global muscle function (Comerford and Mottram, 2012) progressed within cognitive, associative and autonomous stages of motor relearning (Shumway-Cook and Woolacott, 2001). The exercise dosage used, complemented with daily home-based exercises, appears to be in agreement with a recent systematic review on the effects of therapeutic exercise to restore the timing of stabilizers' muscle onset of activation (Crow et al., 2011). However, research evidence such as this is only a guide, and the specific dosage of each of Hugo's exercises was then based on assessment of his performance. Commonly, clinicians will base dosage judgements regarding load and number of repetitions on the quality of the exercise performance and the point where the quality begins to deteriorate or the patient beings to 'lose control'. In Hugo's case, this judgement was assisted by the use of external feedback. This biofeedback was used in these two sessions to facilitate Hugo's planning–control framework optimization by stimulating and complementing his planning and intrinsic feedback mechanisms with electromyographic and kinematic biofeedback on knowledge of performance during specific therapeutic exercises. Practice of the exercises first with biofeedback ensured that Hugo would develop a correct motor plan that would enhance his correctness and accuracy with each exercise at home when the external biofeedback was not available (Glover, 2004). Although the percentage of muscle activation was based on research recommendations, the actual dosage of repetitions was based on assessment in the clinic and identification of the number of repetitions Hugo could perform correctly before his pattern deteriorated.

Clinical Reasoning Commentary:

The theoretical rationale guiding the approach to exercise is based on a range of resources, including contemporary research-informed views regarding muscle control and scapular dyskinesis (Kibler et al., 2013), the functional stability retraining promoted by Comerford and Mottram (2001) and the motor relearning theory and research from Shumway-Cook and Woolacott (2001). Although theory and research have provided a framework to the approach taken and the specific percentage of muscle activation sought (i.e. upper trapezius normalized activity less than 15% and lower trapezius greater than 20%), the dosage of repetitions was still tailored to Hugo's actual performance.

Appointment 2 (1 Week Later)
Re-Assessment

Hugo reported a mild decrease in his symptoms and an increase in functioning, manifest as improvement in his daily activities. All the other outcomes results were maintained.

With the help of the electromyographic and three-dimensional kinematic systems, Hugo's performance on Exercises 2 and 3 were re-assessed, and both were effectively accomplished with less than 15% of upper trapezius normalized activity and more than 20% for the lower trapezius with a good scapula kinematic motion, resulting in an 8/10 kinematic success score for both exercises. Hugo also highlighted that he felt a noticeable decrease in the level of concentration required and judged his rate of perceived exertion as 'moderate' compared with the last visit. When asked how regularly he did his home exercises and attended to his shoulder girdle posture, he reported doing the exercises once a day at the prescribed dosage but admitted to forgetting to correct his posture as the days went by. Re-assessment of his performance doing the roll down on the wall exercise revealed correct dissociation of his thoracic spine with good, relaxed breathing.

Given these results, the following goals were agreed for this week:

1. Continue the scapula cognitive-stage training exercises, emphasizing movements from different postural orientations and positions toward the neutral zone (and maintaining this position) through the co-activation of both lower trapezius and serratus anterior in low-load exercises.
2. Begin associative-stage training by progressively integrating the lower trapezius and serratus anterior co-activation with upper trapezius fibres, and simultaneous coordination with the glenohumeral muscles, during shoulder multi-planar movements below 30 degrees of arm elevation.

- Exercise 1: Scapula V-slide sitting in front of a table – In a sitting position with both arms supported on a table elbow-height and forearms parallel to each other, Hugo was asked to slide both his scapula in the same 'V' form as on the previous exercises and add shoulder protraction while sliding the forearms over the table and back. Between each repetition, Hugo was instructed to move his scapulae in a random manner and then stop, and then the exercise was repeated from that new position, thereby providing practice of the 'V' retraction/depressions from multiple starting positions. Physioplux muscle levels were set as follows: upper trapezius 10%, lower trapezes 15% and serratus anterior 10% of their normalized activity. A correct performance was defined as Hugo being able to move his left scapula to the identified scapulothoracic neutral zone by recruiting and maintaining below the upper trapezius activity level and above both lower trapezius and serratus anterior levels while protracting his shoulder. Hugo achieved a success score of 8/10, with noticeable difficulty maintaining the lower trapezius activity.
- Exercise 2: Wall push-up plus – Exercise 1 principles were applied to a standard push-up to which a full shoulder protraction was added to the end of the push-up, with Hugo in a standing position, arms parallel to each other and to the floor, with his hands on the wall. A success score of 7/10 was obtained.
- Exercise 3: Scapula V-slide plus shoulder movements (<30 degrees) – In a standing position, Hugo was asked again to slide both his scapula in the same 'V' form, as with the previous exercises, and while maintaining the muscles' activity levels set for Exercise 1, consecutively raise his arm in the frontal, scapula and sagittal planes to a maximum of 30 degrees at a comfortable self-selected speed. Because this is within the scapula setting phase during humeral elevation tasks (Dvir and Berme, 1978), a narrow tolerated error of 5 degrees for the scapula coordinates was set for the three-dimensional kinematic biofeedback system. Hugo graded his perceived effort during this exercise as 'moderate' to 'light' and ended with a success score of 9/10.
- Exercise 4: Scapula V-slide plus shoulder isometric contractions – In a sitting position, Hugo was encouraged to reproduce scapulae V-slide motion while maintaining the scapulothoracic neutral zone (with a kinematic tolerance error of 5 degrees and equal electromyographic levels described in Exercise 1) and while isometrically contracting his glenohumeral muscles against alternated low-load manual resistance to flexion/extension, abduction/adduction and internal/external rotation. With a classified perceived exertion of 'somewhat-hard' to 'hard', Hugo finished with a success score of 7/10.

Exercises 1, 2 and 3 were performed through four sets of 10 repetitions each, and Exercise 4 through four sets of 10 repetitions of 10 seconds each, with a minimum rest period between repetitions and a maximum of 30 seconds of rest between sets. For Exercise 4, Hugo was allowed to extend the inter-set rest period to 60 seconds if needed. Toward the end of this session, Hugo was required to perform the last sets of each exercise without the external kinematic and EMG feedback.

The home-based program was as follows:

- Roll down in free standing: Hugo was asked to perform the roll down on the wall exercise but now in free standing. He was asked to focus on thoracic spine movement dissociation and avoid engaging the lumbar spine. Exercise dosage was set to at least once a day, 3 sets × 10 repetitions.
- Scapula V-slide plus shoulder-resisted movements (< 30 degrees) – To continue challenging scapulothoracic awareness and control while integrating stabilizer and mobilizer muscles in simple multi-planar activities, Hugo was asked to perform repetitions of Exercises 3 and 4 (against a wall for isometric resistance) at least once a day, 4 sets × 10.
- Correction of shoulder girdle alignment was again highlighted as important during repetitive tasks and maintaining postures. Interacting with the computer was identified by Hugo as the daily activity where he spent most of his time. Hugo was impressively engaged and motivated with his rehabilitation, further evidenced by his own idea to develop an 'annoying' code that would randomly change his laptop screen brightness as a strategy of external biofeedback to cue him to periodically check, and if necessary, correct, his shoulder girdle posture.
- Gym activity: For the next week, Hugo was encouraged to move from his three-times-per-week cardio training to lower extremity strength-training exercises. With three sessions fully dedicated to lower extremity training, Hugo was cautioned to take care with less obvious but still intensive glenohumeral loading activities that could aggravate his shoulder, such as loading a leg press (or other) machine with heavy weight plates or the use of excessive weight in a lying leg curl machine that could inadvertently cause extra grip force and 'cheating' with the upper extremity near the fully flexed knee curl position. Other lower extremity exercises that would more directly load his shoulders, such as the deadlift or squats, should be avoided for now. Additionally, Hugo was encouraged to use machines rather than free weights so that he would gain additional control during the execution, and if needed, he could immediately and safely suspend the exercise without having to control the free weights while struggling with his symptoms.

Reasoning Question:

5. How does your use of EMG and kinematic biofeedback relate to the motor-learning principles you referred to earlier?

Answer to Reasoning Question:

This session intended to build on motor skills practiced thus far and further challenge the cognitive stage through Hugo's scapulothoracic neutral zone awareness by using a variety of postural challenges during multi-planar movements while ensuring the co-activation of both lower trapezius and serratus anterior in low-load exercises. For example, Exercise 2 was specifically chosen to challenge Hugo's scapula stabilizers' activity while minimizing upper trapezius activity. Hugo's main difficulty was to avoid excess upper trapezius activity that has been demonstrated to occur at the expense of serratus anterior activity, as described in the literature, when performing this exercise (Ludewig et al., 2004). Given Hugo's results indicating that new neuromuscular skills were being slowly acquired, we also began associative stage training by progressively integrating the lower trapezius and serratus anterior co-activation with upper trapezius and simultaneous coordination with the glenohumeral muscles during shoulder multi-planar movements below 30 degrees of arm elevation. Hugo had clear difficulties in coordinating scapula kinematics and simultaneously exerting glenohumeral multi-planar force. This may have been due to Hugo's high-load strength-training history that preferentially biased the effectiveness of his neuromuscular control to high loads, thereby leaving him less effective at controlling low-load directional stability challenges.

Different authors have proposed several models of skill acquisition and motor (re)learning. One popular and now-classic model is centred on three cumulative and sequential stages labelled cognitive, associative and autonomous stages (Fitts and Posner, 1967). The first stage is characterized by the awareness of a specific activity or skill to be performed and how it should be performed. The second stage aims to start incorporating and refining multi-joint movements toward a specific pattern. During the autonomous stage, it is expected that a specific activity or skill becomes automatic. In this last stage, a low degree of cognitive processing is expected, allowing for multi-tasking and secondary attention to the environment. Augmented or external sources of feedback can be of great value in the first two stages of motor relearning. In the cognitive stage, both the external kinematic and EMG

Continued on following page

feedback were used to enhance Hugo's knowledge and awareness of how he was performing specific motor skills and his rate of success in achieving the agreed result. In the early associative-stage exercises, the use of both biofeedback systems also allowed him to ensure if he was achieving the correct scapula position with the desired levels of muscle activity while recruiting glenohumeral mobilizer muscles. This complementary and merged information proved to be of great value, not only by providing Hugo with additional information to the self-generated information from its sensory or internal feedback loops but also as a source of quantification of the knowledge of performance and result for the therapist based on which clinically informed decisions were made.

Appointment 3 (1 Week Later)

Re-Assessment

Two weeks after his first visit, Hugo's functioning level continued to improve, and his symptoms were now only exacerbated when applying additional pressure passively at the end of the glenohumeral flexion and abduction movements. Scapula neuromuscular control was seen via EMG for the first time in a feedforward pattern, and a general increase in muscle strength was evident on manual muscle testing. Both scapula orientation values at rest and during flexion and abduction were also seen for the first time inside the non-impaired published values (except scapula upward rotation, which was still decreased). Hugo reported he had completed all home-based prescribed exercises twice daily. After some hours, he successfully developed the code necessary to randomly alter his laptop brightness and was using that cue regularly to check and correct his shoulder girdle alignment as planned. His shoulder girdle posture was clearly benefiting from his reported adherence, with both of his glenohumeral joints less anteriorly positioned relative to the imaginary plumb line.

Again, with the aid of both EMG and kinematic systems, Hugo's performance on the scapula V-slide plus shoulder-resisted movements (<30 degrees) home exercise was re-assessed. Using the set muscle and kinematic parameters from last week's visit, Hugo reached a 9/10 success score with a perceived 'light' effort, corroborating Hugo's subjective report of improvement.

This session aimed to continue the associative-stage work begun last week: integrating the lower trapezius and serratus anterior co-activation with upper trapezius and simultaneous coordination with the glenohumeral muscles during shoulder multi-planar movements above 30 degrees of arm elevation.

- Exercise 1: Scapula V-slide plus shoulder movements (>30 degrees) – Using last week's Exercise 3 instructions, Hugo was asked to now elevate his arm to 90 degrees in the frontal, scapular and sagittal planes at a comfortable self-selected speed. Hugo graded his perceived effort during the first two sets of this exercise as 'moderate' and as 'light' for the last two sets, and he ended with a success score of 9/10.
- Exercise 2: Scapula V-slide plus shoulder-resisted movements (>30 degrees) (Fig. 27.6) – To Exercise 1, we added elastic resistance using a Thera-band that was able to increase Hugo's perceived effort to 'moderate' at 90 degrees of arm elevation. A success score of 7/10 was obtained.
- Exercise 3: Scapula V-slide plus shoulder isometric contractions – In a sitting position, Hugo was encouraged to reproduce the scapulae V-slide motion, maintain the scapulo-thoracic neutral zone (with a kinematic tolerance error of 5 degrees and equal electro-myographic levels described in last week's Exercise 1) while isometrically contracting his glenohumeral muscles against alternated low-load manual resistance to flexion/extension, abduction/adduction and internal/external rotation. With a classified perceived exertion of 'moderate' to 'somewhat-hard', Hugo finished with a success score of 8/10.
- Exercise 4: Knee push-up plus – From a standard push-up position, but with both knees on the ground, Hugo was asked to fully protract his shoulders at the end of the push-up. The action should be pain-free and executed at a comfortable self-selected speed, similar to last week's wall push-up plus exercise. A success score of 8/10 was obtained with a 'moderate' perceived exertion.
- Exercise 5: Scapula V-slide plus dynamic hug – While standing against the wall with both knees slightly flexed, feet hip-width apart and off the wall, elbows flexed, arms

Fig. 27.6 Scapula V-slide plus shoulder-resisted movements (>30 degrees) in the scapular plane.

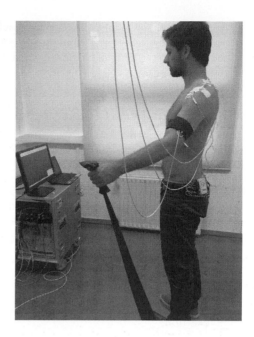

abducted at 60 degrees and internally rotated at 45 degrees, Hugo was asked to slide both scapulae in the same 'V' form and simulate a hugging action by horizontally flexing his arms until his hands touched each other, then to slowly return to the starting position. A success score of 9/10 was obtained with a light to moderate perceived exertion.

All exercises were performed using last week's dosage. The previous calculations for the scapulothoracic neutral zone when the arm is by the side were used for the target scapula orientation of the initial exercises. However, these calculations cannot be used for target scapula orientation when raising the arm. For this, a statistical regression model (de Groot and Brand, 2001) was implemented that, based on angles of humeral elevation, plane of elevation and shoulder girdle starting position, creates a 'normative' (i.e. to non-impaired individuals) reference (+/–5 degrees of error) for judging where the scapula should be (i.e. target scapula orientation) through humeral elevation. Hugo only had access to kinematic external feedback in sets 1 and 3, with feedback for sets 2 and 4 only available for the therapist to monitor Hugo's exercise performance and to access his success scores. This was done to minimize biofeedback dependency over Hugo's own internal feedback mechanisms. The main goal of this session was to push the complexity of the associative-stage training and bring it as close as possible to Hugo's bench-press exercise mechanics, with good scapulothoracic control and reduced rate of perceived exertion.

Re-assessment after in-clinic training revealed Hugo's clear improvements in coordinating his scapula kinematics and simultaneously exerting glenohumeral multi-planar force, evident from both his final success scores and from his rate of perceived exertion.

The home-based program was as follows:

- Scapula V-slide plus shoulder-resisted movements (>30 degrees) and the dynamic hug – To continue promoting the integrating of scapula stabilizer activity into multi-planar low-load and progressively high-load challenges, Hugo was asked to perform repetitions of Exercises 1 and 5 at least once a day, 4 sets × 10.
- Correction of shoulder girdle alignment – Hugo was asked to continue to use the laptop brightness cue he developed to check and then, as needed, modify his posture. With this, he was asked to note if he felt he had been in an incorrect posture for a long time before the stimulus or if he felt that he was periodically correcting his shoulder girdle posture anyway without the benefit of the screen stimulus.
- Gym activity: Hugo was encouraged to continue his gym activity. To maintain the three-times-per-week and avoid an exclusive and monotonous lower extremity training, we agreed to splitting the lower extremity workout into two, interspersed with a cardio

day. I urged Hugo to include the knee push-up plus and the elbow push-up plus exercises in his mat core exercises and to integrate his transversus abdominis and core abdominal muscle training he had already been doing as part of his previous gym training into these exercises.

Appointment 4 (1 Week Later)
Re-Assessment

At his fourth visit, Hugo was extremely motivated and confident with his progress. For the first time, he reported no symptoms during the last week. Both active and passive glenohumeral flexion and abduction range of movement were pain-free, and the muscle strength results were all tested as 5/5. SPADI and DASH scores continued to identify functional improvement. Hugo's scapular neuromuscular control from last week was maintained with a feedforward pattern, and for the first time, all scapulothoracic values during flexion and abduction were seen inside the expected values. When posture was assessed by observation, both of his glenohumeral joints were now almost aligned with the imaginary plumb line. Neer and Hawkins-Kennedy Impingement Tests were negative for pain provocation. A success score of 10/10 was obtained when re-assessing Hugo's performance during the scapula V-slide plus dynamic hug exercise, with a perceived 'very light' exertion.

Based on these results, the aim of this session was to continue working on function-related movements, with expected transfer of learning from the motor skills acquired in first two stages of motor relearning. For this purpose, his gym activities were (1) fragmented into less complex, achievable movements that were progressively trained while maintaining the activation of the stabilizers, and (2) challenging Hugo to maintain the activation of the scapula stabilizers during non-gym occupational and recreational activities.

- Exercise 1: Dynamic hug – equal to last week's Exercise 5.
- Exercise 2: Standard push-up plus and dumbbell bench press – Hugo was asked to perform a standard push-up or a dumbbell bench press, and when reaching full elbows' extension, to add a full shoulder protraction.
- Exercise 3: Dumbbell shoulder press – From a sitting-upright position with both dumbbells in front of the shoulders, Hugo was asked to push them above his head until his elbows were almost fully extended, then to slowly return to the initial position.
- Exercise 4: Multi-planar shoulder-resisted movements – This was to be performed similarly to last week's Exercise 2 but now with the arm elevated to 120 degrees. Additionally, resisted internal and external shoulder-rotation exercises were also performed with the arm at 0 degrees of flexion and elbow against the trunk.

All exercises were performed using last week's dosage and using the same statistical model to predict scapular target orientation during the exercises, with a tolerated error of 5 degrees. In this session, Hugo only had access to kinematic biofeedback in the first 10 repetitions. Dumbbells were used in Exercises 2 and 3 because they tend to increase exercise complexity throughout neuromuscular control and challenge coordination. By adding weights, Exercise 2 and 3 intensities were set to 'light' to 'moderate' for the first two sets and 'somewhat-hard' to 'hard' for the last two to effectively activate the lower trapezius and serratus anterior over the upper trapezius (Andersen et al., 2012). A success scored was obtained in all executions.

From the outcome results of this visit, Hugo effectively achieved all discharge criteria: pain 0/10 using the VNRS and with an overall function score below 2.67/100 for DASH and 3.66/100 for SPADI. The described physical therapy management facilitated a clinically significant increase in function, with a magnitude-of-function gain higher than 10.2 points and 13 points for the DASH and SPADI questionnaires, respectively. Scapula alignment and neuromuscular control and glenohumeral strength were now within their defined expected values. Only the sport-related score was still higher than expected due to the 'mild difficulty' (score 2/5) reported in 'playing your sport as well as you would like' and 'spending your usual amount of time practicing your sport'. We both agreed that it would be a matter of a week or so for him to confidently return to his normal gym routine.

The home-based program was as follows:

- Hugo was encouraged to incorporate the scapula V-slide form in all his upper extremity exercises and concentrate on neuromuscular control before increasing the exercises' intensity.
- Hugo was asked to maintain his shoulder girdle posture awareness and avoid long periods in the same position.

Both should be accomplished without the need for any type of external biofeedback. A follow-up visit was set for 3 months from now.

Appointment 5 (3 Months Later)

Primary and secondary outcome and special tests results for Hugo's five appointments are presented in Table 27.2. Differences in Hugo's scapulothoracic motion when compared to average normative values from non-impaired subjects (Lawrence et al., 2014) during arm abduction and flexion tasks at 30 degrees and 90 degrees of humerothoracic elevation measured over the five appointments are presented in Fig. 27.7. In this follow-up visit, Hugo reported no symptoms since appointment 4. All shoulder physiological movements were pain-free, muscle strength was maintained at 5/5 and all special tests were negative. Lower trapezius and serratus anterior onset activation were in a feedforward pattern, and scapulothoracic orientation values were maintained within published values. For the first time, SPADI and DASH scores were 0. Hugo reported he was regularly doing three-times-per-week gym training and that he found he was 'unconsciously' correcting his posture, mainly while seated (i.e. during classes). A success score of 10/10 was obtained when re-assessing Hugo's performance in the following exercises: scapula V-slide in prone, scapula V-slide in sitting, scapula V-slide sitting in front of a table, knee push-up plus, standard push-up plus, wall push-up plus, scapula V-slide plus shoulder movements (<30 degrees), scapula V-slide plus shoulder movements (>30 degrees), scapula V-slide plus dynamic hug, scapula V-slide plus dynamic hug exercise. All exercises were executed with a reported perceived 'very light' exertion. Table 27.2 gives an overview of the primary and secondary outcome and special test results assessed on weeks 1, 2, 3 and 4 and at the 3-month follow-up.

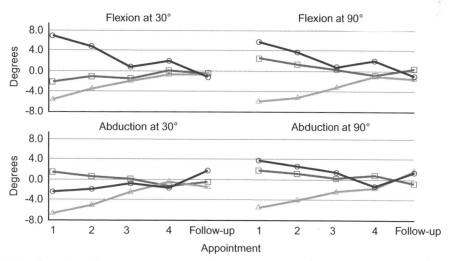

Fig. 27.7 Illustrating differences in Hugo's scapulothoracic motion when compared to average normative values from non-impaired subjects (Lawrence et al. 2014) during arm abduction and flexion tasks at 30 degrees and 90 degrees of humerothoracic elevation measured over the five appointments. Hugo initially demonstrated patterns of excessive scapular internal rotation (line with circle), decreased upward rotation (line with triangle) and slightly decreased posterior tilt (line with square) at the first appointment, with relative normalization of each of these dyskinesias over the course of the five appointments.

TABLE 27.2

OVERVIEW OF THE PRIMARY AND SECONDARY OUTCOMES AND SPECIAL TEST RESULTS ASSESSED AT WEEKS 1, 2, 3 AND 4 AND 3-MONTH FOLLOW-UP

	Pain	Function			Scapula Alignment	Scapula Neuromuscular Control		Scapula Kinematics		Muscle Strength		Special Tests	
	Worst	DASH Overall	DASH Sport	SPADI	Dif	Feedback	Feedforward	Abduction Dif	Flexion Dif	Scapulothoracic	Glenohumeral	Hawkins	Neer
Week 1	5/10	28.3/100	56.2/100	19.5	3.2	SA	LT	3,5/3,7	4,9/4,7	4/4	4/5/4+	+	+
Week 2	4/10	20/100	50/100	16.3	2.8	SA	LT	2,5/2,6	3,1/3,4	4/4	4/5/4+	+	+
Week 3	3/10	15.8/100	43.7/100	5.9	2.2		LT/SA	1,1/1,4	1,4/1,4	5/4+	4+/5/4+	+*	+*
Week 4	0/10	2.5/100	12.5/100	2.7/100	1.6		LT/SA	1,1/1,3	0,9/1,3	5/5	5/5/5	–	–
Follow-up	0/10	0/100	0/100	0/100	1.9		LT/SA	1,2/1,3	0,8/1,0	5/5	5/5/5	–	–

*Special tests only exacerbate symptoms in the end of range of movement (ROM) + additional pressure.
DASH, Disabilities of the Arm, Shoulder and Hand; Dif, mean difference between Hugo's scapulothoracic values and normative from non-impaired subjects (in degrees) at 30 degrees/90 degrees humerothoracic elevation; LT, lower trapezius; SA, serratus anterior; SPADI, Shoulder Pain and Disability Index.

Reasoning Question:

6. Please discuss your assessment of Hugo's progress and also your opinion of the variable time patients generally require given the varied extent of pain, physical impairment, body awareness and motivation patients present.

Answer to Reasoning Question:

Looking at the summary Table 27.2 and Fig. 27.7, we can conclude that Hugo had a positive response to treatment. In a recent systematic review of response to physiotherapy treatment for musculoskeletal shoulder pain (Chester et al., 2013), only two prognostic factors consistently demonstrated an association with physiotherapy outcome (i.e. pain, patient-rated functional outcomes, among others): duration of shoulder pain and baseline function. Based on this systematic review and on Hugo's initial assessment results, I predicted Hugo was likely to respond positively to physiotherapy treatment, not only because of his overall low baseline disability score that is associated with a better functional outcome but also because of his short duration of symptoms that is associated with a better outcome. I believe Hugo's level of body awareness due to his regular sport activity and his high level of motivation were also decisive for the success of this intervention focused on the movement system. Although I still think that Hugo's strength-training history did not enable him to quickly adapt and model his neuromuscular control to react against low-load directional stability challenges, I am deeply convinced that his broad sport-related and kinetic history led him to a level of body awareness and control that, with specific training, enabled him to adapt quickly to the motor-control learning tasks he was given.

Clinical Reasoning Commentary:

The systematic review cited regarding predicting response to physiotherapy treatment for musculoskeletal shoulder pain (Chester et al., 2013) identified only two consistent prognostic factors. However, as discussed in Chapter 1, other prognostic considerations that also should be considered at the level of the individual patient broadly include the nature and extent of patients' problem(s) and their ability and willingness to make the necessary changes (e.g. lifestyle, psychosocial contributing factors, physical contributing factors) to facilitate recovery or improved quality of life.

Clues will be available throughout the subjective and physical examination and the ongoing management, including the following:

- Patient's perspectives and expectations (including readiness, motivation and confidence to make changes)
- External incentives (e.g. return to work) and disincentives (e.g. litigation, lack of employer support)
- Extent of activity/participation restrictions
- Nature of problem (e.g. systemic disorder such as rheumatoid arthritis versus local ligamentous such as ankle sprain)
- Extent of 'pathology' and physical impairments
- Social, occupational and economic status
- Dominant pain type present
- Stage of tissue healing
- Irritability of the disorder
- Length of history and progression of disorder
- Patient's general health, age and pre-existing disorders

REFERENCES

Andersen, C., Zebis, M., Saervoll, C., Sundstrup, E., Jakobsen, M., Sjøgaard, G., et al., 2012. Scapular muscle activity from selected strengthening exercises performed at low and high intensities. J. Strength Cond. Res. 26 (9), 2408–2416.

Aruin, A.S., Latash, M.L., 1995. Directional specificity of postural muscles in feed-forward postural reactions during fast voluntary arm movements. Exp. Brain Res. 103, 323–332.

Bae, Y.H., Lee, G.C., Shin, W.S., et al., 2011. Effect of motor control and strengthening exercises on pain, function, strength and the range of motion of patients with shoulder impingement syndrome. J. Phys. Ther. Sci. 23 (4), 687–692.

Barth, J.R.H., Burkhart, S.S., de Beer, J.F., 2006. 2004 The Bear-Hug test: a new and sensitive test for diagnosing a subscapularis tear. Arthroscopy 22 (10), 1076–1084.

Başkurt, Z., Başkurt, F., Gelecek, N., Özkan, M.H., 2011. The effectiveness of scapular stabilization exercise in the patients with subacromial impingement syndrome. J. Back Musculoskelet. Rehabil. 24, 173–179.

Burkhart, S.S., Morgan, C.D., Kibler, W.B., 2000. Shoulder injuries in overhead athletes. The 'dead arm' revisited. Clin. Sports Med. 19, 125–158.

Chester, R., Shepstone, L., Daniell, H., Sweeting, D., Lewis, J., Jerosch-Herold, C., 2013. Predicting response to physiotherapy treatment for musculoskeletal shoulder pain: a systematic review. BMC Musculoskelet. Disord. 14, 203.

Comerford, M.J., Mottram, S.L., 2001. Functional stability re-training: principles and strategies for managing mechanical dysfunction. Man. Ther. 6 (1), 3–14.

Comerford, M., Mottram, S., 2012. Kinetic Control: The Management of Uncontrolled Movement, first ed. Churchill Livingstone, Edinburgh.

Crow, J., Pizzari, T., Buttifani, D., 2011. Muscle onset can be improved by therapeutic exercise: a systematic review. Phys. Ther. Sport 12 (4), 199–209.

de Groot, J.H., Brand, R., 2001. A three-dimensional regression model of the shoulder rhythm. Clin. Biomech. 16 (9), 735–743.

Delp, S.L., Anderson, F.C., Arnold, A.S., Loan, P., Habib, A., John, C.T., et al., 2007. OpenSim: open-source software to create and analyze dynamic simulations of movement. IEEE Trans. Biomed. Eng. 54 (11), 1940–1950.

Dvir, Z., Berme, N., 1978. The shoulder complex in elevation of the arm: a mechanism approach. J. Biomech. 1, 219.

Ekstrom, R.A., Donatelli, R.A., Soderberg, G.L., 2003. Surface electromyographic analysis of exercises for the trapezius and serratus anterior muscles. J. Orthop. Sports Phys. Ther. 33 (5), 247–258.

Fitts, P.M., Posner, M.I., 1967. Human Performance. Brooks/Cole Pub. Co., Belmont, CA.

Gerber, C., Krushell, R.J., 1991. Isolated rupture of the tendon of the subscapularis muscle: clinical features in 16 cases. J. Bone Joint Surg. Br. 73B, 389–394.

Glover, S., 2004. Separate visual representations in the planning and control of action. Behav. Brain Sci. 27 (1), 3–78.

Haik, M.N., Alburquerque-Sendín, F., Camargo, P.R., 2014. Reliability and minimal detectable change of 3-dimensional scapular orientation in individuals with and without shoulder impingement. J. Orthop. Sports Phys. Ther. 44 (5), 341–349.

Hawkins, R.J., Kennedy, J.C., 1980. Impingement syndrome in athletes. Am. J. Sports Med. 8, 151–158.

Karduna, A.R., McClure, P.W., Michener, L.A., Sennett, B., 2001. Dynamic measurements of three-dimensional scapular kinematics: a validation study. J. Biomech. Eng. 123, 184–190.

Kendall, F., McCreary, E., Provance, P., 1993. Upper extremity and shoulder girdle strength tests. In: Kendall, F., McCreary, E., Provance, P. (Eds.), Muscles: Testing and Function, With Posture and Pain, fourth ed. Williams and Wilkins, Baltimore, Maryland, pp. 235–298.

Kibler, W.B., Ludewig, P.M., McClure, P.W., et al., 2013. Clinical implications of scapular dyskinesis in shoulder injury: the 2013 consensus statement from the 'scapular summit'. Br. J. Sports Med. 47, 877–885.

Kim, S.H., Ha, K.I., Ahn, J.H., Kim, S.H., Cho, H.J., 2001. Biceps Load Test II: a clinical test for SLAP lesions of the shoulder. Arthroscopy 17 (2), 160–164.

Lawrence, R.L., Braman, J.P., Laprade, R.F., Ludewig, P.M., 2014. Comparison of 3-dimensional shoulder complex kinematics in individuals with and without shoulder pain, part 1: sternoclavicular, acromioclavicular, and scapulothoracic joints. J. Orthop. Sports Phys. Ther. 44 (9), 636–645.

Leal, S., Cavalheiro, L., 2001. Constant Score and Shoulder Pain and Disability Index (SPADI) – Cultural and linguistic adaptation. [thesis]. Portugal: School of Technology and Healthcare of the Coimbra Polytechnic Institute.

Lewis, J.S., 2009. Rotator cuff tendinopathy/subacromial impingement syndrome: is it time for a new method of assessment? Br. J. Sports Med. 43, 259–264.

Ludewig, P.M., Cook, T.M., 2000. Alterations in shoulder kinematics and associated muscle activity in people with symptoms of shoulder impingement. Phys. Ther. 80, 276–291.

Ludewig, P.M., Hoff, M.S., Osowski, E.E., Meschke, S.A., Rundquist, P.J., 2004. Relative balance of serratus anterior and upper trapezius muscle activity during push-up exercises. Am. J. Sports Med. 32 (2), 484–493.

Ludewig, P.M., Reynolds, J.F., 2009. The association of scapular kinematics and glenohumeral joint pathologies. J. Orthop. Sports Phys. Ther. 39 (2), 90–104.

Lui, S.H., Henry, M.H., Nuccion, S.L., 1996. A prospective evaluation of a new physical examination in predicting glenoid labral tears. Am. J. Sports Med. 24 (6), 721–725.

MacDermid, J.C., Ghobrial, M., Quiron, K.B., et al., 2007. Validation of a new test that assesses functional performance of the upper extremity and neck (FIT-HaNASA) in patients with shoulder pathology. BMC Musculoskelet. Disord. 8, 42.

Magarey, M.E., Jones, M.A., 2003. Dynamic evaluation and early management of altered motor control around the shoulder complex. Man. Ther. 84, 195–206.

Magarey, M.E., Jones, M.A., 2003a. Specific evaluation of the function of force couples relevant for stabilization of the glenohumeral joint. Man. Ther. 8 (4), 247–253.

Magarey, M.E., Jones, M.A., 2003b. Dynamic evaluation and early management of altered motor control around the shoulder complex. Man. Ther. 8 (4), 195–206.

Mottram, S.L., 1997. Dynamic stability of the scapula. Man. Ther. 2, 123–131.

Neer, C.S., Welsh, R.P., 1977. The shoulder in sports. Orthop. Clin. North Am. 8, 583–591.

O'Brien, S.J., Pagnani, M.J., Fealy, S., McGlynn, S.R., Wilson, J.B., 1998. The active compression test: a new and effective test for diagnosing labral tears and acromioclavicular joint abnormality. Am. J. Sports Med. 26 (5), 610–614.

Roy, J.S., Moffet, H., McFadyen, B.J., et al., 2009. Impact of movement training on upper limb motor strategies in persons with shoulder impingement syndrome. Sports Med. Arthrosc. Rehabil. Ther. Technol. 1, 8.

Santos, J., Gonçalves, R., 2006. Cultural adaptation and validation of Portuguese version of the Disabilities of the Arm, Shoulder and Hand – DASH. [thesis]. Portugal: School of Technology and Healthcare of the Porto Polytechnic Institute.

Scheibel, M., Magosch, P., Pritsch, M., Lichtenberg, S., Habermeyer, P., 2005. The Belly-Off sign: a new clinical diagnostic sign for subscapularis lesions. Arthroscopy 21 (10), 1229–1235.

Seth, A., Matias, R., Veloso, A., Delp, S., 2016. A biomechanical model of the scapulothoracic joint to accurately capture scapula kinematics during shoulder movements. PLoS ONE 11 (1).

Shumway-Cook, A., Woolacott, J., 2001. Motor learning and recovery of function. In: Shumway-Cook, A., Woolacott, J. (Eds.), Motor Control: Theory and Practical Applications, second ed. Lippincott, Philadelphia.

Smart, K., Blake, C., Staines, A., Thacker, M., Doody, C., 2012. Mechanisms-based classifications of musculoskeletal pain: Part 3 of 3: symptoms and signs of nociceptive pain in patients with low back (+/-leg) pain. Man. Ther. 17, 352–357.

Struyf, F., Nijs, J., Mollekens, S., et al., 2013. Scapular-focused treatment in patients with shoulder impingement syndrome: a randomized clinical trial. Clin. Rheumatol. 32, 73–85.

Worsley, P., Warner, M., Mottram, S., Gadola, S., Veeger, H.E., Hermens, H., et al., 2013. Motor control retraining exercises for shoulder impingement: effects on function, muscle activation, and biomechanics in young adults. J. Shoulder Elbow Surg. 22 (4), 11–19.

Wu, G., van der Helm, F.C.T., Veeger, H.E.J.D., et al., 2005. ISB recommendation on definitions of joint coordinate systems of various joints for the reporting of human joint motion-Part II: shoulder, elbow, wrist and hand. J. Biomech. 38, 981–992.

28

Acute Exacerbation of Chronic Low Back Pain With Right-Leg Numbness in a Crop Farmer

Christopher R. Showalter • Darren A. Rivett • Mark A. Jones

Subjective Examination

Bob was a 52-year-old crop farmer. He was happily married and the father of two teenage children. Bob routinely worked 12- to 14-hour days on his 1800 acres, operating various pieces of equipment and machinery, which primarily involved prolonged sitting while operating the equipment. The sitting was interspersed with attaching and detaching heavy implements from the machines and occasional lifting of loads as heavy as 125 lb. His lifestyle was essentially sedentary for long hours, and he did not play any sports or perform any regular exercise.

Bob was referred to our clinic at the insistence of his friend, a previous patient of the clinic, and began the first session by stating, 'I'm here to see if anything can be done about my back problem'. He said he felt our consultation would 'probably not help much', as his regular chiropractor was unable to help with the pain. It was put to Bob that there was no harm in obtaining a second opinion, and he agreed to continue. He explained that he had been having low back pain (LBP) and some numbness in the right leg for 12 weeks.

Area, Nature and Type of Pain

Bob described his pain as 6/10 (on a numerical pain rating scale) throughout the day on most days, which increased to 8/10 at night. His pain was worse in the morning (8–9/10). He reported 'deep, sharp, biting' pain and a 'tight pulling' in the right lower back and pointed to the area of L4–L5 on the right. He also reported numbness in the right anterior thigh and the lateral and posterior calf, as well as a feeling of weakness or 'giving way' in his right leg (Fig. 28.1).

Bob generally retired to bed around 10.00 pm after taking 750 mg of acetaminophen (nonopioid analgesic), 15 mg of oxycodone (opioid analgesic) and 5 mg of prednisone (steroidal anti-inflammatory) that had been prescribed by his primary care physician 2 days earlier. He usually preferred to sleep on his back, but in recent months he had found he could only get comfortable lying on his left side. He usually awoke at approximately 2.00 am with 8/10 pain and took more acetaminophen and oxycodone. Bob reported he could not find a comfortable position in bed to get back to sleep, so he tried to sleep in a reclining chair to avoid waking his wife. He slept fitfully and finally awoke in the morning around 6.00 am with 8–9/10 pain and feeling stiff, like his 'back is rusty'. He continued the drug regime three more times throughout the day, including before bed, as the pain became more intense. Bob was concerned with the amount and type of medications he felt he was 'forced to take to remain working'. He was particularly concerned at the prospect of becoming addicted to oxycodone.

Pain Behavior and Irritability

Bob reported that his LBP was at its worst (8–9/10) in the morning upon waking. He reported that he was able to reduce the morning pain with a hot shower, medications and

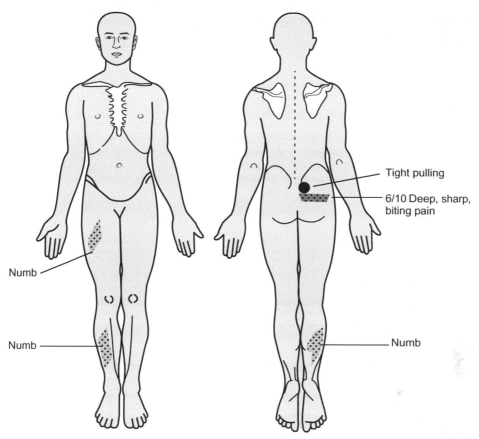

Fig. 28.1 Body chart depicting symptoms.

'getting moving' soon afterward. The LBP varied throughout the day, although it was generally a 6/10, and became worse with prolonged postures of inactivity, including sitting in tractors or cultivator machinery for more than 30 minutes or standing for more than 15 minutes. Once elevated, the pain took approximately 1 hour to settle back to baseline levels, provided he discontinued static sitting and standing postures and 'kept his back moving' with slow gentle walking. Bob took his medications as prescribed but often self-prescribed an additional 750 mg of acetaminophen two to three times a day when his pain was elevated. He felt the need to keep moving and get his lower back 'lubricated' to feel better. As a consequence of his pain behavior, Bob had modified his workday schedule to involve sitting for no more than 30 minutes and standing for no more than 15 minutes. These activities were broken up with periods of slowly walking short distances, for approximately 2–3 minutes. This eased his pain to 4/10, but the relief was short-lived. This schedule was significantly affecting his productivity at work.

Reasoning Question:

1. Can you please outline what your thoughts were at this early stage of the consultation? In particular, can you comment on the type of the pain in this case?

Answer to Reasoning Question:

The key nature of Bob's disorder was disability. His disorder was substantially affecting his lifestyle, sleep and ability to work and provide for his family. This was evident in that he reported he had increasing trouble climbing in and out of trucks, tractors and cultivators due to the 'weakness and feeling of giving way' in his right leg. Bob reported that relatively simple tasks seemed to take greater effort and increase his pain as he performed them. This resulted in his further need to take medication.

Continued on following page

The kind of pain Bob reported had components of both a nociceptive patho-mechanical (stiff-dominant) type of pain and a nociceptive patho-inflammatory (pain-dominant) type of pain (Maitland, 2005a). Mechanical nociceptive pain is typically characterized by pain with movements, particularly toward the end of range, and the pain of a mechanical problem limits normal range. Mechanical pain and range of movement often improve with active or passive movement and are generally worse at the end of the day. Mechanical pain is normally produced by tissue that is compressed, stretched or tightened beyond its usual limits. It may awaken the patient at night and usually subsides rapidly after a change in sleeping position, upon which the patient returns to sleep quickly.

Patho-inflammatory nociceptive pain is usually characterized by pain in the early to mid-range of movement and is exacerbated with some movements, unless the movement is in a particular preferred direction. Inflammatory pain may be chemically mediated, centrally evoked or both. Inflammatory pain is usually worse after rest or inactivity, particularly first thing in the morning after sleep. Inflammatory pain may awaken the patient at night, who often has difficulty returning to sleep, in spite of repeated attempts to alter sleeping position.

Bob exhibited characteristics of both kinds of pain, with inflammatory pain predominating at this time.

Reasoning Question:

2. It appears Bob's condition is quite irritable. Can you please discuss your reasoning processes with respect to this and how you planned to modify your physical examination as a result?

Answer to Reasoning Question:

Maitland (2005a) described the concept of irritability as the patient's response to movement in terms of three interrelated factors: (1) how much activity, or how vigorously a certain activity is performed; (2) how much symptom provocation is evoked; and (3) the duration for the symptoms to return to baseline levels. The inherent value of the concept of irritability is that it guides the vigor of both the physical examination and the subsequent treatment of the patient. A patient with an irritable presentation may require a modified physical examination whereby not all movements and tests are performed, and only essential components of movement are examined. The patient must be properly instructed not to move beyond the first onset of the pain (P1). Similarly, the therapist may not wish to fully reproduce the patient's pain, as doing so may lead to exacerbation of symptoms that will take some time to settle back to baseline levels or may lead to termination of the examination or potentially mask other examination results. Treatment in the management of an irritable presentation may also need to be modified to use only a limited number of bouts of intervention, performed briefly, and in early to mid-range of available pain-free movement. A bout of intervention is the amount of time taken to apply a specific intervention (i.e. 30 seconds). Thus, irritable presentations often respond to short bouts (20–30 seconds) and a limited number of bouts (two or three) at any given treatment session. Attempting to achieve greater gains in the early management of an irritable problem may lead to exacerbation of symptoms and regression from the previous session's gains in pain, range of movement (ROM) and function. A useful heuristic is to consider that 'all problems are considered irritable until proven otherwise'. This concept helps to ensure that patients are not overly examined or treated on day 1. The true degree of irritability becomes more evident at treatment 2, during which specific questioning is directed to the patient regarding his or her symptom response: (1) immediately following treatment, (2) a few hours after treatment, (3) during sleep hours, (4) first thing in the morning and (5) upon return for treatment. This information allows for a more in-depth understanding of the true irritability.

Bob's condition was irritable, as was evidenced by his report of relatively short periods of sitting or standing resulting in increased pain that remains at an elevated level for some time, even up to 1 hour. The concept of irritability has been shown to have moderate inter-rater reliability (Barakatt et al., 2009a). It has been suggested that validated measures of LBP characteristics in current clinical use, such as the Roland-Morris Disability Questionnaire, may adequately capture Maitland's concept of irritability (Barakatt et al., 2009b). A 2012 randomized controlled trial (RCT; Cook et al., 2012a) found that in patients with LBP, the presence of irritability at the initial evaluation was a negative prognostic indicator across the domains of (1) Oswestry Disability Index, (2) numerical pain rating scale, (3) reported rate of recovery and (4) total visits and days in care.

Clinical Reasoning Commentary:

As discussed in Chapter 1, the three main types of pain musculoskeletal clinicians need to be able to assess for and recognize are nociceptive pain (with and without inflammation), neuropathic pain and maladaptive central nervous system (CNS) sensitization, or nociplastic pain (e.g. Gifford et al., 2006; IASP, 2017; Nijs et al., 2014; Wolf, 2011). The description of Bob's pain provided here is consistent with a nociceptive-dominant 'pain type'.

The analysis regarding irritability informs the hypothesis category judgements regarding 'precautions and contraindications to physical examination and treatment'. As discussed in Chapter 1, and consistent with this answer, this clinical judgement informs the following:

- Whether a physical examination should be carried out at all (versus immediate referral for further medical consultation/investigation) and if so, the extent of examination that can be safely performed that will minimize the risk of aggravating the patient's symptoms
- Whether specific safety tests are indicated (e.g. cervical arterial dysfunction testing, neurological examination, blood pressure/heart rate, instability tests, etc.)
- Whether any treatment should be undertaken (versus referral for further consultation/investigation)
- The appropriate dose/strength of any physical interventions planned

Aggravating and Easing Factors

Bob reported that the factors that aggravated his condition included sitting, bending backward and standing. His pain could occasionally be relieved by bending forward while sitting or walking for short periods. Although these movements might reduce his pain slightly, they provided only short-term relief.

Past and Present History

Bob had received chiropractic treatment monthly for approximately 18 years. He generally had visited the chiropractor once per month but sometimes more depending on how his back was feeling. The treatment had routinely comprised thrust manipulation to his lumbar, thoracic and cervical spinal areas. He had not been instructed in any post-treatment care or home exercise program. He felt that the chiropractor gave him some relief that lasted for 2–3 days, but he wondered why his back never seemed to get better to the point that he was pain-free.

Bob stated that he had a 'bad manipulation' in the lumbar spine approximately 4 years ago, resulting in significant LBP and 2 weeks of total bed rest. He felt his back 'has never felt the same since'. He changed chiropractors at that time and continued with monthly treatment.

Twelve weeks prior, Bob started to experience increased intensity of LBP and the onset of numbness in his right leg. There was no event to precipitate these changes. Bob sought chiropractic treatment two to three times per week for 8 weeks with two different chiropractors. Bob had discontinued these chiropractic treatments for the 4 weeks prior to his consultation for physical therapy and had seen his primary care physician 2 days earlier because the pain had become 'unbearable' and the numbness seemed to be getting worse. The physician ordered medications and magnetic resonance imaging (MRI) of the lumbar spine.

Medication and Special Questions

Bob took 20 mg of prednisone four times daily (QID), 750 mg of acetaminophen QID, and 15 mg of oxycodone QID for his LBP. Bob took no other medications and had no general health problems or red flags. He denied any symptoms of spinal cord compression or cauda equina syndromes. No prior imagery of the spine was available.

Imaging

An MRI scan had been ordered but not performed due to the cost involved.

Self-Report Questionnaires

Bob completed a number of self-report forms, with the following results at baseline prior to treatment:

- Numerical pain rating scale (NPRS): Current pain 6/10; 'Worse in morning (8/10)' (Interpretation: moderate pain)
- Modified Oswestry Disability Index (Modified ODI): 56% (Interpretation: severe disability)

- Fear-Avoidance Beliefs Questionnaire (Work subset) (FABQW): 24/42 (Interpretation: some degree of fear and avoidance beliefs shown by the patient)

Reasoning Question:

3. Were there any psychosocial issues that you considered relevant in this case? If so, how may these impact on the overall diagnosis, management and prognosis?

Answer to Reasoning Question:

Bob was the epitome of the stoic farmer. He was willing to endure pain, with minimal complaining, to get his work done. He was eager for pain relief and to get on with his life. He was concerned about potential drug addiction and further deteriorating LBP that would adversely impact his farming and hence his family's financial security. There was no evidence of secondary benefit or yellow flags attributable to his condition. There was a barrier to overcome from the onset of the initial examination, with Bob expressing skepticism about the potential value of physical therapy intervention given that multiple chiropractic visits had not helped. I made it a deliberate point early in our first treatment to explain that the two disciplines are different and that my intention was to not only offer him pain relief through treatments but also strategies to deal with his pain when he was at work and, most importantly, specific strategies and home exercises that he could perform to maximize his rehabilitation and potentially minimize further deterioration and the need for further physical therapy or other care.

Another barrier to overcome was the 18-year treatment history with emphasis on the patient passively submitting to interventions performed upon him, with little advice regarding home care of his spine or the value of general or specific exercises for the low back. The important role of the patient as a collaborative decision-maker in the rehabilitative process would be required to be emphasized as well as the value of a regular exercise program.

Important components of Bob's treatment would therefore need to address his concerns about his condition, educate him in the nature of his condition, empower and encourage him to adopt strategies for self-treatment and emphasize the inherent value of his positive mental attitude and motivation to improve his situation.

Reasoning Question:

4. Can you discuss your clinical hypotheses following the subjective examination? Was there any particular structure you used as a means of planning the physical examination?

Answer to Reasoning Question:

Many therapists using the 'Maitland-Australian concept' find it valuable to 'filter' the subjective data from the patient history through the eight clinical hypothesis categories (Jones and Rivett, 2004) as a valuable aid in planning the physical examination. This intermediate and ongoing step allows for reflection on the pertinent clinical data and an opportunity to plan the physical examination appropriately. The clinical hypotheses confirmed, modified, denied, or newly formed in this step are tested in the physical examination. The eight categories in relation to this case are presented in the following subsections.

1. Capabilities and Restrictions

Capabilities:

- Can drive machinery for up to 30 minutes
- Can recognize onset of increasing symptoms, then discontinue working and walk briefly to prevent further increase in pain
- Able to modify schedule to get most of daily work done

Restrictions:

- Cannot drive machinery longer than 30 minutes
- Modified work schedule causing longer hours at work to complete all daily duties
- Unable to sleep through the night in a bed

Recognizing these capabilities and restrictions allows the therapist and patient to collaboratively set realistic benchmarks for re-assessment and both short- and long-term goals, and furthermore, it promotes using functional measures of overall improvement in terms that are meaningful to the patient.

2. Patient Perspectives

Sacket described evidence-based medicine, also known as evidence-based practice (EBP), as the 'the integration of best available research evidence WITH clinical expertise AND patient values' (Sackett, 1998).

Bob was highly motivated and had strong prognostic indicators in his favor. Skepticism regarding the role and potential effectiveness of physical therapy was an early barrier to overcome. Patient education and developing a collaborative relationship between therapist and patient was an important early goal with this patient. It was important to encourage Bob to become involved in the decision-making process regarding his condition and to stimulate his active participation in the rehabilitation of the disorder. Particular emphasis needed to be made to empower him to understand the value of self-treatment and an ongoing appropriate exercise regime.

3. Mechanisms of Symptom Production

- Peripheral symptoms of lumbar origin were present.
- Central symptoms were unclear at the time.
- Autonomic symptoms were unclear at the time.
- Negative affective symptoms appeared unlikely at the time.

4. Sources of Symptoms

There was evidence of both mechanical and inflammatory pain. The potential likely tissue sources were as follows: lumbar disc, nerve root impingement, compression and/or adhesion, spondylosis and osteoarthritis (OA) of the lumbar vertebrae and zygapophyseal (facet) joints, neurodynamic abnormalities, muscle spasm, tightness, weakness and functional spinal instability (motor control dysfunction).

5. Contributing or Predisposing Factors

Contributing factors were as follows: ergonomic design of various machinery used, time frames spent in specific postures, nature of farm work (prolonged sitting, heavy lifting, long hours).

Predisposing factors were as follows: poor posture, sedentary lifestyle and lack of regular exercise.

6. Precautions and Contraindications to Physical Therapy Examination and Treatment

Bob had an irritable presentation; thus, it was important to limit the initial physical examination to essential components only, limit vigor and carefully monitor symptoms. No other precautions or contraindications were found.

The stability of the disorder was unknown at this time. It was appropriate to be prudently careful until more information was known about Bob's condition and, in particular, his response to initial treatment. As previously stated, irritability was assumed to be a significant factor until proven otherwise.

7. Management

Bob had experienced numerous treatments of thrust manipulation over many years; therefore, it was reasonable to consider the potential for iatrogenic (intervention-induced) spinal segmental laxity in ligamentous, capsular and other structures. Thrust manipulation was unlikely to be offered at this time. The patient denied any prior advice or prescription of exercises designed for lumbar mobility, pain relief or segmental stabilization and neuromuscular control. It was likely that Bob had compromised motor control of his lumbar spine stability due to numerous factors already identified, namely, sedentary work, lack of routine exercises and so forth.

8. Prognosis

Bob exhibited certain characteristics that were positive prognostic indicators overall. He was gainfully self-employed, was in a stable and loving relationship, was in good general health, had a positive personality and sincerely desired to get well and get on with life and the farm work he enjoyed.

There were also negative prognostic indicators. These included the severity and chronicity of his condition, which seemed to be progressive in nature and displayed peripheral symptoms of spinal origin, an ODI score of 56% indicating severe disability and an FABQW score of 24/42. As previously stated, irritability was a negative prognostic indicator across a number of domains (Cook et al., 2012a).

Reasoning Question:

5. Your subjective examination gave you a means of planning your physical examination. Can you discuss more specifically the purpose of your physical examination and perhaps how the Maitland approach is utilized in this part of the assessment?

Answer to Reasoning Question:

Within the context of the Maitland concept, the purpose of the physical examination was as follows:

- Confirm, reject or modify clinical hypotheses developed during the subjective examination.
- Develop new hypotheses during the physical examination.
- Establish movements to be used as benchmarks for subsequent re-assessment.
- Reproduce the patient's 'comparable sign'.
- Identify potential treatment techniques.

Geoffrey Maitland first described the concept of the comparable sign (CS) in 1971 (Maitland, 1971) as 'reproduction of the patient's pain with movement', which he further refined in 1991 (Maitland, 1991) as, 'The aim of physical examination is to provoke, with test movements, either an abnormal

Continued on following page

response in an appropriate [anatomical] site, or, when suited to the disorder, reproduce the symptoms'. Comparable sign is one of the core tenets of the Maitland approach to manual therapy. The test movements Maitland referred to in his writings include active physiological movements, passive physiological movements, passive accessory movements and any spontaneous movement the patient can perform to affect his or her symptoms. Thus, CSs are physical examination findings related to the patient's chief complaint that are reproduced during examination and subsequent treatment. These findings include observed abnormalities of movement, postures or motor control deficits, abnormal responses to movement, static deformities and abnormal joint assessment findings. The CS is most commonly accompanied by the patient's verbal report and confirmation of symptoms of the patient's primary complaint. The CS has been shown to have construct validity (Cook et al., 2015). The concept of the CS is a valuable component of a clinical decision-making process. Within-session and between-session changes in the CS after the second visit have a significant association with positive outcomes for pain and ODI at discharge. A 2-point change (or better) in pain is associated with a 50%, or greater, reduction in ODI at discharge (Cook et al., 2012b).

Clinical Reasoning Commentary:

The hypothesis categories framework was initially proposed by Jones (1987) and has continued to evolve through professional discussion. As highlighted in Chapter 1, it is not necessary or even appropriate to stipulate a definitive list of clinical judgements all clinicians must consider, as this would only stifle the independent and creative thinking important to the evolution of our professions. However, a minimum list of categories of decisions that can/should be considered is helpful to those learning and reflecting on their clinical reasoning because it provides them with initial guidance to understand the purpose of their questions and physical assessments, encourages breadth of reasoning beyond diagnosis and creates a framework in which clinical knowledge can be organized as it relates to decisions that must be made (i.e. diagnosing, understanding patients' perspectives, determining therapeutic interventions, establishing rapport/therapeutic alliance, collaborating, teaching, prognosis and managing ethical dilemmas). The hypothesis categories presented and discussed in Chapter 1 have been modified slightly since the Jones and Rivett (2004) publication.

With respect to the Maitland concept, many of the key principles embedded in contemporary clinical reasoning theory emanated from his concept (see Jones [2014]). Maitland always insisted on a systematic and comprehensive patient examination that, in his words, 'enables you to live the patient's symptoms over 24 hours'. All patient information regarding the problem, its effects on the patient's life and the associated physical impairments found on physical examination had to be analyzed with the aim of 'making features fit'. Patient treatments were never recipes or protocols; rather, specific treatments were based on thorough analysis of the subjective (i.e. patient interview) and physical findings combined with knowledge of research, clinical patterns, treatment strategies that had been successful for similar presentations and systematic re-assessment of all interventions. Although Maitland did not refer to this process of information gathering, analysis, decision-making, intervention and re-assessment as clinical reasoning, it clearly was a structured and logical approach in line with contemporary clinical reasoning theory. Consistent with the aim of contemporary EBP, his 'Brick Wall' concept emphasized consideration of both research and experienced-based evidence, with the research providing a general guide, and the patient's unique presentation determining how that research was applied and ultimately the specific interventions to trial. In particular, he cautioned about over-focusing on pathology that can present differently in different patients and may be asymptomatic. When Maitland still practiced and taught, pain science theory was considerably less developed than now, with much of the understanding then relating to the original gate-control theory of pain and the effects of different treatment modalities, including manual therapy. Similarly, assessment and management of psychosocial factors in musculoskeletal practice have evolved considerably to being more explicit and more structured, with greater appreciation of the influence that distress from psychosocial factors can have on patients' pain and disability. However, when you consider the following direct quote from Maitland, his reference to 'personal commitment (empathy) to understand what the person (patient)' is a direct acknowledgment of the importance of understanding psychosocial factors, simply expressed in different terms with less explicit assessment strategies than we now teach:

The Maitland concept requires open-mindedness, mental agility and mental discipline linked with a logical and methodical process of assessing cause and effect. The central theme demands a positive personal commitment (empathy) to understand what the person (patient) is enduring. The key issues of 'the concept' that require explanation are personal commitment, mode of thinking, techniques, examination and assessment. (Maitland, 1987, p. 136)

Physical Examination
Observation

Bob was examined in a pair of shorts. In standing with feet shoulder-width apart, decreased lumbar lordosis and bilateral paravertebral muscle wasting were observed. A slight shift to the left (contralateral to the right-sided pain) was observed in standing. Shoulder height, scapular position, arm position, gluteal folds, popliteal creases and Achilles tendon alignment were all within normal limits (WNL). The right upper limb showed slightly more muscle hypertrophy than the left (Bob was right-handed). Muscle development was WNL in both lower limbs.

Neurological Examination

Resting pain prior to examination was 6/10. Testing was performed in supine without pillows. The left leg was WNL. On the affected (right) limb, deep tendon reflexes (DTRs) were 1+ at the patellar ligament (indicating potential L4 involvement) and WNL at the Achilles (S1). Sensation testing was performed with eyes closed, and the patient reported when he could feel sensation. Sensation loss was reported as a percentage of normal compared to the other limb. Light touch sensation was tested using cotton swabs, and deficits were found in the anterolateral thigh at 60% sensation, lateral tibia at 60% sensation and the lower calf displaying 80% sensation. These deficits in a dermatomal pattern were suggestive of involvement of the L4 and L5 nerve roots, respectively. Resisted movement was used to test motor function, and resisted knee extension was 4/5 implicating L3 and L4. No atrophy, increased resting tone, or pathological reflexes were observed in either limb, and Babinski signs and clonus were negative bilaterally, ruling out upper-motor-neuron involvement.

Active Physiological Movements

The patient was properly instructed to immediately report any feelings, sensations, symptoms and, particularly, LBP that he experienced during any test movements. He was instructed to not proceed with any movement beyond the initial onset of his pain (P1). Resting pain was 6/10.

Prior to testing active physiological movements, (R) glide correction of the (L) shift deformity was performed in standing. Glide correction involves gently gliding the shoulders to the right while pulling the pelvis to the left, while avoiding any lateral flexion, and evaluating symptom response.

Glide correction in neutral flexion/extension immediately increased his LBP from a 6/10 to 7/10, and his lumbar paraspinal musculature began to spasm. Glide correction in slight extension immediately increased pain from 6/10 to 8/10, with increased spasm. Glide correction in slight lumbar flexion did not affect his pain levels or cause spasm, and he moved more freely and smoothly. The shift was slightly improved upon return to standing (Fig. 28.2).

Active physiological lumbar movements were performed in standing and produced significant findings. Lumbar flexion was limited to 60% range, with pain increasing from 6/10 to 7/10. Extension was limited to 20% range, with pain increasing to 8/10, and right lateral flexion was severely limited (<10% range) and rapidly increased his pain to 9/10. Left lateral flexion did not affect his pain, and Bob felt a 'strong stretch' over the right flank/hip area. Lumbar rotation was tested sitting astride the corner of the treatment table with feet comfortably resting on the floor. Right lumbar rotation was 50% range and produced 7/10 pain. Left rotation was 80% range and produced 7/10 pain. 'Asterisk signs' may be assigned to any significant movements the therapist feels would be valuable to monitor at subsequent visits to determine the patient's response to treatment. Lumbar flexion, extension and right rotation were deemed to be appropriate asterisk signs in this case.

As previously stated, Bob's condition was judged to be considered irritable. Symptoms were therefore continuously and diligently monitored throughout movement testing.

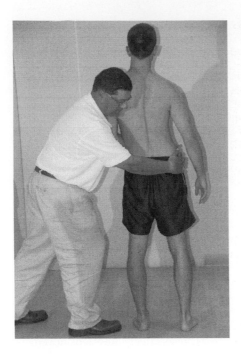

Fig. 28.2 Right side-glide correction of the left lateral shift deformity.

Sufficient rest (sometimes up to 3 minutes) was allowed, as needed, between movements and tests to allow pain to return to baseline levels. Bob was directed not to move further beyond the first onset of pain (P1), and this was reiterated throughout testing. No overpressures or quadrant testing were performed secondary to irritability.

Step Test

For this test, Bob stood with feet shoulder-width apart to ensure equal bilateral loading of the lower limbs. The unaffected limb was placed on a step (approximately 8 inches high). Bob then bent forward, flexing the lumbar spine, with the unaffected hip and knee in approximately 60 degrees of flexion, and symptom response was noted. The test was repeated with the affected foot placed on the step. The clinical reasoning underlying this test is that the foot on the step places the knee and hip in relative flexion, such that when lumbar flexion occurs, the sciatic nerve and lumbosacral plexus are not under significant tension compared with the sciatic nerve on the straight leg side.

Potential interpretations of the results of this test include the following:

1. Reproduction or increase in CS leg pain with the straight leg likely implicates both the sciatic nerve and lumbar motion segment somatic structures (e.g. lumbar disc[s]).
2. Reproduction or increase in CS pain with the flexed leg likely implicates primarily the lumbar motion segment somatic structures (as the sciatic nerve and plexus are not under tension).
3. Reduction or decrease in leg pain in the flexed leg implicates primarily the sciatic nerve, potentially rules out lumbar somatic structures and implicates mechanosensitivity in the course of the sciatic nerve and its lumbosacral nerve roots as potential sources of symptoms.

Bob performed the 'step test' in standing and experienced a reduction in both his 'deep, sharp, biting' LBP and his 'tight pulling sensation' with the affected leg in slight hip and knee flexion. These results tend to negate a lumbar somatic source and implicate sciatic nerve mechanosensitivity and potential foraminal encroachment or nerve root adhesion as mechanical causes for his pain. The 'step test' has not undergone rigorous evaluation and validation. The test makes intuitive sense considering anatomic characteristics and potential pathological mechanical mechanisms.

Passive Physiological Movements

Passive physiological testing allows for appreciation of patient response to intersegmental movements without the impact of muscle contraction or gravity. Passive physiological movements of the lumbosacral spine can be performed in supine, prone and side-lying depending on the patient's presentation and position of comfort and the specific movements to be examined. Passive physiological test movements to be performed on Bob were chosen from meaningful active physiological test results and were all performed in side-lying, which allows the patient to be relatively relaxed (Bob was most comfortable lying on his left side). The side-lying position also allows the therapist to passively assess movements of lumbar flexion, extension, rotation, lateral flexion and combined movements without the need to lift or hold the weight of the patient or the patient's limbs. Passive physiological intervertebral movements (PPIVMs) of the lumbar spine have been shown to have a very high specificity of 0.98 and 0.99 for extension and flexion, respectively, in identifying hypomobility (Abbott et al., 2005).

The relevant results were as follows:

- Flexion 80% range and decreased pain to 5/10, with a report of 'pulling' in the right L4–L5 area.
- Extension, 25% range increased pain to 7/10.
- Lateral flexion (R) 20% range, increased pain to 8/10, firm end feel; lateral flexion (L) 60% range, reduced pain to 4/10, report of 'strong stretch' over the L4–L5–S1 area, springy end feel.
- (R) rotation was 70% range, reduced pain to 4/10 and had a firm end feel, particularly at palpation over the L4, L5 and S1 area.
- (L) rotation was 85% range and produced 7/10 pain.

Palpation and Passive Accessory Intervertebral Movements (PAIVMs)

Bob was examined in prone. Resting pain was 6/10, and no sweating or redness was visible. The (R) L2–S1 area appeared slightly warmer than the surrounding areas. The paraspinal muscles exhibited wasting and had a tonic low-grade spasm at rest. (L) unilateral posteroanterior (UPA) PAIVMs were unremarkable for T12 to S1. Central posteroanterior (CPA) showed significant hypomobility at L3, L4 and L5 and increased pain locally to 7/10. (R) UPAs were most remarkable at both L3 and L4 (most significant), with marked hypomobility detected early in range, and reproduced the low back pain to 8/10. Both were comparable signs. Transverse PAIVMs to the (L) or (R) were unremarkable and did not affect pain. (R) UPA at L4 was deemed an asterisk sign (Fig. 28.3).

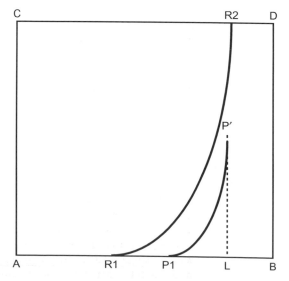

Fig. 28.3 Initial right L4 unilateral posteroanterior movement diagram.
A = point in range at which you choose to start (must be defined for each movement diagram)
B = end of "normal" range of movement for general population
AC = represents the Quality or Intensity of the factors being plotted where A = absence of the factor and C = maximum quality or intensity of the factor to which the examiner is prepared to subject the patient.
For R = Resistance then R2 at C = maximum resistance to movement.
For P = Pain then P2 at C = maximum pain the examiner is willing to provoke.
For S = Spasm then S2 at C = maximum spasm.
BD = completes the movement diagram
L = limit of movement
P1 is the position in range of the onset of pain
R1 is the point in range where an increased resistance to movement is first felt
R2 is the point where no further movement is possible due to resistance
P' is the amount of pain the patient reports when the limit is R2
Behaviour of resistance through range – shape of R1 – R2 line
Behaviour of pain through range – shape of P1 – P' line

Neurodynamic Testing

Straight leg raise (SLR) was performed in supine. Resting pain was 6/10. The unaffected (L) leg moved freely, R1 (first onset of resistance) was at approximately 50 degrees of hip flexion, R2 (maximum resistance) was found at approximately 100 degrees and slight pull was reported in the posteromedial hamstrings, with no report of change in LBP. Sensitization with ankle dorsiflexion and hip medial rotation or adduction increased tension but did not affect symptoms. SLR on the (R) had onset of R1 at approximately 30 degrees of hip flexion, with immediate reproduction of the LBP to 8/10. Sensitization with ankle dorsiflexion immediately increased resistance and pain to 9/10. Hip medial rotation and adduction could not be tolerated at 30 degrees of hip flexion but were tolerated at 20 degrees, and both increased pain to 8/10, with a marked increase in resistance (Fig. 28.4).

SLR of the unaffected leg did not affect the LBP symptoms. This 'well leg raise' test is purported to rule in a herniated nucleus pulposus and is reported to have sensitivity ranging from 0.23 to 0.43, specificity from 0.88 to 1.00, positive likelihood ratios (+LRs) from 1.91 to 14.3 and negative likelihood ratios (–LRs) from 0.59 to 0.86 (Cook and Hegedus, 2013). The negative findings of this test tended to rule out a discogenic source of Bob's pain.

Modified slump testing was performed in (L) side-lying. Thoraco-lumbar flexion was the first component introduced and increased LBP to 7/10. Addition of cervical flexion increased LBP to 8/10. Gentle addition of SLR immediately increased LBP to 9/10 at the first onset of movement, approximately 10 degrees of hip flexion. Further slump testing was discontinued. Pain subsided to resting 6/10 in 3 minutes. The slump test has been shown to have a sensitivity of 0.91, specificity of 0.70, +LR of 3.03, and –LR of 0.13 in ruling in neuropathic pain (Urban and MacNeill, 2015). The results of this test implicated the somatosensory system, including the lumbar nerve roots.

Femoral nerve neurodynamic testing (passive knee flexion) was performed in (L) side-lying with the thoraco-lumbar spine in neutral. Anterior thigh numbness was reproduced at approximately 50 degrees of knee flexion with the hip in neutral. Addition of thoraco-lumbar flexion and subsequent cervical flexion both further decreased the perception of sensation in the anterior thigh and medial knee.

Functional Instability Testing

Transverse abdominis and lumbar multifidus motor control were assessed in supine, prone and four-point kneeling. Bob exhibited very poor motor control of both muscle groups in isolation and during attempted co-contraction. Both muscle groups exhibited late and poorly timed spontaneous recruitment during co-contraction. During isolated attempts at

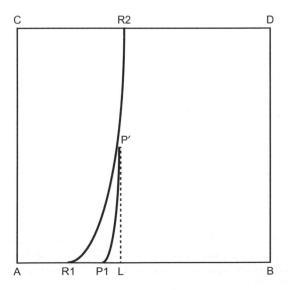

Fig. 28.4 Initial right straight leg raise movement diagram.

contraction, both muscle groups exhibited poor recruitment and weak contractions. Recruitment was only marginally improved with facilitation through palpation, tapping, visualization and use of co-contraction.

Reasoning Question:

6. What were your clinical hypotheses following the physical examination? Can you comment on your prognosis for this patient?

Answer to Reasoning Question:

Bob's clinical presentation suggested the presence of mixed mechanical and inflammatory pain that is irritable in nature, causing moderate disability. There appeared to be some psychosocial impediments to successful management, including stated skepticism of the potential value of physical therapy intervention and resignation to suffer with his pain and impairment, which he perceived to be intractable. Bob also stated that his prior spinal care had concentrated on the application of thrust manipulation without follow-up exercises or advice to remain active. Therefore, he may have had an ingrained perception that his role was largely passive in the care of his spine, not offering input and independently doing little for spine mobility and motor control between treatment sessions. Bob exhibited a familiar clinical pattern of peripheral neuropathic symptoms suggesting a right L4 nerve root source (potential adhesion and/or compression) resulting in some compromise of reflexes, sensation, motor function and limited SLR and slump indicative of neurodynamic involvement. The nerve root pathology may be related to local tissue damage and subsequent healing, including excessive scar tissue formation around the nerve root or in or near the L4–L5 neural foramen following the 'bad manipulation' 4 years prior.

Orthopedic manual therapy management is indicated, and the prognosis is good, provided Bob is engaged and educated regarding his condition and can be convinced to take active responsibility for the self-care he can administer to minimize his current disability and future exacerbations.

Management
Treatment 1 (Day 1)

As previously stated, Bob's presentation was deemed to be irritable and had to be considered as such until proven otherwise. Therefore, the initial assessment was carefully and gently performed with constant feedback from Bob regarding pain and other symptoms. Nonetheless, the assessment itself had the potential to exacerbate symptoms. Therefore, initial treatment on day 1 was kept to a minimum and localized to one segment of the spine.

Bob was placed in prone, and treatment consisted of UPA movements at L4 (the most comparable PAIVM). Grade III UPA at L4 was performed in three bouts of 1 minute each. Grade III oscillatory mobilizations are large amplitude and occur up to 50% between R1 and R2 positions in range. Resting pain of 6/10 was reduced to 5/10.

Re-assessment of asterisk signs revealed the following:

- Lumbar flexion was approximately 75% range, pain 5/10 (60% initially with pain 7/10).
- Extension remained unchanged at approximately 20%, but pain was not increased with extension (increased to 8/10 initially).
- (R) rotation was 60% range, with pain remaining at 5/10 (initially 50% and 7/10 pain).

Bob was advised that the assessment and treatment may cause exacerbation of symptoms. He was instructed to monitor symptoms and to return for treatment the following day. A large ice pack was applied to the lumbar spine for 20 minutes to minimize any post-treatment soreness.

Treatment 2 (Day 2)

Bob was questioned regarding symptom responses post-treatment. He reported slight LBP improvement to 5/10 that lasted for 3 hours post-treatment. He went to bed and took his medications as usual and reported his familiar overnight pattern, with his pain worst in the morning at 8–9/10. He stated that although the pain levels were the same in the morning, his back felt that it was 'moving more freely'. Resting pain levels were 6/10.

Physical examination findings of asterisk signs were as follows:

- Lumbar flexion was approximately 75% range, with pain at 6/10.
- Extension remained unchanged at approximately 20%, with pain increased to 7/10 (increased to 8/10 initially).
- (R) rotation was 60% range, with pain remaining at 5/10 (initially 50% and 7/10 pain).

Treatment consisted of grade III+ UPA at L4 in five bouts of 1 minute each. Grade III+ oscillatory mobilizations are large amplitude and occur at 50%–75% between R1 and R2 positions in range. Resting pain of 6/10 was reduced to 4/10.

Re-assessment of asterisk signs revealed the following:

- Lumbar flexion was approximately 75% range, with pain at 4/10 (was 7/10).
- Extension remained unchanged at approximately 20%, with pain at 6/10 (was 7/10).
- (R) rotation was 60% range, with pain remaining at 5/10.

Right lumbar rotation was introduced in (L) side-lying. The rotational movement was focused to the L3/L4 level using PPIVMs to set the level into rotation. Bob's spine was positioned initially in neutral and then (R) rotated by rotating the shoulders (R) from above until the L3 spinous process was palpated, rotating completely until it was unable to rotate further relative to the L4 spinous process, indicating that available L4/L5 rotation had been taken up. The lower leg was kept comfortably straight while the upper leg was then positioned to adjust the amount of flexion or extension in the lower lumbar spine via the movement of the pelvis. This was determined by palpation of gapping in the interspinous space between L3 and L4. The initial position used was slight lumbar flexion (Fig. 28.5).

Grade III (R) rotations were performed for three bouts of 2 minutes, and symptoms were closely monitored. There was a slight increase in LBP in the first minute of the first bout, but it quickly subsided as available rotational movement increased.

Re-assessment of asterisk signs revealed the following:

- Resting pain 4/10 (from 6/10).
- Flexion was 75% range at 4/10 (was 75% and 4/10).
- Extension was 20% at 4/10 (was 20% at 4/10).
- (R) rotation was 70% range at 4/10 (previously 50% range at 5/10 pain).
- SLR was re-assessed on the right and had onset of R1 at approximately 40 degrees of hip flexion (prior was 30 degrees), with immediate reproduction of the LBP to 7/10 (prior was 8/10). Sensitization with ankle dorsiflexion immediately increased resistance and pain to 8/10 (prior was 9/10).

A large ice pack was applied to the lumbar spine for 20 minutes to minimize any post-treatment soreness. A home exercise program was initiated, with Bob instructed to rest comfortably on his bed, lying on his back with his hips and knees comfortably flexed to approximately 60 degrees, keeping the soles of his feet resting on the bed. Bob was instructed to gently and slowly rock his knees from side to side to impart gentle lumbar rotation. He was specifically advised to only rock his knees in the pain-free range and to avoid the point in range where his LBP began (P1). Bob was instructed to perform these exercises for 5 minutes every hour (when possible) and immediately before going to sleep.

Fig. 28.5 Right rotation in slight lumbar flexion.

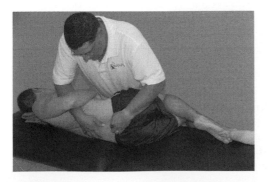

He was further instructed to gently attempt these exercises should he awaken in the middle of the night as he normally does.

Treatment 3 (Day 4)

Bob returned to the clinic, reporting that his LBP remained at the 4/10 for the remainder of the day and evening after the last treatment. He also reported that although he awoke at around 2 am with his usual pain but at a reduced level of 6/10, he was able to reduce the pain and get back to sleep, remaining in his bed, by using the lumbar rotation home exercises. This morning, he was surprised to awake with only 6/10 compared the usual 8–9/10 he experienced prior to treatment. Bob had discontinued the prednisone and oxycodone but was still using 750 mg of acetaminophen before retiring to bed and throughout the day as needed. Resting pain was 4/10.

Physical examination asterisk sign findings were as follows:

- Lumbar flexion was approximately 80% range, with pain at 5/10.
- Extension improved to 35%, with pain increased to 6/10.
- (R) rotation was 70% range, with pain at 5/10.
- Palpation of UPA over L4 increased pain to 6/10 later in resistance, that is, to the right of previous positions on the movement diagram and thus further into resistance as the segment was pain-free through a greater ROM.

Clearing or 'Ruling Out' Adjacent Areas

LBP can be referred from structures other than the lumbar spine. Potential symptom provocation from other associated areas was not assessed prior to treatment 3 because the irritable nature of Bob's disorder indicated the need for a modified clinical examination, and thus additional testing was precluded until irritability was determined and subsequently controlled in prior treatment sessions.

The hip joint was cleared or 'ruled out' by performing bilateral hip quadrant testing with overpressure (Maitland, 2005a). Both hips were mildly hypomobile in flexion, adduction, and internal rotation but did not reproduce Bob's comparable sign. The hip quadrant test has not been rigorously studied, but a component of the overall quadrant test, known as the scour test, has been. The scour test involves the clinician performing a sweeping compression and rotation from external rotation to internal rotation while the hip is held in flexion and adduction. This test has been reported to have a sensitivity of 0.62, specificity of 0.75, +LR of 2.4 and –LR of 0.51 (Sutlive et al., 2008); it is therefore a useful screen to rule out the hip as the source of Bob's symptoms.

The sacroiliac joint (SIJ) can also refer pain to the lumbar spine and lower limb. The SIJ was cleared using a cluster of four tests evaluated by Laslett et al. (2005) which have been shown to have a sensitivity of 0.94 and specificity of 0.78. The tests used included the thigh thrust, distraction, sacral thrust and compressions tests. All tests were negative for producing Bob's pain (CS) and thus effectively ruled out the SIJ as the source of the symptoms.

Treatment 3 on day 4 consisted of grade IV+ UPA at L4 in five bouts of 1 minute each. Grade IV+ oscillatory mobilizations are small amplitude and occur at 50%–75% between R1 and R2 positions in range.

Re-assessment of asterisk signs revealed the following:

- Resting pain of 5/10 was reduced to 2/10.
- Lumbar flexion was approximately 80% range, with pain at 3/10 (previously 5/10).
- Extension 40%, with pain at 3/10 (was 35% and 6/10).
- (R) rotation was 70% range, with pain at 3/10 (previously 6/10 pain).

Right lumbar rotations were repeated in (L) side-lying. The rotational movement was focused to the L3/L4 level using PPIVMs to set the level into rotation as described in the prior treatment. The position was modified to increase the amount of lumbar flexion by placing the spine in more relative flexion. Left lateral flexion was also introduced by placing pillows between the table and the lumbar spine. Grade IV+ (R) rotations were performed for three bouts of 2 minutes, and symptoms were closely monitored.

Re-assessment of asterisk signs revealed the following:

- Resting pain was 2/10 (from 5/10); (R) rotation was 90% range at 2/10 (previously 80% range at 5/10 pain); flexion was 75% range at 2/10 (previously 70% at 5/10).
- SLR was re-assessed on the right and had onset of R1 at approximately 50 degrees of hip flexion (previously 30 degrees), with immediate reproduction of the LBP to 5/10 (previously 8/10). Sensitization with ankle dorsiflexion immediately increased resistance and pain to 6/10 (previously 9/10). Hip medial rotation and adduction were tolerated at 50 degrees of hip flexion (previously 30 degrees) but were tolerated to 30 degrees, and both increased pain to 5/10 (previously 9/10), with a slight increase in resistance (previously a marked increase in resistance).

A large ice pack was again applied to the lumbar spine for 20 minutes to minimize any post-treatment soreness. Bob was asked to demonstrate his home exercise program, and it was found to be correctly performed. The exercise was modified to induce some lumbar flexion by adding a new exercise where Bob would pull alternate knees to his chest 10 times each while concentrating on gentle breathing and relaxing his back. Bob was instructed to continue hourly exercises by performing the alternate knees-to-chest exercises and then the knee rocking lumbar rotation exercises.

Treatment 4 (Day 6)

Bob returned to the clinic, reporting that his LBP remained at 2/10 for the remainder of the day and evening after the last treatment. He also reported that he slept well throughout the night without waking. On the morning of his consultation, his pain upon waking was 2/10. Resting pain was 2/10.

Physical examination of asterisk signs findings revealed the following:

- Lumbar flexion was approximately 80% range, with pain at 3/10.
- Extension improved to 50%, with pain increased to 3/10.
- (R) rotation was 80% range, with pain at 3/10.
- Palpation of UPA over L4 increased pain to 3/10 later in resistance, that is, to the right of previous positions on the movement diagram and thus further into resistance as the segment was pain-free through a greater ROM.

Treatment consisted of grade IV++ UPA at L4 in five bouts of 1 minute each. Grade IV++ oscillatory mobilizations are small amplitude and occur at 75%–100% between R1 and R2 positions in range. Resting pain of 2/10 was reduced to 0/10 (abolished).

Re-assessment of asterisk signs revealed the following:

- Lumbar flexion was approximately 80% range, with pain at 2/10 (previously 80% and 3/10).
- Extension was 70%, with pain at 2/10 (previously 50% and 3/10).
- (R) rotation was 90% range, with pain at 2/10 (previously 80% and 3/10).

Right lumbar rotations were repeated in (L) side-lying. The rotational movement was focused to the L3/L4 level using PPIVMs to set the level into rotation as described in previous treatments. The position was modified to increase the amount of lumbar flexion and to introduce left lateral flexion by the introduction of pillows between the table and the lumbar spine as previously described. In addition, the right leg was allowed to rest hanging off the table and allowed to fall gently toward the floor to enhance tension upon and potential excursion, or 'flossing', of the sciatic nerve in the lateral neural foramen in the SLR position. Grade IV++ (R) rotations were performed for three bouts of 2 minutes, and symptoms were closely monitored (Fig. 28.6).

Re-assessment of asterisk signs revealed the following:

- Resting pain was 1/10 (from 2/10).
- Flexion was 90% range, with 1/10 pain (previously 80% at 2/10).
- Extension was 70%, with 2/10 pain.
- (R) rotation was 90% range, with 1/10 pain (previously 90% range at 2/10 pain).

Fig. 28.6 Right lumbar rotation in lumbar flexion and left side-bend (lateral flexion) with right leg in partial straight leg raise position hanging off the table.

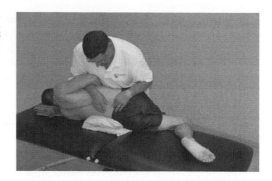

- SLR was re-assessed on the right and had onset of R1 at approximately 70 degrees of hip flexion (previously 50 degrees), with immediate reproduction of the LBP to 1/10 (previously 2/10). Sensitization with ankle dorsiflexion slightly increased resistance and pain to 3/10 (previously 6/10). Hip medial rotation and adduction were tolerated at 60 degrees of hip flexion (prior was 50 degrees), and both increased pain slightly to 3/10 (previously 6/10), with a slight increase in resistance (previously a marked increase in resistance).

Right SLR with gentle 'flossing' was performed in the same modified left side-lying (right rotation) position used for the rotational mobilizations (including lumbar flexion and left lateral flexion) as described previously. SLR was held at 70 degrees of hip flexion while passive dorsiflexion mobilizations grade IV+ (small amplitude at 50%–75% of the R1, R2 range) were used to impart tension through the sciatic nerve for three bouts of 1 minute each.

Re-assessment of asterisk signs revealed the following:

- Resting pain was 0/10 (from 2/10).
- Flexion was 90% range, with 0/10 pain (previously 80% at 1/10).
- Extension was 75%, with 1/10 pain (was 70% with 2/10).
- (R) rotation was 95% range, with 1/10 pain (previously 90% range at 1/10 pain).

Lumbar multifidus control was examined first in standing, then prone and then in quadruped (four-point kneeling). Resting spasm was absent, and Bob was able to perform isolated contractions of the multifidi, but these fatigued easily within 5 seconds. Bob tolerated the quadruped position well. Multifidi recruitment exercises were added to the home program as follows: Bob was instructed to assume the quadruped position and straighten his right arm and left leg simultaneously and hold the positions for 3 seconds. He was instructed to concentrate on keeping his pelvis and low back absolutely still during the 3-second hold. He was then to swap arms and legs and hold for another 3 seconds. Bob's ability to perform the movements and holds was checked for accuracy. He did exhibit some arm and leg wobbling and slight movement of the pelvis. Bob was instructed to perform the exercises with holds five times to each side at least five times a day, concentrating on keeping his pelvis and low back still and stable. Bob was advised to discontinue the new exercises and to call me if he had any increase in symptoms either during or after the exercises.

The lumbar rotation and flexion home exercise program was reviewed and found to be well tolerated and performed correctly. Lumbar extension exercises were added to the program, to be performed in prone or standing to improve extension mobility. The exercises were prescribed to be performed with at least five extensions, only to onset of symptoms, two to three times per day. Bob was instructed to discontinue the new exercises if they caused any increase in symptoms. Bob was rescheduled to return in 1 week.

Treatment 5 (Day 14)

Bob returned to the clinic, reporting that his LBP remained at the 2/10 for the remainder of the day and evening after the last treatment. In the previous week, he had experienced pain going up as high as 3/10 on occasion but noted that the knee rocking and knees-to-chest exercises were able to control the pain and allow him to continue to function. He also reported that he slept through the night without waking since the last treatment. Bob reported that his leg numbness was better and that he had more confidence in his leg not 'giving way'. On the morning of the consultation, his pain upon waking was 1/10. Bob had discontinued acetaminophen and was now relieved to be medication-free. Pain was 1/10 at the beginning of the treatment.

Bob completed a number of self-report forms prior to treatment, with the following results:

- NPRS: Current pain 1/10, worst in the evening at 2/10 (Interpretation: minimal pain)
- Modified ODI: 14% (Interpretation: minimal disability)
- FABQW: 4/42 (Interpretation: Minimal degree of fear and avoidance beliefs shown by the patient)

Neurological testing was performed in supine without pillows. The left leg was WNL. On the affected (right) limb, DTRs were 1+ at the patellar ligament (prior was 1+) and WNL at the Achilles (S1). Sensation testing was performed with eyes closed and Bob reporting when he could feel sensation. Sensation loss was reported as a percentage of normal compared to the other limb. Light touch sensation was tested using cotton swabs, and deficits were found in the anterolateral thigh at 90% sensation (prior was 60%) and lateral tibia at 80% sensation (prior was 60%), with the lower calf displaying normal sensation (prior was 80%). Resisted movement was used to test motor function, and all movements were WNL (resisted knee extension was 4/5 prior). No atrophy, increased resting tone, or pathological reflexes were observed in either limb, and Babinski signs and clonus were negative bilaterally (unchanged from prior testing).

Physical examination asterisk sign findings were as follows:

- Lumbar flexion was approximately 90% range, with 1/10 pain.
- Extension improved to 90%, with pain increased to 2/10.
- (R) rotation was 90% range, with pain at 1/10.
- UPA over L4 increased pain was at 90% range, with pain at 1/10.

Treatment consisted of grade IV++ UPA at L4 in five bouts of 1 minute each. Grade IV++ oscillatory mobilizations are small amplitude and occur at 75%–100% between R1 and R2 positions in range. Resting pain of 1/10 was reduced to 0/10 (abolished).

Re-assessment of asterisk signs revealed the following:

- Lumbar flexion was 100% range, with pain at 1/10.
- Extension was 90%, with pain at 1/10.
- (R) rotation was 95% range, with pain at 1/10 (Fig. 28.7).

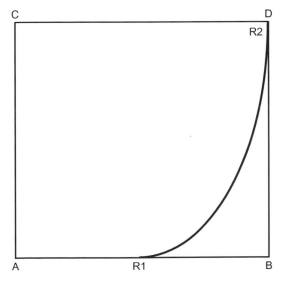

Fig. 28.7 Right L4 unilateral posteroanterior movement diagram.

Right lumbar rotations were repeated in (L) side-lying as per the prior treatment including flexion, lateral flexion and the right leg hanging off the table in the SLR position. Grade IV++ (R) rotations were performed for three bouts of 2 minutes, and symptoms were closely monitored.

Re-assessment of asterisk signs revealed the following:

- Lumbar flexion was approximately 95% range, with pain at 0/10.
- Extension improved to 95%, with pain increased to 1/10.
- (R) rotation was 95% range, with pain at 0/10.
- UPA over L4 was 100% range, with pain at 0/10.
- SLR was re-assessed on the right and had onset of R1 at approximately 90 degrees of hip flexion (previously 70 degrees), with slight reproduction of the LBP to 1/10 (previously 1/10). Sensitization with ankle dorsiflexion slightly increased resistance and pain to 1/10 (previously 3/10). Hip medial rotation and adduction were tolerated at 90 degrees of hip flexion (prior was 60 degrees), and both increased pain slightly to 1/10 (previously 3/10), with a slight increase in resistance (previously a marked increase in resistance).

SLR with gentle flossing was performed in the same modified left side-lying position used for the rotational mobilizations (including lumbar flexion and left lateral flexion as described previously and as per the earlier treatment). SLR was held at 90 degrees of hip flexion while passive dorsiflexion mobilizations grade IV+ (small amplitude at 50%–75% of the R1, R2 range) were used to impart tension or excursion through the sciatic nerve for three bouts of 1 minute each.

Re-assessment of asterisk signs revealed the following:

- Resting pain was 0/10.
- Flexion was 100% range, with pain at 0/10 (previously 95% at 0/10 pain).
- Extension was 95%, with pain at 0/10 (previously 95% with 1/10).
- (R) rotation was 100% range, with pain at 0/10 (previously 95% range at 0/10 pain).
- SLR was 100 degrees, with no LBP, a slight sensation of pulling in the posterior thigh with dorsiflexion, adduction and internal rotation sensitization (Fig. 28.8).

Lumbar multifidus control was reevaluated in quadruped. Bob was able to perform the alternate arm and leg positions without limb wobble and with very slight pelvic movement. Bob was advised to continue with the knees-to-chest flexion and knee rocking rotation exercises and prone or standing lumbar extension twice daily (morning and evening) to maintain flexibility and as needed to control pain. Bob was again advised that the quadruped exercises for fine motor control of the spine were very important – not only for keeping his spine functioning properly and pain-free but, more importantly, to potentially prevent

Fig. 28.8 Final straight leg raise movement diagram.

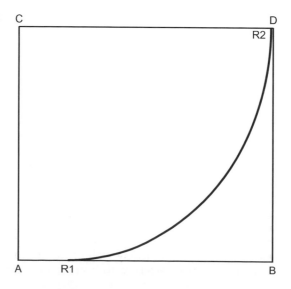

reoccurrence of his symptoms. Bob was advised to continue these exercises at least twice daily until further advised. Bob was encouraged to consider starting a regular exercise regime.

Treatment 6 (Day 30)

Bob returned to the clinic, reporting that he had been mostly pain-free for the previous 2 weeks. In the past week, he had experienced pain going up as high as 2/10 on occasions, but he noted that the knee rocking and knees-to-chest exercises were able to control the pain and allow him to continue to function. He also reported that he had continued to sleep normally. Bob was pain-free at the beginning of the treatment.

Bob completed a number of self-report forms prior to treatment, with the following results:

- NPRS: Current pain 0/10, worst pain 2/10 (Interpretation: minimal pain)
- Modified ODI: 0% (Interpretation: no disability)
- FABQW: 0/42 (Interpretation: no fear and avoidance beliefs shown by the patient)

Physical examination asterisk sign findings were as follows:

- Lumbar flexion was approximately 100% range, with pain at 0/10.
- Extension was 100% range, with pain at 1/10.
- (R) rotation was 100% range, with pain at 0/10.
- UPA over L4 was pain-free with 100% range.

Active physiological testing was performed in standing, and all movements were WNL, including the application of gentle overpressure, except for extension with 1/10 local pain. PAIM assessment of the lumbar spine was performed using CPAs, UPAs and transverse movements from T10 to S1. All were pain-free with range WNL.

Lumbar multifidus control was re-evaluated in quadruped. Bob was able to perform the alternate arm and leg positions without limb or pelvic wobble. The exercises were modified to include simultaneous arm and leg perturbation movements, such as spelling the letters of the alphabet or making concentric circles, to further challenge fine-tuned segmental spinal control. Bob was advised to increase the intensity of the exercises by performing 30 repetitions per side, with 5 seconds of perturbations per side, twice daily. Bob was again advised of the importance of the exercises to maintain normal function and prevent further exacerbations. Lumbar flexion, rotation and extension exercises were maintained at the level of at least twice a day or for pain relief as needed.

Treatment 7 (Day 70)

Bob returned to the clinic, reporting that he had been mostly pain-free for the previous 6 weeks. A tabular summary of the changes in Bob's presentation (indices, comparable signs and asterisk signs) over the course of treatment is presented in Table 28.1.

He had experienced occasional, fleeting pain of 1/10. Sleep had been normal, and he was medication-free and pain-free upon presentation. Bob completed the self-report questionnaires (NPRS, Modified ODI and the FABQW), and all were scored as 0.

Active physiological testing was performed in standing, and all movements were WNL, including the application of gentle overpressure. PAIVM assessment of the lumbar spine was performed using CPAs, UPAs and transverse movements from T10 to S1. All were pain-free with range WNL. The neurological examination was normal, including DTRs, sensation and motor function. SLR was normal and similar to the unaffected side.

Lumbar multifidus control was reevaluated in quadruped. Bob was able to perform the alternate arm and leg positions with excellent control and without any aberrant movements. Bob was again advised of the importance of the exercises to maintain normal function and prevent further exacerbations. It was suggested that Bob continue the exercises twice daily as a regular routine. Lumbar flexion, rotation and extension exercises were advised to be maintained at a frequency twice a day or for pain control and mobility as needed. Bob was discharged from therapy with the advice to return if symptoms should increase or if he required further advice with his exercise regime.

TABLE 28.1

SUMMARY OF CHANGES IN BOB'S PRESENTATION OVER THE COURSE OF HIS TREATMENT

	Initial	Post Rx	Rx 2	Post Rx	Rx 3	Post Rx	Rx 4	Post Rx	Rx 5	Post Rx	Rx 6	Post Rx	Rx 7
	Day 1	Rx	Day 2	Rx	Day 4	Rx	Day 6	Rx	Day 14	Rx	Day 30	Rx	Day 70
Pain (NPRS) (0–10)													
At rest	6		5		4		2		0		0		0
Worst	8		8		6		2		1		0		0
ODI	56%						14%		0%		0%		0%
FABQW	24						4		2		0		0
Asterisk signs (%)		Pain											
APMs													
Flexion	60	7	75	6	80	5	80	2	90	1	100	0	100
Extension	20	8	20	7	35	6	50	3	90	2	100	0	100
Rotation	50	7	60	5	70	5	80	3	90	1	100	0	100
PAIVMs		Pain											
L4 UPA													
Range (%)	10	8	25	4	60	4	80	2	90	1	100	0	100
SLR (%)													
Range	30	8	40	7	50	6	70	5	90	1	100	1	100
DF sens.	9		6		6		3		1		1		0
Lumbar motor control	Poor		Not Tested		Not Tested		Poor		Moderate		Moderate		Excellent

APLMs, Active physiological lumbar movements; *DF sens.*, dorsiflexion sensitivity; *FABQW*, Fear-Avoidance Beliefs Questionnaire (Work subset); *NPRS*, numerical pain rating scale; *ODI*, Oswestry Disability Index; *PAIVMs*, passive accessory intervertebral movements; *Rx*, treatment; *SLR*, straight leg raise; *UPA*, unilateral posteroanterior.

Reasoning Question:

7. Bob scored reasonably highly on the self-report questionnaires prior to treatment, yet he made an excellent recovery. Were you surprised by the time frame and extent of his recovery given the level of disability suggested by those tools?

Answer to Reasoning Question:

The time frame and extent of Bob's recovery were not surprising, even given his moderately high baseline levels of pain, disability and fear-avoidance beliefs using validated indexes. The indices are valuable tools to evaluate various factors at a given point in time. As the patient's clinical situation changes, repeat indices measure relevant change since the prior measurements. Clinically, it is quite common to see significant reductions in pain and irritability following initial treatments focused on the response of the CS to appropriate mobilization treatment. Within a few treatments, pain and irritability were controlled and subsequently reduced. Thus, Bob exhibited typical improvements in pain scores, reduced disability and an associated change in fear-avoidance and beliefs. Later treatment sessions focused on restoration of normal pain-free motion and development of greater spinal segmental control. Repeat measures from the indices exhibited a predictable improvement based on Bob's improving pain, function and fear of movement.

Reasoning Question:

8. You identified some potential barriers to recovery in this case and commented that you needed to address Bob's concerns about his condition, emphasize the value of his positive mental attitude and empower him. Were there any particular counselling or other strategies other than exercise that you used to help address these barriers and motivate Bob?

Answer to Reasoning Question:

Bob presented with a number of potential negative and positive beliefs and attitudes that needed to be dispelled and reinforced, respectively, during treatment to engage him to actively participate in management to minimize the potential for re-occurrence of his condition. The first significant negative belief was evidenced by Bob's unsolicited statement during the initial consultation that 'PT would probably not help much, as his regular chiropractor was unable to help with the pain'. The strategy adopted was not to challenge his skepticism but rather to offer him a second opinion and teach him strategies to independently minimize his pain and remain functional at work. Bob would decide the value of physical therapy care for himself. His erroneous belief was naturally dispelled over time as initial treatments provided him with pain relief, more hours of uninterrupted sleep and greater function at work. A second unstated barrier to rehabilitation was Bob's lengthy history of seeking care for his back whereby his condition was treated by a clinician with little or no active participation from Bob. Once pain relief and improved function had been demonstrated in early clinical sessions and, more importantly, augmented by his specific home exercise program to relieve pain and maintain mobility, Bob was able to realize the value of self-care and active participation in his recovery. Bob was engaged to become a collaborator in treatment decision-making and progression. In this way, Bob was empowered to take greater control of his condition and his future well-being.

Bob's greatest assets were his positive mental attitude and strong motivation to reduce his pain and improve his function at work to provide for his family. Bob also expressed a rational fear of potential opioid addiction. Fortunately, Bob's opioid and steroid prescriptions expired during the period that he was beginning to experience significant pain relief and improved function, and thus he was relieved to realize that he could manage his pain independently and function without prescription medication. Bob was the epitome of the stoic farmer willing to endure pain with minimal complaining to get the job done. The strategy adopted was to tap into Bob's pragmatic, highly motivated nature and to explain the role of physical therapy intervention and the importance of his active self-management in terms he could easily understand. Bob used particular language that included his back feeling 'rusty' and needing to 'get his back moving' and 'lubricated'. This same terminology was used in questioning him about his back throughout his recovery. The importance of routine exercises to maintain spinal mobility and motor control was described to Bob in terms of keeping his back 'lubricated and strong'.

Presumed pathological processes were explained in mechanical terms that Bob could easily understand. The concept of an adhered lumbar nerve root was explained using the analogy of a clutch cable traversing through a small hole in the firewall of a vehicle and activating the clutch mechanism. If the clutch cable was getting stuck at the firewall, the mechanism would not operate correctly. Thus, the intention of treatment was explained to Bob in terms of opening up the hole in the firewall (the lateral neural foramen) to allow the clutch cable (nerve root) to move freely and restore function. A lengthy patho-anatomical discussion, using complex medical terminology, would likely have been less effective in explaining Bob's condition and enabling him to understand and participate in the collaborative clinical decision-making process.

Clinical Reasoning Commentary:

Apparent in the answer to Reasoning Question 7, and evident throughout Bob's management, is that significant emphasis was placed on re-assessing a range of physical impairments and self-report disability measures. Although re-assessment of disability, for example, via the questionnaires used for Bob, is essential to ensure changes monitored in physical impairments translate to meaningful changes in activity and participation, the detail attended to when re-assessing physical impairments (e.g. changes in movement diagrams) enabled greater sensitivity to detect change and guide treatment progression. Management may be informed by research and prior experience, but it should still be seen as a hypothesis to be tested through critical and thorough re-assessment.

Patient education, particularly addressing attitudes and beliefs judged to be unhelpful to recovery and important to minimizing recurrence, needs to be tailored to individual patients, with respect to both the basis of their beliefs and to who they are (e.g. personality, temperament and even worldview). That is, as discussed in Chapter 1, individualizing education requires 'reasoning about teaching': reasoning associated with the planning, execution and evaluation of individualized and context-sensitive teaching, including education for conceptual understanding (e.g. medical and musculoskeletal diagnosis, pain), education for physical performance (e.g. rehabilitative exercise, postural correction, sport technique enhancement) and education for behavioural change. Getting to know Bob, the stoic farmer, and tapping into his language when explaining treatments, combined with using successful self-management to reinforce his role, are good examples of individualized and targeted teaching informed by patient-specific reasoning.

REFERENCES

Abbott, J.H., McCane, B., Herbison, P., Moginie, G., Chapple, C., Hogarty, T., 2005. Lumbar segmental instability: a criterion-related validity study of manual therapy assessment. BMC Musculoskelet. Disord. 6, 56. https://doi.org/10.1186/1471-2474-6-56.

Barakatt, E.T., Romano, P.S., Riddle, D.L., Beckett, L.A., 2009a. The reliability of Maitland's irritability judgments in patients with low back pain. J. Man. Manip. Ther. 17 (3), 135–140.

Barakatt, E.T., Romano, P.S., Riddle, D.L., Beckett, L.A., Kravitz, R., 2009b. An exploration of Maitland's concept of pain irritability in patients with low back pain. J. Man. Manip. Ther. 17 (4), 196–205.

Cook, C., Learman, K., Showalter, C., O'Halloran, B., 2015. The relationship between chief complaint and comparable sign in patients with spinal pain: an exploratory study. Man. Ther. 20 (3), 451–455. http://doi.org/10.1016/j.math.2014.11.007.

Cook, C.E., Hegedus, E.J., 2013. Orthopedic Physical Examination Tests: An Evidence Based Approach, second ed. Pearson, Boston, MA.

Cook, C.E., Learman, K.E., O'Halloran, B.J., Showalter, C.R., Kabbaz, V.J., Goode, A.P., et al., 2012a. Which prognostic factors for low back pain are generic predictors of outcome across a range of recovery domains? Phys. Ther. 93 (1), 32–40. http://doi.org/10.2522/ptj.20120216.

Cook, C.E., Showalter, C., Kabbaz, V., O'Halloran, B., 2012b. Can a within/between-session change in pain during reassessment predict outcome using a manual therapy intervention in patients with mechanical low back pain? Man. Ther. 17 (4), 325–329. http://doi.org/10.1016/j.math.2012.02.020.

Gifford, L., Thacker, M., Jones, M.A., 2006. Physiotherapy and pain. In: McMahon, S.B., Koltzenburg, M. (Eds.), Wall and Melzack's Textbook of Pain, fifth ed. Elsevier, Philadelphia, pp. 603–617.

IASP Taxonomy, 2017. IASP Publications, Washington, D.C., viewed December 2017, http://www.iasp-pain.org/Taxonomy.

Jones, M.A., 1987. The clinical reasoning process in manipulative therapy. In: Dalziel, B.A., Snowsill, J.C. (Eds.), Proceedings of the Fifth Biennial Conference of the Manipulative Therapists Association of Australia. Melbourne, VIC, Australia, pp. 62–69.

Jones, M.A., 2014. Clinical reasoning: from the Maitland Concept and beyond. In: Hengeveld, E., Banks, K. (Eds.), Maitland's Vertebral Manipulation, Management of Neuromusculoskeletal Disorders – Volume One, eighth ed. Churchill Livingstone/Elsevier, Edinburgh, pp. 14–82.

Jones, M.A., Rivett, D.A., 2004. Clinical Reasoning for Manual Therapists. Butterworth Heinemann, Edinburgh.

Laslett, M., Aprill, C.N., McDonald, B., Young, S.B., 2005. Diagnosis of sacroiliac joint pain: validity of individual provocation tests and composites of tests. Man. Ther. 10 (3), 207–218. https://doi.org/10.1016/j.math.2005.01.003.

Maitland, G.D., 1971. Examination of the lumbar spine. Aust. J. Physiother. 17 (1), 5–11. http://doi.org/10.1016/S0004-9514(14)61102-8.

Maitland, G.D., 1987. The Maitland concept: assessment, examination, and treatment by passive movement. In: Twomey, L.T., Taylor, J.R. (Eds.), Clinics in Physical Therapy. Physical Therapy for the Low Back. Churchill Livingstone, New York, pp. 135–155.

Maitland, G.D., 1991. Peripheral Manipulation, third ed. Elsevier, Butterworth Heinemann, Edinburgh.

Maitland, G.D., 2005a. Peripheral Manipulation, fourth ed. Elsevier, Edinburgh.

Maitland, G.D., 2005b. Vertebral Manipulation, seventh ed. Elsevier, Edinburgh.

Nijs, J., van Wilgen, C.P., Lluch Girbés, E., et al., 2014. Applying modern pain neuroscience in clinical practice: criteria for the classification of central sensitization pain. Pain Physician 17, 447–457.

Sackett, D.L., 1998. Evidence-based medicine. Spine 23 (10), 1085–1086.

Sutlive, T.G., Lopez, H.P., Schnitker, D.E., Yawn, S.E., Halle, R.J., Mansfield, L.T., et al., 2008. Development of a clinical prediction rule for diagnosing hip osteoarthritis in individuals with unilateral hip pain. J. Orthop. Sports Phys. Ther. 38 (9), 542–550. https://doi.org/10.2519/jospt.2008.2753.

Urban, L.M., MacNeil, B.J., 2015. Diagnostic accuracy of the slump test for identifying neuropathic pain in the lower limb. J. Orthop. Sports Phys. Ther. 45 (8), 596–603. http://doi.org/10.2519/jospt.2015.5414.

Wolf, C.J., 2011. Central sensitization: implication for diagnosis and treatment of pain. Pain 152, 2–15.

29

Physical Therapy Chosen Over Lumbar Microdiscectomy: A Functional Movement Systems Approach

Kyle A. Matsel • Kyle Kiesel • Gray Cook • Mark A. Jones

Subjective Examination

Chuck is a 28-year-old male who presented to the clinic with a diagnosis of low back pain. Chuck reported that he injured his low back in a rear-end motor vehicle accident (MVA) 8 weeks prior. As a result of the MVA, Chuck began having significant low back pain with left lower extremity symptoms that he reported extended from his low back centrally to the sacral region, left buttock and left posterior leg, including the full dorsal and plantar surfaces of his foot and toes (Fig. 29.1). He presented with no major red flags such as numbness, pins and needles, cauda equina or spinal cord–associated symptoms, and no symptoms in the right leg or upper body.

Immediately post-accident, Chuck was taken to the local hospital, where initial emergency room radiographs were negative for fractures, and he was referred to a neurosurgeon for consultation. Magnetic resonance imagining (MRI) revealed a two-level lumbar disc herniation at L4/L5 and L5/S1. Chuck was given the option at that time to attempt physical therapy or proceed with surgical intervention to address the herniated discs that were considered to be the cause of his pain and associated work-activity limitations.

Chuck is a mechanic by profession and is on his feet on concrete most of the day. No modified duty or work restrictions were suggested by the referring physician. As a mechanic, Chuck was required to lift parts, squat down to work on cars and stand for prolonged periods of time. Chuck was not currently engaged in a fitness program; however, he had previously participated in weight lifting for exercise and wished to return to this in the future. Given the nature of his work, Chuck decided to attempt physical therapy before resorting to a lumbar microdiscectomy operation. Screening questions for potential psychosocial issues (i.e. yellow flags) regarding Chuck's understanding of his problem, his beliefs regarding management, stressors in his life and his level of coping all suggested these were not a problem in his case.

At the initial examination Chuck reported a current pain rating via the visual analogue scale (VAS) of 5/10; however, he stated that the pain could reach 8/10 at its worst by the end of the workday. He reported no significant past medical history and no previous orthopaedic surgeries. Chuck's pain increased with prolonged standing and walking and appeared to decrease with sitting and stretching of his low back by bending forward. Other spinal movements (e.g. twisting) and lower limb movements (e.g. hip, knee) were not a problem. He reported no significant difficulties with sleeping through the night and noted his preferred sleeping position was side-lying with his knees pulled up toward his chest.

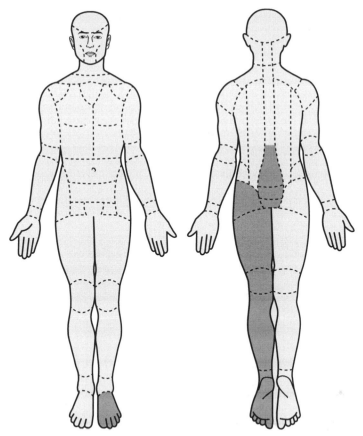

Fig. 29.1 Body chart illustrating area of Chuck's symptoms.

Reasoning Question:

1. What were your hypotheses at this stage regarding dominant 'pain type' (nociceptive, peripheral neuropathic, nociplastic)?

Answer to Reasoning Question:

At this point, it appeared that Chuck's presentation was consistent with a nociceptive-dominant pattern based on the mechanical nature of the symptoms and apparent lack of yellow flags. Symptoms were relatively localized to the lumbar spine and left posterior lower extremity, with no widespread areas of symptoms or inconsistent patterns of provocation that are typically associated with nociplastic pain (e.g. Smart et al., 2012a, 2012c). On the other hand, the area of posterior leg pain and confirmed multi-level disc herniation was potentially consistent with a peripheral neuropathic type of pain problem (e.g. Smart et al., 2012b; Treede et al., 2008), and as such, a neurological examination would be important to help in differentiation. However, the inclusion of the full plantar surface of the foot and toes in his pain pattern is atypical for compromise of a single nerve root and may instead reflect a peripheral nerve compromise.

Reasoning Question:

2. At this stage, did you have any hypotheses regarding potential 'sources of symptoms' (nociception) and 'pathology' for Chuck's symptoms, and were there any 'precautions to the physical examination and treatment' identified from the clinical picture thus far?

Answer to Reasoning Question:

With a multi-level disc herniation confirmed by MRI and radiating symptoms down the lower extremity, we might expect Chuck would have reported some relief from lumbopelvic extension postures or movements. In contrast, Chuck reported movements and postures involving flexion as pain relieving. Because this is not the typical presentation for a pain-provoking discogenic lesion, it is reasonable to hypothesize that the herniations may have been asymptomatic. Any structure, somatic or neural, within the area of symptoms could have been a source of nociception. However, given that Chuck's provocation of symptoms was associated with lumbopelvic extension-oriented posture and movement (e.g. standing

Continued on following page

and walking) and that his symptoms were eased with flexion activities (e.g. sitting and bending forward), plus neither hip or knee movements were affected, it is also reasonable to hypothesize that the source(s) of nociception was located within the lower lumbar spine and/or sacroiliac joint. The lack of overt neurological symptoms (e.g. numbness, pins and needles, weakness) suggested that frank nerve root compression was unlikely, although a neurological examination would be required to test this further, and thus compromise of a nerve root and/or peripheral nerve remained a possibility.

Although potential sources of nociception will be tested further in the physical examination, operating under the assumption that the herniated discs were not the pain generators and that no other overt pathology was evident, the focus of reasoning shifted to movement-pattern dysfunction maintaining nociception. That is, the MVA was likely responsible for initial nociception from the lumbar spine and possibly neural tissues. In response to the pain, the CNS will alter the motor control (timing) of the inner core muscles (Hodges et al., 2013). If the inner core muscles (multifidus, transversus abdominis, pelvic floor, diaphragm) are delayed in their activation, a more global response of the larger force-producing muscles will occur. This is called a 'high-threshold strategy' (Cholewicki et al., 2002) and involves a global co-contraction of erector spinae, rectus abdominis and the external obliques, which is thought to protect the painful region from further injury. A high-threshold strategy is ideal for situations where the system is under high load; however, it is not necessary under less stressful situations. The increased compressive forces that occur through the spine due to the co-contraction of the erector spinae and rectus abdominis muscles may be generating and maintaining nociception and, therefore, Chuck's symptoms. The physical examination will also be used to identify any dysfunctions in movement and control and, if present, what specifically is the cause of any dysfunction.

With respect to precautions that should be taken, although it appears that the herniated discs may be chronic and asymptomatic in nature, exercises that are known to increase disc pressure and potentially cause irritation of the disc or adjacent structures will need to be avoided. For example, loaded lumbar flexion with rotation exercises that may stress the disc will not be a part of the treatment plan, especially if an increase in peripheralization of symptoms in the lower extremity occurs.

Clinical Reasoning Commentary:

Musculoskeletal clinicians need to be able to reason on multiple levels and across multiple categories of decisions (i.e. hypothesis categories). With a hypothesis regarding 'Pain type' as nociceptive dominant and/or neuropathic based on the clinical pattern of symptom area, behaviour and history, combined with equivalent negative findings for nociplastic pain, reasoning regarding 'sources of symptoms' (nociception) and 'pathology' is appropriate. A case is made against a discogenic 'source' despite the radiological evidence of pathology. The possibility of neuropathic and other tissue sources is kept open with plans for further testing in the physical examination, and the clinical reasoning has expanded to include potential 'contributing factors' in the form of 'movement pattern dysfunction' maintaining Chuck's symptoms and disability. The clinical reasoning throughout this portion of the answer reflects the balanced reasoning that musculoskeletal clinicians are required to undertake between 'sources of symptoms', 'pathology' and 'impairments', as discussed in Chapter 1.

On yet another level of reasoning, 'precautions to physical examination and treatment' are identified with respect to both pathology (i.e. disc herniation) and symptom behaviour (i.e. peripheralization).

Physical Examination

Posture

- Mild increased lumbar lordosis

Neurological Examination

- Normal sensation to light touch
- Normal strength through all myotomes
- Normal reflexes at the patellar tendon (L3) and Achilles tendon (S1) levels.

Selective Functional Movement Assessment (SFMA)

Assessment findings are reported according to the SFMA categorizations of 'functional and non-painful', 'functional and painful', 'dysfunctional and non-painful' and 'dysfunctional and painful', with clarification of the dysfunction in parentheses and SFMA categorization of dysfunction highlighted in italics (App. 29.1; Cook, 2010):

- Cervical flexion = functional and non-painful
- Cervical extension = functional and non-painful

Name: **Date:**   **Total score:**

Cervical flexion   ☐ Painful
☐ Can't touch sternum to chin
☐ Excessive effort and/or lack of motor control

Cervical extension   ☐ Painful
☐ Not within 10 degrees of parallel
☐ Excessive effort and/or lack of motor control

Cervical rotation   ☐ Painful right   ☐ Painful left
☐ Right   ☐ Left   Nose not in line with mid-clavicle
☐ Right   ☐ Left   Excessive effort and/or appreciable asymmetry or lack of motor control

Pattern #1 – MRE   ☐ Painful right   ☐ Painful left
☐ Right   ☐ Left   Does not reach inferior angle of scapula
☐ Right   ☐ Left   Excessive effort and/or appreciable asymmetry or lack of motor control

Pattern #2 – LRF   ☐ Painful right   ☐ Painful left
☐ Right   ☐ Left   Does not reach spine of scapula
☐ Right   ☐ Left   Excessive effort and/or appreciable asymmetry or lack of motor control

Multisegmental flexion   ☐ Painful
☐ Cannot touch toes
☐ Sacral angle < 70 degrees
☐ Non-uniform spinal curve
☐ Lack of posterior weight shift
☐ Excessive effort and/or appreciable asymmetry or lack of motor control

Multisegmental extension   ☐ Painful
☐ UE does not achieve or maintain 170
☐ ASIS does not clear toes
☐ Spine of scapula does not clear heels
☐ Non-uniform spinal curve
☐ Excessive effort and/or lack of motor control

Multisegmental rotation   ☐ Painful right   ☐ Painful left
☐ Right   ☐ Left   Pelvis rotation < 50 degrees
☐ Right   ☐ Left   Shoulders rotation < 50 degrees
☐ Right   ☐ Left   Spine/pelvic deviation
☐ Right   ☐ Left   Excessive knee flexion
☐ Right   ☐ Left   Excessive effort and/or lack of symmetry or motor control

Single leg stance   ☐ Painful right   ☐ Painful left
☐ Right   ☐ Left   Eyes open < 10 seconds
☐ Right   ☐ Left   Eyes closed < 10 seconds
☐ Right   ☐ Left   Loss of height
☐ Right   ☐ Left   Excessive effort or lack of symmetry or motor control

Overhead deep squat   ☐ Painful right   ☐ Painful left
☐ Loss of UE start position
☐ Tibia and torso are not parallel or better
☐ Thighs do not break parallel
☐ Loss of sagittal plane alignment: Right_____ Left_____
☐ Excessive effort, weight shift, or motor control

App. 29.1   Selective Functional Movement Assessment (SFMA) form. One of 15 forms or flowcharts used in the SFMA to diagnose movement dysfunction as either a primary mobility problem or a primary stability/motor-control problem.
(Reproduced with kind permission from Functional Movement Systems.)
Key:
ASIS = anterior superior iliac spine
LRF = lateral rotation flexion
MRE = medial rotation extension
UE = upper extremity

- Cervical rotation = functional and non-painful bilaterally
- Upper extremity pattern 1 = functional and non-painful bilaterally
- Upper extremity pattern 2 = functional and non-painful bilaterally
- Multisegmental flexion = dysfunctional (restricted range of movement [ROM]) and non-painful
- Multisegmental extension = dysfunctional (restricted ROM) and painful (lumbar spine)
- Multisegmental rotation = dysfunctional (restricted ROM) and non-painful bilaterally
- Single leg stance = dysfunctional (loss of lumbar-pelvic starting position and excessive exertion in maintaining single leg stance) and non-painful bilaterally
- Overhead deep squat = dysfunctional (loss of upper extremity flexion and inability of the hips to break parallel) and non-painful
- SFMA scoring (App. 29.2) = 56% total dysfunction.

Multisegmental flexion 'breakout' (App. 29.3) (Cook, 2010):

- Standing unilateral (weight-bearing on right side) forward bend = dysfunctional (unable to touch toes) and non-painful bilaterally
- Long sitting toe touch = dysfunctional (unable to touch toes) and non-painful
- Active straight leg raise test = dysfunctional (restricted mobility – 35 degrees) and non-painful bilaterally

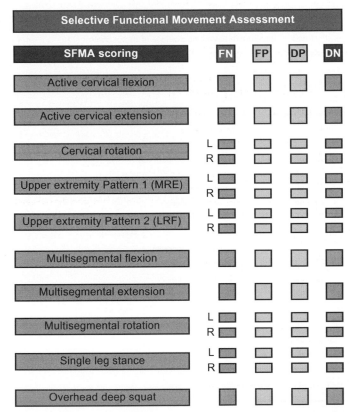

App. 29.2 Selective Functional Movement Assessment (SFM) scoring illustrating the categorical and checklist score sheets for the seven top-tier movements of the SFMA. Scoring: there are 50 total possible checks on the list. Every dysfunction gets one check. The total number of checks is added up and divided by 50 and multiplied by 100 to get a percentage of total dysfunction.
(Reproduced with kind permission from Functional Movement Systems.)
Key:
DN = dysfunctional and non-painful
DP = dysfunctional and painful
FN = functional and non-painful
FP = functional and painful
LRF = lateral rotation flexion
MRE = medial rotation extension

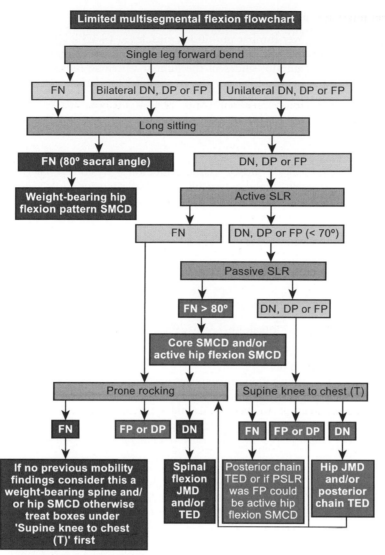

App. 29.3 Multisegmental flexion 'breakout' flowchart illustrating the systematic reduction of a global movement pattern into its regional components.
(Reproduced with kind permission from Functional Movement Systems.)
Key:
DN = dysfunctional and non-painful
DP = dysfunctional and painful
FN = functional and non-painful
FP = functional and painful
JMD = joint mobility dysfunction
SLR = straight leg raise
SMCD = stability motor-control dysfunction
supine knee to chest (T) = supine knees to chest holding thighs
TED = tissue extensibility dysfunction

- Passive straight leg raise test = dysfunctional (restricted mobility – 40 degrees) and non-painful bilaterally with no reproduction of leg pain = *'bilateral posterior chain tissue extensibility dysfunction'* (Cook, 2010)
- Supine knees to chest holding thighs test – functional (full hip flexion joint mobility) and non-painful
- Prone rock ('child's pose') lumbar spine flexion test = dysfunctional (limited joint movement with non-uniform spinal curve) and non-painful = *'lumbar flexion mobility dysfunction'*

Local biomechanical assessment of lumbar spine:

- Tender to palpation over lumbar multifidus muscles at L4/L5 level bilaterally
- Tender to palpation over lumbar erector spinae muscles left > right bilaterally
- Central posterior to anterior glides of the lumbar vertebrae indicated no hypomobile segments (i.e. no evidence of *'lumbar flexion joint mobility dysfunction'*).

Multisegmental extension 'breakout' (App. 29.4A–C) (Cook, 2010):

- Flexion/abduction/external rotation (FABER) test = negative (functional and non-painful) bilaterally
- Modified 'Thomas test'
  Positive for rectus femoris muscle tissue limitation – dysfunctional (restricted) and non-painful bilaterally. Inability to achieve full hip extension ROM with < 90 degrees of passive knee flexion indicated a *'bilateral anterior chain tissue extensibility dysfunction'* (Cook, 2010).
  Negative for tensor fascia lata and iliopsoas muscle tissue limitations bilaterally
- Prone press-up = dysfunctional and painful (increased low back pain and left leg pain)
- Latissimus dorsi length test with hips flexed = dysfunctional (unable to achieve full shoulder flexion) and non-painful
- Latissimus dorsi length test with hips extended = dysfunctional (shoulder flexion ROM did not change) and non-painful

Multisegmental rotation 'breakout' (App. 29.5A–D) (Cook, 2010):

- Seated rotation test = dysfunctional (limited active ROM – 35 degrees right and left) and non-painful bilaterally
- Lumbar locked external rotation unilateral extension/rotation test = dysfunctional (limited active ROM – 35 degrees right and left) and non-painful bilaterally
- Lumbar locked internal rotation unilateral extension/rotation test = dysfunctional (limited active ROM – 35 degrees right and left; limited passive ROM – 40 degrees left and right) and non-painful bilaterally = *'bilateral thorax joint mobility dysfunction'* (Cook, 2010)
- Seated right hip internal rotation ROM (with hips in 90 degrees flexion)
  Active = 20 degrees; passive = 35 degrees (non-painful *'motor-control dysfunction'*; Cook, 2010)
- Seated left hip internal rotation ROM (with hips in 90 degrees flexion)
  Active = 30 degrees; passive = 40 degrees (functional and non-painful)
- Seated bilateral hip external rotation ROM (with hips in 90 degrees flexion)
  Active = 40 degrees; passive = 50 degrees (functional and non-painful)
- Prone bilateral hip internal rotation ROM (with hips in 0 degrees extension)
  Active = 30 degrees; passive = 40 degrees (functional and non-painful)
- Prone right hip external rotation ROM (with hips in 0 degrees extension)
  Active = 40 degrees; passive = 50 degrees (functional and non-painful)
- Prone left hip external rotation ROM (with hips in 0 degrees extension)
  Active 35 degrees; passive = 50 degrees (non-painful *'motor-control dysfunction'*; Cook, 2010)
- Seated tibial internal and external rotation test:
  Active internal rotation = 20 degrees bilaterally (functional and non-painful)
  Active external rotation = 20 degrees bilaterally (functional and non-painful)

Single leg stance 'breakout' (ankle flowchart in App. 29.6) (Cook, 2010):

- Heels walk = functional and non-painful
- Toes walk – functional and non-painful

Rolling assessments:

- Upper extremity and lower extremity supine-to-prone rolling = dysfunctional (lacks segmental control) and non-painful bilaterally = *'fundamental flexion pattern motor control dysfunction'* (Cook, 2010)

Text continued on p. 541

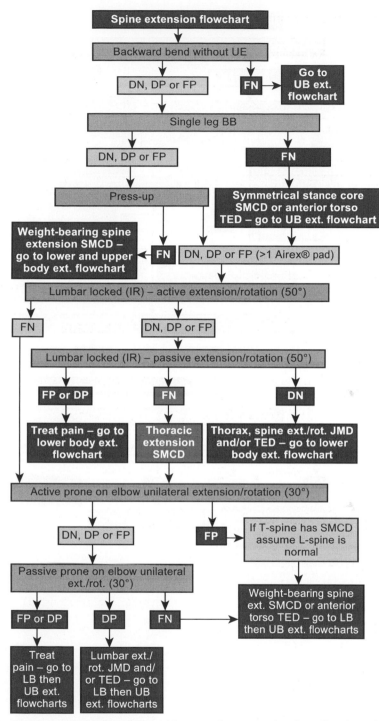

App. 29.4 (A) Spine extension flowchart. Multisegmental extension 'breakout' flowcharts illustrating the systematic reduction of a global movement pattern into its regional components.
(Reproduced with kind permission from Functional Movement Systems.)
Key:
BB = backward bend
DN = dysfunctional and non-painful
DP = dysfunctional and painful
ext. = extension
FN = functional and non-painful
FP = functional and painful
IR = internal rotation
JMD = joint mobility dysfunction

LB = lower body
L-spine = lumbar spine
rot. = rotation
SMCD = stability motor-control dysfunction
TED = tissue extensibility dysfunction
T-spine = thoracic spine
UB = upper body
UE = upper extremity

Continued on following page

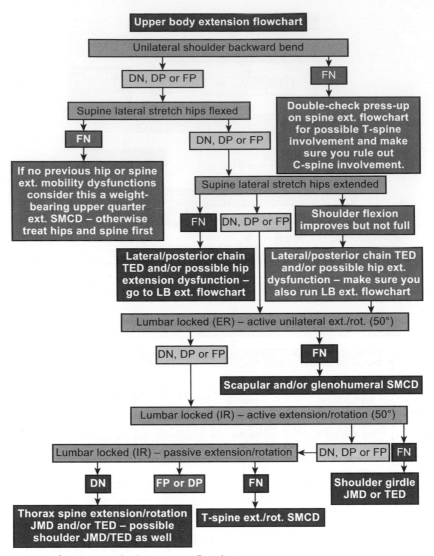

App. 29.4, cont'd (B) Upper body extension flowchart.
Key:
C-spine = cervical spine
DN = dysfunctional and non-painful
DP = dysfunctional and painful
ER = external rotation
ext. = extension
FN = functional and non-painful
FP = functional and painful
IR = internal rotation
JMD = joint mobility dysfunction
LB = lower body
rot. = rotation
SMCD = stability motor-control dysfunction
TED = tissue extensibility dysfunction
T-spine = thoracic spine
UB = upper body

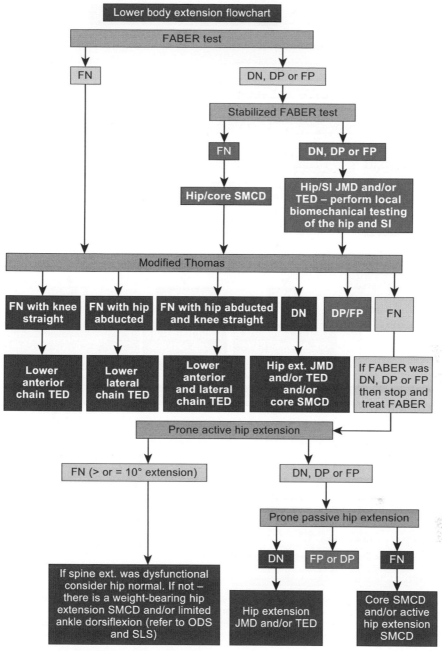

App. 29.4, cont'd (C) Lower body extension flowchart.
Key:
DN = dysfunctional and non-painful
DP = dysfunctional and painful
ext. = extension
FABER = flexion/abduction/external rotation
FN = functional and non-painful
FP = functional and painful
JMD = joint mobility dysfunction
ODS = overhead deep squat
SI = sacroiliac
SLS = single leg stance
SMCD = stability motor-control dysfunction
TED = tissue extensibility dysfunction

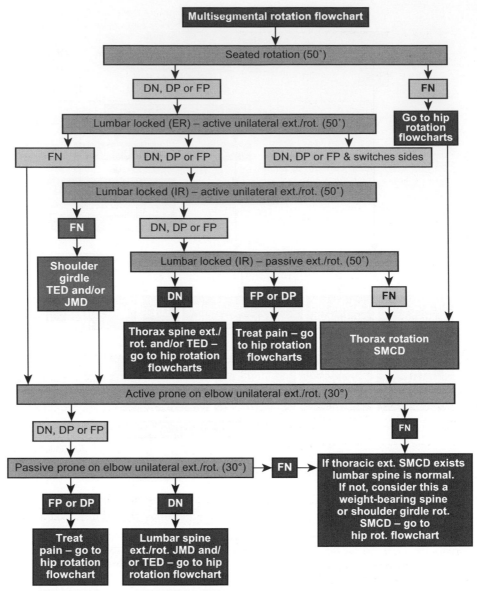

App. 29.5 (A) Spine: limited multisegmental rotation flowchart. Multisegmental rotation 'breakout' flowcharts (spine, hip internal rotation, hip external rotation, tibial rotation) illustrating the systematic reduction of a global movement pattern into its regional components.
(Reproduced with kind permission from Functional Movement Systems.)
Key:
DN = dysfunctional and non-painful
DP = dysfunctional and painful
ER = external rotation
ext. = extension
FN = functional and non-painful
FP = functional and painful
JMD = joint mobility dysfunction
IR = internal rotation
rot. = rotation
SMCD = stability motor control dysfunction
TED = tissue extensibility dysfunction

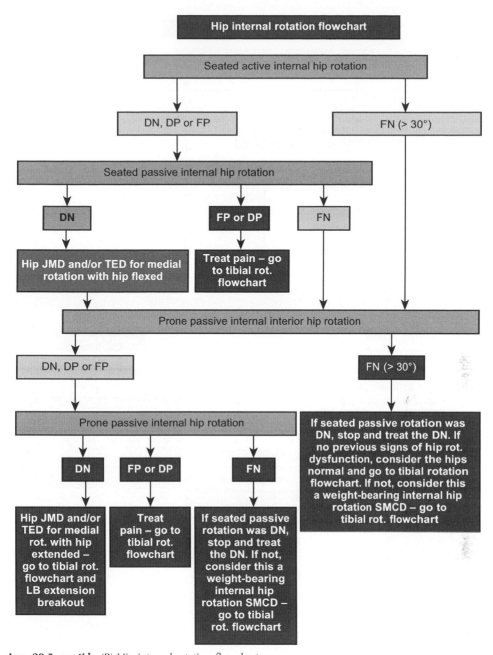

App. 29.5, cont'd (B) Hip internal rotation flowchart.
Key:
DN = dysfunctional and non-painful
DP = dysfunctional and painful
FN = functional and non-painful
FP = functional and painful
JMD = joint mobility dysfunction
LB = lower body
rot. = rotation
SMCD = stability motor-control dysfunction
TED = tissue extensibility dysfunction

Continued on following page

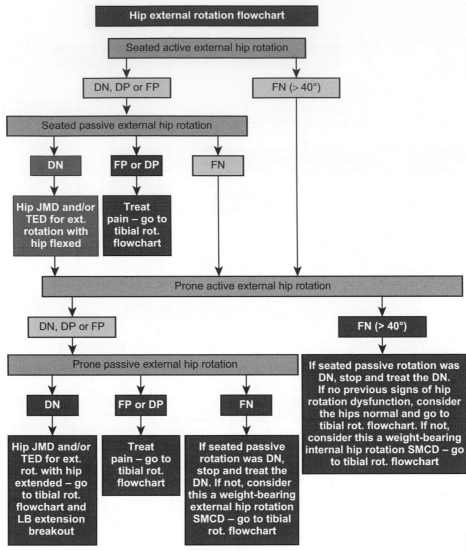

App. 29.5, cont'd (C) Hip external rotation flowchart.

Key:

DN = dysfunctional and non-painful

DP = dysfunctional and painful

ext. = extension

FN = functional and non-painful

FP = functional and painful

JMD = joint mobility dysfunction

rot. = rotation

SMCD = stability motor-control dysfunction

TED = tissue extensibility dysfunction

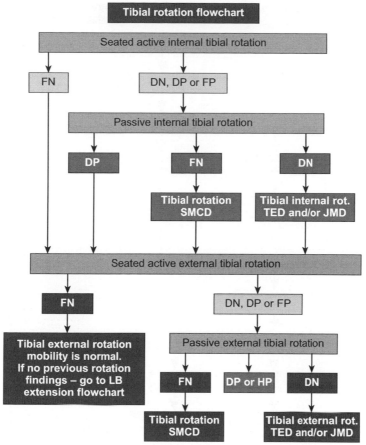

App. 29.5, cont'd   (D) Tibial rotation flowchart.
Key:
DN = dysfunctional and non-painful
DP = dysfunctional and painful
FN = functional and non-painful
FP = functional and painful
JMD = joint mobility dysfunction
LB = lower body
rot. = rotation
SMCD = stability motor-control dysfunction
TED = tissue extensibility dysfunction

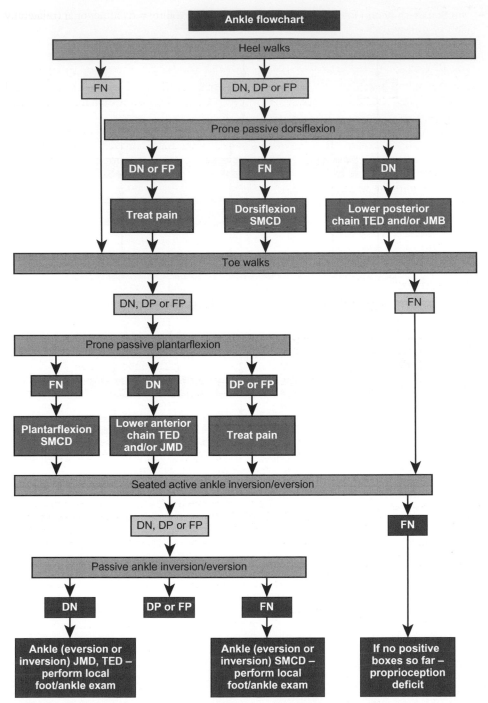

App. 29.6 Single leg stance 'breakouts' ankle flowchart illustrating the systematic reduction of a global movement pattern into its regional components.
(Reproduced with kind permission from Functional Movement Systems.)
Key:
DN = dysfunctional and non-painful
DP = dysfunctional and painful
ext. = extension
FN = functional and non-painful
FP = functional and painful
JMD = joint mobility dysfunction
rot. = rotation
SMCD = stability motor-control dysfunction
TED = tissue extensibility dysfunction

- Upper extremity and lower extremity prone-to-supine rolling = dysfunctional (bilaterally painful in low back)

Special tests:

- Lumbar repeated-movement testing performed in standing and prone/supine lying:
  - Repeated-movement testing for lumbar extension performed both in standing and prone lying resulted in increased low back pain and left lower extremity pain, with no centralization.
  - Repeated-movement testing for lumbar flexion in standing resulted in pain-intensity reduction and centralization from foot to knee after 10 repetitions. Two more sets of 10 repetitions of repeated flexion in standing were performed, with pain centralization occurring to the left hip.
- Sacroiliac joint provocation tests:
  Distraction = negative
  Compression = negative
  Thigh thrust = negative
  Sacral thrust = negative
  Gaenslen's = negative

Summative problems list:

- Bilateral upper posterior chain tissue extensibility dysfunction
- Bilateral thorax joint mobility dysfunction
- Lumbar flexion tissue extensibility dysfunction
- Bilateral anterior chain tissue extensibility dysfunction
- Right hip internal rotation motor control dysfunction with hips in flexion
- Left hip external rotation motor control dysfunction with hips in extension
- Fundamental flexion pattern motor control dysfunction

Reasoning Question:

3. Please discuss your general rationale underpinning your choice and order of physical examination assessments, highlighting your reasoning specific to Chuck's findings.

Answer to Reasoning Question:

From the subjective and objective data, Chuck did not tolerate lumbar extension, as demonstrated by increased pain intensity and peripheralization down the left lower extremity. Conversely, Chuck tolerated lumbar flexion well and further experienced a centralization effect with the repeated flexion motion.

In accordance with the repeated lumbar flexion model advocated by McKenzie (Long et al., 2004), the SFMA top-tier screening results also indicated that the multisegmental flexion pattern was the most dysfunctional and a non-painful pattern. In order to facilitate lumbar flexion to centralize the lower extremity symptoms and begin functional repatterning of the flexion movement pattern, the breakout examination was performed.

To determine why Chuck could not complete the multisegmental flexion pattern, the movement was assessed again under a new condition where the bilateral weight-bearing nature of the movement was changed to a unilateral weight-bearing task. This test is performed by having the patient lift one heel and bear nearly 100% of his weight on the other side while the forward bending movement is repeated. If the pattern becomes functional during this test, it would suggest either an asymmetry exists and/or there is a hip and spine weight-bearing motor-control dysfunction. This was the case with Chuck, as he demonstrated during multisegmental flexion with his left heel raised (i.e. weight-bearing on the right-side) that he was unable to complete the toe-touching movement.

The next step was to reduce the weight-bearing requirements to further break down the movement to its dysfunctional parts. This test was done by performing a forward bending movement without the demands of lower extremity weight-bearing (that is, a sit-and-reach type movement) to determine whether the mobility to complete the movement was present and whether the stability/motor control was not. If Chuck had been able to complete the movement while meeting the three requirements of a sacral angle of at least 80 degrees, a uniform sagittal spinal curve and touching his toes, a diagnosis of a weight-bearing hip motor control dysfunction could have been made because removing the weight-bearing demands of the lower extremity would have allowed for completion of the pattern. However, for the 'multisegmental flexion non-weight-bearing' exercise (i.e. sit and reach), Chuck was unable to complete the toe-touching movement.

Continued on following page

Because a diagnosis still could not be made, the next step was to examine each part of the pattern to determine where the dysfunction lay. In order to complete the multisegmental flexion pattern according to our criteria (Cook, 2010), Chuck would need to have demonstrated at least 70 degrees on straight leg raise (hip flexion with the knee and ankle in neutral), adequate hip joint mobility and adequate spinal flexion mobility. The first test to check the 'parts' of Chuck's multisegmental flexion dysfunction was the active straight leg raise test. The test is performed actively while controlling for potential substitution strategies, such as flexion or external rotation of the opposite hip. If the active test does not yield the required 70 degrees, then the test is performed passively. Passively, we look for 80 degrees. If the passive straight leg raise is less than 80 degrees, and the hip joint demonstrates adequate flexion, a movement-oriented diagnosis of '*posterior chain tissue extensibility dysfunction*' can be made, as was the case with Chuck, whose passive straight leg raise was symmetrical but measured to be 40 degrees bilaterally.

The next step to complete the diagnostic process for the dysfunctional multisegmental flexion pattern was to check spinal flexion mobility. This was done through the prone rock/child's pose test, where Chuck was asked to sit back with his hips going to his heels and to try to get his chest to his thighs. The clinician assesses for spinal flexion mobility, as well as for the presence of a 'uniform spinal curve' in the sagittal plane. This test requires judgement from the clinician to determine whether adequate spinal flexion is present and whether the movement is coming from an adequate distribution throughout the spine, rather than predominantly from an area of hypermobility. In Chuck's case, he demonstrated reduced lumbar spine mobility, resulting in a movement dysfunction diagnosis of 'lumbar spine flexion tissue extensibility dysfunction'. Although the lumbar spine did not demonstrate adequate flexion mobility, the posterior-to-anterior glides of the spine were considered to be normal, thus rendering 'soft tissue restriction' as the diagnosis.

Reasoning Question:

4. As highlighted in Chuck's findings, impairments in function, movement and control can be symptomatic or asymptomatic. Please discuss your reasoning regarding likely physical 'contributing factors' to Chuck's pain and disability.

Answer to Reasoning Question:

As identified through the top-tier SFMA testing, Chuck had both a dysfunctional movement problem and a painful one. Multisegmental lumbar flexion was significantly limited; however, it did not provoke symptoms. This was not the case for the multisegmental extension pattern, which was both limited and provoked Chuck's concordant symptoms. As tempting as it may seem to directly target the painful pattern, in this case, multisegmental extension, our choice for regaining Chuck's function and alleviating his symptoms will be to target the multisegmental flexion pattern. This is due to the concept that pain can alter motor control in unpredictable ways (Hodges and Tucker, 2011). Therefore, prescribing corrective exercises which are painful may or may not be productive. By correcting the flexion pattern first, the likelihood of provoking pain with corrective strategies is much less.

After breaking down the multisegmental flexion pattern, it was found that the contributing factors restricting the pattern were limited tissue extensibility of the posterior chain muscles (hamstrings, gluteals) and Chuck's inability to flex his lumbar spine. These mobility deficits were hypothesized to limit the ability of afferent information to effectively and efficiently reach the CNS. The limited extensibility of the posterior chain muscles, due to length and/or muscle tone, was likely a function of the limited mobility and also the altered motor control in the spine. For example, if motor control is delayed, the brain will likely recruit other neighbouring muscles to act as core stabilizers or limit range of movement as a protective response. Although this response is protective in nature, it is a compensatory altered movement pattern that must be restored to normality.

Although multisegmental extension was painful, the pattern was broken down in order to identify any mobility limitations that could be easily improved to allow for the opportunity for better reflexive motor control. Through the breakout examination, it was determined that Chuck's extension pattern was limited by decreased mobility in his thoracic spine and restricted hip extension ROM. The inability of the joints above and below the lumbar spine (i.e. thoracic spine and hips) to extend essentially places much greater stress on the lumbar spine in order to achieve a given quantity of movement. The lumbar spine's natural tendency is to be a stable joint complex; however, in Chuck's case, it was now in a situation where it had to move excessively, which created excessive shear forces and produced pain. Pain might further alter motor control, and neighbouring joints might lose more mobility to compensate – and the vicious cycle would continue.

Clinical Reasoning Commentary:

The physical examination assessments and associated explained reasoning reflect functional and impairment-focused diagnostic reasoning attending to both motor control and movement impairments, as well as symptom provocation. Commencing with functional multisegmental assessments (see App. 29.1), dysfunctional patterns are differentiated further through a range of 'breakout' assessments designed to identify control and movement sources of the dysfunction (e.g. lower extremity 'posterior chain tissue extensibility' and lumbar spine 'posterior soft tissue restriction' contributing to multisegmental flexion dysfunction; decreased thoracic spine and hip mobility contributing to the multisegmental extension dysfunction, with the hip extension dysfunction attributed to 'bilateral anterior chain tissue extensibility dysfunction'). Also evident in the physical examination assessments completed was further 'testing' of previous hypotheses regarding potential 'sources of symptoms' (i.e. nociception) and 'impairments' through neurological examination, lumbar spine postero-anterior accessory intervertebral movement assessment for mobility and symptom provocation, posterior lumbar muscle palpation, selective hip and knee assessment and sacroiliac joint-provocation tests. This is important because hypotheses formulated through the subjective examination need to be tested in the physical examination. To only assess the dominant functional impairments and not explore and 'disprove' other potential impairments and sources of symptoms may lead to errors of reasoning, such as confirmation bias. Although musculoskeletal clinicians adopt varying approaches to their assessment, a systematic and thorough assessment, as evident here, enables common and unique combinations of impairment to be uncovered for both treatment and re-assessment.

Treatment (First Appointment)

Treatment commenced with an explanation of the examination findings and recommendation for therapy, including the importance of Chuck's participation in home exercise. In regard to the herniated discs, Chuck was educated that his symptoms were not consistent with the typical presentation for a discogenic pain generator. It was explained that the examination findings indicated that numerous mobility deficits in the spine and hips were placing increased stress on his lumbar spine. Furthermore, the increased muscle spasm in his low back muscles was likely acting as a protective response to prevent further injury. Because prolonged standing at work increased Chuck's pain, he was advised to sit down every 20–30 minutes to take stress off his back. This would reduce the symptoms down his leg and allow him to not hurt as much by the end of the workday. In addition, Chuck was advised to avoid sleeping on his stomach at night in order to allow him to get more productive rest. Three physical interventions were then introduced:

1. Supine pistol-grip mid-thoracic spine manipulation (Karas and Olson Hunt, 2014)
- Re-assessed passive lumbar locked internal rotation unilateral extension/rotation test: thoracic spine mobility was judged visually to improve from 40 to 50 degrees bilaterally, making it 'functional and non-painful' in the SFMA classification.
2. Bilateral contract-relax proprioceptive neuromuscular facilitation (PNF) stretching of left and right hamstring muscles (with instruction in a home exercise: static hamstring stretching at the doorway; Fig. 29.2)
- Re-assessed passive straight leg raise test: ROM improved from 40 to 60 degrees bilaterally, indicating better posterior chain tissue extensibility; however, it remained 'dysfunctional and non-painful'.
3. Upper extremity and lower extremity supine-to-prone-flexion rolling exercise (Fig. 29.3) and a diaphragmatic breathing exercise progressed from supine lying to the half-kneeling posture
- Following these exercises, upper and lower extremity supine-to-prone-flexion rolling patterns remained dysfunctional (due to perceived increased exertion still being present) and non-painful; however, the patterns were much improved.

Fig. 29.2 Static hamstring stretching at the doorway.

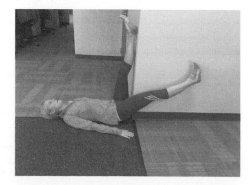

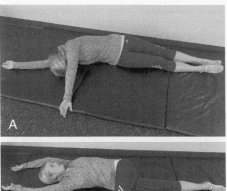
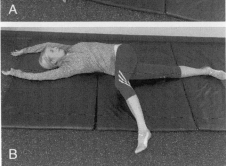

Fig. 29.3 (A) Upper extremity supine-to-prone-flexion rolling exercise. (B) Lower extremity supine-to-prone-flexion rolling exercise.

Reasoning Question:

5. Please discuss your rationale for the specific impairments you treated and the procedures you used.

Answer to Reasoning Question:

The treatment rationale was driven by the assessment process. The movement-oriented diagnoses from the problem list were prioritized, and the most appropriate treatment to address each problem was performed. Initially, the emphasis was on restoring appropriate mobility of the spine and posterior chain extensibility (i.e. hamstrings). Restoring mobility potentially allows for improved processing of afferent information by the CNS. As identified through the breakout examinations, Chuck lacked full thoracic spine ROM that may have obligated his lumbar spine to give up a degree of motor control as compensation for the immobility higher in the spine. Therefore, restoring thoracic mobility through a high-velocity, low-amplitude manipulation was a major priority to set the stage for enhancing lumbar motor control.

As verified through objective testing, Chuck's symptoms were improved with flexion, and on that basis, the initial plan also included restoring the multisegmental flexion pattern. The breakout examination of multisegmental flexion showed a posterior chain tissue extensibility dysfunction due to limited passive straight leg raise bilaterally. Contract-relax PNF hamstring stretching made an immediate change to the passive straight leg raise, and hence that improvement can be inferred to be related to a change in tone of the hamstrings. The excessive tone in the hamstrings was likely protective in nature due to pain and lack of inner core motor control. In order to reinforce the gains in mobility as a function of the tone reduction in the posterior chain, an isolated hamstring stretch was then provided as a home exercise.

The next step following the improvement in mobility of the thoracic spine and of the posterior chain was to begin motor control re-patterning. Chuck's breathing pattern was assessed in supine lying and revealed a dysfunctional apical pattern. Following cueing to utilize more of a diaphragmatic breathing pattern, which should contribute to engaging inner core motor control, the breathing pattern was then sequentially progressed through the neurodevelopmental postures as follows: first supine lying, then prone lying, quadruped, tall kneeling and finally half-kneeling.

In order to grade the severity of Chuck's motor control dysfunction, upper body and lower body supine-to-prone-lying rolling patterns were assessed. Rolling is one of the most fundamental movement patterns learned early on in the neurodevelopmental process. Inability to roll indicates a very basic motor control limitation (Hoogenboom et al., 2009). We began with supine-to-prone-lying rolling in order to facilitate a more flexion-based pattern, as opposed to prone-to-supine-lying rolling, which is more extension based. Because extension movements were painful and increased Chuck's symptoms, they were not assessed.

Clinical Reasoning Commentary:

Treatment at the first appointment commenced with patient education addressing the important issue of the pathological diagnosis Chuck had been given by his referring physician, as well as an explanation of the key physical impairments found in the assessment that were likely contributing to his persistent symptoms. Although Chuck was judged not to have any overt yellow flags, including unhelpful beliefs or fears regarding his diagnosis, conflicting information from different health professionals can contribute to patient confusion and stress, and therefore providing an explanation that incorporates the medical diagnosis is important.

The three physical treatment interventions used at the first appointment were re-assessed for their effect. The focus and extent of outcome re-assessment constitute an un-researched area of practice and likely vary considerably across approaches and clinicians. From a reasoning perspective, what is essential is that key impairments are critically re-assessed so that effects of different interventions on the targeted impairment, as well as others to establish relationships between impairments, are monitored to guide treatment progression.

Appointment 2 (1 Week Later)

Subjectively, Chuck no longer reported any lower extremity symptoms, and his pain was now isolated to the low back region only. Prolonged standing and walking continued to increase his low back pain, which still worsened by the end of the working day.

On physical examination, the following was observed:

- The multisegmental flexion pattern was still dysfunctional and non-painful; however, the quality and quantity of the movement pattern had improved by 50%.
- Passive straight leg raise was improved bilaterally from 40 to 60 degrees.
- The multisegmental extension pattern remained dysfunctional and painful, with no change in provocation of pain in the low back; however, there was no report of any leg pain. Extension mobility was unchanged.

The second treatment session continued PNF contract-relax hamstring muscle stretching to improve posterior chain extensibility. Static doorway hamstring stretching as a home exercise was reviewed and continued as a reinforcement strategy for improving posterior chain extensibility.

Trigger-point dry needling to the lumbar multifidus muscles at the L4/L5 segment was performed to address local tissue extensibility dysfunction evident in lumbar flexion.

Re-assessment demonstrated the following:

- Local tenderness to palpation of lumbar multifidus muscles had decreased following needling.
- Prone rock (child's pose) lumbar flexion test had improved, with a more uniform lumbar spinal curve (although still dysfunctional and non-painful).
- Multisegmental extension had increased 50% in extension mobility, with a subjective report of decreased pain (still dysfunctional and painful).

Chuck now demonstrated functional upper body and lower body supine-to-prone rolling patterns. Competency with fundamental flexion motor control (as per the improved rolling patterns) was considered to now permit stability demands to be progressed in a higher, weight-bearing developmental posture. The rolling patterns were progressed to 'quadruped mountain climbers' (Fig. 29.4) to pattern core stability/motor control with the hips in weight-bearing posture and while still emphasizing lumbar flexion. In a fitness setting, the mountain climber exercise is typically performed quickly to challenge endurance. As a corrective strategy, Chuck was instructed to perform the mountain climber exercise slowly

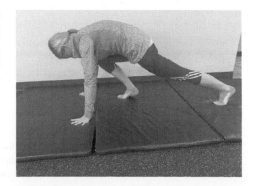

Fig. 29.4 'Quadruped mountain climbers' exercise emphasizing core stability/motor control with the hips in weight-bearing while still emphasizing lumbar flexion. Begin in push-up position. While keeping body in a straight line, bring one knee up to chest and set foot down, and then return to starting position. Alternate legs.

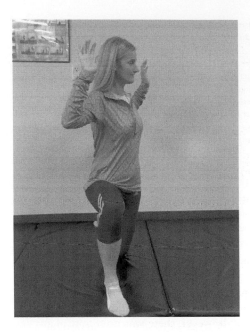

Fig. 29.5 'Half-kneeling rotations' exercise to challenge hip internal and external rotation motor control while simultaneously challenging thoracic spine mobility. Maintain a tall posture in half kneeling by keeping hips forward and shoulders back. Hold arms above head and rotate to one side and then the other, staying tall and keeping hips forward.

to maintain lumbar flexion throughout the entire exercise. Twenty repetitions were performed on each leg.

Half-kneeling static stability with diaphragmatic breathing was also much improved relative to the last session. Static stability was progressed to more dynamic stability by prescribing 'half-kneeling rotations' (Fig. 29.5) to challenge hip internal and external rotation motor control while simultaneously challenging thoracic spine mobility. Chuck required cueing to maintain an upright posture and to not allow the front knee to drop into valgus. Twenty repetitions were performed on each side. Chuck was to perform his home exercise program (static doorway hamstring stretching, mountain climbers and half-kneeling rotations) twice per day.

Appointment 3 (1 Week Later)

Subjectively, Chuck's low back pain had decreased from 5/10 to 2/10 on the VAS at its worst. He reported much less pain with standing and walking, but his low back pain continued to be at its worst toward the end of the working day.

Physical re-assessment revealed the following:

- Multisegmental flexion – functional and non-painful
- Active straight leg raise – improved to 70 degrees bilaterally; 'functional and non-painful'
- Multisegmental extension – dysfunctional (restricted ROM) and non-painful
  - Thomas Test – dysfunctional (restricted rectus femoris muscle length) and non-painful bilaterally, indicating 'limited anterior chain tissue extensibility'
  - Passive lumbar locked internal rotation unilateral spine extension/rotation – still functional and non-painful bilaterally, indicating full thoracic spine joint mobility
  - No tenderness to palpation of lumbar erector spinae muscles bilaterally
  - Mild tenderness to palpation over lumbar multifidus muscles at L4/L5
- Multisegmental rotation – dysfunctional (limited thoracic and hip ROM) and non-painful but with the pattern now improved 50%

Treatment

The third appointment treatment consisted of trigger-point dry needling to the lumbar multifidus muscle as a 'reset' (i.e. when manual intervention invokes acceptable change in ROM and primes the neuromusculoskeletal system for corrective exercise) for the lumbar flexion '*tissue extensibility dysfunction*'. Prone rock (child's pose) lumbar flexion was re-assessed after the needling and now demonstrated a uniform sagittal spinal curve indicating functional and non-painful lumbar flexion. Chuck also no longer reported tenderness to palpation over the lumbar multifidus muscles at L4/L5.

The 'Brettzel' stretch (Fig. 29.6) was given as a reinforcement for thoracic spine mobility and hip flexor static stretching. In order to perform the Brettzel stretch, the patient begins in side-lying with the top thigh flexed to 90 degrees of hip flexion to lock the lumbar spine. The patient grabs the ankle of the opposite leg and passively extends the hip. Finally, the patient rotates the thorax, attempting to lay the scapula flat on the ground.

Because multisegmental extension was now pain-free, stability/motor control patterning was progressed to incorporate extension through instruction in quadruped diagonals (Fig. 29.7). Quadruped mountain climber and half-kneeling rotation exercises were respectively progressed to push walkout and half-kneeling chops with resistance tubing (Figs 29.8 and 29.9).

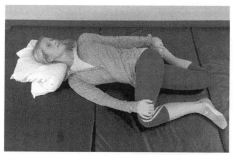

Fig. 29.6 The 'Brettzel stretch' exercise is a re-enforcement for thoracic spine mobility and hip flexor static stretching. Lie on your side with your neck supported in a neutral position. Draw your knee up toward your chest close to your body. The angle between your thigh and knee should be less than 90 degrees. Reach back with your other leg, bringing your thigh as far behind your body as possible. Then bend back knee as much as possible by grabbing your ankle. Do not proceed until both legs are locked up. The next step is to rotate shoulders and head toward the ceiling, trying to lay your back on the ground. Once in this position, use deep diaphragmatic breathing to increase the stretch as the muscles relax.

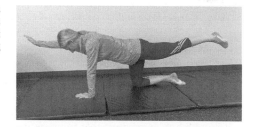

Fig. 29.7 'Quadruped diagonals'. Place your hands directly under your shoulders and knees under hips in an all-fours position. Extend your left arm and right leg in a straight line at the same time while maintaining balance. Repeat on other side.

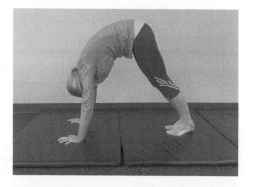

Fig. 29.8 'Push-up walkout' exercise. The push-up walkout begins by having the individual standing with feet shoulder-width apart. Bend over so that your hands hit the floor; bend at the knees if needed. Then walk your hands out as far as possible, keeping a stable back and not hyperextending. Walk the hands back toward the feet and return to standing position.

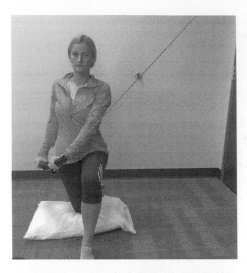

Fig. 29.9 'Half-kneeling chops' exercise. Begin in half kneeling with the leg closest to the wall in the up position. Hip, knee and ankle should all be at 90 degrees. Kneel tall and reach upward at an angle toward the band. Pull the band down across the chest and rotate slightly while maintaining balance and good upright posture.

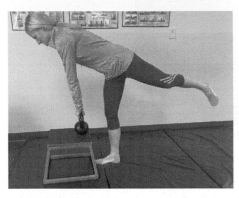

Fig. 29.10 Single leg deadlifting with an 8-kg kettlebell

Fourth Appointment (1 Week Later)

Subjectively, Chuck reported he no longer had any low back or leg pain. Prolonged standing and walking were now pain-free and felt normal.

Physical re-assessment findings were as follows:

- Multisegmental flexion – functional and non-painful
- Multisegmental extension – functional and non-painful
- Multisegmental rotation – dysfunctional (limited thoracic and hip rotation ROM) and non-painful, but the pattern had improved by approximately 75% bilaterally.
- Single leg stance pattern – functional and non-painful bilaterally
- Overhead deep squat pattern – dysfunctional (loss of shoulder flexion) and non-painful. Chuck's hips were now able to break parallel with no sagittal plane deviations, improving the pattern overall by about 50%.

Chuck was now asymptomatic, and his dysfunction as measured by the SFMA scoring tool (App. 29.2) had improved from 56% dysfunctional at initial evaluation to 20% 4 weeks later. Because Chuck was now asymptomatic and demonstrating good progress on the SFMA, the next level of movement-oriented tasks was performed: the Functional Movement Screen (FMS) (Table 29.1). The FMS is recommended to be used near discharge to screen for asymmetries and major movement limitations (Kiesel et al., 2014). The reliability of the FMS is well established (Frohm et al., 2012; Gribble et al., 2013; Minick et al., 2010; Teyhen et al., 2012). FMS (scored on the best of three repetitions) showed no 0 scores, which is indicative of pain; no 1 scores, indicating inability to perform a pattern; and no asymmetries. That is, Chuck was able to perform each of the movement patterns with normally accepted compensatory strategies.

For treatment, Chuck's stability motor-control exercises were upgraded to include single leg deadlifting with an 8-kg kettlebell and a full Turkish getup exercise (Figs 29.10 and

TABLE 29.1

FUNCTIONAL MOVEMENT SCREEN (FMS) RECOMMENDED FOR USE NEAR DISCHARGE TO SCREEN FOR MAJOR MOVEMENT LIMITATIONS THAT MAY STILL EXIST AND REPRESENT POTENTIAL RISK FACTORS FOR EITHER RECURRENCE OF THE RECENTLY RESOLVED PROBLEM OR DEVELOPMENT OF ADDITIONAL PROBLEMS

Pattern	Score
Overhead deep squat	2
Hurdle step	2
Inline lunge	2
Shoulder mobility	2
Active straight leg raise	2
Trunk stability push-up	3
Rotary stability	2

Chuck's total score = 15/21

0 = pain with movement

1 = inability to perform the movement pattern

2 = acceptable performance of movement pattern with compensation

3 = acceptable performance of movement pattern without compensation

Score is based on the best of three trials.

FMS Pattern Descriptions:

- Overhead deep squat – Place a dowel overhead, with the instep of the feet in line with the axilla and toes pointed straight ahead. Descend into the deepest squat possible while trying to maintain the dowel overhead and keeping the feet straight ahead.
- Hurdle step – Measure the height of the client's tibia from the top center of the tibial tuberosity to the foot using the FMS dowel. Adjust the hurdle height to correlate with the measured tibial height. The client stands behind the center of the hurdle with toes touching the base, feet together and the dowel across the shoulders. The client steps over the hurdle step and touches the heel on the ground while maintaining a tall spine. The client then returns to the leg starting position and repeats on the contralateral side.
- Inline lunge – The client's tibial height is measured from the top center of the tibial tuberosity to the floor using the FMS dowel. The dowel is placed behind the client's back in contact with the head, thoracic spine and sacrum. The client's hand opposite the front foot should be the hand grasping the dowel at the cervical spine. The other hand grasps the dowel at the lumbar spine. The client lowers the back knee to touch the board behind the heel of the front foot and returns to starting position, maintaining a vertical spine.
- Shoulder mobility – The client's hand length must be obtained by measuring the distance from the distal wrist crease to the tip of the longest finger with the FMS dowel. The client stands with feet together with thumbs tucked inside of a closed fist. The client reaches simultaneously with one fist behind the neck while the other reaches behind the back. The hands should remain fisted and move in one smooth motion. Measure the distance between the two closest points of the hands. Repeat on the contralateral side.
- Active straight leg raise – The client begins in supine with the hands by the client's sides with the palms up. Knees are together, and the feet are in a neutral position. Find the point between the ASIS and the joint line of the knee, and place the FMS dowel perpendicular to the ground at this position. The client maintains the knee and ankle position while the test leg is up. The opposite leg remains in contact with the ground. Repeat on the opposite side.
- Trunk stability push-up – Begin in the prone position with arms extended. Men and women have different starting points in relation to the hand position. Men begin with their thumbs at the chin level, whereas women begin with the thumbs at the shoulder level. The client performs a push-up from this position, trying to lift the body as one unit.
- Rotary stability – The client begins in the quadruped posture with the FMS board between the knees. The client flexes the shoulder while extending the ipsilateral hip at the same time and then brings elbow to knee while remaining inline over the board. This is performed on both sides. If the client is unable to meet the passing criteria, the test is repeated by flexing the shoulder and extending the contralateral hip in order to perform a diagonal pattern.

Total Possible = 21

29.11). The 'Turkish getup' is a total-body exercise that increases core stabilization and overall strength. The movement is very complex and requires upper body strength to maintain a weight overhead, shoulder stability, hip and gluts strength to raise the body off the floor and tremendous core strength. Chuck was to continue with this home exercise program as instructed and was discharged from physical therapy.

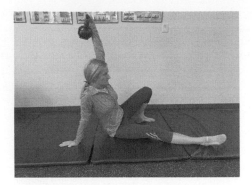

Fig. 29.11 Full Turkish getup exercise.

Reasoning Question:

6. How does your use of the FMS for Chuck, and also for musculoskeletal risk screening in general, both guide exercise prescription for asymptomatic clients and inform your hypothesis of 'prognosis'?

Answer to Reasoning Question:

At this point, Chuck was asymptomatic, and pain was not provoked with any of the top-tier SFMA movement patterns (see App. 29.1). Therefore, a higher degree of motor control testing was needed. For that, the FMS (see Table 29.1) was utilized. The FMS is used for individuals who are not in current pain and do not have any known musculoskeletal disorders. In rehabilitation, most patients are entering into our care with pain; however, upon discharge, the pain has usually been resolved. This is an excellent time to perform the FMS, just prior to discharge and once the symptoms have been alleviated.

Asymmetries and motor-control dysfunctions follow closely behind previous injury as factors associated with increased risk of future injury (Butler et al., 2013; Garrison et al., 2015; Lehr et al., 2013; Plisky et al., 2006; Teyhen et al., 2015). A poor score on the FMS due to lack of quality movement patterns and/or asymmetries indicates an increased risk of future injury (Kiesel et al., 2014; O'Conner et al., 2011). Chuck's FMS testing revealed no pain, asymmetries or limitations in movement quality outside of acceptable compensatory standards. Due to demonstrating no relevant body-movement limitations, it was hypothesized that Chuck had a good prognosis and that he should be able to return to weight lifting and other fitness activities without any fear of reinjury.

The FMS results can provide a guide to exercise prescription when transitioning back to fitness. For example, Chuck's previously dysfunctional multisegmental flexion pattern was analyzed further and found to be due to his '*limited posterior chain extensibility*'. For this, prescribing a single leg deadlifting pattern under load will consolidate the improvement in this movement by using his hip flexion and hip extension mobility in a closed-kinetic-chain position to facilitate greater stability. Similarly, each dysfunction identified in an FMS screening must be analyzed to determine the cause of the dysfunction. Exercise prescription for mobility and/or motor control is then tailored to the specific causes identified.

Clinical Reasoning Commentary:

Minimization of symptom and disability recurrence, as well as injury prevention for healthy individuals generally, requires a good understanding of psychological, social, environmental and physical risk factors. Broadly speaking, a patient's prognosis for recurrence or exacerbation is determined by the nature and extent of the patient's problem(s) and the patient's ability and willingness to make the necessary changes (i.e. to address lifestyle, psychosocial and physical contributing factors). Thoroughness in assessment and clinical reasoning and skills in teaching, motivating and empowering patients are all essential to success.

ACKNOWLEDGEMENTS

Special thanks to Dr Franny Enzler PT, DPT, SCS, CSCS, for modelling in all exercise photographs for this case.

REFERENCES

Butler, R.J., Contreras, M., Burton, L., Plisky, P.J., Kiesel, K.B., 2013. Modifiable risk factors predict injuries in firefighter during training academies. Work 46 (1), 11–17.

Cholewicki, J., Greene, H.S., Polzhofer, G.K., Galloway, M.T., Shah, R.A., Radebold, A., 2002. Neuromuscular function in athletes following recovery from a recent acute low back injury. J. Orthop. Sports Phys. Ther. 32 (11), 568–575.

Cook, E., 2010. Movement. On Target Publishing, Aptos, CA.

Frohm, A., Heijne, A., Kowalski, J., Svensson, P., Myklebust, G., 2012. A nine-test screening battery for athletes: a reliability study. Scand. J. Med. Sci. Sports 22 (3), 306–315.

Garrison, M., Westrick, R., Johnson, M.R., Benenson, J., 2015. Association between the functional movement screen and injury development in college athletes. Int. J. Sports Phys. Ther. 10 (1), 21–28.

Gribble, P.A., Brigle, J., Pietrosimone, B.G., Pfile, K.R., Webster, K.A., 2013. Intrarater reliability of the functional movement screen. J. Strength Cond. Res. 27 (4), 978–981.

Hodges, P.W., Coppieters, M.W., MacDonald, D., Cholewicki, J., 2013. New insight into motor adaptation to pain revealed by a combination of modelling and empirical approaches. Eur. J. Pain 17, 1138–1146.

Hodges, P.W., Tucker, K., 2011. Moving differently in pain: a new theory to explain the adaptation to pain. Pain 152 (3 Suppl.), S90–S98.

Hoogenboom, B., Voight, M.L., Cook, E., Gill, L., 2009. Using rolling to develop neuromuscular control and coordination of the core and extremities of athletes. Int. J. Sports Phys. Ther. 4 (2), 70–82.

Karas, S., Olson Hunt, M.J., 2014. A randomized clinical trial to compare the immediate effects of seated thoracic manipulation and targeted supine thoracic manipulation on cervical spine flexion range of motion and pain. J. Man. Manip. Ther. 22 (2), 108–114.

Kiesel, K.B., Butler, R.J., Plisky, P.J., 2014. Prediction of injury by limited and asymmetrical fundamental movement patterns in American football players. J. Sport Rehabil. 23 (2), 88–94.

Lehr, M.E., Plisky, P.J., Butler, R.J., Fink, M.L., Kiesel, K.B., Underwood, F.B., 2013. Field-expedient screening and injury risk algorithm categories as predictors of noncontact lower extremity injury. Scand. J. Med. Sci. Sports 23 (4), 225–232.

Long, A., Donelson, R., Fung, T., 2004. Does it matter which exercise? A randomized trial of exercise for low back pain. Spine 29 (23), 2593–2602.

Minick, K.I., Kiesel, K.B., Burton, L., Taylor, A., Plisky, P., Butler, R.J., 2010. Interrater reliability of the functional movement screen. J. Strength Cond. Res. 24 (2), 479–486.

O'Connor, F.G., Deuster, P.A., Davis, J., Pappas, C.G., Knapik, J.J., 2011. Functional movement screening: predicting injuries in officer candidates. Med. Sci. Sports Exerc.

Plisky, P.J., Rauh, M.J., Kaminski, T.W., Underwood, F.B., 2006. Star excursion balance test as a predictor of lower extremity injury in high school basketball players. J. Orthop. Sports Phys. Ther. 36 (12), 911–919.

Smart, K.M., Blake, C., Staines, A., Thacker, M., Doody, C., 2012a. Mechanisms-based classifications of musculoskeletal pain: part 1 of 3: symptoms and signs of central sensitisation in patients with low back (+/-leg) pain. Man. Ther. 17, 336–344.

Smart, K.M., Blake, C., Staines, A., Thacker, M., Doody, C., 2012b. Mechanisms-based classifications of musculoskeletal pain: part 2 of 3: symptoms and signs of peripheral neuropathic pain in patients with low back (+/-leg) pain. Man. Ther. 17, 345–351.

Smart, K.M., Blake, C., Staines, A., Thacker, M., Doody, C., 2012c. Mechanisms-based classifications of musculoskeletal pain: part 3 of 3: symptoms and signs of nociceptive pain in patients with low back (+/-leg) pain. Man. Ther. 17, 352–357.

Teyhen, D.S., Plisky, P.J., Kiesel, K.B., Butler, R.J., Goffar, S.L., Rohn, D., 2015. Factors associated with predicting time-loss injuries in active duty soldiers. APTA Combined Sections Meeting. Indianapolis, IN.

Teyhen, D.S., Shaffer, S.W., Lorenson, C.L., et al., 2012. The functional movement screen: a reliability study. J. Orthop. Sports Phys. Ther. 42 (6), 530–540.

Treede, R.D., Jensen, T.S., Campbell, J.N., Cruccu, G., Dostrovsky, J.O., Griffin, J.W., et al., 2008. Neuropathic pain: redefinition and a grading system for clinical and research purposes. Neurology 70, 1630–1635.

30

A 30-Year History of Left-Sided 'Chronic Sciatica'

Alan J. Taylor • Roger Kerry • Darren A. Rivett

Geoff, a 53-year-old male, presented for assessment of chronic left-leg discomfort and numbness, which he had suffered since his mid-20s. He had been referred by a physiotherapy colleague, who confessed to being bemused by the patient's presentation. Geoff worked as a self-employed builder and enjoyed cycling in his spare time, as well as competing in triathlons.

Subjective Examination

On examination, Geoff was very lean and fit (he still rode a bicycle daily between 15 and 80 km) and reported no comorbidities, although he had suffered occasional intermittent low back pain over the last 10–15 years associated with work tasks involving bending, lifting or carrying. He was not taking any medications and had no significant past medical or family history, although he reported a recent 'cardiac ablation for a heart arrhythmia' performed 18 months previously.

History of Present Complaint

Geoff recounted that the onset of his left-leg symptoms was over 30 years ago, and he recalled feelings of left-leg discomfort, weakness and numbness which were manifest when he was cycling (he was a competitive cyclist at the time). He had no low back pain associated with the symptoms at the time of onset. Geoff recalled his back symptoms later developed in his 30s–40s which he related to the manual nature of his job. Cycling presently still provoked his left-leg symptoms. The pain, weakness and numbness were now reported as being non-specific in terms of distribution (see Fig. 30.1), along with a general feeling of fatigue in the limb. He described that the symptoms would begin in the buttock and hindquarter, then 'creep' into the thigh, eventually affecting the whole leg and foot. The numbness was most noticeable in the foot.

On consulting his general practitioner, Geoff was given a diagnosis of 'sciatica'. He was then referred to a physiotherapist, who agreed with this diagnosis, and early management was implemented involving a wide variety of mechanical and manual techniques. These ranged from spinal thrust manipulation to various prescribed exercises. His failure to respond to these physiotherapy treatments led Geoff to visit other manual therapists, including osteopaths and chiropractors. Nonetheless, his condition remained completely unchanged.

Twenty years following the onset of his symptoms, Geoff was categorized under the 'chronic pain' label. He went through a process of pain management, counselling, cognitive-behavioural therapy and various combinations of other pain therapies. None of the described interventions or management strategies proved to be successful.

A recent magnetic resonance imaging (MRI) scan confirmed disc protrusions at L4/L5/S1, with mild impingement on the neural tissue at these same levels. Geoff subsequently underwent spinal injections over the last 12 months, which again had made little or no difference in his condition.

All in all, he considered that his overall condition was unimproved, if not worsening, noting, 'I've tried it all, nothing works … and I reckon it's getting steadily worse'.

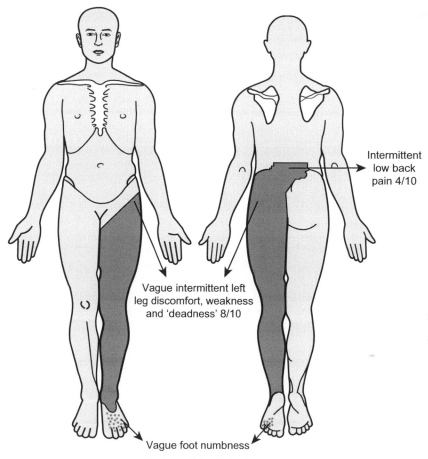

Fig. 30.1   Geoff's body chart.

From a psychosocial perspective, Geoff reported that he was in a stable relationship, had no underlying psychological issues, engaged in regular exercise and had learnt to 'cope', adopting a stoical attitude to his condition. However, he reported remaining frustrated by his condition and his inability to cycle at the same level as his 'mates of the same age', and he described being 'left behind in the hills' as particularly frustrating. He displayed an element of dismissal for some of the explanations he had received of why he was still in pain, and he retained the opinion that 'something was wrong'. He indicated that this was why he continued to search for an answer and pay privately for ongoing consultations.

Reasoning Questions:

1. Can you please provide your initial impressions of Geoff's presentation at this stage of the consultation? In particular, what were your thoughts on his lack of responsiveness to all previous interventions?

Answer to Reasoning Question:

The key elements of Geoff's presentation at this time were the long and protracted history, the description of the symptoms (e.g. fatigue, weakness), the exercise-induced nature of the early and current presenting symptoms (induced by cycling) and the failure to respond to any type of intervention. Pattern recognition at this stage, based on previous work in this field, was suggestive of a possible vascular origin of the pain and other leg symptoms (Taylor and George, 2001; Peach et al., 2012). The failure to respond to previous treatments/interventions is a common feature of such cases and is in fact a reason to consider a vascular assessment, particularly when an exercise-induced element is a feature of the presentation. Geoff's cardiac comorbidity was also potentially a related risk factor, but this seemed unlikely.

Continued on following page

From a broader perspective, there was the possibility of a concomitant chronic non-specific low back pain disorder with distal referral, either from somatic or nerve root structures. However this hypothesis was not supported by the examinations of the previous clinicians.

Clinical Reasoning Commentary:

Practitioners generate hypotheses early in the patient encounter, and it is clearly evident in this answer that pattern recognition, that is, a type of fast or inductive thinking (system 1; see Chapter 1), has been automatically employed. As further exemplified in this response, pattern recognition is highly dependent on prior clinical experiences (both direct, personal experiences and those gleaned from other practitioners) with similar presentations and on the recognition of limited but key clinical cues. In this instance, the protracted history, the type of symptoms described, the lack of responsiveness to numerous prior neuromusculoskeletal interventions and, most importantly, the persistent exercise–symptom relationship are all examples of such critical clinical features that form a pattern.

Symptom Pattern

Geoff explained that he used a pulse monitor for cycling and could predict more or less the exact onset of the symptoms related to his heart rate. His symptoms would initially develop in his left buttock at or around 135 beats per minute (bpm); if he continued to elevate his heart rate via increased effort, such as by climbing a hill or cycling harder on the flat terrain, then the symptoms would develop further into the leg, which would concomitantly feel weak or fatigued. He described it as though he was 'cycling with one leg' and that his 'leg goes dead'. There was no reported relationship between his back pain and his leg symptoms experienced during exercise.

On a visual analogue score (VAS), Geoff indicated his discomfort varied between 0 and 8 out of 10 but that he could control it via the modification of effort linked to his heart rate. As Geoff explained, he only needed to 'ease off' to just below 135 bpm, and all of the symptoms would disappear. In fact, he was able to ride below the threshold of 135 bpm for hours without the onset of any noticeable symptoms. He denied any residual post-ride/effort symptoms.

Symptoms were now also being experienced in 'normal or everyday' effort-related activities, such as pushing a wheelbarrow or climbing stairs. This had only been noticed by Geoff over the last year.

When asked what he expected of his visit to our clinic, Geoff indicated he was seeking a second opinion. In his view, the pain was clearly exercise induced (in the patient's own words: 'from day one, I explained that the pain only came on when I exercised'). The overall impression at this stage was that Geoff was a very stoical 'coper' who, rather than suffering stress or fear and demonstrating avoidance behaviour, was quite simply frustrated with his condition and had a genuine desire to be more active.

Reasoning Questions:

2. Did this further information about the exercise-related onset of Geoff's symptoms cause you to modify any of the hypotheses you may have previously been entertaining, such as the 'pain type', the 'sources of nociception and associated pathology', or 'contributing factors to the development and maintenance of the problem'?

Answer to Reasoning Question:

After 30 years of symptoms, it was clear that Geoff fell into the 'chronic pain' category, and there was a very real possibility that his symptoms might have had an element of maladaptive central sensitization (Nijs et al., 2015) or nociplastic pain, which would fit with contemporary thinking with regard to pain science. However, a key factor supporting an ischaemic-induced nociception presentation was the very clear pattern of reproducibility of his symptoms during exercise, which began at age 18 years and remained to the present day. The young age of onset also suggested that a differential diagnosis of spinal stenosis would have been unlikely.

Furthermore, it is well known that some sports participants, most commonly cyclists, may suffer unilateral or bilateral arterial flow limitations, postulated to be linked to 'kinking' of the arteries and a condition called endofibrosis (Peach et al., 2012). Previous clinical experience with similar patients who had suffered 5- and 15-year delays to diagnosis led to prudence being exercised with regard to accepting the central sensitivity hypothesis. It is well recognized that vascular tissue may be a source of pain either from local nociception/pathology or via the mechanism of ischaemia. The pattern of symptoms in this case suggested the latter and indicated the need for further investigation. In addition, Geoff had been non-responsive to a multitude of pain management interventions for neuromusculoskeletal disorders, which further supported the need to investigate the vascular ischaemic hypothesis.

Clinical Reasoning Commentary:

In this answer, diagnostic reasoning with the simultaneous consideration of hypotheses in two categories is evident (nociplastic – 'pain type'; vascular ischaemia or local pathology – 'source of nociception and associated pathology'). Hypotheses regarding pathology are particularly critical for identifying possible sinister and non-musculoskeletal conditions. Notably, red flags, that is, signs and symptoms that may indicate the presence of more serious pathology and systemic or viscerogenic pathology/disease, should elicit consideration of referral for further consultation/investigation, as has been suggested here for Geoff.

Physical Examination

On inspection, Geoff had no apparent deformities or leg-length discrepancies, and a cursory musculoskeletal examination demonstrated full spinal range of motion without any symptom provocation and an entirely normal neurological examination. These tests were performed because it was considered important to scan or check the spinal somatic and neuropathic tissues before moving on to examine other systems. No further musculoskeletal examination was carried out at this point. Instead, it was decided that the session time would be allocated to examining the vascular system.

Vascular Examination

Observation, Palpation and Resting Blood Pressure

Temperature was normal, capillary refill was normal and there were no signs of ischaemia in the lower limbs (e.g. colour or skin changes). Pulses (femoral, popliteal, dorsalis pedis and posterior tibial) were all present and normal for both limbs at rest.

The ankle-brachial pressure index (ABPI) was next tested. ABPI is a non-invasive vascular screening test to identify large-vessel peripheral arterial disease by comparing systolic blood pressure in the ankle to the highest of the brachial systolic blood pressures, which is the best estimate of central systolic blood pressure. This test was indicated both as a baseline measure of resting vascular health and because of the presenting symptoms (Kim et al., 2012).

Repeated and average resting systolic blood pressure values after 15 minutes of resting in supine lying are shown in Tables 30.1 and 30.2. The left resting ABPI was 1.05 (normal), and the right resting ABPI was 1.09 (normal). Values > 1.2 or < 1.0 are considered abnormal, and the lower the value, the greater the magnitude of arterial disease.

TABLE 30.1

LEFT RESTING SYSTOLIC BLOOD PRESSURE VALUES (mmHg)

Left	1	2	3	Average reading
Ankle	145	143	142	143
Brachial	137	132	140	136

TABLE 30.2

RIGHT RESTING SYSTOLIC BLOOD PRESSURE VALUES (mmHg)

Right	1	2	3	Average reading
Ankle	141	145	143	142
Brachial	133	127	130	130

TABLE 30.3

LEFT POST-EXERCISE SYSTOLIC BLOOD PRESSURE VALUES (mmHg)

Left	@1 min	@2 mins	@3 mins	@4 mins	@5 mins
Ankle	70	0	0	106	94
Brachial	202	165	161	164	153
ABPI	0.35	—	—	0.64	0.61

ABPI, Ankle-brachial pressure index.

TABLE 30.4

RIGHT POST-EXERCISE SYSTOLIC BLOOD PRESSURE VALUES (mmHg)

Right	@1 min	@2 mins	@3 mins	@4 mins	@5 mins
Ankle	160	168	166	166	164
Brachial	202	165	161	164	153
ABPI	0.79	1.02	1.03	1.01	1.07

ABPI, Ankle-brachial pressure index.

Exercise Test

Based on the exercise-induced nature of Geoff's symptoms, an exercise test was performed. Before undertaking this, a full explanation was given, and written consent was obtained. The test comprised an incremental ergometer cycling test to full reproduction of the left-leg/left-foot symptoms. This was reached at 7 minutes and 20 seconds at 166 bpm.

The left average resting brachial systolic blood pressure value (136 mmHg) was used as the reference for the exercise test because it was the highest. Geoff's lower limb symptoms affecting the thigh initially, then the whole limb, were reproduced early in the cycle test at around 5 minutes, at the point where his pulse rate reached the reported 135 bpm. He was asked to continue cycling at this rate until the feelings of pain, numbness, weakness and deadness were all consistent with his usual experience. He then returned to the couch, and further blood pressure readings were taken. His ABPI on the left was calculated at 0.35 and on the right at 0.79 at 1 minute post-exercise. His symptoms cleared after 10 minutes of resting in supine lying. Post-exercise systolic pressure readings are detailed in Tables 30.3 and 30.4.

Reasoning Questions:

3. Many therapists would have undertaken further neuromusculoskeletal examination, such as neurodynamic tests or passive accessory movement testing of the spinal joints. Why did you abandon the neuromusculoskeletal examination so early?

Answer to Reasoning Question:

There were three reasons why the neuromusculoskeletal examination was ceased at this point. First, the neuromusculoskeletal system was now a secondary hypothesis to the vascular system based on pattern recognition. Second, the time at this initial consultation did not permit both a full neuromusculoskeletal examination and an assessment (with an exercise test) of the vascular system. Finally, the referring physiotherapist had provided a detailed record of his neuromusculoskeletal assessment, which, when considering the two earlier points and Geoff's protracted history, suggested instead that the remaining consultation time should concentrate on that part of the puzzle that had not previously been investigated (i.e. the vascular system).

Remember, the patient had specifically asked for a second opinion. If there had been the luxury of more time, further neuromusculoskeletal examination would indeed have been undertaken but only after the vascular assessment. There is a very real need for manual therapists to be able to modify the order and priority of their examinations according to the presenting symptoms (Rushton et al., 2014). That was the rationale in this case.

Reasoning Question:

4. How did you interpret the data collected in the vascular examination?

Answer to Reasoning Question:

Both the patient and his wife (who also attended) were warned before the vascular assessment that we might find nothing from the testing, largely based on the very real possibility that his symptoms by now must have a predominant element of central sensitization (Nijs et al., 2015). However, the exercise test findings gave a clear objective indication that Geoff was suffering from an exercise-induced vascular flow limitation of the left lower limb.

Specifically, the presentation was suggestive of significant stenosis of the common iliac artery based on the symptom distribution and the long recovery time (10 minutes). This opinion was informed by the ABPI cutoff point for lower limb flow limitation post-exercise, which is currently set at 0.66 (Peach et al., 2012), whereas Geoff's ABPI was 0.35 for the left lower limb. This reading was, in fact, the lowest post-exercise ABPI value we had ever encountered over many years of testing in this capacity. Geoff's history and vascular assessment were, taken together, suggestive of an advanced and progressive lesion which would require extensive and lengthy surgery to correct. However, after 30 years of symptoms, it remained unknown at this stage what proportion of his symptoms could be ascribed to the vascular system or whether central sensitization was now the predominant feature.

Clinical Reasoning Commentary:

Two types of reasoning priorities have been alluded to in these answers. First, collaborative reasoning, that is, the shared decision-making between Geoff (and his wife) and the clinician as a therapeutic alliance in the setting of consultation goals and priorities (the desire for a second opinion), as well as the interpretation of the examination findings and those accordingly anticipated from the vascular assessment.

Second, the clinician is clearly not simply obtaining information without thinking. In fact, by the end of the subjective examination, the clinician has opinions (hypotheses) in multiple hypothesis categories which enable a judgement about which physical examination procedures are most important to prioritize at this first appointment. Although the physical examination is not limited to hypotheses formulated in the subjective examination, existing hypotheses logically still inform physical testing and prioritizing which tests are most important at the first consultation. Although in this case the physical examination has screened the relevant systems (e.g. neuromusculoskeletal), not every available physical test was deemed necessary for Geoff, and a clear rationale (as opposed to following a rigid routine without reasoning) is evident.

Management

On the basis of the previously reported findings and his worsening condition, it was considered that Geoff was a candidate for a full diagnostic workup by a vascular team. The findings of the consultation were explained to him, and he was referred back to his general practitioner with a report of the findings, as well as a recommendation for him to see a vascular team in his local government health service.

Geoff went on to have a series of vascular tests, including exercise/stress tests, which confirmed our clinic's findings. A magnetic resonance arteriogram (MRA) (Fig. 30.2)

Fig. 30.2 Magnetic resonance arteriogram (MRA) showing subtle end of fibrotic narrowing (arrow) of the left external iliac artery.

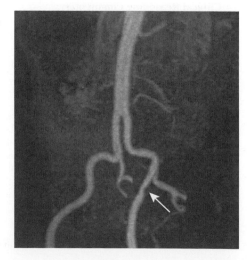

demonstrated extensive stenosis of his common/external iliac artery. He underwent a 5-hour operation involving an endarterectomy and vein grafting. The surgeons found more extensive pathology (endofibrotic narrowing) than the MRA scans had suggested.

Outcome

At 1 year post-surgery, Geoff reported a complete resolution of his leg symptoms and that he had returned to running and cycling. He still suffered occasional low back pain during everyday activity and work.

Reasoning Questions:

5. Geoff had endured decades of discomfort, been misdiagnosed by multiple health professionals and been labelled a 'chronic pain patient' requiring psychological interventions. On reflection, what were the clues in Geoff's presentation that should have alerted these practitioners to the fact that he instead suffered from a vascular abnormality?

Answer to Reasoning Question:

On reflection, the key element for me was that the exercise-induced nature of the presenting symptoms had been consistently overlooked by a series of physicians and other clinicians over the 30-year period of Geoff's presentation. This case highlights that there is a real need for clinicians to be cognizant that vascular flow issues can affect any area of the body at any age. Furthermore, vascular knowledge and the ability to perform a basic vascular examination are key tools in the armory of all competent neuromusculoskeletal practitioners. An exercise-induced nature to presenting symptoms together with key patient symptom descriptors such as limb 'fatigue', 'weakness' or the limb 'going dead' are an indication to prioritize vascular assessment over routine neuromusculoskeletal examination. As always, the take-home message is to *listen to the patient* and to consider all the body systems that may be implicated in such cases.

Reasoning Question:

6. What are your recommendations regarding what the clinician should specifically listen for, and perhaps explicitly screen for, in the subjective examination for potential vascular compromise?

Answer to Reasoning Question:

This case clearly illustrates the necessity to listen to the patient from the outset and to consider the systems which may be implicated by the patient's descriptions. Complaints of exercise-induced symptoms which incorporate descriptors such as 'fatigue', 'tiredness' and 'weakness' in the lower (or upper) limb require clinicians to consider the vascular system in their clinical reasoning. Clear questioning about the nature, distribution and easing strategies may guide the clinician (Table 30.5 may assist the practitioner in recognizing vascular causes of back and leg pain). Commonly, sports participants (if probed) will be able to relate the specific heart rates at which the symptoms commence and ease. This should alert the clinician to consider the vascular system as a source of symptoms and undertake, or refer for, appropriate investigations.

It is essential to be aware that young, fit athletes who do not have vascular risk profiles may present complaining of pain of vascular origin. Geoff's case illustrates just how long this can be overlooked.

Clinical Reasoning Commentary:

By carefully listening to the patient and his story and by exercising unbiased clinical reasoning, the clinician has succeeded where many, many other practitioners have failed. A combination of reflection on similar prior vascular cases leading to the assimilation of a clinical pattern and the avoidance of common errors in reasoning has helped the clinician lead Geoff to an appropriate outcome. In particular, given the 30-year history of 'chronic sciatica', it would have been very understandable if the clinician had not avoided the error of the 'priming' influence of prior information (e.g. diagnosis provided in the referral, MRI findings) or the related error of 'conservatism or stickiness' whereby the initial impression and common diagnosis of sciatica was not revised in the face of subsequent non-supportive information (see Chapter 1). By carefully considering all body systems, such frequent pitfalls, where other practitioners had likely landed, were deftly sidestepped.

The vascular system is sometimes not given due consideration by manual therapists, and this case serves to illustrate the importance of vascular assessment skills and of maintaining an open mind to vascular presentations in the clinic.

TABLE 30.5

VASCULAR CAUSES OF BACK AND LEG PAIN

Condition	Symptom Localization	Behaviour	Clinical Sign	Effect of Body Position	Key Investigation	Patient Profile
Abdominal aortic aneurysm	Silent or low back abdominal/groin pain	Silent or resting pain May present as a mechanical pattern	Palpation Auscultation	May have a mechanical pattern	Duplex U/S MRA CT angiography	Aged 60 + M > F Hypertension Smoker
Aortic stenosis	Bilateral buttock, thigh, calf, foot pain/fatigue/ paraesthesia and exercise intolerance	Exercise-induced symptoms (e.g. walking, slopes, stairs) Eased by rest	Reduced distal pulses after exercise Syncope	—	ABPI Duplex U/S MRA CT angiography	Older age, with risk factors for atherosclerosis
Aortic coarctation	Bilateral buttock, thigh, calf, foot pain/fatigue/ paraesthesia and exercise intolerance	Exercise-induced symptoms (e.g. walking, slopes, stairs) Eased by rest	Reduced distal pulses after exercise	—	ABPI Duplex U/S MRA CT angiography	Congenital, may be discovered at any age, known to affect young sports participants (rare)
Common iliac artery stenosis	Unilateral or bilateral buttock, thigh, calf, foot pain/fatigue/ paraesthesia and exercise intolerance	Exercise-induced symptoms (e.g. walking, slopes, stairs) May manifest during high-intensity exercise/ sports Eased by rest	Reduced distal pulses after exercise	Hip/trunk flexion + exercise may exacerbate symptoms	ABPI Duplex U/S MRA CT angiography	Older age, with risk factors for atherosclerosis Young, fit athletes performing high-intensity exercise
Internal iliac artery stenosis	Low back/hip/ buttock/ gluteal region	Exercise-induced symptoms (e.g. walking, slopes, stairs) Eased by rest Erectile dysfunction (males)	Distal pulses normal	—	Penile-brachial index (males) Duplex U/S MRA CT angiography	Older age, with risk factors for atherosclerosis
External iliac artery endofibrosis	Unilateral OR bilateral thigh, calf, foot pain/ fatigue/paraesthesia and exercise intolerance	Exercise-induced symptoms during high-intensity sport/ activity	Reduced distal pulses after exercise	Hip/trunk flexion + exercise may exacerbate symptoms	ABPI Duplex U/S MRA CT angiography	Young, fit athletes performing high-intensity exercise No vascular risk factors
Popliteal artery entrapment syndrome	Unilateral or bilateral calf, foot pain/fatigue/ paraesthesia and exercise intolerance	Exercise-induced symptoms during high-intensity sport/ activity	Reduced distal pulses after exercise	Loaded ankle plantarflexion/ dorsiflexion may affect symptoms/ pulses	Duplex U/S MRA CT angiography	Older age, with risk factors for atherosclerosis Young, fit athletes performing high-intensity exercise
Compartment syndrome (calf)	Bilateral calf pain/ cramps/tightness (±95% of cases)	Exercise-induced symptoms during high-intensity sport/ activity	Distended tight calf Normal pulses after exercise	—	Intra-compartment pressure measurement	Any age Common in sport/exercise

ABPI, Ankle-brachial pressure index; *CT*, computed tomography; *MRA*, magnetic resonance arteriogram; *U/S*, ultrasound.

REFERENCES

Kim, E.S., Wattanakit, K., Gornik, H.L., 2012. Using the ankle-brachial index to diagnose peripheral artery disease and assess cardiovascular risk. Cleve. Clin. J. Med. 79 (9), 651–661. doi:10.3949/ccjm.79a.11154. Review. PubMed PMID: 22949346.

Nijs, J., Apeldoorn, A., Hallegraeff, H., Clark, J., Smeets, R., Malfliet, A., et al., 2015. Low back pain: guidelines for the clinical classification of predominant neuropathic, nociceptive, or central sensitization pain. Pain Physician 18 (3), E333–E346. Review. PubMed PMID: 26000680.

Peach, G., Schep, G., Palfreeman, R., Beard, J.D., Thompson, M.M., Hinchliffe, R.J., 2012. Endofibrosis and kinking of the iliac arteries in athletes: a systematic review. Eur. J. Vasc. Endovasc. Surg. 43 (2), 208–217. doi:10.1016/j.ejvs.2011.11.019.

Rushton, A., Rivett, D., Carlesso, L., Flynn, T., Hing, W., Kerry, R., 2014. International framework for examination of the cervical region for potential of Cervical Arterial Dysfunction prior to Orthopaedic Manual Therapy intervention. Man. Ther. 19 (3), 222–228. doi:10.1016/j.math.2013.11.005. [Epub 2013 Nov 23]; PubMed PMID: 24378471.

Taylor, A.J., George, K.P., 2001. Exercise induced leg pain in young athletes misdiagnosed as pain of musculoskeletal origin. Man. Ther. 6 (1), 48–52. PubMed PMID:11243909.

SECTION 3

Learning and Facilitating Clinical Reasoning

31

Strategies to Facilitate Clinical Reasoning Development

Nicole Christensen • Mark A. Jones • Darren A. Rivett

Introduction

A common observation among clinicians and their educators about clinical reasoning is that they know it when they see it, and they know it when they don't! The challenge lies in knowing how to facilitate performance improvements when inadequate clinical reasoning is identified. This chapter aims to serve as a resource for all those involved in facilitating the learning of, as well as from, clinical reasoning.

Clinician educators are involved in the facilitation of clinical reasoning development at all levels of formal professional education, from the preparation of learners for first entry to practice to mentoring post-professional clinical students in their advancement toward specialty practice. Individual musculoskeletal practitioners who are committed to continual growth and improvement of their own practice abilities also engage in informal opportunities to facilitate clinical reasoning development throughout their careers, both independently and with colleagues in various practice communities. As such, it is important for all clinicians to develop their skills in the facilitation of clinical reasoning as part of their professional development throughout their careers.

The facilitation of clinical reasoning development in clinician learners results in both short-term and long-term benefits to the learners themselves, their current patients and all those they will work with in their future practice. This is because improving the quality of clinical reasoning not only affects the decisions made by a learner with today's patients but also improves the ability of that clinician to learn from today's experiences and also to apply that new knowledge to clinical reasoning and decision-making with future patients. Clinical reasoning itself and the ability to learn from experiences of reasoning are, in effect, interdependent learning outcomes, with improvement in one enhancing the potential for greater achievement in the other. In this chapter we have grounded our proposed facilitation strategies in current understandings of clinical reasoning in the literature (as presented in Chapter 1) and relevant educational theories.

Describing Clinical Reasoning

Literature describing research-based models of expert practice and the clinical reasoning of experts has been summarized (Christensen et al., 2011; Chapter 1) previously as follows:

- Clinical reasoning involves the interaction of individuals (clinicians, patients and involved others) in a collaborative exchange to achieve a mutually derived understanding of the presenting problem and to negotiate a plan for addressing that problem (Edwards et al., 2004b; Edwards and Jones, 2007; Jones, 2014).
- Clinical reasoning is patient-centered and situated within the context of a biopsychosocial approach to health care (Edwards et al., 2004a; Jensen et al., 2000; Jones, 2014).
- Clinical reasoning involves deductive, inductive and abductive reasoning (Edwards et al., 2004a; Edwards and Jones, 2007; Jones, 2014; Chapter 1).
- Clinical reasoning is characterized by complexity and is nonlinear, essentially cyclical, as it evolves throughout an episode of care (Edwards and Jones, 2007; Jones, 2014; Stephenson, 2004).

- Clinical reasoning plays a central role in critically reflective learning from practice experiences and in the development of clinical expertise (Edwards and Jones, 2007; Higgs and Jones, 2008; Jones, 2014).

Research-based descriptions of novice and less skilled musculoskeletal clinicians' clinical reasoning have also appeared in the literature. For example, in physiotherapy, the clinical reasoning of novices has been broadly characterized as more therapist centered and lacking in collaboration, with less focus on understanding of the patient as a person in favor of a narrower focus on primarily the physical aspects of a patient's presentation (Jensen et al., 1990, 1992; Resnik and Jensen, 2003). Beginning practitioners in their first 2 years of practice have been shown to develop from decision-making characterized as standardized and objectively data driven to more individualized clinical reasoning that is inclusive of the patient's context and narrative (Black et al., 2010; Hayward et al., 2013). Another study of extreme novices in their first year of training described their early clinical reasoning as a rote (checklist-oriented), protocol-driven process, which progressed to more robust reasoning, including both hypothetico-deductive and early pattern-recognition processes, by the time they reached their final year of training when reasoning was being facilitated through case-based decision-making activities in the academic setting (Gilliland, 2014).

These descriptions of novice clinical reasoning support the findings of Christensen et al. (2008a, 2008b, Christensen, 2009), who characterized novice students at the time of professional entry as understanding clinical reasoning to be a deductive, linear process. The clinical reasoning of the novices studied was also found to be lacking in an awareness of the role of collaboration in clinical reasoning and of how to use critical self-reflection as a means to learn from their reasoning experiences (Christensen et al., 2008b). This finding is in stark contrast with the summary description of skilled clinical reasoners provided at the beginning of this section.

Clinical Reasoning and Transformative Learning

Critical reflection on clinical reasoning experiences is described as the vehicle from which clinicians learn from past clinical encounters and for future encounters and through which they build knowledge and eventual expertise (Brookfield, 1986; Edwards and Jones, 2007; Higgs and Jones, 2008; Jensen et al., 2000; Stephenson, 1998). Transformative learning theory (Cranton, 2006; Mezirow, 2009) is a particular branch of reconstructivist learning theory that can provide a foundation for proposed educational strategies for facilitating the learning of, and from, clinical reasoning. Transformative learning is a process of using a prior understanding to construct a new or revised interpretation to guide future action. This learning transforms the learner by expanding the learner's understanding, resulting in knowledge that is more 'inclusive, discriminating, reflective, open and emotionally able to change' (Mezirow, 2009, p. 22). Particularly relevant to our focus on using critical reflection on clinical reasoning experiences as the stimulus for transformative learning is this description of one of its outcomes: 'adults learn to reason for themselves – to advance and reassess reasons for making a judgment – rather than act on the assimilated beliefs, values, feelings and judgments of others' (Mezirow, 2009 p. 23). This type of learning is critical for novice clinicians, who can tend to excessively rely on others' knowledge and judgement when just starting out in practice, but also to more experienced clinicians who sometimes fall into cognitively lazy habits of practice with insufficient critical reflection and reasoning. Expertise in clinical practice can be viewed as a result of excellence in learning from clinical experiences. The facilitation of critical self-reflection on clinical reasoning creates opportunities for challenging clinical knowledge and any potentially unsubstantiated assumptions underlying that knowledge. This type of challenge allows for growth and transformation of existing frames of reference, including theoretical or research-derived and experience-derived knowledge that, through application and testing with a recent clinical experience, may be revealed to have been inadequate.

Capability as a Learning Outcome

Informed by an understanding of the key characteristics of the clinical reasoning of experts and the observable gaps between expert reasoning and the clinical reasoning of novices,

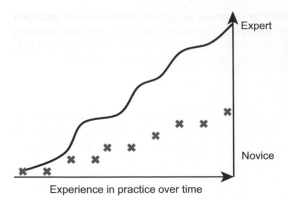

Fig. 31.1 Proposed role of clinical reasoning capability in accelerating the development of expertise. Solid line represents the developmental trajectory of a novice clinician with more capability in clinical reasoning thinking and experiential learning skills. Line of Xs represents the development of a novice with less capability.

Christensen and colleagues (2008a, 2009, 2011; Christensen and Nordstrom, 2013; Christensen and Jensen, 2019) have proposed an approach to facilitating the teaching and learning of clinical reasoning focused on the development of key thinking and experiential learning skills identified in the skilled clinical reasoning of experts. The literature clearly presents a consensus of support for the notion that development of practice-based knowledge through the accumulation and critically reflective processing of clinical experiences is necessary for the development of expertise (Edwards and Jones, 2007; Higgs and Jones, 2008; Jensen et al., 2000, 2019). Although novices cannot simply be 'taught' to be experts, the concept of clinical reasoning capability is grounded in the idea that clinical reasoning capability can be facilitated in clinicians at any point along the continuum from novice to expert practice (Christensen et al., 2008a; Christensen, 2009; Christensen and Jensen, 2019). It is this capability that is thought to contribute to the development of expertise through accumulated clinical experiences (see Fig. 31.1).

The concept of capability in this case is grounded in descriptions in the higher education literature (Stephenson, 1998) in which the term *capability* has been operationally defined as 'the justified confidence and ability to interact effectively with other people and tasks in unknown contexts of the future as well as known contexts of today'. Capability is observed through the following characteristics:

- Confident, effective decision-making and associated actions in practice
- Confidence in the development of a rationale for decisions made
- Confidence in working effectively with others
- Confidence in the ability to navigate unfamiliar circumstances and learn from the experience

In addition to the development of confidence in one's effectiveness as a collaborator and a decision-maker, in both known and unknown contexts, capability is also characterized by a motivation to intentionally develop knowledge through reflective learning in clinical practice (Doncaster and Lester, 2002). These concepts and descriptions of capability can be seen as compatible with characteristics of transformative learners.

Clinical Reasoning Capability

Building on this more general understanding of capability in the educational literature, Christensen and colleagues (2008b, 2009) described clinical reasoning capability as the integration and effective application of thinking and learning skills to make sense of, and learn collaboratively from, clinical experiences. Their model of clinical reasoning capability proposes four key areas of interdependent thinking and experiential learning skills, directly related to descriptions of the thinking and learning skills inherent in the clinical reasoning of expert physiotherapists, including those in musculoskeletal practice. The skills proposed to be linked to the development of excellence as both a clinical reasoner and an experiential learner are **reflective thinking, critical thinking, complexity thinking** and **dialectical thinking** (Christensen et al., 2008a, 2008b; Christensen, 2009; Christensen and Jensen, 2019). Consistent with the literature on capability, which describes it as always evolving as practice contexts that were previously unknown become known (Doncaster and Lester,

2002; Stephenson, 1998), these proposed clinical reasoning capability skills are not intended to represent a comprehensive or definitive list of all aspects of thinking and learning important to developing excellence in clinical reasoning; rather, they include essential, foundational aspects that can be built upon and tailored to all practice contexts.

Reflective Thinking

Reflective thinking is thinking about a situation in order to make sense of it, which involves evaluating the influence of all relevant aspects of the situation and individuals involved (e.g. clinician, patient, clinical setting, resources available, time constraints, etc.). Reflection allows for interpretation of experience; as part of reflection, the thinker comes to know the 'why' of a situation by subjectively and objectively reconsidering the context in order to bring to light the underlying assumptions used to justify beliefs (Mezirow, 2000). When reflective thinking calls into question the adequacy of the clinician's knowledge, learning from the clinical reasoning experience is facilitated as prior knowledge is revised and/or expanded. Schön (1987) describes various moments in time when reflection is integral to making sense of, and eventually improving, the quality of practice experiences: reflection on action, reflection for action and reflection in action. As applied to a clinical reasoning encounter, reflection on action occurs after the clinical action is completed and involves cognitive organization of experiences to make sense of what happened. Reflection for action involves planning for future encounters by thinking back on past experiences. This includes reflecting on the adequacy of the knowledge available to the clinical reasoner during those past encounters, identifying and actively seeking to fill any gaps in existing knowledge, and making links between past experiences and anticipated future events.

Reflection in action occurs in the midst of an experience and allows for modification of clinical reasoning by 'thinking on your feet' in order to best adapt to an emerging understanding of a situation. In order to successfully employ reflection in action to modify decision-making in the moment, a clinician must be able to readily access contextually relevant knowledge from memory. This is also related to metacognition (Higgs et al., 2008; Marcum, 2012; Schön, 1987) – self-awareness and monitoring of one's own thinking while in action – described in Chapter 1 as integral to the facilitation of learning from clinical experiences. Wainwright and colleagues (2010) describe how reflection at different times in relation to a clinical encounter was used by novice and experienced clinicians. Their research findings include the observation that novices less commonly used reflection in action, and when it was used, it focused mainly on the patient's performance. More experienced clinicians reflected in action more often and were focused not only on the patient's performance but also on self-monitoring of their own reasoning in action.

These findings highlight the importance of facilitation of reflection and evaluation of one's reasoning in action as essential to the facilitation of learning from, and developing expertise in, clinical reasoning. In the context of today's complex practice environment, Jensen (2011) recently reinforced this importance to the community of professional teachers and learners:

... It is the reflective ability to understand the context, identify what values may be at risk, and understand the meanings that others see in the situation that is critical. This reflective ability is best learned by moving well beyond reflection on-action to more critical self reflection on students' thinking about their thinking, their metacognitive skills, and their ability to self-regulate and self-monitor. (pp. 1679–1680)

Critical Thinking

Critical thinking, also described in Chapter 1, is intimately linked to reflective thinking and involves intellectual discipline in the process of actively conceptualizing, synthesizing, analyzing and evaluating information; this information can be gathered or generated from observation, experience, interaction, reasoning and reflection, and it serves as a guide toward action (Paul, 1992; Paul and Elder, 2006). In this context, critical thinking is conceived of as a way of thinking about thinking with the intent of questioning and clarifying erroneous assumptions underlying the thinking, and it is a skill that promotes learning from and about thinking. In this way, similar to reflective thinking, critical thinking is also linked to metacognition. There is some recent evidence that a standardized measure of critical thinking abilities in the context of health care, the Health Science Reasoning Test (HSRT), is able to demonstrate significant differences in the critical thinking abilities of novices as compared to clinical specialist physical therapists (Huhn et al., 2011). This finding supports the proposal that more skilled, experienced practitioners have more sophisticated critical thinking skills, which parallels the observation of more sophisticated clinical reasoning skills in expert clinicians. Thus, this also further supports the proposition that because it is a foundational element of skilled clinical reasoning, critical thinking is a key component of clinical reasoning capability. Huhn and colleagues (2011) also suggest that critical thinking is a skill that can and should be explicitly developed in novices as one way to support the development of clinical reasoning skill. Explicit teaching and assessment of critical thinking skills themselves have also been recognized as an essential curricular element for all health professions by an interprofessional group of educators, as stated in a recently published consensus document (Huang et al., 2014).

Hawkins and colleagues (2010) have summarized elements of clinical reasoning linked to interdependent structures present in all thinking, as follows:

Whenever we think, we think for a purpose within a point of view based on assumptions leading to implications and consequences. We use concepts, ideas, and theories to interpret data, facts, and experiences in order to answer questions, solve problems, and resolve issues. (p. 5)

In the context of clinical reasoning capability, critical thinking applies to both the examination and management of a particular patient's clinical presentation and to the critical evaluation of one's own thinking or reasoning used to engage in, interpret and synthesize that patient's clinical information (Christensen et al., 2008b; Christensen, 2009). Critical thinking also makes it possible to bring to light blind spots or gaps in knowledge that may be adversely affecting a clinician's clinical reasoning in a given context. The important role of critical thinking in exploring the potential for biases, incorrect assumptions, inadequate knowledge and erroneous unconscious patterns of interpretation is essential to the concept of demonstrating capability in clinical reasoning.

Complexity Thinking

Complexity thinking is a way of thinking that is grounded in an acknowledgement of the dynamic interdependencies present in systems at work between the many elements and players influencing a given situation (Plsek and Greenhalgh, 2001; Davis et al., 2000). Therefore, complexity thinking is linked to the recognition and consideration of the relative weighting of all relevant internal (within the person) and external (the context in which the person is functioning) factors influencing a given clinical presentation (Christensen et al., 2008b; Christensen and Nordstrom, 2013; Stephenson, 2004). Skilled clinical reasoning has been shown to be in part characterized by this ability to see and appropriately address all influences (both biological and psychosocial) at play in a particular clinical presentation, leading to a mutually agreed-upon plan of care (Edwards et al., 2004a).

Capability in clinical reasoning is also conceived of as being characterized by motivation and skill in learning from clinical experiences (Christensen et al., 2008b; Christensen, 2009). Consistent with a complexity science perspective of learning, clinical experience alone is not enough to cause learning to happen; rather, experience is viewed as a trigger or an opportunity for learning to emerge from interactions with other individuals (Davis and Sumara, 2006). Complexity thinking therefore is also a key element that enables a capable clinician to consider and appreciate the importance and implications of establishing a collaborative relationship with the patient. Collaboration is an essential component of clinical reasoning when conceptualized as a complex, interactive social system through which decisions emerge (Christensen et al., 2008b; Christensen, 2009). This collaborative interaction between participants in clinical reasoning is proposed to be a hallmark of clinical reasoning capability (Christensen et al., 2008b; Christensen, 2009).

Development of an understanding of both the physical or biological aspects of a patient's presentation and the psychosocial and behavioral aspects as being relevant, inseparable and interdependent elements of the health of the complex human beings who are our patients is consistent with clinical reasoning within a biopsychosocial approach to health care and therefore clearly requires complexity thinking. In this way, complexity thinking is also consistent with the dialectical reasoning approach (see Chapter 1) observed in the reasoning of experts (Edwards and Jones, 2007). Interestingly, it has been proposed that facilitating in a learner the recognition of some of the challenges raised by the complexity inherent in a particular situational context (in this case, collaborative clinical reasoning in today's healthcare climate) can in and of itself become a trigger for transformative learning (Alhadeff-Jones, 2012).

Complexity thinking is also necessary to facilitate continuous learning from experiences. Indeed, a complex way of thinking encompasses a perspective that views engaging in reasoning as a potential source of transformative learning, that is, 'a method of learning involving human error and uncertainty…taking into consideration both the individual and collective experiences grounding any activity' (Alhadeff-Jones, 2012, p. 190). In this way, complexity thinking is again closely linked to collaborative clinical reasoning and the learning that can emerge for all involved.

Dialectical Thinking

The clinical reasoning of experts, as described by Edwards and Jones (2007), is characterized by a fluidity of reasoning between deductive thinking and inductive thinking within each of the clinical reasoning strategies (Edwards et al., 2004a). As described in Chapter 1, expert physiotherapists have been shown to dialectically move in their reasoning between contrasting biological and psychosocial poles in a fluid and seemingly effortless manner (Edwards et al., 2004a). This thinking ability is proposed to be necessary for clinicians to develop a holistic understanding of the person who is the patient and the clinical presentation of the patient's problem(s), consistent with a biopsychosocial approach to clinical reasoning (Edwards and Jones, 2007). Development of dialectical thinking allows for clinicians to achieve a more complex and contextual understanding of situations both impacting and impacted by a patient's presentation. Recognition of the interdependence of dialectical thinking and complexity thinking is also key to the promotion of capability in clinical reasoning, as capability includes effectiveness in working with others to achieve collaborative and productive working relationships (Doncaster and Lester, 2002; Stephenson, 1998). The ability to simultaneously perceive and interpret information in terms of its implications for different categories of judgements (e.g. 'hypothesis categories' as discussed in Chapter 1) and to dialectically shift reasoning from one focus (e.g. physical/biological) to another (e.g. psychosocial) is also an advanced reasoning ability that can be developed through practice and assistance.

Making Learning More Likely

How can we use our understanding of the ways in which the clinical reasoning of novices differs from that of experts and the notions of transformative learning and capability in clinical reasoning to better facilitate clinical reasoning development in learners of musculoskeletal practice across all professional education settings? As a complex, abstract practice phenomenon, the teaching and facilitation of learning of clinical reasoning is challenging in both the classroom and clinical education contexts.

Core elements within which educators should frame a transformative learning approach to teaching have been summarized by Taylor (2009) as follows: **promotion of individual experience; engagement in critically reflective dialogue with others; a holistic, contextual awareness; and learning situated in an authentic practice context**. These elements are described as interdependent when put into an educational framework and are thus integrated within the suggested educational strategies described in the following sections.

Making Visible the Invisible: Use of Common Definitions, Language and Models

The first and arguably most important step in facilitating the development of both the thinking and learning skills underpinning skilled clinical reasoning, in both academic classroom and clinical education settings at all educational levels, is to make visible to the learner what is invisible. This can be seen as a form of promoting a contextual awareness of clinical reasoning in a community of learners. The profession of physiotherapy can be seen as an example of what Wenger (1998) describes as a community of practice. The notion of giving an artificially concrete 'form' to abstract, invisible concepts and experiences (such as clinical reasoning) is described by Wenger (1998) as a way in which a community shapes the experiences of its members in order to provide focused attention to experiences in a particular way so as to facilitate new kinds of understanding (i.e. learning). Clinical reasoning is an invisible phenomenon; the actions of those involved (e.g. patient–clinician interactions throughout the examination and ongoing management) provide an external observer (e.g. clinical supervisor or professional colleague) only one perspective from which to infer all of the reasoning happening within and between those individuals. Therefore, clinical reasoning must be able to be made visible in a mutually understood way, dialogue and discussion enabled, critical self-reflection promoted and experiential learning facilitated in order for reasoning development and progression toward expert practice to occur. Indeed, all of the strategies suggested herein build on this fundamental theme of making visible and explicit their links to facilitating clinical reasoning development by way of a common language and framework to enable the development of a mutual understanding within which the learners and facilitators can discuss, critically reflect and promote the development of clinical reasoning capability.

Commonly understood and accepted definitions, models and frameworks of clinical reasoning that enable visualization of all of the aspects of clinical reasoning are essential to this strategy. The dialectical model of clinical reasoning (Edwards and Jones, 2007) and associated clinical reasoning strategies model (Edwards et al., 2004) are two such models that have been described in the literature and are grounded in the study of expert physiotherapists' clinical reasoning, including musculoskeletal clinicians. The 'hypothesis categories' framework is more theoretical but has research evidence for its use (Rivett and Higgs, 1997; Miller, 2009). Each of these is described in detail in Chapter 1. By fostering a learner's awareness of different foci of reasoning (i.e. clinical reasoning strategies) and their interactions, as well as different categories of clinical judgements (i.e. hypothesis categories) and their interactions, while developing the learner's ability to dialectically move in his or her focus of reasoning and categories of judgements, the learner's clinical reasoning capability can be more easily and explicitly facilitated. The development of complex understandings and complexity thinking is facilitated when discussing the different foci of reasoning and categories of judgements, with attention given to the basis and validity of judgements or hypotheses formulated, interdependent relationships between aspects of a patient case and how hypotheses can be further tested. Further complexity is appreciated when analysis and discussion include relevance and weighting of examination and re-assessment findings in the broader context of the patient's life, including the patient's pain or disability experiences, expectations and goals. The ability for learners and educators/facilitators to have access to a commonly understood language of clinical reasoning, embedded in clinical reasoning models and frameworks such as these, assists in their identification of, description of and critical reflection on their clinical reasoning, enabling assessment of reasoning performance, which is needed to facilitate learning of, and from, clinical reasoning.

Using Clinical Reasoning as a Curricular Framework

Once a model of clinical reasoning has been adopted as a 'visible' framework within which learners and facilitators can identify and name various foci of reasoning (i.e. clinical reasoning strategies) and categories of clinical judgements (i.e. hypothesis categories), then use these to critique clinical reasoning performance, the teaching and learning of profession-specific technical skills can be embedded or situated within clinical reasoning as a larger umbrella or learning context (Christensen, 2009; Christensen and Nordstrom, 2013). Clinical reasoning then becomes the foundational context within which to add profession-specific technical knowledge, rather than discussions of associated clinical reasoning serving as intermittent teaching points under the larger umbrella of learning technical skills. This type of curricular structure is not typically found in most entry-level or post-professional educational curricula; these curricula are instead typically organized around the development of technical skills.

An example of using clinical reasoning as the curricular organizing framework is a situation where the focus of learning is on interventions appropriate for a particular array of impairments and/or activity restrictions. This technical skills content could be situated as one example within a larger context of procedural reasoning strategies/considerations for addressing various examples of patient presentations. Another example, this time focused on inductive thinking, is a curriculum that frames the content related to the effective education of patients about injury prevention or wellness within a larger context of narrative reasoning strategies. In this case, the focus would be on understanding the patient's perspective on his or her current situation and the patient's existing attitudes about making health-behavior changes, as well as how this understanding would influence the education of patients in injury prevention and wellness, depending on what the perspective of the individual patient might be. This type of curricular organization might more easily facilitate the building of explicit connections between what students know about how to 'do' musculoskeletal practice and the clinical reasoning and experiential learning processes within which the 'doing' takes place (Christensen and Nordstrom, 2013).

Facilitating Reflection on Hypothetico-Deductive Reasoning and Authentic Pattern Development

The hypothesis categories framework is discussed extensively in Chapter 1. This framework can be used in both academic classroom and clinical education settings to assist learners to develop adequate breadth and depth in hypothesis formation and testing while reasoning through various patient presentations (from paper-based patients to real patients in the clinic). These hypothesis categories have been integrated into clinical reasoning forms, a learning tool originally designed and used by educators in the area of musculoskeletal physiotherapy, which are available online at Appendices 1 & 2. These sorts of forms have been successfully used as a tool to trace and make visible to learners their 'slow', or system 2, analytical thinking and reasoning, as discussed in Chapter 1. The long-version clinical reasoning form particularly promotes learners' consideration of a broad range of factors related to each of the hypothesis categories at key points (end of patient history/subjective examination, end of physical examination, after several appointments), thereby promoting reflection on the evolving reasoning of the practitioner. Completed long clinical reasoning forms provide access to the learner's reasoning, thus making the invisible visible to both the learner and his or her supervisor. When competency is demonstrated, learners can be asked to complete only select portions of the long form and eventually change to the short form that more succinctly focuses on the hypothesis categories. Variations on these forms have been used by clinical reasoning educators in entry-level education as well as post-professional programs internationally, and they have been adapted for clinical areas outside of manual therapy and musculoskeletal practice over the years.

Working through a clinical reasoning form and reflecting on a patient's progression through an episode of care can also then be extended to an exercise that facilitates explicit and conscious development of authentic clinical pattern recognition for future practice. By authentic clinical patterns, we mean patterns that have been derived from a learner's own clinical experiences, thereby facilitating the potential for experiential and potentially transformative learning. After completing an episode of care, the learner can reflect back on key findings from the patient interview, tests and measures, and responses to intervention strategies as related to the various hypothesis categories in order to organize what has been learned from the clinical experience as an authentic, experience-derived clinical pattern in the learner's practice knowledge base. The goal is to facilitate pattern construction that is grounded in sound clinical reasoning and which includes elements of the physical signs and symptoms, in addition to various psychosocial factors and elements of the patient's narrative that, in retrospect, proved to be relevant factors to the patient's presentation and progression. System 1 'fast' thinking, in the extreme form of pattern recognition that is uncritically accepted or adopted without adequate validation, is recognized as one of the more common forms of reasoning errors in medicine (Croskerry, 2009). Critical reflection on the quality of clinical patterns constructed by learners may potentially facilitate quality and accuracy in pattern recognition whereby the learner integrates critically examined new knowledge into his or her future intuitive, system 1 thinking in practice.

Facilitating Critical Self-Reflection Through Focused Questioning

Facilitation of critical self-reflection on clinical reasoning experiences involves dialogue and questioning. Questions are thought to be effective in establishing a dynamic whereby learners can 'figure things out' for themselves as they are facilitated in thinking about, and making explicit to an external audience, their own thinking (Cranton, 2006). The intent is to help learners realize what they know, reasoned about and did well and also to facilitate self-identification of any gaps in knowledge or reasoning skills that can focus efforts for future learning and improved performance. Cranton contends that 'our habitual expectations – what we expect to happen based on what has happened in the past – are the product of experiences, and it is those expectations that are called into question during the trans-formative learning process' (2006 p. 8). By engaging learners with strategic questions to stimulate constructive dialogue, rather than by 'teaching' or 'telling' learners what educators believe they 'need to know', they can be facilitated in constructing new understandings and in revising problematic knowledge that they have recognized as inadequate for their reasoning. Cranton (2009) also reminds us that 'educators who have a goal of facilitating transformative learning in their practice can only set up an environment and create activities that have the potential to challenge participants' habits of mind and engage in critical self-reflection' (pp. 183–184). In other words, the outcome of the learning experience is not dictated by nor guaranteed by the educator; the goal is to foster and support the processes that may lead to transformative learning and that potentially may result in empowering learners as more capable clinical reasoners and learners.

One example of how a learner responding to focused questions can facilitate learning from one's own clinical reasoning experiences was described in the prior section; written learning tools such as the clinical reasoning form help to make explicit for the learner any strengths or deficits in his or her ability to generate, test and validate or negate hypotheses adequately (in this case, guided by the hypothesis categories framework). Critical self-reflection facilitated by a mentor's questioning about areas of strength, areas needing improvement and any knowledge gaps surfaced by a learning tool such as the clinical reasoning form can further facilitate critically reflective learning from this type of intentional, systematic self-reflection.

Another framework that has been used to provide structure for the type of questioning most likely to facilitate critical self-reflection was originally proposed by Mezirow (1991) and further developed by Cranton (2006). Cranton's proposed framework includes questions to promote content reflection (critical examination of the content or description of a problem), process reflection (critical examination of the problem-solving strategies being used) and premise reflection (questioning the validity of underlying assumptions that may have guided thinking or actions). This general framework has since been adapted for use in facilitating critical self-reflection on clinical reasoning (Christensen et al., 2011) and is presented herein. These adaptations served to intentionally focus the learner on elements of clinical reasoning consistent with the dialectical, collaborative, biopsychosocially oriented reasoning models developed by Edwards and colleagues (2004; Edwards and Jones, 2007).

In contrast to a more intense, detailed focus of reflective questioning about each aspect of clinical reasoning as the clinician moves through the phases of the clinical encounter (either in person or via a reflective tool such as the clinical reasoning form), the focus of this framework moves backward from conclusions drawn at the end of an encounter. These reflective questions prompt clinical reasoners to critically evaluate both the accuracy and the quality of the clinical reasoning supporting their conclusions and clinical decisions and facilitate explicit linkages between their reflections and experiential learning. This shift from more detail-focused reflective questioning toward questioning focused on the broader perspective of the quality of their reasoning and its outcomes (i.e. conclusions drawn) can be made once clinical learners have demonstrated proficiency in the more detail-oriented, comprehensive critical examination of their reasoning.

This proposed critical self-reflection framework (Christensen et al., 2011) is intended to be a simple guide to help facilitators orient their questions in four distinct but related areas of focus, as presented in Table 31.1.

The fourth set of questions is focused on making explicit any new understandings for the learner and could include learning that existing knowledge and/or clinical reasoning being reflected on was of high quality. The learning through critical self-reflection should encompass positive validation of the learner's achievements, as well as self-identification of any gaps in knowledge or reasoning skills that can then become the focus of new learning goals in future patient encounters.

TABLE 31.1

QUESTIONING FRAMEWORK TO FACILITATE CRITICAL SELF-REFLECTION

Question's Area of Focus	Supporting Questions
1. What conclusions have been drawn about what the patient's problem is and how it came to be?	• What are the cause-and-effect relationships underlying the patient's presentation? (Focus is on outcomes of all deductive/diagnostic reasoning.) • What is your understanding of the patient's perspectives on their problem? On your working relationship? (Focus is on outcomes of inductive/narrative reasoning.)
2. How did you come to these conclusions?	• How did you empirically validate (i.e. through hypothesis testing) any cause-and-effect relationships you have discovered? (Focus is on evaluating quality of deductive, system 2 thinking.) • How did you determine if you understand the patient's story and perspectives? (Focus is on quality of inductive thinking and verification of its quality through attainment of consensual validation from the patient of learner's interpretations.) • How did you make sure you haven't engaged in any clinical reasoning errors? (Further discussion of common clinical reasoning errors as a tool to assist in critical reflection is provided in the text.)
3. Have you used pattern recognition or intuition? (This question is exploring critical self-reflection on system 1 thinking.)	• Have you made any assumptions that guided your thinking? • What are your assumptions about the way this problem typically presents? • What are your assumptions about this 'type' of patient/person? • How do you know your assumptions were valid? • Do you think any of your assumptions compromised your reasoning?
4. What have you learned?	• What have you learned about your clinical reasoning? • What have you learned by identifying and questioning any assumptions you made? • Will you revise your perspective on anything based on this experience? • How is the knowledge you have gained important for you in the future? Will you think or do anything differently next time?

TABLE 31.2

FACILITATING REFLECTION ON CHARACTERISTICS OF CLINICAL THINKING

Characteristics of Clinical Thinking	Sample Questions to Facilitate Reflection
Clarity, accuracy, precision, relevance and depth: • Considerations of whether the reasoning adequately addresses the underlying complexity of the issue	What do you mean by ____? How could you verify whether or not you got that right? Could you be more specific about your thoughts about ____? Could you explain how this particular aspect of the patient's situation relates to the bigger picture?
Breadth: • Considerations of whether there is a need for another point of view	Did you consider any other ways to explain why the patient is presenting this way before you came to your conclusion? If not, can you think of any now?
Logic and significance: • Determination of the most important aspect to focus on	In reflecting back on all the things you had to think through during this patient encounter, what was the most important? Why?
Fairness: • Self-reflection on potential bias or vested interests that may be influencing reasoning	Do you feel that you were able to maintain your objectivity in this situation? Is it possible that you were influenced in the moment by any automatic assumptions or biases?

Hawkins and colleagues (2010) advocate questioning that focuses on what they term 'universal intellectual standards essential to sound clinical reasoning' (p. 11). This framework, in contrast to the one just described, can be seen in part as more focused on the details of thinking rather than the bigger-picture lessons from an experience, but in reality, it provides a multitude of pathways through which critical thinking and critical self-reflection can be promoted. This involves orienting questions around characteristics of the learner's clinical thinking related to four areas (Hawkins et al., 2010), as summarized in Table 31.2.

Each example of questioning tools and frameworks just presented can also serve to facilitate the assessment of clinical reasoning performance. By teasing out aspects of the quality of clinical reasoning into separate areas, these frameworks can serve to orient and focus areas of strength and weakness when a learner's clinical reasoning is being assessed and can guide future dialogue and development of focused learning goals to address areas of necessary growth.

Facilitating the Questioning of Assumptions

One of the most challenging areas within which to effectively facilitate critical self-reflection on clinical reasoning is that of questioning of assumptions. Learners are often, to some degree, unaware of assumptions or biases that may be influencing their clinical reasoning, presenting an even greater challenge to a facilitator attempting to stimulate learners to self-identify issues with their thinking and reasoning. Brookfield (2012) has offered a learning activity specifically aimed at developing learners' skills in both self-assessing and also neutral questioning skills that is likely to help reveal potential assumptions that influenced an individual's thinking. The activity is called the Critical Conversation Protocol (Brookfield, 2012. pp. 120–127). This type of activity is designed for settings outside of patient care, such as the academic classroom or clinical education settings where there are multiple peer learners. Learners work in small groups (minimum of three learners per group), and each member has a role that fulfills a specific function in each step of the activity. The roles are storyteller, detective(s) and umpire. A summary of the overall activity and specific activities for each role is included in Table 31.3.

	TABLE 31.3

CRITICAL CONVERSATION PROTOCOL ACTIVITY (ADAPTED WITH PERMISSION FROM BROOKFIELD [2012, pp. 120–127])

Step	Activities and Description of Each Team Member's Role
1	• Storyteller tells a story from his or her practice; something that the storyteller remembers because it was frustrating for the storyteller and has left him or her puzzled or uncertain (i.e. a critical incident). • Detective(s) and umpire listen carefully.
2	• Detective(s) ask questions about the incident. Their goal is to understand the incident from multiple perspectives if possible (e.g. from the storyteller's perspective, from the patient's perspective, from another healthcare team member's perspective, from an involved caregiver's perspective) and to uncover any assumptions they think the storyteller might be holding. • Detective(s) are permitted to ask only questions that request information (e.g. 'Can you say more about…?' 'Can you explain why you decided…?'). They must avoid questions that explicitly or implicitly pass judgement, offer opinions or give advice (e.g. 'Why would you think…?' 'Didn't you think…?' 'I would have…'). • Storyteller can ask in return why the detective is asking a particular question, in order to make sure the relevance is clear to all involved. • Umpire serves to keep the question-and-answer exchange consistent with a spirit of mutual inquiry and curiosity (e.g. the umpire may bring to the attention of the detective[s] ways in which their questioning, tone, body language, etc. may evoke defensiveness in the storyteller).
3	• Detective(s) report the assumptions they believe they have heard in the storyteller's descriptions of the incident and in responses to questions they have asked. • The reporting of detective(s) must be in neutral, nonjudgemental language. • No advice is given. The intent is to pose possibilities for the storyteller to consider.
4	• Detective(s) give alternative interpretations of the events described by the storyteller. These alternatives must be plausible and also represent a different perspective on the event than that presented by the storyteller. • The intent is for the detective(s) to speculate about how the learning event might have looked if viewed from another's perspective. • Again, no advice is given. • Storyteller is then allowed to give any further information that might cast doubt on alternative explanations offered. Storyteller can also ask detective(s) to elaborate or provide reasons for why they have come to this alternative perspective.
5	• Detectives can now give any advice they may have. • Storyteller and detective(s) each offer what they have learned from the conversation: what assumptions they realize they missed and needed to explore further; how reflecting on the conversation will affect their future actions. • Umpire gives an overall summary of and feedback on the communication styles of the storyteller and detective(s) and gives his or her impressions of the effectiveness of their interactions with each other. • Umpire also offers an assessment of areas where participants excelled or struggled and gives his or her own opinion or perspective on the story.

It is difficult to examine your own assumptions. As Brookfield (2008, p. 68) highlights, 'to some extent we are all prisoners trapped within the perceptual frameworks that determine how we view our experiences'. Having a second person (through this activity or through reflective discussion with a supervisor or colleague) listen to an individual's reasoning and probe the basis for that reasoning can assist in externalizing implicit perceptions and assumptions that are frequently unrecognized by that individual. In addition to facilitating an individual to come to an awareness of assumption(s) he or she is operating under and to explore whether or not the assumption(s) are well grounded, this type of exercise also facilitates the awareness of other points of view that may be taken to provide a broader or different perspective on troublesome clinical dilemmas.

Facilitating Lateral and Creative Thinking

One of the risks in advocating for a common model of clinical reasoning and for the adoption of the use of common frameworks, such as the hypothesis categories, in facilitating the learning of/from clinical reasoning is that these frameworks might be adopted in a rigid manner, potentially by both educators and learners. Rigidity such as this precludes a healthy process of adaptation and evolution of frameworks as indicated by growth in our collective knowledge and understanding of clinical reasoning and by constantly evolving changes in musculoskeletal practice. Therefore, an important aspect of facilitating learners' capability in clinical reasoning in both familiar and unfamiliar circumstances is the facilitation of creative and lateral thinking skills – the type of thinking that is required to find new alternatives to solve a problem when all existing alternatives have been ineffective. Indeed, as stated by Jensen (2011), 'if we agree with the assumption that professional education is not simply learning to apply knowledge and skill to practice but also to make judgements, often in uncertain conditions, then we need to expand our approach to learning to facilitate creativity and innovation' (p. 1679).

Seasoned educators often observe novices who lack the confidence to try things they have not seen others successfully attempt before them. In order to successfully facilitate learners in developing justified confidence in their ability to reason through any practice situation encountered, we suggest that they must be facilitated in generating previously unconsidered ideas, testing these ideas and evaluating their feasibility and value through trial and error.

Approaches to facilitating creative thinking are grounded in the premise that it is possible to learn and improve skills in coming up with new ideas through specific strategies (De Bono, 2015; James and Brookfield, 2014). De Bono's approach to creativity is through what he terms lateral thinking (De Bono, 2015). Lateral thinking is defined as the process of intentionally restructuring old patterns of thinking in order to create new ones. This is differentiated from vertical thinking, which is described as logical, sequential, linear thinking. Although vertical thinking is essential to inductively recognize clinical patterns and to deductively substantiate those patterns through hypothesis-oriented questioning and physical assessment (i.e. differential diagnosis), lateral thinking is also important to the generation of new insights and discoveries that enable individual practitioners and the broader profession to advance their knowledge and practice. Several lateral thinking strategies are summarized as follows (De Bono, 2015):

- Instead of stopping when a promising approach to a problem has been found, continue to generate as many alternative pathways as possible to become aware of and explore all of the possibilities, and then, if appropriate, consider exploring alternative pathways identified and comparing outcomes with the initial approach taken.
- Don't be too quick to dismiss information as irrelevant (e.g. patient seemingly going off on a tangent in the patient interview) because consideration of information that typically is not considered relevant (in this example, what the patient considers important) may facilitate the reconstruction or expansion of existing patterns.
- Be aware of what is considered the dominant or typical approach to a problem, and intentionally explore other ideas that may have been labeled as 'incorrect' or 'inefficient' solutions, in order to challenge the assumptions underlying current accepted approaches. It is difficult to truly be 'lateral' in your thinking if you cannot first recognize how you have been thinking.

Teaching lateral thinking centers on helping students recognize their current thinking patterns and processes (e.g. interpretations of patient information, diagnostic and management decisions) and encouraging them to think more widely, outside of what might seem obvious and logical to them (De Bono, 2015). This alternative approach then facilitates the learner in recognizing new perspectives that can raise awareness of equally or even more effective approaches to resolving clinical problems. Lateral thinking approaches can be integrated into educational activities in both academic and clinical education contexts to varying degrees. As long as a learner's clinical reasoning is logical and safe, lateral thinking should be encouraged in authentic practice encounters whenever possible. If we only encourage logical thinking and practice within the realm of what is 'known' or substantiated by research evidence, we then limit the variability and creativity of thinking that is important to innovation and the evolution of our practice. Given today's resource limitations and focus on efficiency in many practice settings, when there are limited opportunities to facilitate true lateral thinking in authentic practice settings, it may be more feasible to explore lateral thinking strategies through dialogue only or with peers in role-played clinical situations rather than with actual patients.

James and Brookfield (2014) suggest another activity that can promote creative thinking and the making of unexpected connections between seemingly separate parts of a subject, potentially leading to the development of new and creative approaches. This is the Six Degrees of Separation activity, adapted from a well-known popular game in which participants attempt to link all film references to the actor Kevin Bacon in six steps or less (James and Brookfield, 2014, pp. 198–199). In this version, collaborative creativity is facilitated as groups of peer learners are challenged to plot a viable pathway of connections (in six steps or less) between two seemingly unrelated (at face value) aspects of their theoretical and practice knowledge, such as a mobility impairment of the right metatarsophalangeal joint and left upper trapezius muscle hypertonicity. The members of the group brainstorm together and also can undertake independent research to develop the links; the group votes on the best pathway between the two points. The outcomes of this activity are thought to include promotion in learners of an awareness of multiple perspectives and insights different from their own, their own abilities (and confidence levels) in offering new perspectives of their own and how a group can collaboratively develop a new approach that is likely superior to any one member's individual contributions – this is characteristic of a complex system, requiring complexity thinking to achieve optimal outcomes. This activity and student/supervisor discussions regarding unproven theoretical explanations for patients' problems are examples of 'abductive reasoning', as discussed in Chapter 1. Although abductive reasoning is important, students need to be cautioned that improvement in patient outcomes does not itself validate the theoretical explanation.

Using Knowledge of Clinical Reasoning Errors to Facilitate Self-Reflection

Knowledge of common errors in reasoning described in the literature can provide another framework that can be used to facilitate critical self-reflection on the quality of clinical reasoning. In effect, particular aspects of learners' clinical reasoning can be scanned or audited for incidences of these known types of errors. This audit can be done by the learners themselves or by a learning facilitator who can use the insights gained to guide further facilitatory questioning and dialogue. In this way, these errors can become another sort of diagnostic framework to be used to make visible, identify and name aspects of clinical reasoning that may need to be improved upon.

Many descriptions of various types of errors in thinking and reasoning exist in the literature, and Chapter 1 provides a summary of errors from various sources. Another helpful description is presented by Scott (2009), who summarized clinical reasoning errors in diagnosis as follows:

- Gravitation to a readily available heuristic: acceptance of a diagnosis based on its superficial similarity to another case (related to 'memory bias' in Chapter 1)
- Premature anchoring heuristic: fixation on first impressions that is unaltered with new or conflicting information (related to 'conservatism or stickiness' in Chapter 1)
- Premature closure of reasoning: acceptance of a diagnosis without challenge through adequate consideration of likely alternatives (related to 'priming influence' in Chapter 1; also see the description of confirmation bias later in this section)

Common errors in reasoning related to management include (Scott, 2009) the following:

- Framing effect: being influenced by the perception of relative risk when making a decision, based on whether or not the risk is presented/perceived in positive or negative terms and/or a tendency to avoid versus seek risk

- Commission bias: deciding to do something regardless of evidence that would contradict the decision
- Extrapolation error: inappropriately choosing to apply an option to a situation or individual because it was applied successfully in another dissimilar situation or group

Two additional clinical reasoning bias errors described in the literature and also quite helpful to facilitate the questioning of assumptions in learners are confirmation bias (Klein, 2005) and outcome bias (Sacchi and Cherubini, 2004). Confirmation bias is a tendency to look for, notice and remember only the information that fits with pre-existing expectations (i.e. a favorite hypothesis or clinical pattern). An example of confirmation bias would be when a clinician suspects subacromial impingement as responsible for the signs and symptoms present in a patient with shoulder pain and only performs tests for subacromial impingement. Finding those positive, the clinician fails to include an examination of the cervical spine region as another likely potential source of referred shoulder symptoms. In this way, information that might contradict or negate a presentation associated with subacromial impingement may not be collected (competing hypotheses go untested) or perhaps are devalued or ignored completely. The clinician never considers that the patient may have more than one region or system involved and/or that the shoulder region may not be the source of the problem at all.

Outcome bias is a tendency for an overreliance on outcome information to indicate the accuracy or quality of the clinical reasoning that determined the choice of intervention. Lesser or greater value tends to be placed on the quality of reasoning in situations based on the level of difficulty of the decision-making process for the clinician, without any critical analysis to substantiate this. This is particularly relevant in complex cases where overall poorer prognoses may lead to conclusions that the associated clinical reasoning was poorer than in simple cases with relatively good prognoses, with the latter possibly leading to conclusions about the associated clinical reasoning being of higher quality. For example, a clinician might consult with a patient who reports that her condition has been steadily improving for the prior month. The patient describes that she has improved about 10% per week for the past 4 weeks. At the next visit, the patient reports a 10% improvement after the first visit with the clinician. The clinician would be guilty of outcome bias if he or she concludes that the treatment or advice provided at the first visit was solely responsible (or responsible at all) for the improvement noted because the rate of improvement was exactly the same as that prior to the initial consultation.

Although most of the discussions of clinical reasoning errors in the literature focus on cognitive errors in deductively oriented clinical reasoning, it is important to explicitly acknowledge and screen for clinical reasoning errors in narratively oriented (inductive) clinical reasoning as well (Jones, 2014). These include the following:

- Either no screening of psychosocial factors or assessment that is too superficial
- Judgements based on insufficient assessment:
  - The patient doesn't volunteer personal problems, so the therapist assumes they are not present.
  - The patient alludes to a personal problem (e.g. stress at work/home), and the therapist does not clarify or establish the history and relationship to the clinical presentation.
  - The clinician doesn't clarify if the patient is coping with the problem or how the patient copes.
  - The clinician doesn't explore the effects of the problem on the patient's understanding/beliefs, symptoms, expectations and future prospects, which often leads to superficial judgement.
- The clinician makes a premature judgement regarding psychosocial factors (i.e. after first appointment).
- The clinician views a problem as either a biological problem or a psychosocial problem rather than appreciating that there is always an interaction between body and mind.
- The clinician approaches narrative reasoning judgements like diagnostic reasoning judgements—for example:
  - The clinician assumes there is a standard normative interpretation (e.g. range of movement) that enables a belief or behaviour to be judged 'maladaptive' (e.g. stress, anger, praying, demonstrative pain behaviours).

The Role of Skilled Clinical Mentoring in the Facilitation of Clinical Reasoning

In a study of novice and experienced physical therapists, Wainwright and colleagues (2011) identified mentorship as one of several factors common to both groups that influenced the professional development of decision-making abilities over time. Many of the strategies for facilitating the learning of, and from, clinical reasoning discussed previously are directly applicable to situations where learners are being mentored individually or in small groups in the clinical setting. Less skilled clinical mentors have a tendency to focus mainly on issues related to diagnostic and procedural reasoning, as well as deductive testing of hypotheses, and to give advice about the performance of technical skills, often running out of time to engage with their mentees in dialogue more specifically about clinical reasoning. Often, clinical mentors become mentors based on their clinical abilities or on having completed a program wherein they were mentored, without necessarily having any specific knowledge or training in the practice of mentoring or in the facilitation of clinical reasoning. The knowledge, skills and abilities of mentoring constitute a form of practice in and of themselves; therefore, just as clinicians do, mentors also span the continuum from novice to expert levels of proficiency. Optimal facilitation of a learner's clinical reasoning development will largely rely on promotion of adequate depth and breadth of reflection, through the use of questioning and dialogue as previously described, with intentional facilitation of critical self-reflection across all the clinical reasoning strategies, including deductive and inductive reasoning (Christensen et al., 2011). Mentors likely vary considerably in their ability to achieve this without specific training in the role.

Important to this discussion of the role of skilled clinical mentoring in the facilitation of clinical reasoning is a consideration of the nature of the mentoring relationship itself. Descriptions of mentoring relationships have evolved over time as they have been influenced by adult learning theory, self-directed learning theory and research (Zachary, 2012). Modern depictions of mentoring describe a mutual, facilitated learning relationship where the mentor serves as a resource and stimulus for learning rather than as an expert with all the answers. One aspect of excellent mentoring, therefore, is the establishment of a learning culture wherein acknowledging when one does not 'know' is often more important to role modeling and to facilitating the development of expertise than having all the answers; similarly, mentees must be able to comfortably expose their own gaps in knowledge and skills in order to most optimally facilitate their own learning in practice.

Brookfield (2008) described a common, yet privately held fear experienced by all sorts of teachers and learners: the fear of being found out as an 'imposter' – in this context, due to not knowing enough and not being a skilled enough clinician. Brookfield (2008) suggests that the solution for minimizing this struggle against 'impostership' involves being transparent and acknowledging recognized deficits in knowledge or skills – in effect, neutralizing the fear of being found out by others by self-identifying any gaps in knowledge and proactively taking action to address them (Jones, 2014).

Mentors serve to model what Taylor and Jarecke (2009) describe as a form of 'critical humility' (p. 287). Mentors and mentees, both learners in the relationship, practice an attitude of openness to the discovery that their knowledge is partial and evolving, and yet they remain both committed and confident in existing knowledge and the translation of that knowledge to action in practice (Taylor and Jarecke, 2009). In the context of this chapter, this perspective on the development of mentoring relationships is consistent with facilitating the development of capability in clinical reasoning.

Dialogue has been previously described in this chapter as a primary medium through which to facilitate potentially transformative learning (Cranton, 2006; Mezirow, 2009; Taylor, 2009). Particularly relevant to clinical learning settings where true mentoring relationships can be developed is the understanding of the role of dialogue as not so much 'analytical, point-counterpoint dialogue, but dialogue emphasizing relational and trustful communication' (Taylor, 2009, p. 9). Truly transformative learning requires learners to reveal vulnerabilities and work with the facilitator to, at times, critically examine some very core beliefs and assumptions about themselves as well as others (Mezirow, 2009; Taylor, 2009). In this way, engaging in dialogue within a mentoring relationship must be viewed as more than having analytical conversations about things such as learners' clinical reasoning performances (and other aspects of their practice). Rather, transformative learning is most likely when facilitated within the context of mutual trust whereby the learner is confident that the facilitator is questioning and challenging him or her with the intent of moving the learner toward construction of knowledge, as opposed to destruction of confidence (Brookfield, 1986; Cranton, 2006; Zachary, 2012). Within this type of mutual learning relationship, a learner is able to willingly experience discomfort at times, knowing that the facilitator is working with the intent to identify the learner's 'edge of meaning' (Berger, 2004, p. 338); this is where the learner must come to terms with the limitations of his or her understanding in order to then extend those limits so that new knowledge can emerge. In medicine, a recent systematic review reported that when a mentoring relationship is characterized by emotional safety, support, learner-centeredness, mutual respect and informality, the observed resultant learners' behaviors were independence and a willingness to more deeply reflect, extrapolate and synthesize learning (Davis and Nakamura, 2010).

Unique to authentic clinical education settings are situations where a mentee checks in with a mentor and there may only be a few minutes within which the mentor must interact in order to facilitate the mentee's thinking in action. Medical educators have observed that during clinical consultations, the learner would often present the details of the case first, taking at least half of the time available for the consultation (Neher and Stevens, 2003). The mentor typically would then ask for further specific details about the case and then use the remainder of the time to guide the learner in developing the plan of care. Neher and Stevens (2003) have developed a model of mentoring in this type of situation, in order to make the most of quick clinical consultation conversations. It is designed to be brief, and the recommended sequence of steps is intended to foster the learner's ownership of reasoning through the clinical problem journey. In this way, it allows the mentor to both identify gaps in the learner's knowledge base and to minimize any teaching or advice giving that is deemed necessary for the provision of appropriate patient care at that moment (Neher and Stevens, 2003). The Five Microskills Model focuses on five tasks or skills that a mentor tries to accomplish when discussing a case quickly with a mentee in the midst of a practice encounter:

1. Obtain a commitment from the learner about what he or she thinks is happening with the patient's problem first (instead of a summary of the case so that the mentor can solve the problem).
2. Probe for underlying reasoning (e.g. consider all relevant reasoning strategies and hypothesis categories).
3. Teach/review general concepts, principles and specific knowledge relevant to understanding the case (if needed or if gaps in knowledge have been revealed that are critical to caring for the patient at that juncture).
4. Provide positive feedback about what the learner has done well.
5. Correct errors (as needed in the moment, for the benefit of the patient).

Debriefing retrospectively after completing the patient encounter can then provide the opportunity for the learner to critically reflect on how well the learner 'owned' his or her clinical reasoning in action, and the dialogue can then move into more in-depth critical self-reflection. This type of model can assist mentors in making a 'diagnosis' of the learner's clinical reasoning at that point in time while also ensuring the patient is being cared for appropriately. It also facilitates the learner in reflecting on his or her reasoning in action, which is a skill that we have previously highlighted as a key differentiating factor between novice and more experienced clinicians (Wainwright et al., 2010).

Using Technology to Enhance Opportunities for Clinical Reasoning Development

Various forms of technology are emerging as powerful tools in the facilitation of clinical reasoning development and in the development of experiential learning skills. Simulated clinical encounters with standardized patient actors and simulations with high-fidelity mannequins are becoming more and more common in both the professional-entry education and continuing professional education of clinicians (e.g. Motola et al., 2013). The key to maximizing learning from simulation experiences is the debriefing of the experience with peers and a learning facilitator (e.g. Simon et al., 2010). Although the terminology in the simulation literature varies, the key principles relevant to simulation debriefing are consistent with the descriptions provided previously in this chapter of key characteristics of skilled mentoring in the facilitation of critical self-reflection on clinical reasoning and decision-making. Simulated educational experiences within the professional-entry education of physiotherapists have been shown to be an effective form of clinical preparation of students for authentic clinical practice (Blackstock et al., 2014; Watson et al., 2012). Among the advantages of simulated clinical reasoning experiences are that facilitators are able to suspend the 'action' in order to dialogue with learners to facilitate metacognitive thinking and reflection in action, often in a more in-depth manner than can realistically be achieved when in a real patient care situation. The result can be more frequent and more robust opportunities to capitalize on spontaneous learning opportunities that are completely in context with the clinical scenario being experienced, both in action and on action, immediately after the simulation is concluded.

Other ways of facilitating clinical reasoning with technology in an academic setting include the use of e-learning platforms that provide opportunities for virtual online synchronous (e.g. online video chat platforms where faculty and students dialogue in real time) or asynchronous learning spaces (e.g. discussion boards and wiki activities where participants post written pieces and responses and engage in a dialogue that is not in real time). For example, Snodgrass (2011) describes ways in which wiki activities focused on the collaborative creation of a group patient case presentation can be both an efficient alternative to use of class time for the presentation of content and also effective in facilitating the collaborative presentation and refinement of knowledge as well as the reasoning underlying its development. Along with collaboration, facilitated by the nature of the coordinated group creation of a wiki, critical thinking is also facilitated as students provide each other feedback and work to improve the final wiki product by offering refinements to their peers.

Specific Strategies for Independent Self-Directed Learning

Although many of the strategies we have suggested for optimal facilitation of clinical reasoning development may seem to require both a learner and a learning facilitator, it is possible for learners to adopt many of these same strategies to facilitate their own critical self-reflection. Engaging with others outside of ourselves is more likely to result in the exposure of any blind spots or faulty assumptions we may have as clinical reasoners; however, there are ways to facilitate your own reasoning growth independently as well:

- Just as clinicians must keep current with emerging research evidence and theories related to the technical aspects of their practice, it is important to keep current with emerging research and literature in the area of clinical reasoning through independent reading, study and conference presentations or other continuing professional education opportunities.
- Setting aside a regular, dedicated time for critical self-reflection on selected practice experiences is critical for growth in clinical reasoning. Individuals can engage in self-questioning within the same frameworks as suggested earlier, asking themselves questions about all aspects of their reasoning to identify areas of weakness and potential future learning.
- Recording critical self-reflections in writing over a period of time and then reviewing and reflecting on any patterns noted over time is another way to develop perspective about one's own clinical reasoning. Writing is thought to potentially strengthen the reflective experience because it creates a record of one's thought patterns outside of one's own mind that can then be reflected upon and also shared with others if desired (Taylor, 2009). Strengths and areas of weakness are more easily identified when put in writing and reflected upon after time has passed.
- There is a growing body of resources to facilitate a process of systematic self-study by exploring patient cases available in journal publications, texts, face-to-face continuing

education courses, or online video-recorded 'masterclass'-type demonstrations of expert reasoning. Many of these resources include critical discussion of the clinical reasoning and decision-making involved (synchronously if in a face-to-face course or asynchronously if in a pre-recorded online resource). Clinicians can critically reflect on their reasoning as compared to that presented as part of the case presentation in order to expose potential blind spots or gaps in current research evidence or in their own clinical knowledge.

- Readers of this book's cases (Chapters 6–30) can practice clinical reasoning, and also critical reflection on their own reasoning, by reading and attempting to answer the Reasoning Questions provided in the case studies and by critically considering the authors' answers. This activity should stimulate further critical reflection (of their own reasoning and the reasoning of others) by identifying similarities and differences in the reasoning answers as compared to their own reasoning.

Conclusion

In this chapter we have presented a summary of clinical reasoning and educational research evidence and theory, with the intent of grounding our suggested strategies for facilitating the learning of, and from, clinical reasoning at all levels of professional development. We also hope that readers may be both inspired and facilitated in developing additional well-grounded strategies to share. In this way, we can all contribute to the evolution of clinical reasoning development within our community of practice. The appreciation for new experiences and opportunities to interact with new individuals with unique stories and challenges to be overcome is part of what has inspired many of us to enter musculoskeletal practice. Our ability to enjoy and promote our own opportunities for continuous learning and development in the midst of today's complex practice environment is how we can best contribute to helping ourselves, our professions and those we serve to thrive.

REFERENCES

Alhadeff-Jones, M., 2012. Transformative learning and the challenges of complexity. In: Taylor, E.W., Cranton, P., Associates (Eds.), The Handbook of Transformative Learning: Theory, Research, and Practice. Jossey-Bass Wiley, San Francisco, CA, pp. 178–194.

Berger, J.C., 2004. Dancing on the threshold of meaning: recognizing and understanding the growing edge. JTED 2, 336–351.

Black, L., Jensen, G.M., Mostrom, E., Perkins, J., Ritzline, P.D., Hayward, L., et al., 2010. The first year of practice: an investigation of the professional learning and development of promising novice physical therapists. Phys. Ther. 90, 1758–1773.

Blackstock, F.C., Watson, K.M., Morris, N.R., Jones, A., Wright, A., McMeeken, J.M., et al., 2014. Simulation can contribute a part of cardiorespiratory physiotherapy clinical education: two randomized trials. Simul. Healthc. 8 (1), 32–42.

Brookfield, S.D., 1986. Understanding and Facilitating Adult Learning: A Comprehensive Analysis of Principles and Effective Practices. Jossey-Bass, San Francisco, CA.

Brookfield, S.D., 2008. Clinical reasoning and generic thinking skills. In: Higgs, J., Jones, M., Loftus, S., Christensen, N. (Eds.), Clinical Reasoning in the Health Professions, third ed. Butterworth Heinemann Elsevier, London, pp. 65–75.

Brookfield, S.D., 2012. Teaching Critical Thinking: Tools and Techniques to Help Students Question Their Assumptions. Jossey-Bass Wiley, San Francisco, CA.

Christensen, N., 2009. Development of clinical reasoning capability in student physical therapists. Doctor of Philosophy Thesis. Adelaide, South Australia: University of South Australia. Available at: http://trove.nla.gov.au/work/36257790.

Christensen, N., Jensen, G., 2019. Developing clinical reasoning capability. In: Higgs, J., Jensen, G., Loftus, S., Christensen, N. (Eds.), Clinical Reasoning in the Health Professions, fourth ed. Elsevier, Edinburgh, pp. 427–433.

Christensen, N., Jones, M., Edwards, I., 2011. Clinical reasoning and evidence-based practice. Home Study Course 21.2.1: Current Concepts of Orthopaedic Physical Therapy, 3rd ed. La Crosse, WI: Orthopaedic Section, APTA, Inc.

Christensen, N., Jones, M., Edwards, I., Higgs, J., 2008a. Helping physiotherapy students develop clinical reasoning capability. In: Higgs, J., Jones, M., Loftus, S., Christensen, N. (Eds.), Clinical Reasoning in the Health Professions, third ed. Butterworth Heinemann Elsevier, London, pp. 389–396.

Christensen, N., Jones, M., Higgs, J., Edwards, I., 2008b. Dimensions of clinical reasoning capability. In: Higgs, J., Jones, M., Loftus, S., Christensen, N. (Eds.), Clinical Reasoning in the Health Professions, third ed. Butterworth Heinemann Elsevier, London, pp. 101–110.

Christensen, N., Nordstrom, T., 2013. Facilitating the teaching and learning of clinical reasoning. In: Jensen, G.M., Mostrom, E. (Eds.), Handbook of Teaching and Learning for Physical Therapists, third ed. Butterworth-Heinemann Elsevier, St. Louis, MO, pp. 183–199.

Cranton, P., 2006. Understanding and Promoting Transformative Learning: a Guide for Educators of Adults, second ed. Jossey-Bass Wiley, San Francisco, CA.

Cranton, P., 2009. From tradesperson to teacher: a transformative transition. In: Mezirow, J., Taylor, E.W., Associates (Eds.), Transformative Learning in Practice: Insights from Community, Workplace, and Higher Education. Jossey-Bass Wiley, San Francisco, CA, pp. 182–190.

Croskerry, P., 2009. Clinical cognition and diagnostic error: applications of a dual process model of reasoning. Adv. Health Sci. Educ. Theory Pract 14, 27–35.

Davis, B., Sumara, D., 2006. Complexity and Education: Inquiries Into Learning, Teaching, and Research. Lawrence Erlbaum Associates, Mahwah, NJ.

Davis, B., Sumara, D., Luch-Kapler, R., 2000. Engaging Minds: Learning and Teaching in a Complex World. Lawrence Erlbaum Associates, Mahwah, NJ.

Davis, O.C., Nakamura, J., 2010. A proposed model for an optimal mentoring environment for medical residents: a literature review. Acad. Med. 85 (6), 1060–1066.

De Bono, E., 2015. Lateral Thinking: Creativity Step by Step (Perennial Library). Harper Colophon, New York.

Doncaster, K., Lester, S., 2002. Capability and its development: experiences from a work-based doctorate. Stud High Educ 27, 91–101.

Edwards, I., Jones, M., 2007. Clinical reasoning and expert practice. In: Jensen, G., Gwyer, J., Hack, L., Shepard, K. (Eds.), Expertise in Physical Therapy Practice, second ed. Saunders Elsevier, St. Louis, MO, pp. 192–213.

Edwards, I., Jones, M., Carr, J., Braunack-Mayer, A., Jensen, G.M., 2004a. Clinical reasoning strategies in physical therapy. Phys. Ther. 84, 312–330.

Edwards, I., Jones, M., Higgs, J., Trede, F., Jensen, G., 2004b. What is collaborative reasoning? Adv. Physiother. 6, 70–83.

Gilliland, S., 2014. Clinical reasoning in first- and third-year physical therapist students. J. Phys. Ther. Educ. 28 (2), 64–80.

Hawkins, D., Elder, L., Paul, R., 2010. The Thinker's Guide to Clinical Reasoning. Foundation for Critical Thinking, Tomales, CA.

Hayward, L.M., Black, L.L., Mostrom, E., Jensen, G.M., Ritzline, P.D., Perkins, J., 2013. The first two years of practice: a longitudinal perspective on the learning and professional development of promising novice physical therapists. Phys. Ther. 93, 369–383.

Higgs, J., Fish, D., Rothwell, R., 2008. Knowledge generation and clinical reasoning in practice. In: Higgs, J., Jones, M., Loftus, S., Christensen, N. (Eds.), Clinical Reasoning in the Health Professions, third ed. Butterworth Heinemann Elsevier, London, pp. 163–172.

Higgs, J., Jones, M., 2008. Clinical reasoning and multiple problem spaces. In: Higgs, J., Jones, M., Loftus, S., Christensen, N. (Eds.), Clinical Reasoning in the Health Professions, third ed. Butterworth Heinemann Elsevier, London, pp. 3–17.

Huang, G.C., Newman, L.R., Schwartzstein, R.M., 2014. Critical thinking in health professions education: summary and consensus statements of the Millennium Conference 2011. Teach. Learn. Med. 26 (1), 95–102.

Huhn, K., Black, K., Jensen, G.M., Deutsch, J.E., 2011. Construct validity of the Health Science Reasoning Test. J. Allied Health 40 (4), 181–186.

James, A., Brookfield, S.D., 2014. Engaging Imagination: Helping Students Become Creative and Reflective Thinkers. Jossey-Bass Wiley, San Francisco, CA.

Jensen, G.M., 2011. Learning: what matters most. Phys. Ther. 91, 1674–1689.

Jensen, G.M., Gwyer, J., Shepard, K.F., 2000. Expert practice in physical therapy. Phys. Ther. 80, 28–43.

Jensen, G., Resnick, L., Haddad, A., 2019. Expertise and clinical reasoning. In: Higgs, J., Jensen, G., Loftus, S., Christensen, N. (Eds.), Clinical Reasoning in the Health Professions, fourth ed. Elsevier, Edinburgh, pp. 67–76.

Jensen, G.M., Shepard, K.F., Gwyer, J., Hack, L.M., 1992. Attribute dimensions that distinguish master and novice physical therapy clinicians in orthopedic settings. Phys. Ther. 72, 711–722.

Jensen, G.M., Shepard, K.F., Hack, L.M., 1990. The novice versus the experienced clinician: insights into the work of the physical therapist. Phys. Ther. 70, 314–323.

Jones, M., 2014. Clinical reasoning: from the Maitland concept and beyond. In: Hengeveld, E., Banks, K. (Eds.), Vertebral Manipulation: Management of Musculoskeletal Disorders, vol. 1, eighth ed. Churchill Livingstone, Edinburgh, pp. 14–82.

Klein, J., 2005. Five pitfalls in decisions about diagnosis and prescribing. Br. Med. J. 330, 781–784.

Marcum, J.A., 2012. An integrated model of clinical reasoning: dual-processing theory of cognition and metacognition. J. Eval. Clin. Pract. 18, 954–961.

Mezirow, J., 1991. Transformative Dimensions of Adult Learning. Jossey Bass Publishers, San Francisco, CA.

Mezirow, J., 2000. Learning to think like an adult: core concepts of transformation theory. In: Mezirow, J. (Ed.), Learning as Transformation: Critical Perspectives on a Theory in Progress. Jossey-Bass, San Francisco, CA, pp. 3–33.

Mezirow, J., 2009. Transformative learning theory. In: Mezirow, J., Taylor, E.W., Associates (Eds.), Transformative Learning in Practice: Insights from Community, Workplace, and Higher Education. Jossey-Bass Wiley, San Francisco, CA, pp. 18–31.

Miller, P., 2009. Pattern recognition is a clinical reasoning strategy in musculoskeletal physiotherapy. Master's thesis, The University of Newcastle, Australia.

Motola, I., Devine, L.A., Chung, H.S., Sullivan, J.E., Issenberg, S.B., 2013. Simulation in healthcare education: a best evidence practical guide. AMEE Guide No. 82. Med. Teach. 35 (10), e1511–e1530.

Neher, J.O., Stevens, N.G., 2003. The one-minute preceptor: shaping the teaching conversation. Fam. Med. 35 (6), 391–393.

Paul, R., 1992. Critical Thinking: What Every Person Needs to Survive in a Rapidly Changing World, second ed., revised. Foundation for Critical Thinking, Santa Rosa, CA.

Paul, R., Elder, L., 2006. The Miniature Guide to Critical Thinking: Concepts and Tools, fourth ed. The Foundation for Critical Thinking: Santa Rosa, CA.

Plsek, P.E., Greenhalgh, T., 2001. Complexity science: the challenge of complexity in health care. Br. Med. J. 323, 625–628.

Resnik, L., Jensen, G.M., 2003. Using clinical outcomes to explore the theory of expert practice in physical therapy. Phys. Ther. 83, 1090–1106.

Rivett, D.A., Higgs, J., 1997. Hypothesis generation in the clinical reasoning behavior of manual therapists. J. Phys. Ther. Educ. 11 (1), 40–45.

Sacchi, S., Cherubini, P., 2004. The effect of outcome information on doctors' evaluations of their own diagnostic decisions. Med. Educ. 38, 1028–1034.

Schön, D., 1987. Educating the Reflective Practitioner. Jossey-Bass Inc. Publishers, San Francisco, CA.

Scott, I., 2009. Errors in clinical reasoning: causes and remedial strategies. Br. Med. J. 339, 22–25.

Simon, R., Raemer, D.B., Rudolph, J.W., 2010. Debriefing Assessment for Simulation in Healthcare (DASH)© Rater's Handbook. Center for Medical Simulation, Boston, MA. Available at: https://harvardmedsim.org/_media/ DASH.handbook.2010.Final.Rev.2.pdf. 2010. English, French, German, Japanese.

Snodgrass, S., 2011. Wiki activities in blended learning for health professional students: Enhancing critical thinking and clinical reasoning skills. AJET 27 (4), 563–580.

Stephenson, J., 1998. The concept of capability and its importance in higher education. In: Stephenson, J., Yorke, M. (Eds.), Capability and Quality in Higher Education. Kogan Page, London, pp. 1–13.

Stephenson, R., 2004. Using a complexity model of human behaviour to help interprofessional clinical reasoning. Int. J. Ther. Rehabil. 11, 168–175.

Taylor, E.W., 2009. Fostering transformative learning. In: Mezirow, J., Taylor, E.W., Associates (Eds.), Transformative Learning in Practice: Insights from Community, Workplace, and Higher Education. Jossey-Bass Wiley, San Francisco, CA, pp. 3–17.

Taylor, E.W., Jarecke, J., 2009. Looking forward by looking back: Reflections on the practice of transformative learning. In: Mezirow, J., Taylor, E.W., Associates (Eds.), Transformative Learning in Practice: Insights from Community, Workplace, and Higher Education. Jossey-Bass Wiley, San Francisco, CA, pp. 275–289.

Wainwright, S.F., Shepard, K.F., Harman, L.B., Stephens, J., 2010. Novice and experienced physical therapist clinicians: a comparison of how reflection is used to inform the clinical decision-making process. Phys. Ther. 90 (1), 75–88.

Wainwright, S.F., Shepard, K.F., Harman, L.B., Stephens, J., 2011. Factors that influence the clinical decision making of novice and experienced physical therapists. Phys. Ther. 91 (1), 87–101.

Watson, K.A., Wright, A.B., Morris, N.C., McMeeken, J.D., Rivett, D.A., Blackstock, F.F., et al., 2012. Can simulation replace part of clinical time? Two parallel randomised controlled trials. Med. Educ. 6 (7), 657–667.

Wenger, E., 1998. Communities of Practice: Learning, Meaning, and Identity. Cambridge University Press, Cambridge UK.

Zachary, L.J., 2012. The Mentor's Guide: Facilitating Effective Learning Relationships, second ed. Jossey Bass Wiley, San Francisco, CA.

APPENDIX **1**

Clinical Reasoning Reflection Form

This reflection form from the School of Health Sciences at the University of South Australia can be used to record reflections at the completion of the subjective examination, physical examination and day 1 treatment.

STUDENT .... DATE .... PATIENT'S NAME ....

Perceptions/Analysis

On Completion of the Subjective Examination (S/E)

1. Activity and participation capabilities and restrictions
   Capabilities ....
   ....

   Restrictions ....
   ....

2. Patient perspectives on his or her experience (i.e. psychosocial)
   What is the patient's understanding of the problem? What is the patient's understanding of pain? Could factors such as understanding/beliefs, stress or coping be influencing the patient's clinical presentation? Does the patient appear motivated to engage with therapy, or is the patient seeking passive treatment only? What are the patient's expectations regarding treatment and recovery? What are the patient's goals? Are the patient's expectations and goals realistic and likely to be helpful? Are there any social-factor barriers?
   ....
   ....
   ....

3. Pain type
   Identify the DOMINANT pain type (i.e. nociceptive with or without inflammation, neuropathic, maladaptive central nervous system sensitization/nociplastic) and supporting evidence.
   ....
   ....
   ....

4. Source of symptoms and associated pathology
   Identify potential sources of symptoms (e.g. structures/tissues). What pathological processes may be contributing to the patient's pain (e.g. inflammation, infection, ischemia)? Could structural strain or pathology (e.g. stenosis, tendinosis) be contributing to the patient's pain?
   ....
   ....
   ....

5. Contributing factors
   List any potential contributing factors identified in the subjective examination (e.g. psychosocial, ergonomic/environmental, health comorbidities).
   ....
   ....
   ....

6. Precautions and contraindications
   List any features suggesting caution or contraindication to physical examination or treatment.
   ....
   ....
   ....

7. Day 1 priorities
   Specify your priorities for physical examination on day 1.
   ....
   ....
   ....

Perceptions/Analysis
On Completion of the Physical Examination (P/E)

8. Physical impairments and associated structures/tissues involved
   Identify the main physical impairments that correlate with the patient's activity and participation restrictions. What structures/tissue sources may be contributing to those impairments?
   ....
   ....
   ....

9. Contributing factors
   Are any physical factors (e.g. posture, mobility, movement patterns, awareness/control/strength, fitness) potentially contributing to the patient's condition?
   ....
   ....
   ....

10. Pain type
    Specify the findings from the P/E supporting or not supporting the dominant pain type hypothesized in the S/E.
    ....
    ....
    ....

11. Source of the symptoms and pathology
    Identify potential tissue sources and pathology supported by the P/E.
    ....
    ....
    ....

12. Broad management and specific treatments
    Specify and justify your broad management plan at this stage and the specific treatment(s) you plan for day 1.
    ....
    ....
    ....

13. Assessment, re-assessment, outcome measures
    Identify assessment tools appropriate for this patient to assist your understanding of
    the patient's disability experience and monitoring of outcomes. Identify the key S/E
    and P/E re-assessments you plan to monitor.
    ....
    ....
    ....

14. Explanation/education
    Highlight the focus of the explanation you gave to the patient.
    ....
    ....
    ....

Perceptions/Analysis
On Completion of the Day 1 Treatment

15. Re-assessment
    What are your thoughts following re-assessment of today's treatment?
    ....
    ....
    ....

16. Plans for further assessment
    Identify any further assessments (S/E or P/E) you plan to do.
    ....
    ....
    ....

17. Treatment progression and self-management
    What are your immediate plans for progression of today's treatment?
    ....
    ....
    ....

    What self-management do you plan to suggest, and when will you do so?
    ....
    ....
    ....

18. Prognosis
    Indicate how long you think the problem will take to resolve, and list the positive
    and negative prognostic indicators from the S/E, P/E and response to day 1 treatment.
    Positives..
    ....
    ....

    Negatives...
    ....
    ....

APPENDIX **2**

Clinical Reasoning Reflection Worksheet

This clinical reasoning worksheet from the School of Health Sciences at the University of South Australia can be used to prompt and record the clinician's thinking processes.

NAME .... DATE .... PATIENT'S NAME ....

Please provide a de-identified copy of the patient's body chart with the form.

Clinical Reasoning Based on the Subjective Examination

1. ACTIVITY CAPABILITY/RESTRICTION
   Identify the key abilities and restrictions the patient has in executing activities.
   * Abilities _____
   * Restrictions _____

2. PARTICIPATION CAPABILITY/RESTRICTION
   Identify the key abilities and restrictions the patient has with involvement in life situations (work, family, sport, leisure).
   * Abilities _____
   * Restrictions _____

3. PATIENT'S PERSPECTIVES ON HIS OR HER EXPERIENCE (PSYCHOSOCIAL)
   3.1 What is your assessment of the patient's understanding of the problem? Specifically consider the patient's threat appraisal with respect to his or her beliefs about the problem, what can be done and the future. Do the patient's understanding and threat appraisal present a potential barrier to the patient's recovery?
   _____
   _____
   _____

   3.2 What is your assessment of the patient's feelings (positive and negative) about the problem, its effect on the patient's life and how it has been managed to date? Do any expressed negative feelings present a potential barrier to the patient's recovery?
   _____
   _____
   _____

   3.3 Does the patient have any **explicit coping strategies** (for pain, stress, unhelpful thoughts/emotions), and if so, do they appear to be adaptive or maladaptive? Does the patient convey **any avoidance behaviours** (to activities or participation), and if so, does this appear reasonable for the patient's disability, or is it potentially maladaptive?
   _____
   _____
   _____

3.4 What effect do you anticipate the patient's attitude toward (1) physical exercise and (2) self-management will have on your management?

_____
_____
_____

3.5 Identify one experience from the patient's story that appears representative for the patient, and provide your assessment of what that experience means to the patient.

_____
_____
_____

3.6 What is your assessment of the patient's expectations for physiotherapy? Specifically comment on whether you feel they are appropriate or whether they may reflect maladaptive understanding and emotions that together will need to be addressed in your management.

_____
_____
_____

What are the patient's goals related to the problem(s), the patient's general health management and your specific physiotherapy management? What is your assessment of the patient's goals (e.g. appropriate, if not, why not)?

_____
_____
_____

4. PAIN TYPE

4.1 Identify features from the subjective examination supporting clinical patterns for nociceptive, neuropathic and maladaptive central nervous system sensitization.

Nociceptive Symptoms	Neuropathic Symptoms	Maladaptive Central Nervous System Sensitisation (nociplastic)

4.2 Identify the proportion of pain types you hypothesize in the accompanying pie chart:

5. SOURCES OF SYMPTOMS

5.1 If a nociceptive-dominant pain type is hypothesized, list in order of likelihood all possible sources of nociceptive for each area/component of pain.

If symptoms other than pain present, similarly list possible sources for each type of symptom.

Source	Symptom 1:	Symptom 2:	Symptom 3:	Symptom 4:
Somatic local				
Somatic referred				
Neuropathic				
Vascular				
Visceral				

5.2 Pathology

Are the patient's symptoms associated with a specific process (e.g. Degenerative? Ischaemic? Over-strain? Inflammatory?)? Explain.

_____
_____
_____
_____
_____

Is there a clinical pattern of a specific pathology? Explain.

_____
_____
_____
_____
_____

If there has been overt tissue injury, at what stage of the inflammatory/healing process would you judge the injury to be (e.g. acute inflammatory phase, 0–72 hours; proliferation phase, 72 hours to 6 weeks; remodelling and maturation phase, 6 weeks to several months)?

_____
_____
_____
_____
_____

6. CONTRIBUTING FACTORS

6.1 Based on the subjective examination, are there any contributing factors hypothesized as associated with the development or maintenance of the patient's symptoms, activity and participation restrictions?

- **Hypothesized physical factors based on knowledge of patient's activity levels/fitness, work and lifestyle, sport, medical and neuro-musculoskeletal history** (e.g. biomechanical, muscle length/strength/control, joint mobility, neural mobility, posture, etc.):

  _____

  _____

- **Environmental/ergonomic factors** (workplace setup, etc.):

  _____

  _____

- **Psychosocial factors** (e.g. patient's perspectives/understanding of problem and requirements for recovery/management, feelings regarding problem and its management, attributions, health beliefs and behaviours, social circumstances):

  _____

  _____

- **Health-related factors** (e.g. health-related issues that will affect the symptoms and development of the symptoms):

  _____

  _____

7. THE BEHAVIOUR OF THE SYMPTOMS
   7.1 **Give your interpretation of each of the following:**
   - **Severity**:   _____
     (Symptom 1) Low   High
   - **Severity**:   _____
     (Symptom 2) Low   High
   - **Irritability**: _____
     (Symptom 1) Non-irritable   Very irritable
   - **Irritability**: _____
     (Symptom 2) Non-irritable   Very irritable

   Give an example of irritability.

   _____

   _____

   7.2 **What is the relationship of the patient's activity/participation restrictions and/or symptoms to each other?** (This question is only relevant if more than one activity or participation restriction and/or more than one set of symptoms.)
   - **Behavioural:** Does the current pattern of activity and participation restrictions have a common theme, such as flexion, extension, load, posture or stress related?

     _____

     _____

   - **Behavioural:** Are the different symptoms related in their behaviour (e.g. respond together to aggravating and easing factors)? If so, in what way?

     _____

     _____

   - **Historical:** Are the symptoms, activity and participation restrictions related historically? If so, in what way?

     _____

     _____

7.3 **Provide your interpretation of the contribution of mechanical and/or inflammatory features to the nociceptive component:**

- Inflammatory: _____

  0   10

- Mechanical: _____

  0   10

- List those factors that support your decision.

Inflammatory	*Mechanical*

8. HISTORY OF THE SYMPTOMS

8.1 Give your *interpretation* of the history (present and past) for each of the following:

- **Nature of the onset** (e.g. is it consistent with a particular process, pathology or clinical syndrome, and does it suggest a dominant pain type?)

  _____

  _____

  _____

- **What is the extent of physical impairment and associated tissue damage/change** hypothesized to be present? (e.g. mild versus severe, with supporting evidence; also, does this fit with a predominantly peripherally evoked or centrally mediated process?)

  _____

  _____

  _____

- **What are the implications for the physical examination?** (Specifically, how do your priorities change for the day 1 physical examination?)

  _____

  _____

  _____

- **What is the progression of the presentation since onset?** (better, worse, same, variability/stability)

  _____

  _____

  _____

- **Is the patient's symptom presentation consistent with the history?** (Explain your answer.)

  _____

  _____

  _____

9. HEALTH CONSIDERATIONS, PRECAUTIONS AND CONTRAINDICATIONS TO PHYSICAL EXAMINATION AND MANAGEMENT

   9.1 **Is there anything specific in the patient's answers to the "Medical Screening Questionnaire" (or your abbreviated initial screening) that represents a potential or clear caution/contraindication to your physical examination and management? Specify.**

_____

_____

_____

       Is there anything in your subjective examination questioning that indicates the need for caution in your physical examination or management (e.g. highly irritable/inflammatory condition, rapidly worsening, progressive neurologically, red-flag issues not identified in questionnaire, potential cervical arterial dysfunction, spinal cord or cauda equina compression/ischaemia, weight loss, medications, investigations etc.)? Specify.

_____

_____

_____

   9.2 **If precautions are identified in 9.1, identify what action is indicated** (e.g. medical consultation, specific safety screening such as instability tests, cervical artery tests, etc.).

_____

_____

_____

   9.3 **Does the patient's general health or level of physical fitness indicate the need for consideration of health screening and/or fitness testing?**   **YES/NO**
- If yes, what health screening questionnaire(s) would you consider using?

_____

_____

- What cardiovascular fitness testing would be appropriate?

_____

_____

- What other specific fitness screening tests would be appropriate?

_____

_____

- Is this testing a day 1 priority? Explain your answer.   YES/NO

_____

_____

9.4 **At which points under the following headings will you limit your physical examination?**
  • Circle the relevant description.

Local Symptoms (Consider Each Component)	Referred Symptoms (Consider Each Component)	Dysesthesias	Symptoms of CAD	Visceral or Other System Symptoms
	Short of P1	Short of Production		
Point of onset/ increase in resting symptoms	Point of onset/ increase in resting symptoms	Point of onset/ increase in resting symptoms	Point of onset/ increase in resting symptoms	Point of onset/ increase in resting symptoms
Partial reproduction	Partial reproduction	Partial reproduction		Partial reproduction
Total reproduction	Total reproduction	Total reproduction		Total reproduction

9.5 **Is there any health, red flag or precaution-related reason to limit your examination (separate from your symptom provocation decision noted previously)?**
  Consider your responses to question 9.1 and 9.3 in making your decision.
  • Circle the relevant description:

Active Examination	Passive Examination
• Active movement short of limit • Active limit • Active limit + overpressure • Additional tests	• Passive movement short of R1 • Passive movement into moderate resistance • Passive movement into full overpressure

  • **If you hypothesize a dominant maladaptive central sensitization (nociplastic) pain type in the patient's presentation (e.g. as per pie chart in 4.2), indicate how you will attend to this in your physical examination.**

  _____
  _____
  _____

  • If your hypothesis is a dominant maladaptive central sensitization (nociplastic pain type), what would be your priorities for Day 1?

  _____
  _____
  _____

9.6 **Is a neurological examination necessary?**   **YES/NO**
  • **If so, indicate which neurological structures should be included** (e.g. nerve root, peripheral nerve, spinal cord, cauda equina, cranial nerves).

  _____
  _____

  • Is this examination a day 1 priority? Explain your answer.   **YES/NO**

  _____
  _____

9.7 **If relevant, do you expect a comparable sign(s) to be easy/hard to find** (e.g. are the patient's symptoms **easy** to provoke so likely to be easy to reproduce in the clinic?)?
   - Explain your answer.   **EASY/HARD**

   _____
   _____
   _____
   _____

9.8 **What are the clues (if any) in the subjective examination to any specific treatment techniques or approaches to treatment that may be appropriate** (e.g. a particular movement or position that is pain relieving might form the basis of a mobilizing technique; postural symptoms might indicate need for an endurance program; indications of chronic pain might indicate the need for an educational bias to your management)?
   - Explain your answer.   **YES/NO**

   _____
   _____
   _____
   _____

10. **WRITE OUT YOUR PLAN FOR YOUR PHYSICAL EXAMINATION**
   - Highlight with an asterisk (*) those procedures to be included on day 1.

Functional tests:	
Functional outcome measure:	
Posture:	
Fitness-related tests: • CV tests • Strength/endurance	
Active movements:	
Passive movements: • Physiological • Accessory	
Resistive tests:	
Neurological examination:	
Neurodynamic:	
Soft tissue:	
Motor control:	
Other:	

Perceptions, Interpretations and Implications
Following the Physical Examination and First Treatment

11. Identify the key **PHYSICAL IMPAIRMENTS** from your physical examination that may require **management/re-assessment** (e.g. posture, movement pattern impairments, motor control impairments, soft tissue/joint/muscle/neural mobility/sensitivity, fitness levels, strength/power/endurance).

1.	
2.	
3.	
4.	
5.	
6.	
7.	
8.	
9.	
10.	
11.	
	List any assessments not completed on day 1:

12. **THE SOURCES AND PATHOBIOLOGICAL MECHANISMS OF THE PATIENT'S SYMPTOMS**

    12.1 **List the components of symptoms from section 5 and number in order of likelihood the possible structure(s) at fault for each apparent component. Then identify the supporting and negating evidence from the _PHYSICAL EXAMINATION_ for each structure.**

Component	Possible Structure(s) at Fault	Physical Examination Supporting Evidence	Physical Examination Negating Evidence
e.g. Left mid-cervical pain	• Left PIV joints C2–C5	• Thickened soft tissue over laminae • C2–C5 • Tenderness C2–C5 • Active LF & rotation left limited range	• PPIVMs LF & rotation left C2/ C3–C5/C6 normal ROM

12.2 **List the supporting and negating evidence from the PHYSICAL EXAMINATION for the following pain types and tissue mechanisms:**

	Supporting Evidence	Negating Evidence
Pain type: • Nociceptive • Neuropathic • Maladaptive central nervous system sensitization (nociplastic)		
Motor and other output: • Motor • Signs of autonomic nervous system dysfunction • Potentially maladaptive cognitive and/or affective cues apparent during the physical examination		
Tissue-Healing Mechanisms	*Supporting Evidence*	*Negating Evidence*
If an overt (macro or micro) tissue injury has occurred (e.g. muscle/tendon/ligament/etc.) such that the tissues will go through the understood healing process, identify the features from the physical examination that support the phase of healing:		
Acute inflammatory phase		
Proliferation phase		
Remodelling and maturation phase		

12.3 **What does the physical examination (P/E) suggest regarding tissue health (process, specific pathology, clinical syndrome), and does that fit with your previous tissue health hypothesis from the subjective examination (S/E)?**
   • Explain your answer.   **YES/NO**

_____

_____

_____

_____

12.4 **Based on your full S/E and P/E assessment and analysis, list the favourable and unfavourable prognostic indicators** (consider, for example: pain type and tissue mechanisms, patient perspectives, inflammatory versus mechanical presentation, degree of irritability, nature of onset and progression, effects of previous interventions, medical screening findings, extent of physical impairments and possible contributing factors):

Favourable	*Unfavourable*

12.5 **Based on your assessment of favourable and unfavourable prognostic indicators, indicate whether you feel you/physiotherapy can assist this patient, and state as specifically as you can (e.g. days, weeks, months) how much time or the number of treatments likely to be required.**
  * Able to help?

  _____

  * How much time is required?

  _____

  * Percentage improvement anticipated?

  _____

Implications of Perceptions and Interpretations for Ongoing Management

13. MANAGEMENT

  13.1 **Is there anything about your physical examination findings which would indicate the need for caution in your management? Explain.** YES/NO

  _____
  _____

  13.2 **Does your interpretation of the physical examination findings change the anticipated emphasis of treatment? Explain.** YES/NO

  _____
  _____

  13.3 **What was your management on day 1** (e.g. explanation/advice, exercise, passive mobilization, general exercise, referral for further investigation etc.)?

  _____
  _____

  * Why was this chosen over other options?

  _____
  _____

  * **If passive treatment was used, what was your principal treatment technique(s)?** (Indicate technique, position in which it was performed, grade, dosage.)

  _____
  _____

  * **What physical examination findings support your choice?** (Include in your answer a movement diagram of the most comparable passive movement sign [*most positive passive movement*].)

  _____
  _____
  _____

MOVEMENT DIAGRAM

13.4 **If dynamic management was used, what was your principal focus/starting point?** (Indicate exercise, position in which it was performed/taught, dosage.)

_____

_____

13.5 **If education was your starting point, what was your principal focus?** (Indicate key messages targeted.)

_____

_____

13.6 **What was the effect of your day 1 intervention?**
  • Subjective response:

_____

_____

  • Physical response:

_____

_____

What is your expectation of the patient's response over the next 24 hours?

_____

_____

13.7 **What is your plan and justification of management for this patient?**
  • Overall management plan (e.g. general components of clinical presentation requiring attention)

_____

_____

  • Type of treatment

_____

_____

  • Priorities with treatment

_____

_____

  • Attention to components other than the primary presentation

_____

_____

• Rate of progress, etc.

_____

_____

13.8 **Is attention to the general fitness/cardiovascular health of the patient a priority in your management? Explain.** **YES/NO**

_____

_____

• If so, how do you plan to incorporate this in your overall management?

_____

_____

13.9 **Do you envisage a need to refer the patient to another health provider** (e.g. physician, orthopaedic surgeon, **neurologist**/neurosurgeon, vascular surgeon, endocrinologist, psychologist/psychiatrist, anaesthetist, dietician, Feldenkrais practitioner, Pilates practitioner, gym instructor, etc.)?
   • Explain.

_____

_____

14. **REFLECTION ON PAIN MECHANISMS, SOURCE(S), CONTRIBUTING FACTOR(S) AND PROGNOSIS**

After Third Visit

14.1 **How has your understanding of the patient and the patient's problem(s) changed from your interpretations made following the first session?**

_____

_____

• How have the patient's perceptions of his or her problem and management changed since the first session?

_____

_____

• Are the patient's needs being met?

_____

_____

14.2 **On reflection, what clues (if any) can you now recognize that you initially missed, misinterpreted or under- or over-weighted?**

_____

_____

• What would you do differently next time?

_____

_____

• Have you been able to address all components as indicated in your management plan or advance your treatment at the rate planned? Explain. **YES/NO**

_____

_____

• If not, what barriers have prevented you from advancing your treatment as you planned?

_____

_____

After Sixth Visit

14.3 **How has your understanding of the patient and the patient's problem changed from your interpretation made following the third session?**

_____

_____

- How have the patient's perceptions of his or her problem and management changed since the third session?

_____

_____

- Have the patient's expectations been met?

_____

_____

14.4 **On reflection, what clues (if any) can you now recognize that you initially missed, misinterpreted or under- or over-weighted?**

_____

_____

- What would you do differently next time?

_____

_____

- Have you been able to address all components as indicated in your management plan or advance your treatment at the rate planned? Explain.   **YES/NO**

_____

_____

- If not, what barriers have prevented you from advancing your treatment as you planned?

_____

_____

14.5 **If the outcome is to be short of 100% (i.e. "cured"), at what point will you cease management, and why?**

_____

_____

After Discharge

14.6 **How has your understanding of the patient and the patient's problem changed from your interpretations made following the sixth session?**

_____

_____

- How has the patient's perceptions of his or her problem and management changed since the sixth session?

_____

_____

- How much have you been able to address the patient's concept of self-efficacy, responsibility for self-management and perceptions of the importance of healthy lifestyle in the management of his or her problem?

_____

_____

14.7 **In hindsight, what were the principal source(s) and pathobiological mechanisms of the patient's symptoms?**

_____

_____

_____

_____

• What were the patient's principal health-/fitness-related issues?

_____

_____

• How successful have you been in addressing all components of the patient's problem? Explain.

_____

_____

_____

_____

14.8 **Identify the key subjective and physical features (i.e. clinical pattern) that would help you recognize this presentation in the future.**

                 Subjective   _Physical_

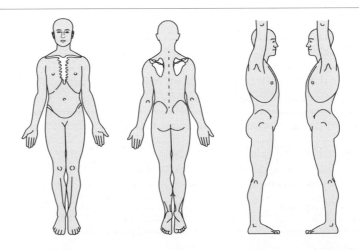

Index

Page numbers followed by "*f*" indicate figures, "*t*" indicate tables, and "*b*" indicate boxes.